ESSENTIAL IMMUNOLOGY

931

SEVENTH EDITION

ESSENTIAL IMMUNOLOGY

Ivan M. Roitt

MA, DSc(Oxon), FRCPath, Hon MRCP (Lond), FRS
*Professor and Head of
Departments of Immunology and Rheumatology Research
University College and Middlesex School of Medicine
University College
London W1P 9PG*

OXFORD

BLACKWELL SCIENTIFIC PUBLICATIONS

LONDON EDINBURGH BOSTON

MELBOURNE PARIS BERLIN VIENNA

© 1971, 1974, 1977, 1980, 1984, 1988, 1991
Blackwell Scientific Publications
Editorial Offices:
Osney Mead, Oxford OX2 0EL
25 John Street, London WC1N 2BL
23 Ainslie Place, Edinburgh EH3 6AJ
3 Cambridge Center, Cambridge
    Massachusetts 02142, USA
54 University Street, Carlton
    Victoria 3053, Australia

Other Editorial Offices:
Arnette SA
2, rue Casimir-Delavigne
75006 Paris
France

Blackwell Wissenschaft
Meinekestrasse 4
D-1000 Berlin 15
Germany

Blackwell MZV
Feldgasse, 13
A-1238 Wien
Austria

First published 1971
Reprinted 1972 (twice), 1973 (twice)
Second edition 1974, Reprinted 1975
Third edition 1977, Reprinted 1978, 1979
Fourth edition 1980, Reprinted, 1982, 1983
Fifth edition 1984
Sixth edition 1988, Reprinted 1988
Reprinted with corrections 1989
Seventh edition 1991

Spanish editions 1972, 1975, 1978, 1982, 1988
Italian editions 1973, 1975, 1979, 1986
Portuguese editions 1973, 1976
French editions 1975, 1979
Dutch editions 1975, 1978, 1982
Japanese editions 1976, 1978, 1982, 1986, 1988
German editions 1977, 1984, 1988
Polish edition 1977
Greek editions 1978, 1988
Slovak edition 1981
Indonesian edition 1985
Russian edition 1988
ELBS editions 1977, 1982, 1988 (Reprinted 1991)

Set by Setrite Ltd, Hong Kong
Printed and bound by
Dah Hua Printing Press Co Ltd, Hong Kong

DISTRIBUTORS

Marston Book Services Ltd
PO Box 87
Oxford OX2 0DT
(*Orders*: Tel. 0865 791155
          Fax: 0865 791927
          Telex: 837515)

USA
    Mosby-Year Book, Inc.
    11830 Westline Industrial Drive
    St Louis, Missouri 63146
    (*Orders*: Tel: 800 633−6699)

Canada
    Mosby-Year Book, Inc.
    5240 Finch Avenue East
    Scarborough, Ontario
    (*Orders*: Tel: 416 298−1588)

Australia
    Blackwell Scientific Publications (Australia) Pty Ltd
    54 University Street
    Carlton, Victoria 3053
    (*Orders*: Tel: 03 347−0300)

British Library
Cataloguing in Publication Data

Roitt, Ivan M. (Ivan Maurice) *1927−*
    Essential immunology. —7th ed.
    1. Medicine. Immunology
    I. Title
    616.079

    ISBN 0-632-02877-7

CONTENTS

CONTENTS

10 · IMMUNITY TO INFECTION
I—Adversarial strategies

11 · IMMUNITY TO INFECTION
II—Prophylaxis and Immunodeficiency

12 · HYPERSENSITIVITY

vii

13 · TRANSPLANTATION

14 · AUTOIMMUNE DISEASES
I—Scope and Aetiology

15 · AUTOIMMUNE DISEASES
II—Pathogenesis, Diagnosis and
Treatment

PREFACE

Dear Reader; Like the previous editions of *Essential Immunology*, this 7th edition is concerned primarily with teaching and, to that end, much effort has gone into ensuring that the concepts evolve in a logical way and are presented lucidly and that there is an abundance of visual material to aid comprehension. Although the last edition was almost entirely re-written, you just cannot stop these Immunologists from making exciting new advances so that radical additions have had to be made, including around 70 new illustrations.

Undoubtedly, the advances in molecular biology have had an outstanding impact on the subject through the provision of recombinant molecules, further understanding of gene regulation, and the availability of transfected cells and transgenic animals as model systems, and wherever appropriate these have been taken fully into account.

Major advances in the following areas have been treated in depth:
- Novel structure of class I, and by implication class II, major histocompatibility complex molecules, their relationship to presentation of processed antigen peptides to T-cell receptors and the cell biology of antigen processing
- T-cell receptors and recognition of heat shock proteins
- The positive selection for self-MHC and negative selection of auto-reactive cells in the thymus
- The frequent occurrence of programmed cell death
- Events in the germinal centres of secondary lymphoid follicles leading to proliferation, isotype switch, somatic mutation and memory cell production
- Different processes in B- and T-cell affinity maturation
- The increased complexity of the cytokine network and difference in cytokine secretion in response to different infections
- Vaccines based on new microbial vectors for genes which confer immunity
- Peptide vaccines
- Use of mice with severe combined immunodeficiency to recreate human immunological processes
- New models, therapies and understanding of AIDS
- Genetically engineered antibodies
- Use of anti-CD4 and CD8 to induce tolerance in the adult
- Update on CD and HLA nomenclature
- Natural auto- and anti-microbial antibodies produced by CD5 positive cells

I very much hope you will enjoy reading this new edition.

Sincerely,
Ivan M. Roitt

ACKNOWLEDGEMENTS

I have a special debt of gratitude to Fritz Melchers and his team of editors, and the publishers Springer-Verlag, Berlin, who allowed me to view the manuscripts for volume VII of *Progress in Immunology* covering the 7th International Congress of Immunology before the printed version was published. As a result it was possible to include more up-to-date material from the world-leading contributors in the present edition. It is with great pleasure that I express my thanks to J. Brostoff, A. Cooke, H.M. Geysen, F.C. Hay, P.G. Isaacson, D.K. Male, J.H.L. Playfair, J. Taverne and N. Woolf for invaluable discussions. I am indebted also to my co-editors, J. Brostoff and D.K. Male, the publishers Gower Medical Publishing Ltd. and the following individuals for permission to utilize or modify their figures which have appeared in *Immunology*: J. Brostoff and A. Hall for Figs 1.14 and 12.6, J. Horton for Fig. 9.24, P. Lydyard and C. Grossi for Figs 3.1 and 3.10, G. Rook for Figs 10.1 and 10.6, J. Taverne for Fig. 10.15 and Table 10.2.

Mike Rubens has maintained his vigorous professional creativity in the design work on the figures, and Mary-Clare Swatman and John Robson have provided the friendly and effective editing one has come to expect and appreciate from Blackwell's. Christine Meats continued to be a terrific secretary and my wife maintained her loving support despite the occasional irrascible lapse by the long-suffering author.

USER GUIDE

Throughout the illustrations standard forms have been used for commonly-occurring cells and pathways. A key to these is given in the figure below.

THE BASIS OF IMMUNOLOGY
I – Innate Immunity

We live in a potentially hostile world filled with a bewildering array of infectious agents (figure 1.1) of diverse shape, size, composition and subversive character which would very happily use us as rich sanctuaries for propagating their 'selfish genes' had we not also developed a series of defence mechanisms at least their equal in effectiveness and ingenuity (except in the case of many parasitic infections where the situation is best described as an uneasy and often unsatisfactory truce). It is these

defence mechanisms which can establish a state of immunity against infection (Latin *immunitas*, freedom from) and whose operation provides the basis for the delightful subject called 'Immunology'.

Aside from ill-understood constitutional factors which make one species innately susceptible and another resistant to certain infections, a number of non-specific anti-microbial systems (e.g. phagocytosis) have been recognized which are '*innate*' in the sense that they are not intrinsically affected by

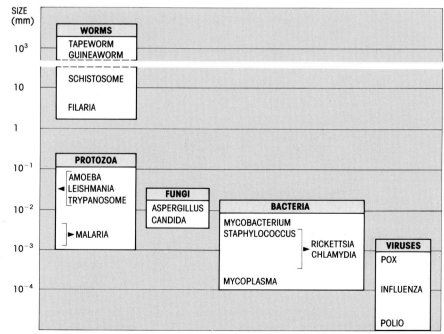

Figure 1.1. *The formidable range of infectious agents which confront the immune system. Although not normally classified as such because of their lack of a cell wall, the mycoplasmas are included under bacteria for convenience. Fungi adopt many forms and approximate values for some of the smallest forms are given.*

prior contact with the infectious agent. We shall discuss these systems and examine how, in the state of *specific acquired immunity*, their effectiveness can be greatly increased.

Barriers against infection

The simplest way to avoid infection is to prevent the micro-organisms from gaining access to the body (figure 1.2). The major line of defence is of course the skin which, when intact, is impermeable to most infectious agents; when there is skin loss, as for example in burns, infection becomes a major problem. Additionally, most bacteria fail to survive for long on the skin because of the direct inhibitory effects of lactic acid and fatty acids in sweat and sebaceous secretions and the low pH which they generate. An exception is *Staphylococcus aureus* which often infects the relatively vulnerable hair follicles and glands.

Mucus, secreted by the membranes lining the inner surfaces of the body, acts as a protective barrier to block the adherence of bacteria to epithelial cells. Microbial and other foreign particles trapped within the adhesive mucus are removed by mechanical stratagems such as ciliary movement, coughing and sneezing. Among other mechanical factors which help protect the epithelial surfaces, one should also include the washing action of tears, saliva and urine. Many of the secreted body fluids contain bactericidal components, such as acid in gastric juice, spermine and zinc in semen, lacto-peroxidase in milk and lysozyme in tears, nasal secretions and saliva.

A totally different mechanism is that of microbial antagonism associated with the normal bacterial flora of the body. These suppress the growth of many potentially pathogenic bacteria and fungi at superficial sites by competition for essential nutrients or by production of inhibitory substances. To give one example, pathogen invasion is limited by lactic acid produced by particular species of commensal bacteria which metabolize glycogen secreted by the vaginal epithelium. When protective commensals are disturbed by antibiotics, susceptibility to opportunistic infections by *Candida* and *Clostridium difficile* is increased. Gut commensals may also produce colicins, a class of bactericidins which bind to the negatively charged surface of susceptible bacteria and insert a hydrophobic helical hairpin into the membrane; the molecule then undergoes a 'Jeckyl and Hyde' transformation to become completely hydrophobic and form a voltage-dependent channel in the membrane which kills by destroying the cell's energy potential. Even at this level, survival is a tough game.

If micro-organisms do penetrate the body, two main defensive operations come into play, the destructive effect of soluble chemical factors such as bactericidal enzymes and the mechanism of phagocytosis—literally 'eating' by the cell.

Phagocytic cells kill micro-organisms

'Professional' phagocytes

The engulfment and digestion of micro-organisms is assigned to two major cell types recognized by Metchnikoff at the turn of the century as *micro-* and *macrophages*.

The polymorphonuclear neutrophil

This cell, the smaller of the two, shares a common haemopoietic stem cell precursor with the other formed elements of the blood and is the dominant white cell in the bloodstream. It is a non-dividing short-lived cell with a multilobed nucleus and an array of granules which are virtually unstained by histological dyes such as haematoxylin and eosin, unlike those structures in the closely related eosinophil and basophil (figures 1.3 and 1.5). The neutrophil granules are of three types: the primary

Figure 1.3. continued

were very kindly provided by Mr M. Watts of the Dept of Haematology, Middlesex Hospital Medical School; (c) was kindly supplied by Prof. J.J. Owen, (g) by Drs P. Lydyard and G. Rook, (h) by Dr Meryl Griffiths and (k) by Prof. N. Woolf.

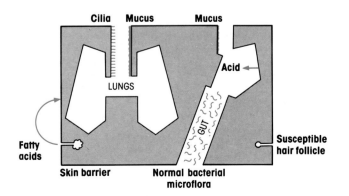

Figure 1.2. *The first lines of defence against infection: protection at the external body surfaces.*

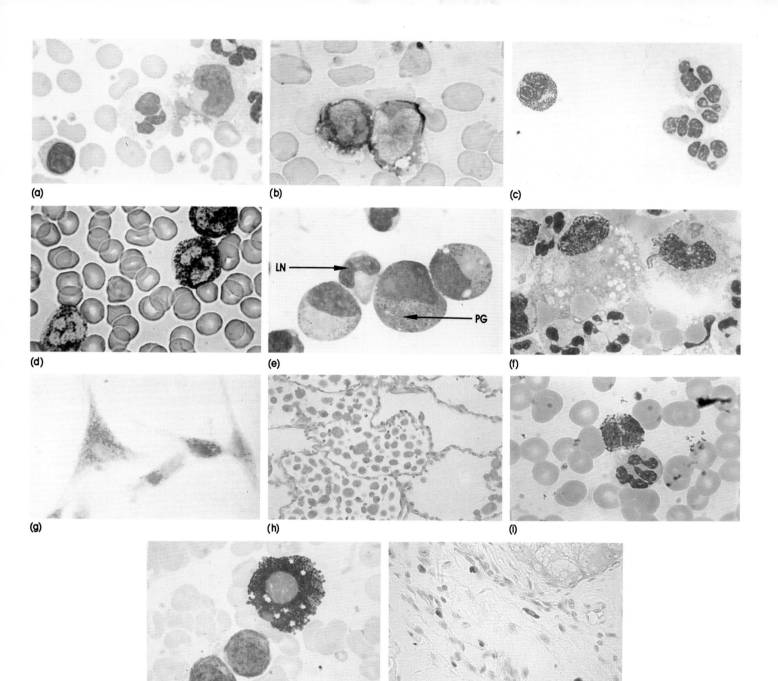

Figure 1.3. *Cells involved in innate immunity. (a) Monocyte, showing 'horseshoe-shaped' nucleus and moderately abundant pale cytoplasm. Note the three multilobed polymorphonuclear neutrophils and the small lymphocyte (bottom left). Romanowsky stain. (b) Two monocytes stained for non-specific esterase with α-naphthyl acetate. Note the vacuolated cytoplasm. The small cell with focal staining at the top is a T-lymphocyte. (c) Four polymorphonuclear leucocytes (neutrophils) and one eosinophil. The multilobed nuclei and the cytoplasmic granules are clearly shown, those of the eosinophil being heavily stained.*
(d) Polymorphonuclear neutrophil showing cytoplasmic granules stained for alkaline phosphatase. (e) Early neutrophils in bone marrow. The primary azurophilic granules (PG) originally clustered near the nucleus, move towards the periphery where the neutrophil-specific granules are generated by the Golgi apparatus as the cell matures. The nucleus gradually becomes lobular (LN). Giemsa.

(f) Inflammatory cells from the site of a brain haemorrhage showing the large active macrophage in the centre with phagocytosed red cells and prominent vacuoles. To the right is a monocyte with horseshoe-shaped nucleus and cytoplasmic bilirubin crystals (haematoidin). Several multilobed neutrophils are clearly delineated. Giemsa. (g) Macrophages in monolayer cultures after phagocytosis of mycobacteria (stained red). Carbol-Fuchsin counterstained with Malachite Green. (h) Numerous plump alveolar macrophages within air spaces in the lung. (i) Basophil with heavily staining granules compared with a neutrophil (below). (j) Mast cell from bone marrow. Round central nucleus surrounded by large darkly staining granules. Two small red cell precursors are shown at the bottom. Romanowsky stain. (k) Tissue mast cells in skin stained with Toluidine Blue. The intracellular granules are metachromatic and stain reddish purple. Note the clustering in relation to dermal capillaries. The slides from which illustrations (a), (b) (d), (e), (f), (i) and (j) were reproduced

azurophilic granule containing myeloperoxidase, some lysozyme and a family of cationic proteins; the secondary 'specific' granules holding lactoferrin, lysozyme and a B_{12}-binding protein; and tertiary granules akin to the conventional lysosomes with acid hydrolases. The abundant glycogen stores can be utilized by glycolysis enabling the cells to function under anaerobic conditions.

The macrophage

These cells derive from bone marrow promonocytes which, after differentiation to blood monocytes, finally settle in the tissues as mature macrophages where they constitute the *mononuclear phagocyte system* (figure 1.4). They are present throughout the connective tissue and around the basement membrane of small blood vessels and are particularly concentrated in the lung (alveolar macrophages), liver (Kupffer cells), and lining of spleen sinusoids and lymph node medullary sinuses where they are strategically placed to filter off foreign material. Other examples are mesangial cells in the kidney glomerulus, brain microglia and osteoclasts in bone. Unlike the polymorphs, they are long-lived cells with significant rough-surfaced endoplasmic reticulum and mitochondria (figure 1.5) and whereas

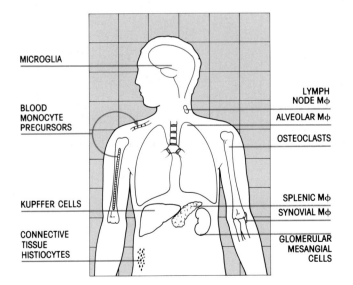

Figure 1.4. *The mononuclear phagocyte system (previously included with endothelial cells and polymorphs under the term 'the reticuloendothelial system' or RES). Promonocyte precursors in the bone marrow develop into circulating blood monocytes which eventually become distributed throughout the body as mature macrophages (Mϕ) as shown. The other major phagocytic cell, the polymorphonuclear neutrophil, is largely confined to the bloodstream except when recruited into sites of acute inflammation.*

the polymorphs provide the major defence against pyogenic (pus-forming) bacteria, as a rough generalization it may be said that macrophages are at their best in combating those bacteria (figure 1.3g), viruses and protozoa which are capable of living within the cells of the host.

Phagocytosis

Before phagocytosis can occur, the microbe must first adhere to the surface of the polymorph or macrophage, an event mediated by some rather primitive recognition mechanism likely to involve carbohydrate elements. Depending on its nature, a particle attached to the surface membrane may initiate the ingestion phase by activating an actin—myosin contractile system which extends pseudopods around the particle (figures 1.6 and 1.7); as adjacent receptors sequentially attach to the surface of the microbe, the plasma membrane is pulled around the particle just like a 'zipper' until it is completely enclosed in a vacuole (phagosome; figures 1.6 and 1.8). Events are now moving smartly and within one minute the cytoplasmic granules fuse with the phagosome and discharge their contents around the imprisoned micro-organism (figure 1.8) which is subject to a formidable battery of microbicidal mechanisms.

Killing

Oxygen-dependent mechanisms

Trouble starts for the invader from the moment phagocytosis is initiated. There is a dramatic increase in activity of the hexose monophosphate shunt generating NADPH. This is utilized ultimately to reduce molecular oxygen bound to a unique plasma-membrane cytochrome (cyt b_{-245}) causing a burst of oxygen consumption. As a result, oxygen is converted to superoxide anion, hydrogen peroxide, singlet O_2 and hydroxyl radicals, all of which are powerful microbicidal agents. Furthermore, the combination of peroxide, myeloperoxidase and halide ions constitutes a potent halogenating system capable of killing both bacteria and viruses (table 1.1).

Oxygen-independent mechanisms

It can also be seen from table 1.1 that the dismutation of superoxide consumes hydrogen ions and raises the pH gently so allowing the family of cationic

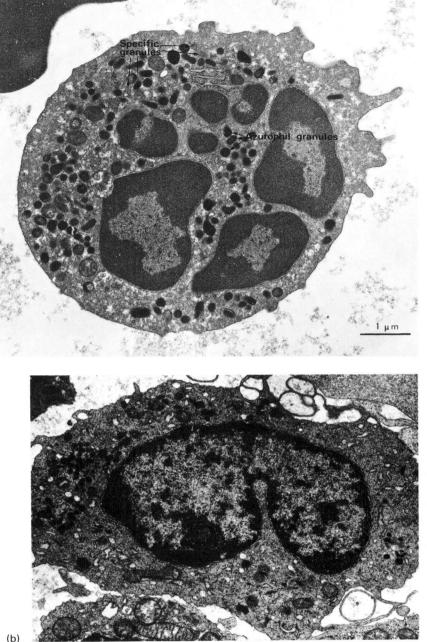

Specific granules

Azurophil granules

1 μm

(a)

Figure 1.5. *Ultrastructure of phagocytic cells. (a) Neutrophil. The multi-lobed nucleus and cytoplasmic granules are well displayed. (Courtesy of Dr D. McLaren.) (b) Monocyte (× 10 000). 'Horseshoe' nucleus. Phagocytic and pinocytic vesicles, lysosomal granules, mitochondria and isolated profiles of rough-surfaced endoplasmic reticulum are evident.*

(b)

proteins to function optimally. Although not fully characterized yet, they damage bacterial membranes both by neutral proteinase (cathepsin G) action and by direct transfer to the microbial surface of a protein which increases bacterial permeability, cationic proteins of high molecular weight, and the so-called defensins. Low pH, lysozyme and lactoferrin constitute bactericidal or bacteriostatic factors which are oxygen independent and can function

under anaerobic circumstances. Finally, the killed organisms are digested by hydrolytic enzymes and the degradation products released to the exterior (figure 1.7).

By now, the reader may be excused a little smugness as she or he shelters behind the impressive anti-microbial potential of the phagocytic cells. But there are snags to consider; our formidable array of weaponry is useless unless the phagocyte can (i)

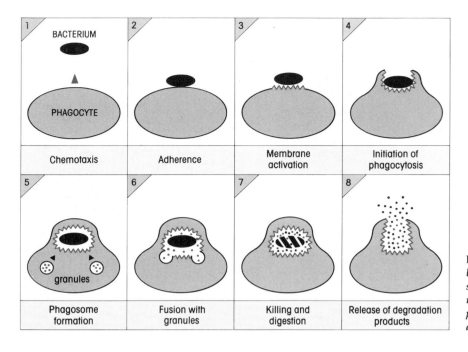

1	2	3	4
BACTERIUM / PHAGOCYTE			
Chemotaxis	Adherence	Membrane activation	Initiation of phagocytosis

5	6	7	8
granules			
Phagosome formation	Fusion with granules	Killing and digestion	Release of degradation products

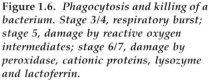

Figure 1.6. *Phagocytosis and killing of a bacterium. Stage 3/4, respiratory burst; stage 5, damage by reactive oxygen intermediates; stage 6/7, damage by peroxidase, cationic proteins, lysozyme and lactoferrin.*

6

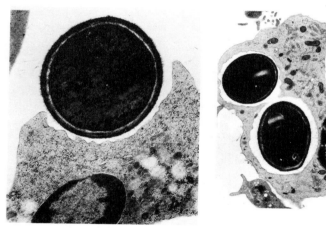

(a)   (b)

Figure 1.7. *Adherence and phagocytosis. (a) Phagocytosis of* **Candida albicans** *by a polymorphonuclear leucocyte (neutrophil). Adherence to the surface initiates enclosure of the fungal particle within arms of cytoplasm. Lysosomal granules are abundant but mitochondria are rare (× 15 000). (b) Phagocytosis of C. albicans by a monocyte showing near completion of phagosome formation (arrowed) around one organism and complete ingestion of two others (× 5000). (Courtesy of Dr H. Valdimarsson.)*

'home onto' the micro-organism, (ii) adhere to it, and (iii) respond by the membrane activation which initiates engulfment. Some bacteria do produce chemical substances such as the peptide formyl. met. leu. phe. which directionally attract leucocytes, a process known as chemotaxis; some organisms do adhere to the phagocyte surface and some do spontaneously provide the appropriate membrane initiation signal. However, our teeming microbial adversaries are continually mutating to produce new species which may outwit the defences by doing none of these. What then? The body has solved these problems with the effortless ease that comes with a few million years of evolution by developing the complement system.

Complement facilitates phagocytosis

Complement and its activation

Complement is the name given to a complex series of some 20 proteins which, along with blood clotting, fibrinolysis and kinin formation, forms one of the triggered enzyme systems found in plasma. These systems characteristically produce a rapid, highly amplified response to a trigger stimulus

6

Fig 1

CHAPTER 1

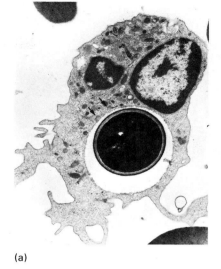
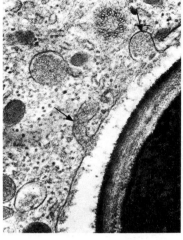

Figure 1.8. *Phagolysosome formation. (a) Neutrophil 30 minutes after ingestion of* C. albicans. *The cytoplasm is already partly degranulated and two lysosomal granules (arrowed) are fusing with the phagocytic vacuole. Two lobes of the nucleus are evident (× 5000). (b) Higher magnification of (a) showing fusing granules discharging their contents into the phagocytic vacuole (arrowed). (× 33 000; courtesy of Dr H. Valdimarsson.)*

(a)   (b)

OXYGEN-DEPENDENT MECHANISMS:

Glucose + NADP$^+$	$\xrightarrow[\text{shunt}]{\text{hexose monophosphate}}$	pentose phosphate + NADPH	$\left.\begin{array}{c} \\ \\ \end{array}\right\}$ O$_2$ burst + generation of superoxide anion
NADPH + O$_2$	$\xrightarrow{\text{cytochrome b}_{-245}}$	NADP$^+$ + **O$_2^-$**	
2O$_2^-$ + 2H$^+$	$\xrightarrow[\text{dismutation}]{\text{spontaneous}}$	**H$_2$O$_2$** + **^{1}O$_2$**	$\left.\begin{array}{c} \\ \\ \end{array}\right\}$ Spontaneous formation of further microbicidal agents
O$_2^-$ + H$_2$O$_2$	$\xrightarrow{}$	**.OH** + OH$^-$ + **^{1}O$_2$**	
H$_2$O$_2$ + Cl$^-$	$\xrightarrow{\text{myeloperoxidase}}$	**OCl$^-$** + H$_2$O	$\left.\begin{array}{c} \\ \\ \end{array}\right\}$ Myeloperoxidase generation of micro-bicidal molecules
OCl$^-$ + H$_2$O	$\xrightarrow{}$	**^{1}O$_2$** + Cl$^-$ + H$_2$O	
2O$_2^-$ + 2H$^+$	$\xrightarrow[\text{dismutase}]{\text{superoxide}}$	O$_2$ + H$_2$O$_2$	$\left.\begin{array}{c} \\ \\ \end{array}\right\}$ Protective mechanisms used by host + many microbes
2H$_2$O$_2$	$\xrightarrow{\text{catalase}}$	2H$_2$O + O$_2$	

OXYGEN-INDEPENDENT MECHANISMS:

Low mol. wt defensins Cathepsin G High mol. wt cationic proteins Bactericidal permeability increasing protein	Damage to microbial membranes
Lysozyme	Splits mucopeptide in bacterial cell wall
Lactoferrin	Deprives proliferating bacteria of iron
Proteolytic enzymes Variety of other hydrolytic enzymes	Digestion of killed organisms

Table 1.1. *Anti-microbial systems in phagocytic vacuoles. Microbicidal species in bold letters. O$_2^-$, superoxide anion; ^{1}O$_2$, singlet (activated) oxygen; OH, hydroxyl free radical.*

mediated by a cascade phenomenon where the product of one reaction is the enzymic catalyst of the next.

Some of the complement components are designated by the letter 'C' followed by a number which is related more to the chronology of its discovery than to its position in the reaction sequence. The most abundant and the most pivotal component is C3 which has a molecular weight of 195 kDa and is present in plasma at a concentration of around 1.2 mg/ml.

The C3 cleavage mechanism

Under normal circumstances, an internal thiolester bond in C3 becomes activated at a very slow rate either through reaction with water or with trace amounts of a plasma proteolytic enzyme to form a reactive intermediate, either the split product C3b, or a functionally similar molecule designated C3i or $C3(H_2O)$. In the presence of Mg^{++}, this can complex with another complement component, factor B, which then undergoes cleavage by a normal plasma enzyme (factor D) to generate C3bBb. Note that conventionally, a bar over a complex denotes enzymic activity and that on cleavage of a complement component, the larger product is generally given the suffix 'b' and the smaller 'a'.

C3bBb has an important new enzymic activity: it is a 'C3 convertase' which can split C3 to give C3a and C3b. We will shortly discuss the important biological consequences of C3 cleavage in relation to microbial defences, but under normal conditions there must be some mechanism to restrain this process to a 'tick-over' level since it can also give rise to more C3bBb, that is, we are dealing with a potentially runaway positive-feedback circuit (figure 1.9). As with all potentially explosive triggered cascades, there are powerful regulatory mechanisms.

The control of C3b levels

In solution, the C3bBb convertase is unstable and factor B is readily displaced by another component,

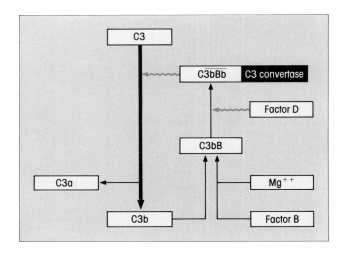

Figure 1.9. *The C3 convertase loop.* 〜〜〜〜➤ *represents an activation process. The horizontal bar above a component designates its activation.*

factor H, to form a complex which is susceptible to attack by the C3b inactivator, factor I (figure 1.10; further discussed on p. 240). The inactivated iC3b is biologically inactive and undergoes further degradation by proteases in the body fluids.

Activation of the C3 cleavage mechanism

A number of micro-organisms can activate the C3bBb convertase to generate large amounts of C3 cleavage products by stabilizing the enzyme on their (carbohydrate) surfaces thereby protecting the C3b from factor H. Another protein, properdin, acts subsequently on this bound convertase to stabilize

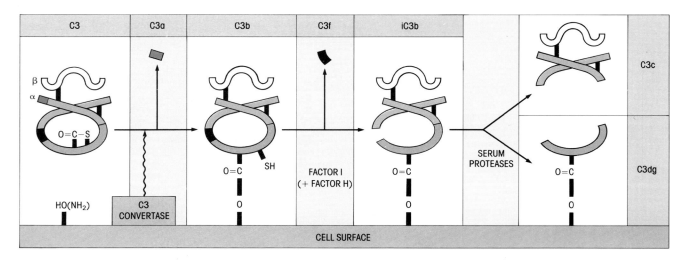

Figure 1.10. *Structural basis for the cleavage of C3 by C3 convertase and its binding to ·OH or ·NH$_2$ groups at the cell surface through exposure of the internal thiolester bonds.*

Further cleavage leaves a smaller fragment, C3d, attached to the membrane. (Based essentially on Law S.K.A. & Reid K.B.M. (1988) **Complement,** *figure 2.4, IRL Press, Oxford.)*

it even further. As C3 is split by the surface membrane-bound enzyme, it undergoes conformational change and its potentially reactive internal thiolester bond becomes exposed and binds covalently to hydroxyl or amino groups available at the microbial cell surface (figure 1.10). Each catalytic site thereby leads to the deposition of large numbers of C3b molecules on the micro-organism. This series of reactions leading to C3 breakdown provoked directly by microbes has been called '*the alternative pathway*' of complement activation (figure 1.11).

The post-C3 pathway

Recruitment of a further C3b molecule into the $\overline{C3bBb}$ enzymic complex generates a C5 convertase which activates C5 by proteolytic cleavage releasing a small polypeptide, C5a, and leaving the large C5b

fragment loosely bound to C3b. Sequential attachment of C6 and C7 to C5b forms a complex with a transient membrane binding site and an affinity for the β-peptide chain of C8. The C8α chain sits in the membrane and directs the conformational changes in C9 which transform it into an amphipathic molecule capable of insertion into the lipid bilayer (cf. the colicins, p. 2) and polymerization to an annular 'membrane attack complex' (MAC; figures 1.12 and 2.3). This forms a transmembrane channel fully permeable to electrolytes and water, and due to the high internal colloid osmotic pressure of cells, there is a net influx of Na$^+$ and water frequently leading to lysis.

Complement has a range of biological functions

These can be grouped conveniently under three headings:

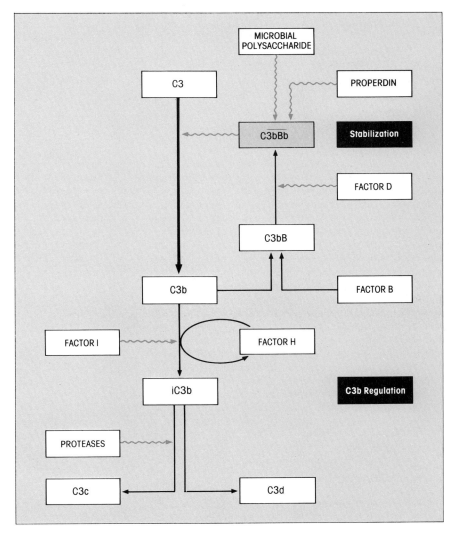

Figure 1.11. *Microbial activation of the alternative complement pathway by stabilization of the $\overline{C3bBb}$ enzyme, and its control by factors H and I. Although in phylogenetic terms this is the oldest pathway, it was discovered after a separate pathway to be discussed in the next chapter, and so has the confusing designation 'alternative'.*

9

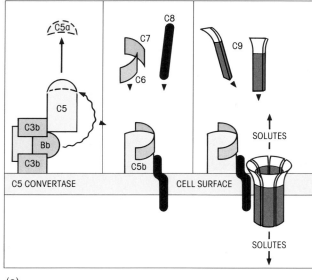

(a)

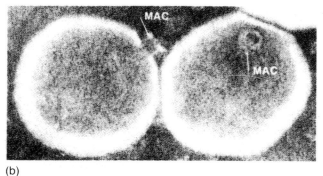

(b)

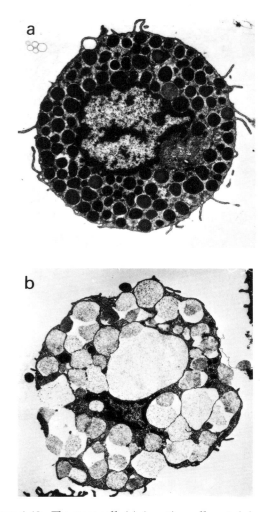

a

b

Figure 1.12. *Post C3 pathway generating C5a and the C5b−9 membrane attack complex (MAC). (a) Cartoon of molecular assembly. The conformational change in C9 protein structure which converts it from a hydrophilic to an amphipathic molecule (bearing both hydrophobic and hydrophilic regions) can be interrupted by an antibody raised against linear peptides derived from C9; since the antibody does not react with the soluble or membrane-bound forms of the molecule, it must be detecting an intermediate structure transiently revealed in a deep-seated structural rearrangement.*
(b) Electron micrograph of a membrane C5b−9 complex incorporated into liposomal membranes clearly showing the annular structure. The cylindrical complex is seen from the side inserted into the membrane of the liposome on the left, and end-on in that on the right. Although in itself a rather splendid structure, formation of the annular C9 cylinder is probably not essential for cytotoxic perturbation of the target cell membrane, since this can be achieved by insertion of amphipathic C9 molecules in numbers too few to form a clearly defined MAC. (Courtesy of Prof. J. Tranum-Jensen and Dr S. Bhakdi.)

Figure 1.13. *The mast cell. (a) A resting cell containing many membrane-bound granules containing pre-formed mediators. (b) A triggered mast cell. Note that the granules have released their contents and are morphologically altered, being larger and less electron dense. Although most of the altered granules remain within the circumference of the cell, they are open to the extracellular space. (Electron micrographs × 5400; courtesy of Drs D. Lawson, C. Fewtrell, B. Gomperts and M. Raff: from* **J. Exp. Med.** *1975, 142, 391.)*

organisms to the cell surface (discussed more fully on p. 205).

2 Biologically active fragments

C3a and C5a, the small peptides split from the parent molecules during complement activation, have several important actions. Both act directly on phagocytes, especially neutrophils, to stimulate the respiratory burst associated with production of oxygen metabolites and to enhance the expression of surface receptors for C3b and iC3b. Also, both are 'anaphylatoxins' in that they are capable of trig-

1 Adherence reactions

Phagocytic cells have receptors for C3b and iC3b which facilitate the adherence of C3b-coated micro-

gering mediator release from mast cells (figures 1.3 and 1.13) and their circulating counterpart the basophil (figure 1.3), a phenomenon of such relevance to our present discussion that I have presented details of the mediators and their actions in figure 1.14; note in particular the chemotactic properties of these mediators and their effects on blood vessels. In its own right, C5a is a potent neutrophil chemotactic agent and has a striking ability to act directly on the capillary endothelium to produce vasodilatation and increased permeability, an effect which seems to be prolonged by leukotriene B_4 released from activated mast cells, neutrophils and macrophages.

3 Membrane lesions

As described above, the insertion of the membrane attack complex into a membrane may bring about cell lysis. Providentially, complement is relatively inefficient at lysing the cell membranes of the autologous host due to the presence of control proteins.

The complement-mediated acute inflammatory reaction

We can now put together an effectively orchestrated defensive scenario initiated by activation of the

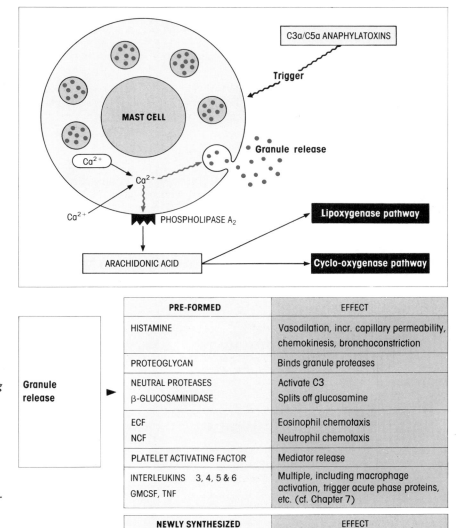

Figure 1.14. *Mast cell triggering leading to release of mediators by two major pathways: (i) release of pre-formed mediators present in the granules, and (ii) the metabolism of arachidonic acid produced through activation of a phospholipase. Intracellular* Ca^{++} *and cAMP are central to the initiation of these events but details are still unclear. Mast cell heterogeneity is discussed on p. 254. (ECF = eosinophil chemotactic factor; NCF = neutrophil chemotactic factor. Chemotaxis refers to directed migration of granulocytes up the concentration gradient of the mediator while chemokinesis describes randomly increased motility of these cells.)*

PRE-FORMED	EFFECT
HISTAMINE	Vasodilation, incr. capillary permeability, chemokinesis, bronchoconstriction
PROTEOGLYCAN	Binds granule proteases
NEUTRAL PROTEASES	Activate C3
β-GLUCOSAMINIDASE	Splits off glucosamine
ECF	Eosinophil chemotaxis
NCF	Neutrophil chemotaxis
PLATELET ACTIVATING FACTOR	Mediator release
INTERLEUKINS 3, 4, 5 & 6 GMCSF, TNF	Multiple, including macrophage activation, trigger acute phase proteins, etc. (cf. Chapter 7)

NEWLY SYNTHESIZED	EFFECT
LEUKOTRIENES C_4, D_4 (SRS-A) LEUKOTRIENE B_4	Vasoactive, bronchoconstriction, chemotaxis and/or chemokinesis
PROSTAGLANDINS THROMBOXANES	Affect bronchial muscle, platelet aggregation and vasodilation

Granule release → (PRE-FORMED)

Lipoxygenase pathway → (LEUKOTRIENES)
Cyclo-oxygenase pathway → (PROSTAGLANDINS)

alternative complement pathway (see figure 1.15).

In the first act, C3bBb is stabilized on the surface of the microbe and cleaves large amounts of C3. The C3a fragment is released but C3b molecules bind copiously to the microbe. These activate the next step in the sequence to generate C5a and the membrane attack complex (although many organisms will be resistant to its action).

A central role for the mast cell

The next act sees C3a and C5a, together with the mediators they trigger from the mast cell, acting to recruit polymorphonuclear neutrophils and further plasma complement components to the site of microbial invasion. The relaxation induced in arteriolar walls causes increased blood flow and dilatation of the small vessels while contraction of capillary endothelial cells allows exudation of plasma proteins. Under the influence of the chemotaxins, neutrophils slow down and the surface adhesion molecules they are stimulated to express cause them to marginate to the walls of the capil-

laries where they pass through gaps between the endothelial cells (diapedesis) and move up the concentration gradient of chemotactic factors until they come face to face with the C3b-coated microbe. Adherence to the neutrophil C3b-receptors then takes place, C3a and C5a at relatively high concentrations in the chemotactic gradient activate the respiratory burst and, hey presto, the slaughter of the last act can begin!

The processes of capillary dilatation (redness), exudation of plasma proteins and also of fluid (oedema) due to hydrostatic and osmotic pressure changes, and accumulation of neutrophils are collectively termed *the acute inflammatory response*.

And an important job for the macrophage?

Although not yet established with the same confidence that surrounds the role of the mast cell in acute inflammation, the concept seems to be emerging that the tissue macrophage may mediate a parallel series of events with the same final end result. Non-specific phagocytic events and certain

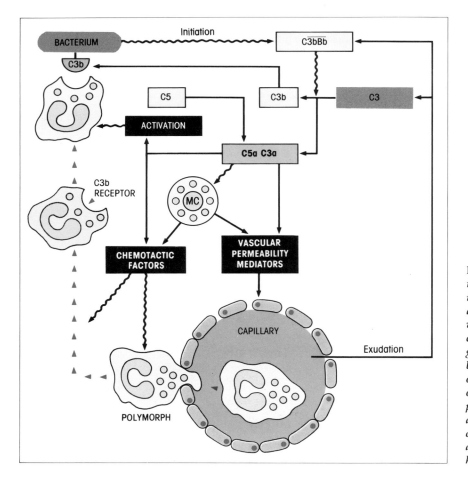

Figure 1.15. *The defensive strategy of the acute inflammatory reaction initiated by bacterial activation of the alternative C pathway. Directions: start with the activation of the C3bBb C3 convertase by the bacterium, notice the generation of C3b (which binds to the bacterium), C3a and C5a and recruitment of mast cell mediators, follow their effect on capillary dilatation and exudation of plasma proteins and their chemotactic attraction of polymorphs to the C3b-coated bacterium and triumph in their adherence and final activation for the kill.*

12

bacterial toxins such as the lipopolysaccharides (LPS) can activate macrophages, but the phagocytosis of C3b-opsonized microbes and the direct action of C5a generated through complement activation are guaranteed to goad the cell into copious secretion of mediators of the acute inflammatory response (figure 1.16).

Of these, the cytokines interleukin-1 and tumour necrosis factor up-regulate the expression of adhesion molecules for neutrophils on the surface of endothelial cells and promote the secretion of a neutrophil activation peptide (NAP-1). The polymorphonuclear neutrophils themselves are attracted by a potent neutrophil chemotactic factor (NCF) and leukotriene B_4. The latter also increases capillary permeability, an effect greatly enhanced by the co-secretion of prostaglandin E_2. Thus, under the stimulus of complement activation, the macrophage provides a pattern of cellular events which reinforce the mast-cell-mediated pathway leading to acute inflammation—yet another of the body's fail-safe redundancy systems (often known as the 'belt and braces' principle).

Humoral mechanisms provide a second defensive strategy

Turning now to those defence systems which are mediated entirely by soluble factors, we recollect that many microbes activate the complement system and may be lysed by the insert of the membrane attack complex. The spread of infection may be limited by enzymes released through tissue injury which activate the clotting system. Of the soluble bactericidal substances elaborated by the body, perhaps the most abundant and widespread is the enzyme lysozyme, a muramidase which splits the exposed peptidoglycan wall of susceptible bacteria (cf. figure 10.1).

Acute phase proteins

A number of plasma proteins collectively termed *acute phase proteins* show a dramatic increase in concentration in response to infection or tissue injury. These include C-reactive protein (CRP), serum amyloid A protein, α_1-anti-trypsin, α_2-macroglobulin, fibrinogen, caeruloplasmin, C9 and factor B.

As an example, during an infection, microbial products such as endotoxins stimulate the release of interleukin-1 (IL-1) which is an endogenous pyrogen (incidentally capable of improving our general defences by raising the body temperature) and IL-6. These in turn act on the liver to increase the synthesis and secretion of CRP to such an extent that its plasma concentration may rise 1000-fold.

Human CRP is composed of five identical polypeptide units non-covalently arranged as a cyclic

13

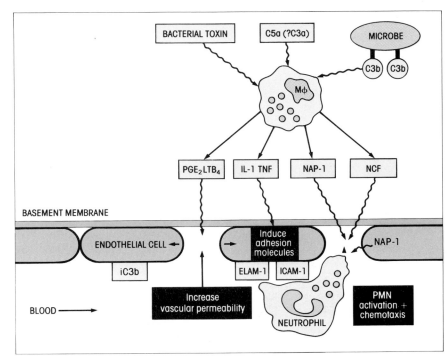

Figure 1.16. *Stimulation by complement components induces macrophage secretion of mediators of the acute inflammatory response. Blood neutrophils stick to the adhesion molecules on the endothelial cell and use this to provide traction as they force their way between the cells, through the basement membrane (with the help of secreted elastase) and up the chemotactic gradient. During this process they become progressively activated by NAP-1. (NAP-1, neutrophil activating peptide; NCF, neutrophil chemotactic factor; PGE$_2$, prostaglandin E$_2$; LTB$_4$, leukotriene B$_4$; IL-1, interleukin-1; TNF, tumour necrosis factor; ELAM-1, endothelial cell leucocyte adhesion molecule; ICAM-1, intercellular adhesion molecule.)*

pentamer. This class of protein has been around in the animal kingdom for some time since a closely related homologue, limulin, is present in the haemolymph of the horseshoe crab, not exactly a close relative of *Homo sapiens*. A major property of CRP is its ability to bind, in a Ca-dependent fashion, to a number of micro-organisms which contain phosphorylcholine in their membranes, the complex having the useful property of activating complement (by the classical and not the alternative pathway with which we are at present familiar). This results in the deposition of C3b on the surface of the microbe which thus becomes opsonized (i.e. 'made ready for the table') for adherence to phagocytes.

Another opsonin of the same ilk is the Ca-dependent mannose-binding protein which can attach to the surface carbohydrates of certain micro-organisms and then activate the classical complement sequence. Interest in the molecule conglutinin has perked up recently with the demonstration, first, that it is found in humans and not just in cows, and second, that it can bind to *N*-acetyl glucosamine; being polyvalent, this implies an ability to coat bacteria with C3b by cross-linking the available sugar residue in the complement fragment with the bacterial proteoglycan. Although it is not clear whether conglutinin is a member of the acute phase protein family, I mention it here because it embellishes the general idea that the evolution of lectin-like molecules which bind to microbial rather than self-polysaccharides and which can then hitch themselves to the complement system, provides a useful form of protection for the host against a number of infectious agents.

Interferons

These are a family of broad-spectrum anti-viral agents present in birds, reptiles and fishes as well as the higher animals, and first recognized by the phenomenon of viral interference in which an animal infected with one virus resists superinfection by a second unrelated virus. Different molecular forms of interferon have been identified, all of which have been gene cloned. There are at least 14 different α-interferons (IFNα) produced by leucocytes while fibroblasts, and probably all cell types, synthesize IFNβ. We will keep a third type (IFNγ), which is not directly induced by viruses, up our sleeves for the moment.

Cells synthesize interferon when infected by a virus and secrete it into the extracellular fluid whence it binds to specific receptors on uninfected neighbouring cells. The bound interferon now exerts its anti-viral effect in the following way. At least two genes are thought to be derepressed in the interferon-treated cell allowing the synthesis of two new enzymes. The first, a protein kinase, catalyses the phosphorylation of a ribosomal protein and an initiation factor necessary for protein synthesis, so greatly reducing mRNA translation. The other catalyses the formation of a short polymer of adenylic acid which activates a latent endonuclease; this in turn degrades both viral and host mRNA.

Whatever the precise mechanism of action ultimately proves to be, the net result is to establish a cordon of uninfectable cells around the site of virus infection so restraining its spread. The effectiveness of interferon *in vivo* may be inferred from experiments in which mice injected with an antiserum to murine interferons could be killed by several hundred times less virus than was needed to kill the controls. However, it must be presumed that interferon plays a significant role in the recovery from, as distinct from the prevention of, viral infections.

As a group, the interferons may prove to have a wider biological role than the control of viral infection. It will be clear, for example, that the induced enzymes described above would act to inhibit host cell division just as effectively as viral replication. The interferons may also modulate the activity of other cells such as the natural killer (NK) cells, to be discussed in the following section.

Extracellular killing

Natural killer (NK) cells

Viruses lack the apparatus for self-renewal so it is essential for them to penetrate the cells of the infected host in order to take over its replicative machinery. It is clearly in the interest of the host to find a way to kill such infected cells *before* the virus has had a chance to reproduce. NK cells appear to do just that when studied *in vitro*.

They are large granular lymphocytes (figure 2.6a) with a characteristic morphology (figure 2.7b). They are thought to recognize structures on high molecular weight glycoproteins which appear on the surface of virally infected cells and which allow them to be differentiated from normal cells. This recognition occurs through receptors on the NK cell surface which bring killer and target into close opposition. Activation of the NK cell ensues and leads to polarization of granules between nucleus and target within minutes and extracellular release of their contents into the space between the two cells.

Perhaps the most important of these is a *perforin* or *cytolysin* bearing some structural homology to C9; like that protein, but without any help other than from Ca^{2+}, it can insert itself into the membrane of the target, apparently by binding to phosphorylcholine through its central amphipathic domain. It then polymerizes to form a transmembrane pore with an annular structure, comparable to the complement membrane attack complex. Whereas C9-induced cell lysis involves initial damage to outer membranes followed later by nuclear changes, NK cells kill by *apoptosis* (programmed cell death) in which one sees very rapid nuclear fragmentation effected by a Ca-dependent endonuclease which acts on the vulnerable DNA between nucleosomes to produce the 200 kb 'nucleosome ladder' fragments; only afterwards can one detect release of ^{51}Cr-labelled cytoplasmic proteins through defective cell surface membranes. Thus, although perforin and C9 appear to produce comparable membrane 'pores', this dramatic difference in killing mechanisms has led to some doubt concerning the precise role of the perforin molecules. It has certainly been claimed that antibodies made against the cytolysin inhibit this extracellular killing. The granules also contain lymphotoxin (tumour necrosis factor β) and two serine esterases which can function as NK cytotoxic factors but the time course of their action casts some doubt over the primacy of their role in NK-mediated lysis. Chondroitin sulphate A, a protease-resistant highly negatively charged proteoglycan, is also present and may subserve the function of protecting the NK cell from autolysis by its own lethal agents (figure 1.17).

The various interferons augment NK cytotoxicity and since interferons are produced by virally infected cells, we have a nicely integrated feedback defence system.

Eosinophils

Large parasites such as helminths cannot physically be phagocytosed and extracellular killing by eosinophils would seem to have evolved to help cope with this situation. These polymorphonuclear

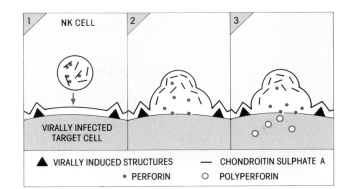

Figure 1.17. *Extracellular killing of virally infected cell by natural killer (NK) cell (following diagram by Tschopp J. & Conzelmann A. In **Immunology Today** 1986, 7, 135). As the NK receptors bind to the surface of the virally infected cell, the granules release perforin molecules extracellularly; these polymerize to form transmembrane channels which bring about lysis of the target. Tschopp & Conzelmann have shown that chondroitin sulphate A binds to and inactivates the perforin particularly at the low pH within the granule and suggest that as the granule discharges, the higher pH dissociates the perforin which then acts to lyse the target cell.*

'cousins' of the neutrophil have distinctive granules which stain avidly with acid dyes (figure 1.3) and have a characteristic appearance in the electron microscope (figure 10.16). A major basic protein (MBP) is localized in the core of the granules while an eosinophilic cationic protein together with a peroxidase have been identified in the granule matrix. Other enzymes include arylsulphatase B, phospholipase D and histaminase. They have surface receptors for C3b and on activation produce a particularly impressive respiratory burst with concomitant generation of active oxygen metabolites. As if that were not enough, it has recently been demonstrated that one of the granule proteins can produce a transmembrane plug in the target membrane like C9 and the NK perforin.

Most helminths can activate the alternative complement pathway, but although resistant to C9 attack, their coating with C3b allows adherence of eosinophils through their C3b receptors. If this contact should lead to activation, the eosinophil will launch its extracellular attack which includes the release of MBP and especially the cationic protein which damages the parasite membrane.

THE BASIS OF IMMUNOLOGY
II – Specific Acquired Immunity

The need for specific immune mechanisms

Our microbial adversaries have tremendous opportunities through mutation to evolve strategies which evade our innate immune defences. For example, most of the *successful* parasites activate the alternative complement pathway and bind C3b, yet eosinophils which adhere are somehow not triggered into offensive action. The same holds true for many bacteria while some may so shape their exteriors as to avoid complement activation completely. The body obviously needed to 'devise' defence mechanisms which could be dovetailed individually to each of these organisms no matter how many there were. In other words *a very large number* of specific immune defences needed to be at the body's disposal. Quite a tall order!

Antibody — the specific adaptor

Evolutionary processes came up with what can only be described as a brilliant solution. This was to fashion an adaptor molecule which was intrinsically capable not only of activating the complement system *and* of stimulating phagocytic cells, but also of sticking to the offending microbe. The adaptor thus had three main regions, two concerned in communicating with complement and the phagocytes (the biological functions) and one devoted to

binding to an individual micro-organism (the external recognition function). In most biological systems like hormones and receptors, and enzymes and substrates, recognition usually occurs through fairly accurate complementarity in shape allowing the ligands to approach so close to each other as to permit the normal intermolecular forces to become relatively strong. In the present case, each adaptor would have a recognition portion complementary in shape to some micro-organism to which it could then bind reasonably firmly. The part of the adaptor with biological function would be constant, but for each of hundreds of thousands of different organisms, a special recognition portion would be needed.

Thus the body has to make hundreds of thousands, or even millions, of adaptors with different recognition sites. The adaptor is of course the molecule we know affectionately as *antibody* (figure 2.1).

Antibody initiates a new complement pathway ('classical')

Antibody, when bound to a microbe, will link to the first molecule in the so-called classical complement sequence, C1q. This molecule is polyvalent with respect to antibody binding and consists of a central collagen-like stem branching into six peptide chains each tipped by an antibody-binding subunit (resembling the blooms on a bouquet of flowers). C1q is associated with two further subunits, C1r and C1s, in a Ca^{++} stabilized trimolecular complex

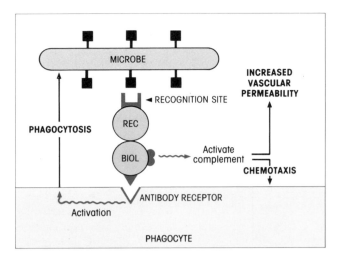

Figure 2.1. *The antibody adaptor molecule. The constant part with biological function (BIOL) activates complement and the phagocyte. The portion with the recognition unit for the foreign microbe (REC) varies from one antibody to another.*

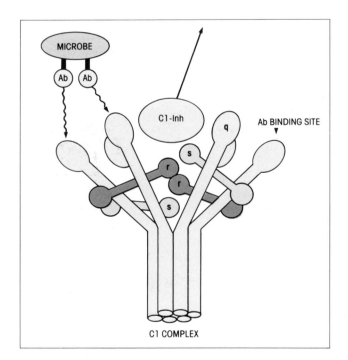

Figure 2.2. *Activation of the classical complement pathway. C1 is composed of C1q associated with the flexible rod-like Ca-dependent complex, $C1r_2-C1s_2$ (⬤—⬤—r—⬤—⬤); s and r indicate potential serine protease active sites) which interdigitate with the six arms of C1q, either as indicated or as 'W' shapes on the outer side of these arms. The C1-inhibitor normally prevents spontaneous activation of $C1r_2-C1s_2$. If the complex of a microbe or antigen with antibodies attaches to two or more of the globular Ab-binding sites on C1q, the molecule presumably undergoes conformational change which releases the C1-Inh and activates $C1r_2-C1s_2$.*

(figure 2.2). Changes in C1q consequent upon binding the antigen−antibody complex bring about the sequential activation of proteolytic activity in C1r and then C1s.

Both these molecules contain repeats of a 60 amino acid unit folded as a globular domain and referred to as a short consensus repeat (SCR) or more recently as a complement control protein repeat (CCP) since it is a characteristic structural feature of several proteins involved in control of the complement system. As a consequence of antibody binding to C1q, C1s acquires protease activity. The next component in the chain C4 (unfortunately components were numbered before the sequence was established) now binds to C1 through these €CPs and is cleaved enzymatically by C1s. As expected in a multi-enzyme cascade, several molecules of C4 undergo cleavage, releasing a small C4a fragment and revealing a nascent but labile internal thiolester

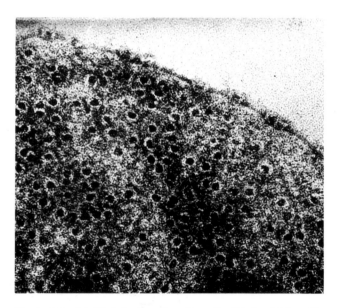

Figure 2.3. *Multiple lesions in cell wall of* **Escherichia coli** *bacterium caused by interaction with IgM antibody and complement. (Human antibodies are divided into five main classes, immunoglobulin M — shortened to IgM — IgG, IgA, IgE and IgD, which differ in the specialization of their 'rear ends' for different biological functions such as complement activation or mast cell sensitization.) Each lesion is caused by a single IgM molecule and shows as a 'dark pit' due to penetration by the 'negative stain'. This is somewhat of an illusion since in reality these 'pits' are like volcano craters standing proud of the surface, and are each single 'membrane attack' complexes. Comparable results may be obtained in the absence of antibody since the cell wall endotoxin can activate the alternative pathway in the presence of higher concentrations of serum. Magnification × 400 000. (Courtesy of Drs R. Dourmashkin and J.H. Humphrey.)*

bond in the residual C4b like that in C3 (cf. figure 1.10) which may then bind either to the antibody-C1 complex or the surface of the microbe itself. Note that C4a, like C5a and C3a, has anaphylatoxin activity, although feeble and 4b resembles C3b in its opsonic activity.

In the presence of Mg^{++}, C2 can complex with the C4b to become a new substrate for the C1s; the resulting product C4b2b now has the vital C3 convertase activity required to activate C3 with the same specificity as the C3bBb generated by the alternative pathway. From then on things march along exactly in parallel to the post-C3 pathway with one molecule of C3b added to the C4b2b to make it into a C5-splitting enzyme with eventual production of the membrane attack complex (figure 2.3). Just as the alternative pathway C3 convertase is controlled by factors H and I, so the breakdown of C4b2b is brought about by either a C4 binding protein (C4bp) or a cell surface C3b receptor (CR1) in the presence of factor I.

The similarities between the two pathways are set out in figure 2.4 and show how antibody can supplement and even improve on the ability of the innate immune system to initiate acute inflammatory reactions. Antibody provides yet a further bonus in this respect; the class known as immunoglobulin E (see legend to figure 2.3) can sensitize mast cells through binding to their surface so that combination with antigen triggers mediator release independently of C3a or C5a, adding yet more flexibility to our defences.

Complexed antibody activates phagocytic cells

I drew attention to the fact that many C3b-coated organisms adhere to phagocytic cells yet avoid provoking their uptake. If small amounts of antibody are added the phagocyte springs into action. It does so through the recognition of two or more antibody molecules bound to the microbe, using specialized receptors on the cell surface.

A single antibody molecule complexed to the micro-organism is not enough because it cannot cause the cross-linking of antibody receptors in the phagocyte surface membrane which is required to activate the cell. There is a further consideration connected with what is often called 'the bonus effect of multivalency'; for thermodynamic reasons, which will be touched on in Chapter 4, the associ-

19

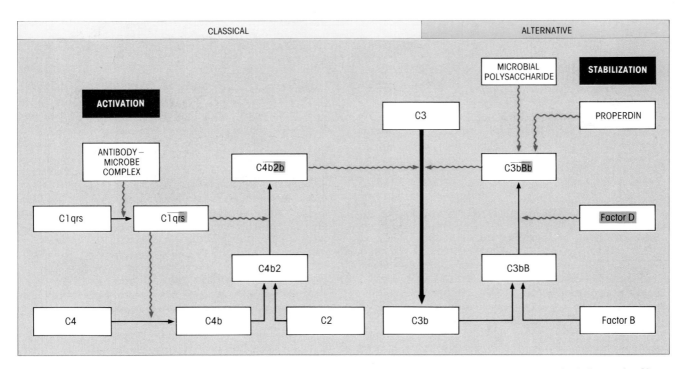

Figure 2.4. *Comparison of the alternative and classical complement pathways. The classical pathway with odd exceptions such as C-reactive protein, is antibody dependent, the alternative pathway is not. The molecular unit with protease activity is highlighted. Beware confusion with nomenclature. The large C2 fragment which forms the C3 convertase is often labelled as C2a but to be consistent with C4b, C3b and C5b, it seems more logical to call it C2b.*

ation constant of ligands which use several rather than a single bond to react with receptors is increased geometrically rather than arithmetically. For example, three antibodies bound close together on a bacterium could be attracted to a macrophage a thousand times more strongly than a single antibody molecule (figure 2.5).

Cellular basis of antibody production

Antibodies are made by lymphocytes

The majority of resting lymphocytes are small cells with a darkly staining nucleus due to condensed chromatin and relatively little cytoplasm containing the odd mitochondrion required for basic energy provision. Figures 2.6 and 2.7 compare the mor-

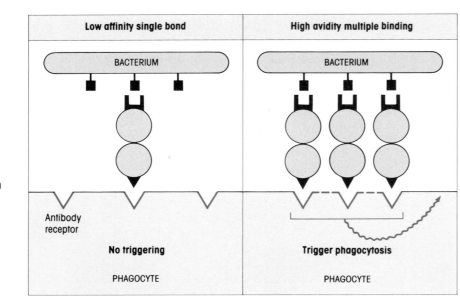

Figure 2.5. *Binding of bacterium to phagocyte by multiple antibodies gives strong association forces and triggers phagocytosis by cross-linking the surface receptors for antibody.*

Facing page

Figure 2.6. *Cells involved in the acquired immune response. (a) Small lymphocytes. Condensed chromatin gives rise to heavy staining of the nucleus. The cell on the bottom is a typical resting granular T-cell with a thin rim of cytoplasm. The upper nucleated cell is a large granular lymphocyte (LGL); it has more cytoplasm and azurophilic granules are evident. Isolated platelets are visible. B-lymphocytes range from small to intermediate in size and lack granules. Giemsa stain. (b) Small agranular T-cells stained with non-specific esterase showing Gall bodies (each a cluster of primary lysosomes associated with a lipid droplet) which appear as characteristic cytoplasmic dot(s), stained for non-specific esterase; compare with diffuse distribution in cytoplasm of monocyte at side. (c) T-lymphocytes from buffy coat stained with a monoclonal anti-T using the alkaline phosphatase immunoenzymatic method (cf. figure 5.21). Note the single unstained non-T lymphocyte on the bottom. (d) Transformed lymphocytes (lymphoblasts) following stimulation of lymphocytes in culture with a polyclonal activator. The large lymphoblasts with their relatively high ratio of cytoplasm to nucleus may be compared in size with the isolated small lymphocyte. One cell is in mitosis. May–Grunewald–Giemsa. (e) Identification of lymphocytes by rosette formation with red cells visualized in U.V. light after staining with Acridine Orange which makes the lymphocyte nucleus fluorescent green. T-cell rosettes are formed by spontaneous*
binding to sheep erythrocytes. B-cell rosettes are developed through binding of IgG-coated erythrocytes to specific cell surface receptors. (f) Immunofluorescent staining of B-lymphocyte surface immunoglobulin using fluorescein-conjugated (■) anti-Ig. Provided the reaction is carried out in the cold to prevent pinocytosis, the labelled antibody cannot penetrate to the interior of the viable lymphocytes and reacts only with surface components. Patches of aggregated surface Ig are seen which are beginning to form a cap in the right-hand lymphocyte. During cap formation, submembranous myosin becomes redistributed in association with the surface Ig and induces locomotion of the previously sessile cell in a direction away from the cap. (g) Plasma cells. The nucleus is eccentric. The cytoplasm is strongly basophilic due to high RNA content. The juxta-nuclear lightly stained zone corresponds with the Golgi region. May–Grunewald–Giemsa. (h) Plasma cells stained to show intracellular immunoglobulin using a fluorescein-labelled anti-IgG (green) and a rhodamine-conjugated anti-IgM (red). (i) Langerhans cells in human epidermis in leprosy, increased in the subepidermal zone, possibly as a consequence of the disease process. Stained by the immunoperoxidase method with S-100 antibodies. Material for (a), (b) and (c) was kindly supplied by Mr M. Watts of the Dept. Haematology, Middlesex Hospital Medical School, (d), (e) and (f) by Dr P. Lydyard, (g) and (h) by Prof. C. Grossi and (i) by Dr Marian Ridley.

20

CHAPTER 2

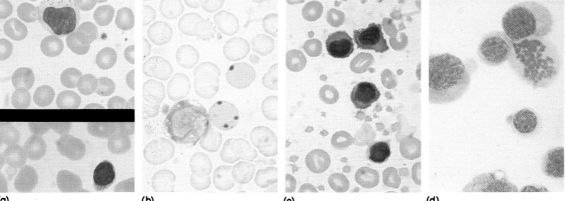

(a)   (b)   (c)   (d)

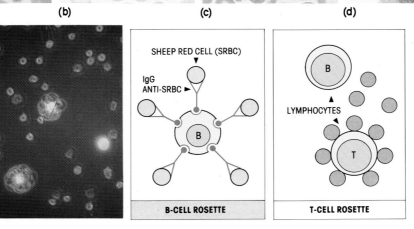

(e)

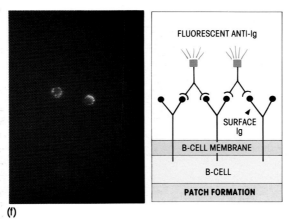

(f)

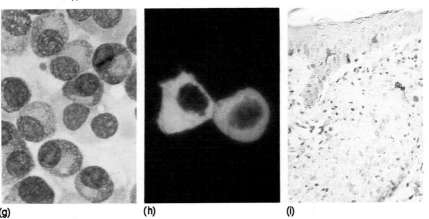

(g)   (h)   (i)

SPECIFIC ACQUIRED IMMUNITY

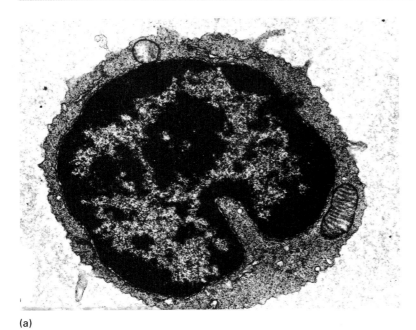

(a)

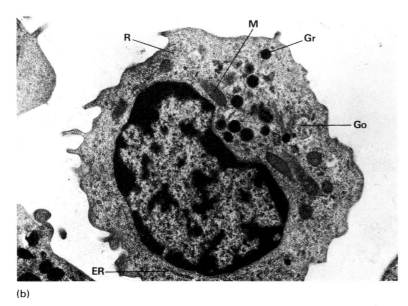

(b)

Figure 2.7. *(a) Small agranular T-lymphocyte. Indented nucleus with condensed chromatin, sparse cytoplasm: single mitochondrion shown and many free ribosomes but otherwise few organelles (× 13 000). B-lymphocytes are essentially similar with slightly more cytoplasm and occasional elements of rough-surfaced endoplasmic reticulum. (b) Large granular lymphocyte (× 7500). The more abundant cytoplasm contains several mitochondria (M), free ribosomes (R) with some elements of rough-surfaced endoplasmic reticulum (ER), prominent Golgi apparatus (Go) and characteristic membrane-bound electron-dense granules (Gr). The nuclear chromatin is less condensed than that of the agranular T-cell. (Courtesy of Drs A. Zicca and C.E. Grossi.)*

phology of these cells with that of the minority population of large granular lymphocytes which includes the NK set referred to in Chapter 1.

The central role of the small lymphocyte in the production of antibody was established largely by the work of Gowans. He depleted rats of their lymphocytes by chronic drainage of lymph from the thoracic duct by an indwelling cannula, and showed that they had a grossly impaired ability to mount an antibody response to microbial challenge. The ability to form antibody could be restored by injecting thoracic duct lymphocytes obtained from another rat. The same effect could be obtained if,

before injection, the thoracic duct cells were first incubated at 37°C for 24 hours under conditions which kill off large and medium sized cells and leave only the small lymphocytes. This shows that the small lymphocyte is necessary for the antibody response.

The small lymphocytes can be labelled if the donor rat is previously injected with tritiated thymidine; it then becomes possible to follow the fate of these lymphocytes when transferred to another rat of the same strain which is then injected with micro-organisms to produce an antibody response (figure 2.8). It transpires that after contact

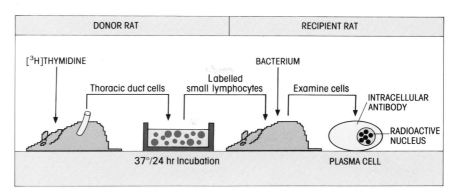

Figure 2.8. *Labelled small lymphocytes become antibody-forming plasma cells when transferred to a recipient rat which is immunized with a bacterium. Transferred cell with radioactive nucleus shown by autoradiography. Intracellular antibody revealed by staining with fluorescent probes (cf. figure 2.6h).*

with the injected microbes, some of the transferred labelled lymphocytes develop into plasma cells (figures 2.6g and 2.9) which can be shown to contain (figure 2.6h) and secrete antibody.

Antigen selects the lymphocytes which make antibody

The molecules in the micro-organisms which evoke and react with antibodies are called *antigens* (*generates anti*bodies). It was originally envisaged that antibodies were derived from some master plastic molecule which could be moulded to the right shape by using the antigen as a template. Stimulated by the ideas of Jerne and Burnet and many others (not forgetting the incredible Ehrlich who foresaw it at the turn of the century, would you believe it?!), we now know that antibodies are formed before antigen is ever seen and that they are *selected for* by antigen.

It works in the following way. Each lymphocyte of a subset called the B-lymphocytes, because they differentiate in the bone marrow, is programmed to make one, and only one, antibody and it places this antibody on its outer surface to act as a receptor. This can be detected by using fluorescent probes and in figure 2.6f one can see the molecules of antibody on the surface of a human B-lymphocyte stained with a fluorescent rabbit antiserum raised against a preparation of human antibodies. Each lymphocyte has of the order of 10^5 antibody molecules on its surface.

When an antigen enters the body, it is confronted by a dazzling array of lymphocytes all bearing different antibodies each with its own individual recognition site. The antigen will only bind to those receptors with which it makes a good fit. Lymphocytes whose receptors have bound antigen receive a triggering signal and develop into antibody-

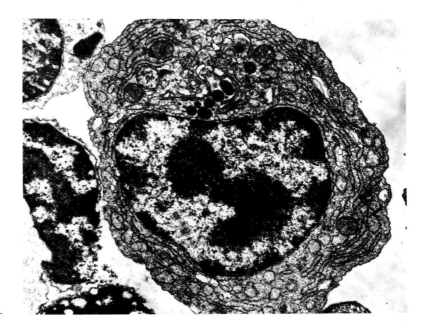

Figure 2.9. *Plasma cell (× 10 000). Prominent rough-surfaced endoplasmic reticulum associated with the synthesis and secretion of Ig.*

SPECIFIC ACQUIRED IMMUNITY

forming plasma cells and since the lymphocytes are programmed to make only one antibody, that secreted by the plasma cell will be identical with that originally acting as the lymphocyte receptor, i.e. it will bind well to the antigen. In this way, antigen selects for the antibodies which recognize it effectively (figure 2.10).

The need for clonal expansion means humoral immunity must be acquired

Because we can make hundreds of thousands, maybe even millions, of different antibody molecules, it is not feasible for us to have too many lymphocytes producing each type of antibody; there just would not be enough room in the body to accommodate them. To compensate for this, lymphocytes which are triggered by contact with antigen undergo successive waves of proliferation (figure 2.6d) to build up a large clone of plasma cells which will be making antibody of the kind for which the parent lymphocyte was programmed. By this system of *clonal selection*, large enough concentrations of antibody can be produced to combat infection effectively (figure 2.11).

The importance of proliferation for the development of a significant antibody response is highlighted by the ability of anti-mitotic drugs to abolish antibody production to a given antigen stimulus completely.

Because it takes time for the proliferating clone to build up its numbers sufficiently, it is usually several days before antibodies are detectable in the serum following primary contact with antigen. The newly formed antibodies are a consequence of antigen exposure and it is for this reason that we speak of the *acquired immune response*.

When we make an antibody response to a given infectious agent, by definition that micro-organism must exist in our environment and we are likely to meet it again. It would make sense then for the immune mechanisms alerted by the first contact with antigen to leave behind some memory system which would enable the response to any subsequent exposure to be faster and greater in magnitude.

Our experience of many common infections tells us that this must be so. We rarely suffer twice from such diseases as measles, mumps, chicken-pox, whooping cough and so forth. The first contact clearly imprints some information, imparts some *memory*, so that the body is effectively prepared to repel any later invasion by that organism and a state of immunity is established.

Secondary antibody responses

By following the production of antibody on the first and second contacts with antigen we can see the basis for the development of immunity. For example, when we inject a bacterial product such as tetanus toxoid into a rabbit, for reasons already discussed, several days elapse before antibodies

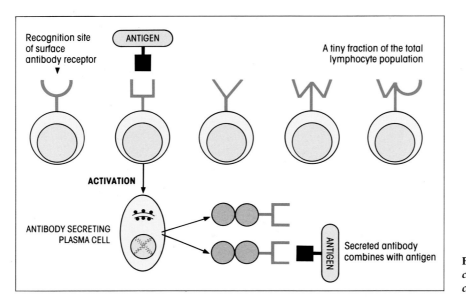

Figure 2.10. *Antigen activates those B-cells whose surface antibody receptors it can combine with firmly.*

24

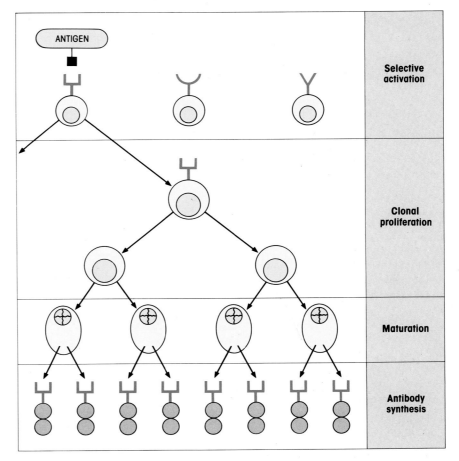

Figure 2.11. *Clonal selection. The cell selected by antigen undergoes many divisions during the clonal proliferation and the progeny mature to give an expanded population of antibody-forming cells. The antibody response is particularly vulnerable to anti-mitotic agents at the proliferation stage.*

can be detected in the blood; these reach a peak and then fall (figure 2.12). If we now allow the animal to rest and then give a second injection of toxoid, the

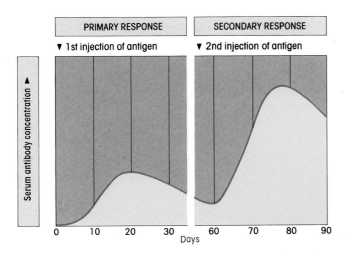

Figure 2.12. *Primary and secondary response. A rabbit is injected on two separate occasions with tetanus toxoid. The antibody response on the second contact with antigen is more rapid and more intense.*

course of events is dramatically altered. Within two to three days the antibody level in the blood rises steeply to reach much higher values than were observed in the *primary response*. This *secondary response* then is characterized by a more rapid and more abundant production of antibody resulting from the 'tuning up' or priming of the antibody-forming system.

With our knowledge of lymphocyte function, it is perhaps not surprising to realize that these are the cells which provide memory. This can be demonstrated by adoptive transfer of lymphocytes to another animal, an experimental system frequently employed in immunology (cf. figure 2.8). In the present case, the immunological potential of the transferred cells is expressed in a recipient treated with X-rays which destroy its own lymphocyte population; thus any immune response will be of donor not recipient origin. In the experiment described in figure 2.13, small lymphocytes are taken from an animal given a primary injection of tetanus toxoid and transferred to an irradiated host which is then boosted with the antigen; a rapid, intense

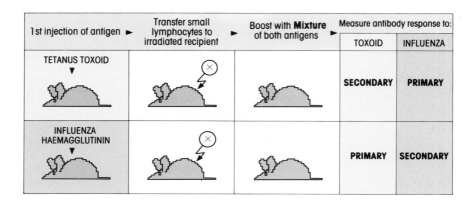

1st injection of antigen ▶	Transfer small lymphocytes to irradiated recipient ▶	Boost with **Mixture** of both antigens ▶	Measure antibody response to:	
			TOXOID	INFLUENZA
TETANUS TOXOID ▼			SECONDARY	PRIMARY
INFLUENZA HAEMAGGLUTININ ▼			PRIMARY	SECONDARY

Figure 2.13. *Memory for a primary response can be transferred by small lymphocytes. Recipients are treated with a dose of X-rays which directly kill lymphocytes (highly sensitive to radiation) but only affect other body cells when they divide; the recipient thus functions as a living 'test-tube' which permits the function of the donor cells to be followed.*

The reasons for the design of the experiment are given in the text. In practice, because of the possibility of interference between the two antigens, it would be wiser to split each of the primary antigen-injected groups into two, giving a separate boosting antigen to each to avoid using a mixture.

production of antibody characteristic of a secondary response is seen. To exclude the possibility that the first antigen injection might exert a *non-specific* stimulatory effect on the lymphocytes, the boosting injection includes influenza haemagglutinin as a control antigen. Furthermore, a 'criss-cross' control group primed with influenza haemagglutinin must also be included to ensure that this antigen is capable of giving a secondary booster response. I have explained the design of the experiment at some length to call attention to the need for careful selection of controls.

The higher response given by a primed lymphocyte population can be ascribed mainly to an expansion of the numbers of cells capable of being stimulated by the antigen (figure 2.14) although we shall see later that there are some qualitative differences in the cells as well.

The specificity of acquired immunity

The establishment of memory or immunity by one organism does not confer protection against another unrelated organism. After an attack of measles we are immune to further infection but are susceptible to other agents such as the polio or mumps viruses. Acquired immunity then shows *specificity* and the immune system can differentiate specifically between the two organisms. A more formal experimental demonstration of this discriminatory power was seen in figure 2.13 where priming with tetanus toxoid evoked memory for that antigen but not for influenza and vice versa.

The basis for this lies of course in the ability of the recognition sites of the antibody molecules to distinguish between antigens; antibodies which react with the toxoid do not bind to influenza and, *mutatis mutandis* as they say, anti-influenza is not particularly smitten with the toxoid.

This ability to recognize one antigen and distinguish it from another goes even further. The individual must also recognize what is foreign, i.e. what is 'non-self'. The failure to discriminate between 'self' and 'non-self' could lead to the synthesis of antibodies directed against components of the subject's own body (*autoantibodies*) which in principle could prove to be highly embarrassing. On purely theoretical grounds it seemed to Burnet and Fenner that the body must develop some mechanism whereby 'self' and 'non-self' could be distinguished, and they postulated that those circulating body components which were able to reach the developing lymphoid system in the perinatal period could in some way be 'learnt' as 'self'. A permanent unresponsiveness or tolerance would then be created so that as immunological maturity was reached there would normally be an inability to respond to 'self' components. As we shall see later, these predictions have been amply verified.

Vaccination

Nearly 200 years ago, Edward Jenner carried out the remarkable studies which mark the beginning of immunology as a systematic subject. Noting the pretty pox-free skin of the milkmaids, he reasoned

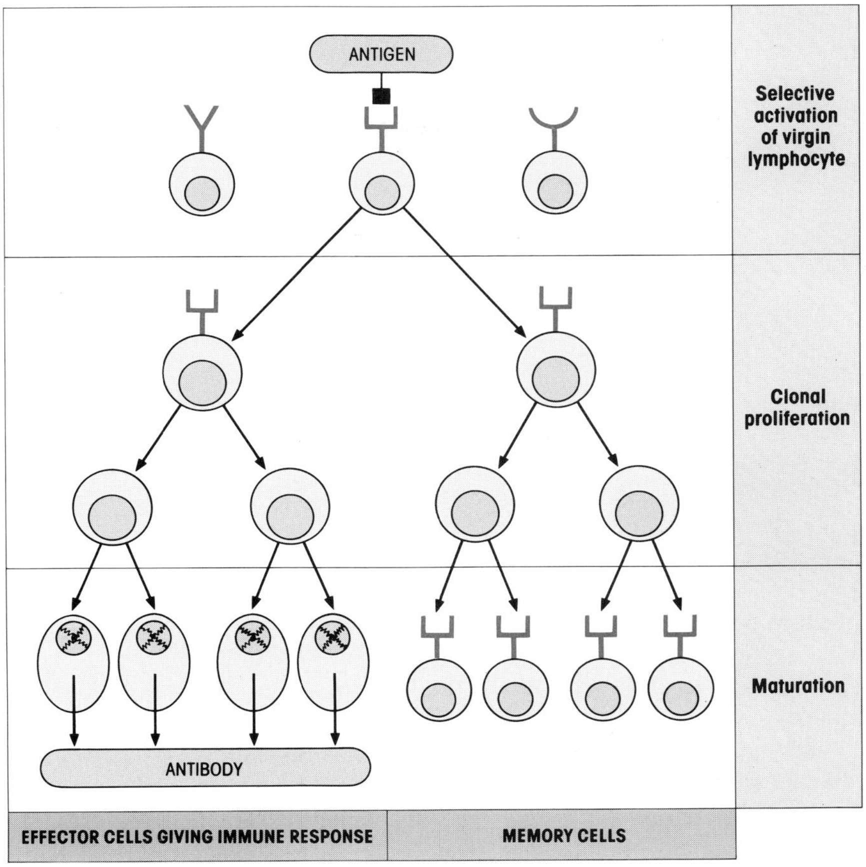

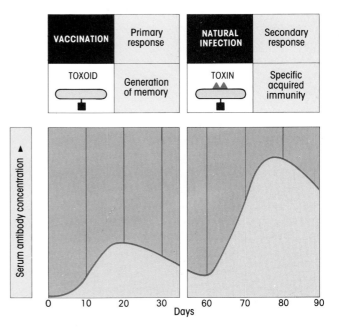

Figure 2.14. *The cellular basis for the generation of effector and memory cells after primary contact with antigen. A fraction of the progeny of the original antigen-reactive lymphocytes become non-dividing memory cells and others the effector cells of humoral or, as we shall see subsequently, cell-mediated immunity. Memory cells require fewer cycles before they develop into effectors and this shortens the reaction time for the secondary response. The expanded clone of cells with memory for the original antigen provides the basis for the greater secondary relative to the primary immune response. Priming with low doses of antigen can often stimulate effective memory without producing very adequate antibody synthesis.*

27

that deliberate exposure to the pox virus of the cow, which is not virulent for the human, might confer protection against the related human small-pox organism. Accordingly, he inoculated a small boy with cowpox and was delighted—and I hope relieved—to observe that he was now protected against a subsequent exposure to smallpox (what would today's ethical committees have said about that?!). By injecting a harmless form of a disease organism, Jenner had utilized the specificity and memory of the acquired immune response to lay the foundations for modern vaccination (Latin *vacca*, cow).

The essential strategy is to prepare an innocuous form of the infectious organism or its toxins which still substantially retains the antigens responsible for establishing protective immunity. This has been done by using killed or live attenuated organisms, purified microbial components or chemically modified antigens (figure 2.15).

Figure 2.15. *The basis of vaccination illustrated by the response to tetanus toxoid. Treatment of the bacterial toxin with formaldehyde destroys its toxicity (associated with ▲▲) but retains antigenicity. Exposure to toxin in a subsequent natural infection boosts the memory cells producing high levels of neutralizing antibody which are protective.*

SPECIFIC ACQUIRED IMMUNITY

Cell-mediated immunity protects against intracellular organisms

Many micro-organisms live inside host cells where it is impossible for humoral antibody to reach them. Obligate intracellular parasites like viruses *have* to replicate inside cells; facultative intracellular parasites like mycobacteria and leishmania can replicate within cells, particularly macrophages, but *don't have to*; they like the intracellular life because of the protection it affords. A totally separate acquired immunity system has evolved to deal with this situation based on a distinct lymphocyte subpopulation made up of T-cells, designated thus because, unlike the B-lymphocytes, they differentiate within the milieu of the thymus gland. Because they are specialized to operate against cells bearing intracellular organisms, T-cells only recognize antigen when it is on the surface of a body cell. Accordingly, its surface receptors, which are different from the antibody molecules used by B-lymphocytes, recognize antigen *plus* a surface marker which informs the T-lymphocyte that it is making contact with another cell. These cell markers belong to an important group of molecules known as the major histocompatibility complex (MHC) identified originally through their ability to evoke powerful transplantation reactions in other members of the same species.

Lymphokine-producing T-cells help macrophages to kill intracellular parasites

These organisms only survive inside macrophages through their ability to subvert the innate killing mechanisms of these cells. None the less, they cannot prevent the macrophage from processing small antigenic fragments (possibly of organisms which have spontaneously died) and placing them on the host cell surface. A subpopulation of T-lymphocytes called T-helper cells, if primed to that antigen, will recognize and bind to the combination of antigen with class II MHC molecules on the macrophage surface and produce a variety of soluble factors called *lymphokines*. These include γ-interferon and other macrophage activating factors which switch on the previously subverted microbicidal mechanisms of the macrophage and bring about the death of the intracellular micro-organisms (figure 2.16).

Killing of virally infected cells by cytotoxic T-cells

We have already discussed the advantage to the host of killing virally infected cells before the virus begins to replicate and have seen that large granular lymphocytes with NK activity (p. 14) can subserve a cytotoxic function. However, NK cells have a limited range of specificities and in order to improve their efficacy, this range needs to be expanded.

One way in which this can be achieved is by coating the target cell with antibodies specific for the virally coded surface antigens because NK cells have receptors for the constant part of the antibody molecule, rather like phagocytic cells. Thus antibodies will bring the NK cell very close to the target by forming a bridge, and the NK cell being activated by the complexed antibody molecules is able to kill the virally infected cell by its extracellular mechanisms (figure 2.17). This system, termed *'antibody-dependent cell-mediated cytotoxicity'* (ADCC) is very impressive when studied *in vitro* but it has proved difficult to establish to what extent it operates within the body.

On the other hand, a subset of cytotoxic T-cells has evolved for which there is evidence of *in vivo* activity. These cells have a very wide range of antigen specificities because they clonally express a large number of different surface receptors similar to, but not identical with, the surface antibody receptors on the B-lymphocytes. Again, each lymphocyte is programmed to make only one receptor and, like the T-helper cell, recognizes antigen only in association with a cell marker, in this case class I MHC molecules (figure 2.17). Through this recognition of surface antigen, the cytotoxic cell comes into intimate contact with its target and administers the 'kiss of death'. It also releases γ-interferon which would help to reduce the spread of virus to adjacent cells, particularly in cases where the virus itself may prove to be a weak inducer of IFNα or β.

In an entirely analogous fashion to the B-cell, T-cells are selected and activated by combination with antigen, expanded by clonal proliferation and mature to give T-helper and cytotoxic T-effectors together with an enlarged population of memory cells. Thus both T- and B-cells provide specific acquired immunity with a variety of mechanisms which in most cases operate to extend the range of effectiveness of innate immunity and confer the valuable advantage that a first infection prepares us to withstand further contact with the same micro-organism.

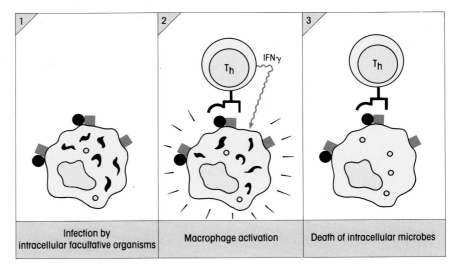

Figure 2.16. *Intracellular killing of micro-organisms by macrophages activated by lymphokines released from T-helpers binding to surface microbial antigen (●) complexed with class II MHC molecules (■).*

1	2	3
Infection by intracellular facultative organisms	Macrophage activation	Death of intracellular microbes

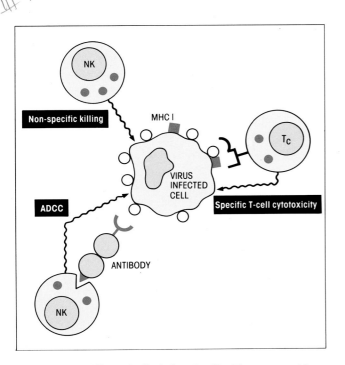

Figure 2.17. *Killing virally infected cells. The non-specific killing mechanism of the NK cell can be focused on the target by antibody to produce antibody-dependent cell-mediated cytotoxicity (ADCC). The cytotoxic T-cell homes onto its target specifically through receptor recognition of surface antigen in association with MHC class I molecules.*

Immunopathology

The immune system is clearly 'a good thing', but like mercenary armies, it can turn to bite the hand that feeds it, and cause damage to the host.

Thus where there is an especially heightened response or persistent exposure to exogenous antigens, tissue damaging or *hypersensitivity* reactions may result. Examples are allergy to grass pollens, blood dyscrasias associated with certain drugs, immune complex glomerulonephritis occurring after streptococcal infection, and chronic granulomas produced during tuberculosis or schistosomiasis.

In other cases, the ability to maintain non-reactivity against self-components may break down giving rise to a wide variety of diseases with an *autoimmune* component, such as thyrotoxicosis, myasthenia gravis and many of the rheumatological disorders.

Another immunopathological reaction of some consequence is *transplant rejection* where the major histocompatibility complex antigens on the donor graft may well provoke a fierce reaction. Lastly, one should consider the by no means infrequent occurrence of inadequate functioning of the immune system—immunodeficiency. I would like to think that at this stage the reader would have no difficulty in predicting that the major problems in this condition relate to persistent infection, the type of infection being related to the elements of the immune system which are defective.

SUMMARY

Innate immunity

A wide range of innate immune mechanisms operate which do not improve with repeated exposure to infection. Micro-organisms are kept out of the body by the skin, the secretion of mucus, ciliary action, the lavaging action of bactericidal fluids (e.g. tears), gastric acid and microbial antagonism. If penetration occurs, bacteria are destroyed by soluble factors such as lysozyme and by phagocytosis with intracellular digestion.

The main phagocytic cells are polymorphonuclear neutrophils and macrophages. Organisms adhere to their surface, activate the engulfment process and are taken inside the cell where they fuse with cytoplasmic granules. A formidable array of oxygen-dependent and oxygen-independent microbicidal mechanisms then come into play.

The complement system, a multicomponent triggered enzyme cascade, is used to attract phagocytic cells to the microbes and engulf them. The most abundant component, C3, is split by a convertase enzyme formed from its own cleavage product C3b and factor B and stabilized against breakdown caused by factors H and I, through association with the microbial surface. As it is formed, C3b becomes linked covalently to the microorganism. The next component, C5, is activated yielding a small peptide, C5a; the residual C5b binds to the surface and assembles the terminal components C6—9 into a membrane attack complex which is freely permeable to solutes and can lead to osmotic lysis. C5a is a potent chemotactic agent for polymorphs and greatly increases capillary permeability. C3a and C5a act on mast cells causing the release of further mediators such as histamine, leukotriene B4 and tumour necrosis factor (TNF) with effects on capillary permeability and adhesiveness, and neutrophil chemotaxis; they also activate neutrophils. The activated neutrophils bind to the C3b-coated microbes by their surface C3b receptors and may then ingest them. The influx of polymorphs and the increase in vascular permeability constitute the potent anti-microbial *acute inflammatory response* (figure 2.18). Inflammation can also be initiated by tissue macrophages which subserve a similar role to the mast cell, since signalling by bacterial toxins, C5a or by iC3b-coated bacteria adhering to surface complement receptors causes release of TNF, LTB4, PGE$_2$, neutrophil chemotactic factor and a neutrophil activating peptide.

Other humoral defences involve the acute phase proteins such as C-reactive protein.

Recovery from viral infections can be effected by the interferons which block viral replication. Virally infected cells can be killed by large granular lymphocytes with natural killer (NK) activity.

Extracellular killing by C3b-bound eosinophils may be responsible for the failure of many large parasites to establish a foothold in potential hosts.

30

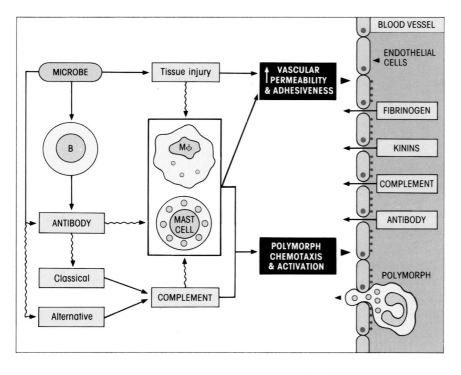

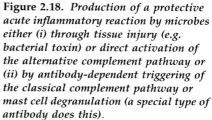

Figure 2.18. *Production of a protective acute inflammatory reaction by microbes either (i) through tissue injury (e.g. bacterial toxin) or direct activation of the alternative complement pathway or (ii) by antibody-dependent triggering of the classical complement pathway or mast cell degranulation (a special type of antibody does this).*

Specific acquired immunity

The antibody molecule evolved as a specific adaptor to attach to micro-organisms which either fail to activate the alternative complement pathway or prevent activation of the phagocytic cells. The antibody fixes to the antigen by its specific recognition site and its constant structure regions activate complement through the classical pathway (binding C1 and generating a C4b2b convertase to split C3) and phagocytes through their antibody receptors. This supplementary route into the acute inflammatory reaction is enhanced by antibodies which sensitize mast cells and by immune complexes which stimulate mediator release from tissue macrophages (figure 2.18).

Antibodies are made by plasma cells derived from B-lymphocytes each of which is programmed to make only one antibody which is placed on the cell surface as a receptor. Antigen binds to the cell with a complementary antibody, activates it and causes clonal proliferation and finally maturation to antibody-forming cells and memory cells. Thus the antigen brings about clonal selection of the cells making antibody to itself. The increase in memory cells after priming means that the acquired secondary response is faster and greater providing the basis for vaccination, using a harmless form of the infective agent for the initial injection.

Another class of lymphocyte, the T-cell, is concerned with control of intracellular infections. Like the B-cell, each T-cell has its individual antigen receptor (although it differs structurally from anti-body) which recognizes antigen and undergoes clonal expansion to form effector and memory cells providing specific acquired immunity. The T-cell recognizes cell surface antigens in association with molecules of the major histocompatibility complex (MHC).

T-helper cells which see antigen with class II MHC on the surface of macrophages, release γ-interferon to activate the macrophage and enable it to kill intracellular parasites. Unlike NK cells, cytotoxic T-cells have the ability to recognize specific antigen plus class I MHC on the surface of virally infected cells which are killed before the virus replicates. They also release γ-interferon which can make surrounding cells resistant to viral spread (figure 2.19).

Although the innate mechanisms do not improve with repeated exposure to infection as do the acquired, they play a vital role since they are intimately linked to the acquired systems by two different pathways which all but encapsulate the whole of immunology. Antibody, complement and polymorphs give protection against most extracellular organisms while T-cells, soluble cytokines, macrophages and NK cells deal with intracellular infections (figure 2.20).

Immunopathologically-mediated tissue damage can occur as a result of (i) inappropriate hypersensitivity reactions to exogenous antigens, (ii) loss of tolerance to self-giving autoimmune disease and (iii) reaction to foreign grafts. Immunodeficiency leaves the individual susceptible to infection.

31

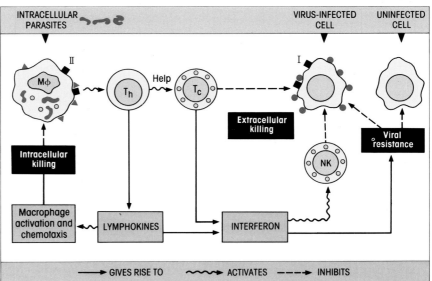

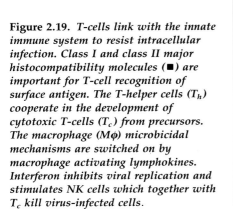

Figure 2.19. *T-cells link with the innate immune system to resist intracellular infection. Class I and class II major histocompatibility molecules (■) are important for T-cell recognition of surface antigen. The T-helper cells (T$_h$) cooperate in the development of cytotoxic T-cells (T$_c$) from precursors. The macrophage (Mφ) microbicidal mechanisms are switched on by macrophage activating lymphokines. Interferon inhibits viral replication and stimulates NK cells which together with T$_c$ kill virus-infected cells.*

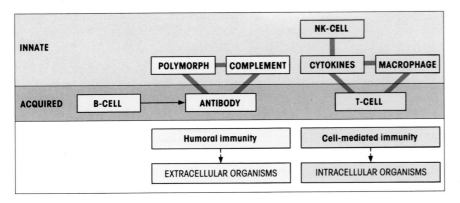

Figure 2.20. *The two pathways linking innate and acquired immunity which provide the basis for humoral and cell-mediated immunity respectively.*

Further reading

Gallin J., Goldstein I. & Snyderman R. (eds) (1987) *Inflammation: Basic Principles and Clinical Correlates.* Raven Press, New York.

Herberman R.B., Reynolds C.W. & Ortaldo J. (1986) Mechanisms of cytotoxicity by NK cells. *Ann. Rev. Immunol.,* 4, 651.

Klein J. (ed.) (1990) *Immunology.* Blackwell Scientific Publications. (An up-to-date, well-written, scholarly tome.)

Law S.K.A. & Reid K.B.M. (1988) *Complement. In Focus Series.* D.K. Male (ed.). IRL Press, Oxford.

Melchers F. *et al.* (eds) (1989) Series of up-to-date articles on complement, mast cells and the role of macrophages in mediating acute inflammation. In *Progress in Immunology* **VII.** Springer-Verlag, Berlin.

Mims C.A. & White D.O. (1984) *Viral Pathogenesis and Immunology.* Blackwell Scientific Publications, Oxford.

Rother K. & Till G.O. (eds) (1988) *The Complement System.* Springer-Verlag, Berlin.

General reading

Herbert W.J., Wilkinson P.C. & Stott D.I. (eds) (1985) *Dictionary of Immunology,* 3rd edn. Blackwell Scientific Publications, Oxford.

Hood L.E., Weissman I.L., Wood W.B. & Wilson J.H. (1984) *Immunology,* 2nd edn. Benjamin/Cummings, California, USA. (A very good, in-depth textbook of fundamental immunology in which concepts are extended by numerous mind-bending problems, many of which are based on original data. Thin on clinical side.)

Male K., Champion B. & Cooke A. (1987) *Advanced Immunology.* Gower Medical Publishing, London.

Playfair J.H.L. (1987) *Immunology at a Glance,* 4th edn. Blackwell Scientific Publications, Oxford. (Very useful for revision.)

Roitt I.M., Brostoff J. & Male D.K. (1989) *Immunology,* 2nd edn. Gower Medical Publishing, London. (An extensively and colourfully illustrated textbook.)

Stites D.P., Stobo J.D. & Wells J.V. (1987) *Basic and Clinical Immunology,* 6th edn. Lange Medical Publications, California. (I find this of most use for reference purposes.)

Historical

Ehrlich P. (1890) *On Immunity with Special Reference to Cell Life.* In *Progress in Immunology* **VII**. Melchers F. *et al.* (eds) Springer-Verlag, Berlin. (Translation of a lecture to the Royal Society (London) on the side-chain theory of antibody formation, showing this man's perceptive genius. A 'must'!)

Humphrey J.H. & White R.G. (1970) *Immunology for Students of Medicine,* 3rd edn. Blackwell Scientific Publications, Oxford. (Dated but scholarly.)

Landsteiner K. (1946) *The Specificity of Serological Reactions.* Harvard University Press (reprinted 1962 by Dover Publications, New York).

Mazumdar P.M.M. (ed.) (1989) *Immunology 1930—1980.* Wall & Thompson, Toronto.

Metchnikoff E. (1893) *Comparative Pathology of Inflammation.* Transl. F.A. & E.H. Starling, Kegan Paul, Trench, Trübner & Co., London.

Parish H.J. (1968) *Victory with Vaccines.* Churchill Livingstone, Edinburgh.

Silverstein A.M. (1989) *A History of Immunology.* Academic Press, San Diego.

Series for the advanced reader

Advances in Immunology (Annual). Academic Press, London.

Ann. Rev. Immunology. Ann Reviews Inc., California.

Immunological Reviews (ed. G. Moller). Munksgaard, Copenhagen.

Progress in Allergy. S. Karger, Basle.

Progress in Immunology. Springer-Verlag, Berlin. (Triennial proceedings of the international congresses in immunology with an up-to-date account of a wide range of subjects.)

Seminars in Immunology. W.B. Saunders, Philadelphia.

Current information

Current Opinion in Immunology. Current Science, London. (Focused highlights of the advances made in the previous year.)

Immunology Today. Elsevier Science Publications, Amsterdam. (The immunologist's 'newspaper'.)

Major journals

Ann. Allergy, Ann. d'Immunologie, Cancer Immunol., Cell, Cell. Immunology, Clin. Allergy, Clin. Exp. Immunology, Clin. Immunol & Immunopath, European J. Immunology, Human Immunol., Immunogenetics, Immunology, Immunopharmacology, Immunotherapy, Infect. & Immunity, Int. Arch. Allergy, J. Allergy Clin. Immunol., J. Autoimmunity, J. Clin. Immunol., J. Clin. Lab. Immunology, J. Exp. Med., J. Immunogenetics, J. Immunology, J. Immunol. Methods, J. Reticuloendoth. Soc., Lancet, Mol. Immunol., Nature, N. Engl. J. Med., Parasitic Immunol., Scand. J. Immunology, Science, Tissue Antigens, Transplantation.

CHAPTER 3

MOLECULES WHICH RECOGNIZE ANTIGEN

THE IMMUNOGLOBULINS

The basic structure is a four-peptide unit

The antibody molecule is made up of two identical heavy and two identical light chains held together by interchain disulphide bonds (figure 3.1). These chains can be separated by reduction of the S—S

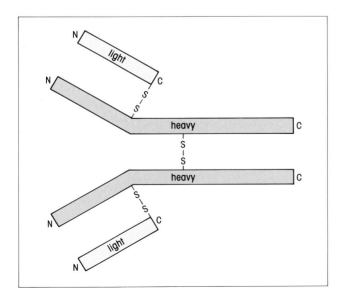

Figure 3.1. *Antibody model with two heavy and two light polypeptide chains held by interchain disulphide bonds. In the diagram the amino-terminal residue (N) is on the left for each chain.*

bonds and acidification. In the most abundant type of antibody, immunoglobulin G, the exposed hinge region is extended in structure due to the high proline content and is therefore vulnerable to proteolytic attack; thus the molecule is split by papain to yield two identical fragments, each with a single combining site for antigen (Fab; *fragment antigen binding*), and a third fragment which lacks the ability to bind antigen and is termed Fc (*fragment crystallizable*). Pepsin strikes at a different point and cleaves the Fc from the remainder of the molecule to leave a large 5S fragment which is formulated as F(ab')$_2$ since it is still divalent with respect to antigen binding just like the parent antibody (figure 3.2).

The location of the antigen combining sites was elegantly demonstrated by a study of purified antibodies to the dinitrophenyl (DNP) group mixed with the compound:

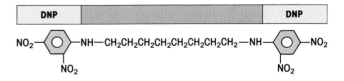

The two DNP groups are far enough apart not to interfere with each other's combination with antibody so that they can bring the antigen combining sites on two different antibodies together end to end. When viewed by negative staining in the electron microscope, a series of geometric forms are observed which represent the different structures to

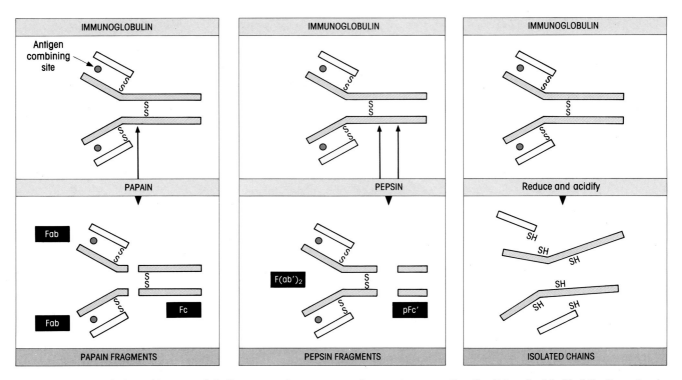

| IMMUNOGLOBULIN | IMMUNOGLOBULIN | IMMUNOGLOBULIN |

Antigen combining site

PAPAIN   PEPSIN   Reduce and acidify

Fab   F(ab')₂
Fab   Fc   pFc'

PAPAIN FRAGMENTS   PEPSIN FRAGMENTS   ISOLATED CHAINS

Figure 3.2. *Degradation of immunoglobulin to constituent peptide chains and to proteolytic fragments showing divalence of pepsin F(ab')$_2$ for antigen binding and univalence of the papain Fab. After pepsin digestion the pFc'* *fragment representing the C-terminal half of the Fc region is formed and is held together by non-covalent bonds. The portion of the heavy chain in the Fab fragment is given the symbol Fd.*

be expected if a Y-shaped hinged molecule with a combining site at the end of each of the two arms of the Y were to complex with this divalent antigen. Triangular trimers, square tetramers and pentagonal pentamers may be readily discerned (figure 3.3). The way in which these polymeric forms arise is indicated in figure 3.4. The position of the Fc fragment and its lack of involvement in the combination with antigen are apparent from the shape of the polymers formed using the pepsin F(ab')$_2$ fragment (figure 3.3e).

Amino acid sequences reveal variations in immunoglobulin structure

For good reasons, the antibody population in any given individual is just incredibly heterogeneous, and this has meant that determination of amino acid sequences was utterly useless until it proved possible to obtain the homogeneous product of a single clone. The opportunity to do this first came from the study of *myeloma proteins*.

In the human disease known as multiple myeloma, one cell making one particular individual im-

munoglobulin divides over and over again in the uncontrolled way a cancer cell does, without regard for the overall requirement of the host. The patient then possesses enormous numbers of identical cells derived as a clone from the original cell and they all synthesize the same immunoglobulin—the myeloma or M-protein—which appears in the serum, sometimes in very high concentrations. By purification of the myeloma protein we can obtain a preparation of an immunoglobulin having a unique structure. Monoclonal antibodies can also be obtained by fusing individual antibody-forming cells with a B-cell tumour to produce a constantly dividing clone of cells dedicated to making the one antibody (cf. figures 2.10 and 7.11).

The sequencing of a number of such proteins has revealed that the N-terminal portions of both heavy and light chains show considerable variability whereas the remaining parts of the chains are relatively constant, being grouped into a restricted number of structures. It is conventional to speak of variable and constant regions of both heavy and light chains (figure 3.5).

Certain sequences in the variable regions show quite remarkable diversity and systematic analysis

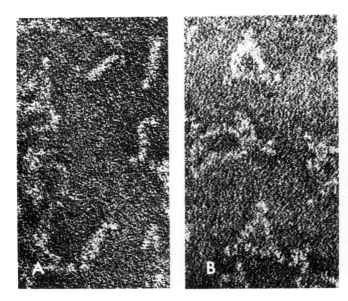

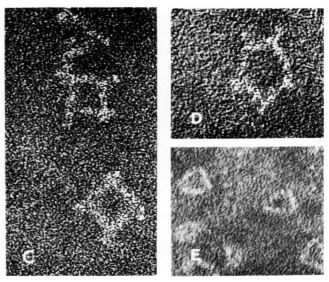

Figure 3.3. (a)–(d) Electron micrograph (× 1 000 000) of complexes formed on mixing the divalent DNP hapten with rabbit anti-DNP antibodies. The 'negative stain' phosphotungstic acid is an electron-dense solution which penetrates in the spaces between the protein molecules. Thus the protein stands out as a 'light' structure in the electron beam. The hapten links together the Y-shaped antibody molecules to form (a) dimers, (b) trimers, (c) tetramers and (d) pentamers (cf. figure 3.4). The flexibility of the molecule at the hinge region is evident from the variation in angle of the arms of the 'Y'.

(e) As in (b); trimers formed using the F(ab')₂ antibody fragment from which the Fc structures have been digested by pepsin (×500 000). The trimers can be seen to lack the Fc projections at each corner evident in (b). (After Valentine R.C. & Green N.M. (1967). J. mol. Biol. 27, 615; courtesy of Dr Green and with the permission of Academic Press, New York.)

37

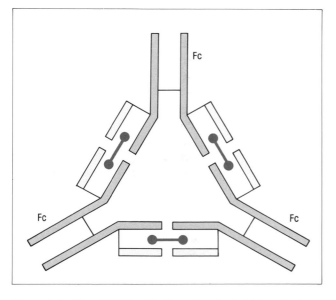

Figure 3.4. Three DNP antibody molecules held together as a trimer by the divalent antigen (●—●). Compare figure 3.3b. When the Fc fragments are first removed by pepsin, the corner pieces are no longer visible (figure 3.3e).

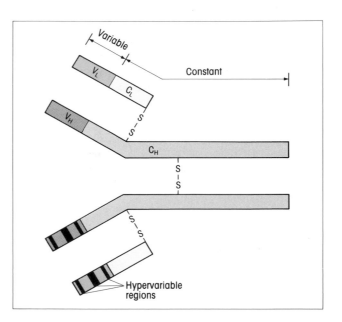

Figure 3.5. Amino acid sequence variability in the antibody molecule. The terms 'V region' and 'C region' are used to designate the variable and constant regions respectively, 'V_L' and 'C_L' are generic terms for these regions on the light chain and 'V_H' and 'C_H' specify variable and constant regions on the heavy chain. As stressed previously, each pair of heavy chains are identical, as are each pair of light chains.

localizes these hypervariable sequences to three segments on the light chain (figure 3.6) and three on the heavy chain.

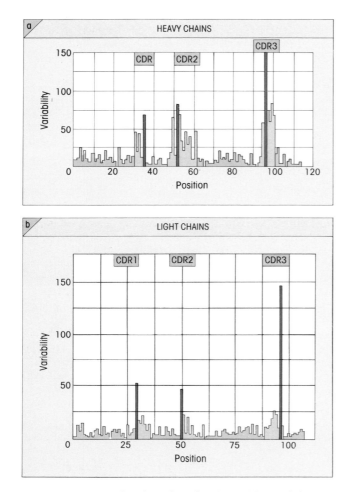

Figure 3.6. *Wu and Kabat plot of amino acid variability in the variable region of immunoglobulin heavy and light chains. The sequences of chains from a large number of myeloma monoclonal proteins are compared and variability at each position is computed as the number of different amino acids found divided by the frequency of the most common amino acid; obviously, the higher the number the greater the variability. The three hypervariable regions (green) in the heavy (a) and light chains (b), usually referred to as Complementarity Determining Regions (CDR), are clearly defined. The intervening peptide sequences are termed framework regions. (Courtesy of Prof. E.A. Kabat.)*

Isotypes

Based upon the structure of their heavy chain constant regions, immunoglobulins are classed into major groups termed *classes* which may be further subdivided into subclasses. In the human, for example, there are five classes: immunoglobulin G (IgG), IgA, IgM, IgD and IgE, They may be differentiated not only by their sequences but also by the

antigenic structures to which these sequences give rise. Thus, by injecting a human IgG myeloma protein into a rabbit, it is possible to raise an antiserum which can be absorbed by mixtures of myelomas of other classes to remove cross-reacting antibodies and which will then be capable of reacting with IgG, but not IgA, IgM, IgD or IgE (figure 3.7).

Since all the heavy chain constant region (C_H) structures which give rise to classes and subclasses are expressed together in the serum of a normal subject, they are termed isotypic variants (table 3.1). Likewise, the light chain constant regions (C_L) exist in isotypic forms known as κ and λ which are associated with all heavy chain isotypes. Because the light chains in a given antibody are identical, immunoglobulins are either κ or λ but never mixed (unless specially engineered in the laboratory). Thus IgG exists as IgGκ *or* IgGλ, IgM as IgMκ or IgMλ, and so on.

Allotypes

This type of variation depends upon the existence of allelic forms (encoded by alleles or alternative genes at a single locus) which therefore provide genetic markers (table 3.1). In somewhat the same way as the red cells in genetically different individuals can differ in terms of the blood group antigen system A, B, O, so the Ig heavy chains differ in the expression of their allotypic groups. Typical allotypes are the Gm specificities on IgG (Gm = *marker on IgG*) which are recognizable by the ability of the individual's IgG to block agglutination of red cells coated with anti-rhesus D bearing the Gm allotype by sera from patients with rheumatoid arthritis containing the appropriate anti-Gm rheumatoid factors (figure 3.8). Allotypic differences at a given Gm locus usually involve one or two amino acids in the peptide chain. Take, for example, the G1m(a) locus on IgG1 (table 3.1). An individual with this allotype would have the peptide sequence: Asp.Glu. Leu.Thr.Lys. on each of his IgG1 molecules. Another person whose IgG1 was a-negative would have the sequence *Glu.* Glu.*Met.*Thr.Lys., i.e. two amino acids different. To date, 25 Gm groups have been found on the γ-heavy chains and a further three (the Km—previously Inv groups) on the κ constant region.

Allotypic markers have also been found on the immunoglobulins of rabbits and of mice using reagents prepared by immunizing one animal with an immune complex obtained with antibodies from

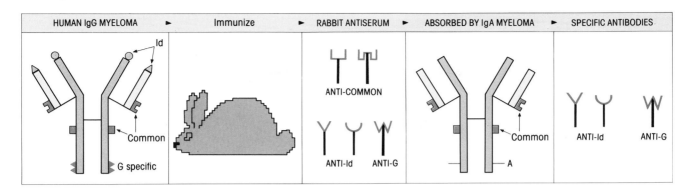

| HUMAN IgG MYELOMA | ► | Immunize | ► | RABBIT ANTISERUM | ► | ABSORBED BY IgA MYELOMA | ► | SPECIFIC ANTIBODIES |

Figure 3.7. *How to use monoclonal myeloma proteins to produce antibodies specific for different Ig structures. The rabbit makes antibodies directed to different parts of the human IgG myeloma. Antibodies to those parts which are common to other Ig classes can be absorbed out with myelomas of those classes leaving antibodies reacting with class-specific G and variable region-specific (idiotype; Id) structures on the original molecule. By the same token, further absorption with other IgG myelomas will remove the common IgG specific antibodies leaving an antiserum directed to the idiotypic determinants alone. (In an attempt to simplify, I have ignored subclasses and allotypes, but the same principles can be extended to generating antisera specific for these variants.) The rabbit produces a mixture of polyclonal antibodies directed against each structural site on the antigen, i.e. they are produced by clones derived from a variety of antigen-specific parent cells which each react stereochemically in a slightly different way with the same structure (cf. p. 67).*

V_H/V_L		C_H/C_L	
IDIOTYPE	ISOTYPE	▬▬	ISOTYPE

▲ Hypervariable
(Ag combining site)

▲ ALLOTYPE

TYPE OF VARIATION	DISTRIBUTION	VARIANT	LOCATION	EXAMPLES
ISOTYPIC	All variants present in serum of a normal individual	Classes Subclasses Types Subgroups Subgroups	C_H C_H C_L C_L V_H/V_L	IgM, IgE IgA1, IgA2 κ, λ λOz^+, λOz^- $V_{\kappa I}$ $V_{\kappa II}$ $V_{\kappa III}$ V_{HI} V_{HII} V_{HIII}
ALLOTYPIC	Alternative forms: genetically controlled so not present in all individuals	Allotypes	Mainly C_H/C_L sometimes V_H/V_L	Gm groups (human) b4, b5, b6, b9 (rabbit light chains) Igh-1ª, Igh-1ᵇ (mouse γ_{2a} heavy chains)
IDIOTYPIC	Individually specific to each immuno-globulin molecule	Idiotypes	Variable regions	Probably one or more hypervariable regions forming the antigen-combining site

Table 3.1. *Summary of immunoglobulin variants.*

another animal of the same species. As in other allelic systems, individuals may be homozygous or heterozygous for the genes encoding the markers; these are expressed co-dominantly and are inherited in simple Mendelian fashion. Take, for example, the b4, b5 allotypes on rabbit light chains: an animal of b⁴b⁴ genotype would express the b4 allotype whereas a rabbit of b⁴b⁵ genotype derived from b⁴b⁴ and b⁵b⁵ parents would express the b4 marker on one fraction and b5 on another fraction of its immunoglobulin molecules.

Idiotypes

We have seen that it is possible to obtain antibodies that recognize isotypic and allotypic variants; it is also possible to raise antisera which are specific for individual antibody molecules and discriminate between one monoclonal antibody and another independently of isotypic or allotypic structures (figure 3.7). Such antisera define the individual determinants characteristic of each antibody, collectively termed the *idiotype* (Kunkel & Oudin). Not

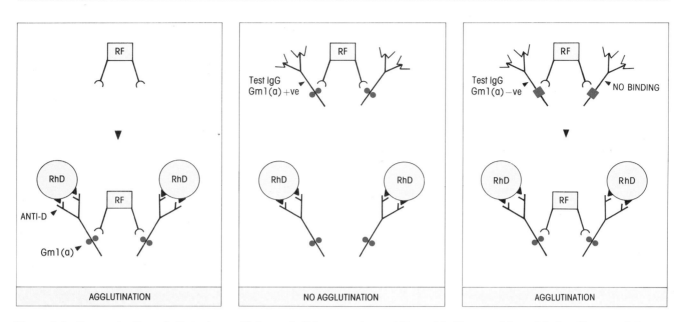

Figure 3.8. *Demonstration of allotypic specificity on IgG by agglutination inhibition. RhD red cells coated with anti-D bearing the allotype, are agglutinated by a rheumatoid arthritis serum selected for the ability of the rheumatoid* factor (RF; anti-IgG) to combine with the allotype. If the test IgG added bears the allotype in question, it will block the combining sites on RF which will no longer be able to agglutinate the red cells.*

surprisingly, it turns out that the idiotypic determinants are located in the variable part of the antibody associated with the hypervariable regions (figure 3.9).

Anti-idiotypes which react with one antibody and no other are said to recognize *private* idiotypes and provide further support for the idea that each antibody has a unique structure. Frequently, antibody molecules of closely similar amino acid structure may, in addition, share idiotypes (e.g. MI04 and Hdex2 in figure 3.9) and we then speak of *public* or *cross-reacting* idiotypes.

Anti-idiotypic sera provide useful reagents for demonstrating the same V region on different heavy chains and on different cells, for identification of specific immune complexes in patients' sera, for recognition of V_L type amyloid in subjects excreting Bence-Jones' proteins, for detection of residual monoclonal protein after therapy and perhaps for selecting lymphocytes with certain surface receptors. The reader will (or should) be startled to learn that it is possible to raise *auto*anti-idiotypic sera since this means that individuals can make antibodies to their own idiotypes. This has quite momentous consequences as will become apparent when we discuss the Jerne network theory in Chapter 8.

Immunoglobulins are folded into globular domains which subserve different functions

Immunoglobulin domains have a characteristic structure

In addition to the *interchain* disulphide bonds which bridge heavy and light chains, there are internal, *intrachain* disulphide links which form loops in the peptide chain. As Edelman predicted, the loops are compactly folded to form globular domains (figure 3.10) which have a characteristic β-pleated sheet protein structure.

Significantly, the hypervariable sequences appear at one end of the variable domain where they form parts of the β-turn loops and are clustered close to each other in space.

The variable domain binds antigen

The clustering of the hypervariable loops at the tips of the variable regions where the antigen binding site is localized (figures 3.3 and 3.4) makes them the obvious candidates to subserve the function of antigen recognition (figure 3.11) and this has been confirmed by X-ray crystallographic analysis of

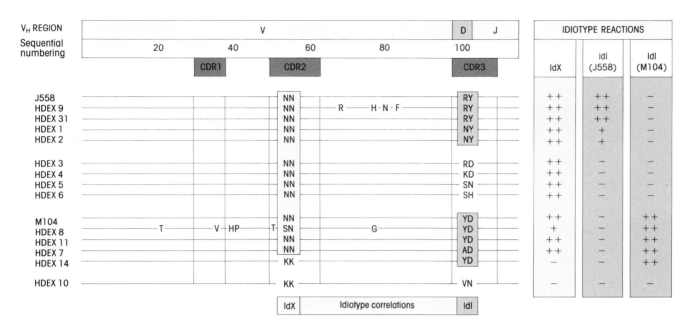

Figure 3.9. *Structural correlates of idiotopes (individual determinants on an idiotype) on antidextran antibodies. Amino acid sequences of variable heavy chain regions of mouse monoclonal antidextran antibodies are shown. All antibodies have λ₁ L chains. Lines indicate identity to the sequence of the first protein, J558; letters (Dayhoff code) show differences or regions correlated with idiotopes (central boxed areas). The cross-reacting idiotope (IdX) is associated with second complementarity determining region (CDR2)* *structures while the private idiotopes (IdI) are features of the CDR3 region in these antibodies. The presence of the idiotopes on each antibody molecule is assessed by reaction with antisera specific for IdX, J558 IdI and M104 IdI (on the right). Cross-reacting idiotopes may also be associated with the CDR3 region in other systems (from J.M. Davie et al. (1986) Ann. Rev. Immunol. 4, 147, with permission. © by Annual Reviews Inc.).*

complexes formed between the Fab fragments of monoclonal antibodies and their respective antigens. The issue has been put beyond doubt by the demonstration that the antigen specificity of a mouse monoclonal antibody could be conferred on a human immunoglobulin molecule by replacing the human hypervariable sequences with those of the mouse (cf. figure 7.12). The sequence heterogeneity of the three heavy and three light chain hypervariable loops ensures tremendous diversity in combining specificity for antigen through variation in the shape and nature of the surface they create. Thus each hypervariable region may be looked upon as an independent structure contributing to the complementarity of the binding site for antigen and one speaks of *complementarity determinants*.

That these variable regions of heavy and light chains both contribute to antibody specificity is suggested by experiments in which isolated chains were examined for their antigen combining power. In general, varying degrees of residual activity were associated with the heavy chains but relatively little

with the light chains; on recombination, however, there was always a significant increase in antigen binding capacity.

Amino acids associated with the combining site can be identified by 'affinity labelling'. In this technique, a hapten (a well-defined chemical grouping to which antibodies can be formed, e.g. DNP in figure 3.3) is equipped with a chemically reactive side-chain which will form covalent links with adjacent amino acids after combination of the hapten with antibody, so labelling residues in the neighbourhood of the combining site. A modification introduced by Porter and his colleagues utilizes a 'flick-knife' principle. The hapten with an azide side-chain combines with its antibody and is then illuminated with ultraviolet light; this converts the azide to the reactive nitrene radical which will covalently link to almost any organic group with which it comes in contact (e.g. figure 3.12). The affinity label binds to both heavy and light chains *in the hypervariable regions*.

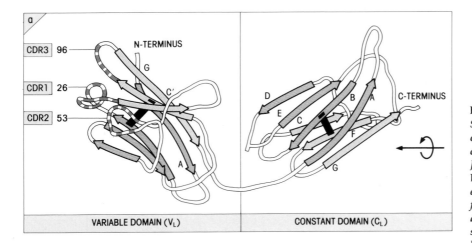

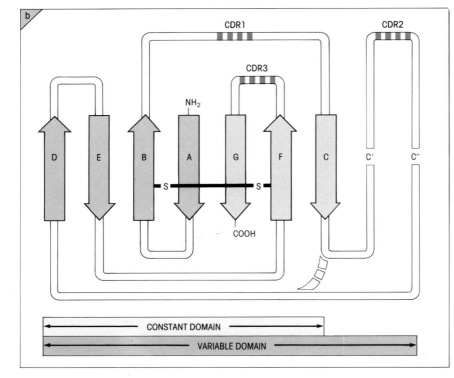

Figure 3.10. *Ig domain structure. (a) Structure of the globular domains of a light chain (from X-ray crystallographic studies of a Bence-Jones' protein by Schiffler et al. (1973) Biochemistry 12, 4620). One surface of each domain is composed essentially of four chains (grey arrows) arranged in an anti-parallel β-pleated structure stabilized by interchain H bonds between the amide CO. and NH. groups running along the peptide backbone, and the other surface of three such chains (green arrows); the dark bar represents the intra-chain disulphide bond. This structure is characteristic of all immunoglobulin domains. Of particular interest is the location of the hypervariable regions (■■■■) in three separate loops which are closely disposed relative to each other and form the light chain contribution to the antigen binding site (cf. figure 3.11). One numbered residue from each complementarity determinant is identified. To generate a Fab fragment (cf. left side figure 3.13c), imagine a V_H-C_H1 segment just like the V_L-C_L in the diagram, rotate it 180° around the axis of the arrow on the right of the figure and lay it on top of V_L-C_L segment (Dr A. Feinstein). (b) Schematic view of folding pattern of constant and variable light-chain domains showing the β-strands (A−G) and the extra sequence C' C" in the variable structure. Lettering and colours as in (a).*

Constant region domains determine secondary biological function

The classes of antibody differ from each other in many respects: in their half-life, their distribution throughout the body, their ability to fix complement and their binding to cell surface Fc receptors. Since the classes all have the same κ and λ light chains, and heavy and light variable region domains, these differences must lie in the heavy chain constant regions.

It has been possible to localize these biological activities to the various heavy chain domains by using myeloma proteins which have spontaneous domain deletions, or enzymic fragments produced by papain (Fc), pepsin (F(ab')₂ and pFc', the C-terminal portion of Fc) and plasmin (Facb from rabbit IgG lacks pFc' but retains the N-terminal half of Fc). Nowadays, of couse, it can all be done by genetically engineered proteins.

A model of the IgG molecule is presented in figure 3.13 which indicates the spatial disposition and interaction of the domains in IgG and ascribes the various biological functions to the relevant structures. In principle, the V region domains form the recognition unit (cf. figure 2.1) and constant

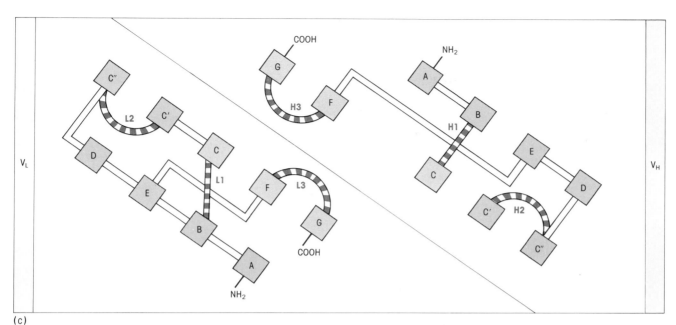

(c)

Fig. 3.10. (continued) *(c) End on view of the β-strands forming the two faces of each domain. The CDR loops (H1-3, L1-3) come out of the plane of the paper towards the reader. Lettering and β-strand colours as in (a).*

43

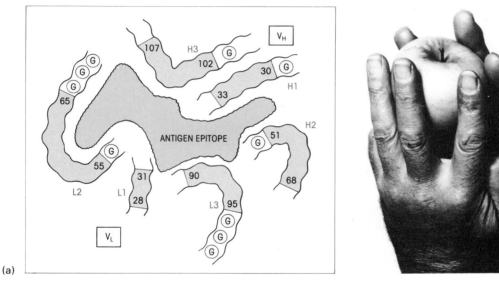

(a)

(b)

Figure 3.11. *The binding site. (a) Idealized two-dimensional representation of an antigen binding site formed by spatial apposition of peptide loops containing the hypervariable regions (hot spots: ▫) on light and heavy chains. Numbers refer to amino acid residues. Glycine residues (◎) are invariably present at the positions indicated whatever the specificity or animal species of the immunoglobulin. They are of importance in allowing peptide chains to fold back and form β-pleated sheet structures which enable the hypervariable regions to lie close to each other (figure 3.10). Wu and Kabat have suggested that the flexibility of bond angle in this amino acid contributes to the effective formation of a binding site. On this basis the greater frequency of invariant glycines on the light chain might indicate that coarse specificity for antigen binding was provided by the heavy chain and 'fine tuning' by the light chain. Through binding to different combinations of hypervariable regions and to different residues within each of these regions, each antibody molecule can form a complex with a variety of antigenic determinants (with a comparable variety of affinities). (b) A simulated combining site for a hapten formed by apposing the three middle fingers of each hand, each finger representing a hypervariable loop. With protein epitopes the area of contact is usually greater and tends to involve more superficial residues (cf. figure 4.5). There appears to be a small repertoire of main chain conformations for at least five of the six CDRs, the particular configuration adopted being determined by a few key conserved residues (Chothia C. et al. (1989) **Nature**, 342, 877). (Photograph by B.N.A. Rice; inspired by A. Munro!)*

MOLECULES WHICH RECOGNIZE ANTIGEN

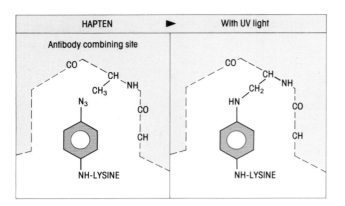

Figure 3.12. *Affinity labelling: the hapten binds to its antibody and the azide group activated by ultraviolet light loses N$_2$ forming a reactive radical which combines with an adjacent amino acid—in this hypothetical example an alanine residue. Analysis of the protein after digestion would show the alanine to be labelled with the hapten and implicate this residue in the combining site. Studies by Fleet G.W.J., Porter R.R. & Knowles J.R. (**Nature 1969, 224, 511**) indicate that the affinity label combines with heavy and light chains in a ratio of approximately 3.5:1 in their particular hapten— antibody combination.*

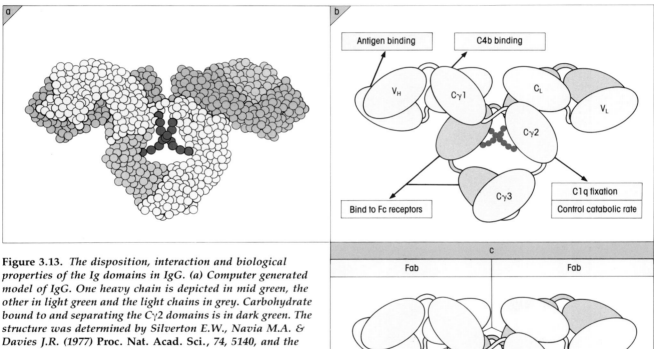

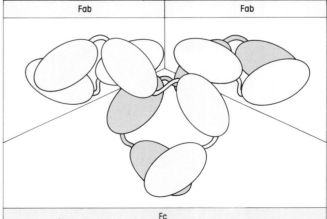

Figure 3.13. *The disposition, interaction and biological properties of the Ig domains in IgG. (a) Computer generated model of IgG. One heavy chain is depicted in mid green, the other in light green and the light chains in grey. Carbohydrate bound to and separating the Cγ2 domains is in dark green. The structure was determined by Silverton E.W., Navia M.A. & Davies J.R. (1977)* **Proc. Nat. Acad. Sci.,** *74, 5140, and the figure generated by computer graphics using R.J. Feldmann's system (Nat. Inst. Health). (b) Diagram based on the model indicating the location of biological function and showing apposing domains making contact through hydrophobic regions (after Dr A. Feinstein). The structures of these contact frameworks are highly conserved, an essential feature if different V$_H$ and V$_L$ domains are to associate in order to generate a wide variety of antibody specificities. These hydrophobic regions on the two complement fixing C$_H$2 (Cγ2) domains are partly masked by carbohydrate and remain independent so allowing the formation of a hinge region which is extremely flexible both with respect to variation in the angle of the Fab fragments and their rotation about the hinge peptide chain. Thus combining sites in IgG can be readily adapted to spatial variations in the presentation of the antigenic epitopes. The combined Cγ2 and Cγ3 domains* bind to Fc receptors on phagocytic cells, NK cells and placental syncytiotrophoblast; also to staphylococcal protein A. (Note the IgG heavy chain is designated γ and the constant region domains Cγ1, Cγ2 and Cγ3.) (c) Relationship of Fab and Fc fragments to these domains.

44

region domains mediate the secondary biological functions.

Immunoglobulin classes and subclasses

The physical and biological characteristics of the five major immunoglobulin classes in the human are summarized in tables 3.2 and 3.3. The following comments are intended to supplement this information.

Immunoglobulin G

Its relative abundance, its ability to develop high affinity binding for antigen and its wide spectrum of secondary biological properties, makes IgG appear as the prime workhorse of the Ig stable. During the secondary response IgG is probably the major immunoglobulin to be synthesized. IgG diffuses more readily than the other immunoglobulins into the extravascular body spaces where, as the predominant species, it carries the major burden of

DESIGNATION	IgG	IgA	IgM	IgD	IgE
Sedimentation coefficient	$7S$	$7S, 9S, 11S$*	$19S$	$7S$	$8S$
Molecular weight	150 000	160 000 and dimer	900 000	185 000	200 000
Number of basic four-peptide units	1	1, 2*	5	1	1
Heavy chains	γ	α	μ	δ	ϵ
Light chains $\kappa + \lambda$	$\kappa + \lambda$	$\kappa + \lambda$	$\kappa + \lambda$	$\kappa + \lambda$	$\kappa + \lambda$
Molecular formula†	$\gamma_2\kappa_2, \gamma_2\lambda_2$	$(\alpha_2\kappa_2)_{1-2}$ $(\alpha_2\lambda)_{1-2}$ $(\alpha_2\kappa_2)_2 S$* $(\alpha_2\lambda_2)_2 S$*	$(\mu_2\kappa_2)_5$ $(\mu_2\lambda_2)_5$	$\delta_2\kappa_2(\delta_2\lambda_2?)$	$\epsilon_2\kappa_2, \epsilon_2\lambda_2$
Valency for antigen binding	2	2,4	5(10)	2	2
Concentration range in normal serum	8–16 mg/ml	1.4–4 mg/ml	0.5–2 mg/ml	0–0.4 mg/ml	17–450 ng/ml‡
% Total immunoglobulin	80	13	6	0–1	0.002
% Carbohydrate content	3	8	12	13	12

Table 3.2. *Physical properties of major human immunoglobulin classes.*
* *Dimer in external secretions carries secretory component—S.*
† *IgA dimer and IgM contain J-chain.*
‡ $ng = 10^{-9} g$.

	IgG	IgA	IgM	IgD	IgE
Major characteristics	Most abundant Ig of internal body fluids particularly extravascular where it combats micro-organisms and their toxins	Major Ig in sero-mucous secretions where it defends external body surfaces	Very effective agglutinator; produced early in immune response — effective first-line defence vs. bacteraemia	Most, if not all, present on lymphocyte surface	Protection of external body surfaces Recruits anti-microbial agents Raised in parasitic infections Responsible for symptoms of atopic allergy
Complement fixation					
Classical	++	–	+++	–	
Alternative	–	±	–	–	
Cross placenta	++	–	–	–	–
Fix to homologous mast cells and basophils	–	–	–	–	++
Binding to macrophages and polymorphs	++	±	–	–	±

Table 3.3. *Biological properties of major immunoglobulin classes in the human.*

MOLECULES WHICH RECOGNIZE ANTIGEN

neutralizing bacterial toxins and of binding to micro-organisms to enhance their phagocytosis.

Activation of the classical complement pathway

Complexes of bacteria with IgG antibody trigger the C1 complex when a minimum of two Fcγ regions in the complex bind C1q (figure 2.2, p. 18). Using site-specific mutagenesis whereby individual amino acids in the Cγ2 domain are altered by manipulation of the heavy chain gene, the binding site for C1q has been localized to three charged residues, glutamic acid 318, lysine 320 and lysine 322 lying on the surface of the protein. Activation of the next component C4 tends to produce attachment of C4b to the Cγ1 domain. Thereafter, release of C3a and C5a leads to the chemotactic attraction of our friendly polymorphonuclear phagocytic cells (cf. p. 2) which adhere to the bacteria through surface receptors for complement and the Fc portion of IgG (Fcγ); binding to the Fc receptor then stimulates ingestion of micro-organisms through phagocytosis. In a similar way, the extracellular killing of target cells coated with IgG antibody is mediated largely through recognition of the surface Fcγ by NK cells bearing the appropriate receptors (cf. p. 14). The thesis that the biological individuality of different immunoglobulin classes is dependent on the heavy chain constant regions, particularly the Fc, is amply borne out in relationship to the activities we have discussed such as transplacental passage, complement fixation and binding to various cell types, where function has been shown to be mediated by the Fc part of the molecule.

The diversity of Fcγ receptors

Since a wide variety of interactions between IgG complexes and different effector cells have been identified, we really should spend a little time looking at the receptors for Fcγ which mediate these phenomena.

Fcγ receptor I (FcγRI) is present on monocytes and to a lesser extent on unstimulate macrophages. It is effective in mediating the extracellular killing of target cells coated with IgG antibody (ADCC; p. 260). Conceivably, it might be concerned with the overall regulation of IgG levels in the body, since the catabolic rate appears to depend directly upon the total IgG concentration and one might speculate that endocytosis of FcγRI which has a high affinity for monomeric IgG could contribute significantly to this degradation. On the other hand, synthesis is largely governed by antigen stimulation, so that in germ-free animals, for example, IgG levels are extremely low but rise rapidly on transfer to a normal environment.

FcγRII is a low affinity receptor present on monocytes, neutrophils, eosinophils, platelets and possibly B-cells. Binding of IgG complexes to platelets provokes thrombosis and occupation of B-cell Fc receptors leads to downregulation of cellular responsiveness, possibly being responsible for the negative feedback effect of IgG on antibody production (cf. p. 154).

Another low affinity receptor FcγRIII found on macrophages, polymorphs, eosinophils and NK cells would seem to be largely responsible for mediating ADCC by NK cells and clearance of immune complexes from the circulation by macrophages. For example, the clearance of IgG coated erythrocytes from the blood of chimpanzees was essentially inhibited by the monovalent Fab fragment of a monoclonal anti-FcγIII (work out why the Fab fragment was used). The mad flurry of gene cloning and sequencing is revealing important similarities between proteins in different cells subserving comparable functions. In this connection, it is quite fascinating that a peptide in the mouse equivalent of human FcγRIII has close homology with the γ-chain from the mast cell FcεRI and the zeta chain of the T-cell receptor complex, to be discussed later. Almost certainly, these represent a family of related proteins sharing a common role in a signal transducing pathway. Thus signals through the receptors are transmitted to initiate phagocytosis in macrophages, to bring out the killer in NK cells, to trigger degranulation in mast cells and to bring about the activation of resting T-lymphocytes.

Alone of the Ig classes, IgG possesses the crucially important ability to cross the human placenta so that it can provide a major line of defence for the first few weeks of a baby's life, and this may be further reinforced by the transfer of colostral IgG across the gut mucosa in the neonate. These transport processes involve translocation of the IgG across the cell-barrier by complexing to an Fcγ receptor. A recent study succeeded in cloning a new FcγRn receptor from the intestinal cells of the rat which transports IgG from mother's milk into the baby (figure 3.14). Note how the direction of transport is achieved by the differential binding of IgG to the receptor at the pH of the lumen versus that at the basal surface. Unlike FcγRI, a member of the Ig super-family (p. 198), FcγRn is an MHC class I molecule associated with β_2-microglobulin.

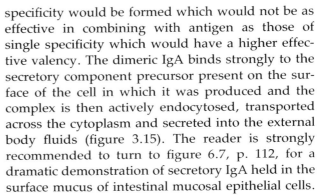

| LUMEN | INTESTINAL CELL | BASAL SURFACE |
| pH 6.0 | | pH 7.4 |

Figure 3.14. *Transport of IgG from maternal milk across the intestinal cells of the baby rat. IgG binds to the receptor (FcγRn) at pH 6.0, is taken into the cell within a clathrin coated vesicle and released at the pH of the basal surface. The directional movement of IgG is achieved by the asymmetric pH effect on Ig-receptor interaction. In the placenta, the receptor does not need to show differential binding because its function is to allow the fetal IgG concentration to rise to that in the maternal circulation. (Based on a diagram by P. Parham (1989)* **Nature,** *337, 118).*

Non-precipitating 'univalent' antibodies

IgG has two combining sites for antigen and there has been a tendency to scoff at claims to have discovered 'univalent' antibodies. Sceptics must now accept that 5–15% of the IgG in all antisera appear to consist of non-precipitating asymmetric molecules with a single effective binding site. The other site is blocked stereochemically by a mannose-rich carbohydrate in the Cγl domain. If one takes an antibody directed to a small molecule such as dinitrophenyl (DNP cf. p. 35), this spatial block by adjacent carbohydrate on binding of DNP linked to a larger carrier protein, can be overcome by distancing the DNP group from the bulky carrier with a spindly carbon chain spacer.

Immunoglobulin A

IgA appears selectively in the sero-mucous secretions such as saliva, tears, nasal fluids, sweat, colostrum and secretions of the lung, genito-urinary and gastro-intestinal tracts where it clearly has the job of defending the exposed external surfaces of the body against attack by micro-organisms. It is present in these fluids as a dimer stabilized against proteolysis by combination with another protein— the secretory component which is synthesized by local epithelial cells and has a single peptide chain of molecular weight 60 000. The IgA is synthesized locally by plasma cells and dimerized intracellularly together with a cysteine-rich polypeptide called J-chain of molecular weight 15 000. If dimerization occurred randomly *after* secretion, dimers of mixed

specificity would be formed which would not be as effective in combining with antigen as those of single specificity which would have a higher effective valency. The dimeric IgA binds strongly to the secretory component precursor present on the surface of the cell in which it was produced and the complex is then actively endocytosed, transported across the cytoplasm and secreted into the external body fluids (figure 3.15). The reader is strongly recommended to turn to figure 6.7, p. 112, for a dramatic demonstration of secretory IgA held in the surface mucus of intestinal mucosal epithelial cells.

IgA antibodies function by inhibiting the adherence of coated micro-organisms to the surface of mucosal cells thereby preventing entry into the body tissues. Aggregated IgA binds to polymorphs and can also activate the alternative (figure 2.4), as distinct from the classical, complement pathway which probably accounts for reports of a synergism between IgA, complement and lysozyme in the killing of certain coliform organisms. Human plasma contains relatively high concentrations of monomeric IgA and its role is still something of a mystery.

Immunoglobulin M

Often referred to as the macroglobulin antibodies because of their high molecular weight, IgM molecules are polymers of five four-peptide subunits each bearing an extra C_H domain. As with IgA, polymerization of the subunits depends upon the presence of J-chain whose function may be to stabilize the Fc sulphydryl groups during Ig synthesis so that they remain available for cross-linking

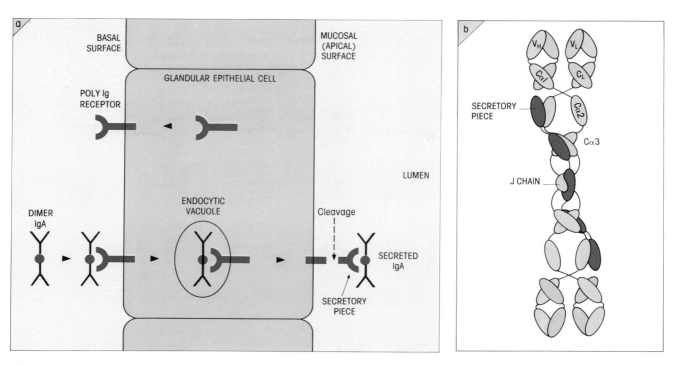

Figure 3.15. *Secretory IgA. (a) The mechanism of IgA secretion at the mucosal surface. The mucosal cell synthesizes an Ig receptor which is inserted into the basal membrane. Dimeric IgA binds to this receptor and is transported via an endocytic vacuole to the apical surface. Cleavage of the receptor releases secretory IgA still attached to part of the receptor termed* **secretory piece.** *Note how the receptor*

cleavage introduces an asymmetry which drives the transport of IgA dimers to the mucosal surface (in quite the opposite direction to the transcytosis of milk IgG in figure 3.14). (b) The structure of secretory IgA showing the domains, the J chain holding the IgA dimer together, and a speculative view of the Ig-like domains of secretory piece.

the subunits to give the structure shown in figure 3.16a. Under negative staining in the electron microscope, the free molecule in solution assumes a 'star' shape but when combined as an antibody with an antigenic surface membrane it can adopt a 'crab-like' configuration (figure 3.16b and c). The theoretical combining valency is of course 10 but this is only observed on interaction with small haptens; with larger antigens the effective valency falls to 5 and this must be attributed to some form of steric restriction due to lack of flexibility in the molecule. IgM antibodies tend to be of relatively low affinity as measured against single determinants (haptens) but, because of their high valency, they bind with quite respectable avidity to antigens with multiple epitopes (bonus effect of multivalency, p. 72).

For the same reason, these antibodies are extremely efficient agglutinating and cytolytic agents and since they appear early in the response to infection and are largely confined to the bloodstream, it is likely that they play a role of particular importance in cases of bacteraemia. The isohaemagglutinins (anti-A, anti-B) and many of the 'natural' antibodies to micro-organisms are usually IgM;

antibodies to the typhoid 'O' antigen (endotoxin) and the 'WR' antibodies in syphilis also are found in this class. IgM would appear to precede IgG in the phylogeny of the immune response in vertebrates.

Monomeric IgM (i.e. a single four-peptide unit) with a hydrophobic sequence stitched into the C-terminal end of the heavy chain to anchor the molecule in the cell membrane, is the major antibody receptor used by B-lymphocytes to recognize antigen (cf. figure 2.10).

Immunoglobulin D

This class was recognized through the discovery of a myeloma protein which did not have the antigenic specificity of IgG, A or M, although it reacted with antibodies to immunoglobulin light chains and had the basic four-peptide structure. The hinge region is particularly extended and although protected to some degree by carbohydrate, it may be this feature which makes IgD, among the different immunoglobulin classes, uniquely susceptible to proteolytic degradation, and account for its short half-life in plasma (2.8 days). An exciting development has

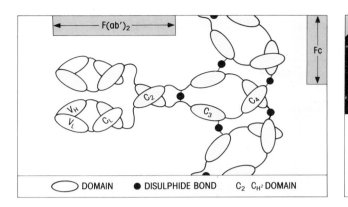

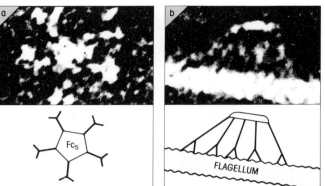

DOMAIN   ● DISULPHIDE BOND   C₂ C_H² DOMAIN

Figure 3.16. *The structure of IgM. The arrangement of domains in one of the five subunits showing how the pentamer is built up through the disulphide linkages between C_H3 and C terminal regions (after Hilschman & Feinstein). Without too much aggravation, I hope the reader will appreciate that the hinge region in IgG (cf. figure 3.13) is replaced by a rigid pair of extra domains (C_H2), while C_H3 and C_H4 domains in IgM are structurally equivalent to the C_H2 and C_H3 regions respectively in IgG. (a) As shown by electron microscopy of a human Waldenström's macroglobulin in free solution adopting a 'star'-shaped configuration. (b) As revealed in an E.M. preparation of*

specific sheep IgM antibody bound to **Salmonella paratyphi** *flagellum where the immunoglobulin has assumed a 'crab-like' conformation in establishing its links with antigen. With the F(ab')₂ arms bent out of the plane of the central Fc₅ region, the C_H3 complement binding domains are now readily accessible to the first component of complement (cf. p. 17). The Fc₅ constellation obtained by papain cleavage can activate complement directly. (Electron micrographs — kindly provided by Dr A. Feinstein and Dr E.A. Munn — are negatively stained preparations of magnification × 2 000 000, i.e. 1 mm represents 0.5 nm.)*

been the demonstration that nearly all the IgD is present, together with IgM, on the surface of a proportion of blood lymphocytes where it seems likely that they may operate as mutually interacting antigen receptors for the control of lymphocyte activation and suppression. The even greater susceptibility of IgD to proteolysis on combination with antigen could well be implicated in such a function.

Immunoglobulin E

Only very low concentrations of IgE are present in serum and only a very small proportion of the plasma cells in the body are synthesizing this immunoglobulin. It is not surprising, therefore, that so far only six cases of IgE myeloma have been recognized compared with tens of thousands of IgG paraproteinaemias. IgE antibodies remain firmly fixed for an extended period when injected into human skin where they are bound with high affinity to the FcεRI receptor on mast cells (figure 3.17). Contact with antigen leads to degranulation of the mast cells with release of preformed vasoactive amines and cytokines, and the synthesis of a variety of inflammatory mediators derived from arachidonic acid. This process is responsible for the symptoms of hay fever and of extrinsic asthma when patients with atopic allergy come into contact with the allergen, e.g. grass pollen.

The main *physiological* role of IgE would appear to be protection of anatomical sites susceptible to trauma and pathogen entry, by local recruitment of plasma factors and effector cells through triggering an acute inflammatory reaction. Infectious agents penetrating the IgA defences would combine with specific IgE on the mast cell surface and trigger the release of vasoactive agents and factors chemotactic for granulocytes, so leading to an influx of plasma IgG, complement, polymorphs and eosinophils (cf. p. 206). In such a context, the ability of eosinophils to damage IgG-coated helminths and the generous IgE response to such parasites would constitute an effective defence.

Immunoglobulin subclasses

Antigenic analysis of IgG myelomas revealed further variation and showed that they could be grouped into four isotypic *subclasses* now termed IgG1, IgG2, IgG3 and IgG4. The differences all lie in the heavy chains which have been labelled γ1, γ2, γ3 and γ4 respectively. These heavy chains show considerable homology and have certain structures in common with each other — the ones which react with specific anti-IgG antisera — but each has one or more additional structures characteristic of its own subclass arising from differences in primary amino acid composition and in interchain disulphide bridging.

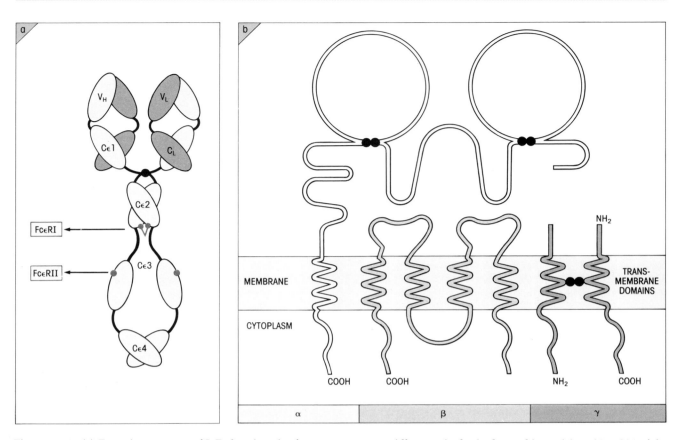

Figure 3.17. *(a) Domain structure of IgE showing site for binding to the high affinity receptor FcεRI on mast cells in the Cε2 domain and to the low affinity receptor FcεRII on inflammatory cells and B-lymphocytes in the Cε3. Note the general similarity in structure to the IgM basic unit in figure 3.16 with the IgG hinge replaced by the extra Cε2 coupled domains, but also the lack of association of the penultimate C-terminal domains (in this case Cε3) which is a consistent feature of all Ig classes. (b) Schematic diagram of the high affinity mast cell receptor for IgE, FcεRI. The α-chain binds* *very avidly to a single site located in positions 301–304 of the Cε2 domain. The seven transmembrane domains cluster together. The two covalently linked γ-chains show considerable homology with FcγRIII and the ζ(zeta)-peptide of the T-cell receptor complex; their role is almost certainly transduction of the signal initiated by FcεRI cross-linking by antigen (cf. figure 12.1, p. 254). The low affinity FcεRII requires the presence of both Cε3 domains for significant binding to IgE. Double black dots represent disulphide links.*

	IgG1	IgG2	IgG3	IgG4
% Total IgG in normal serum	65	23	8	4
Electrophoretic mobility	slow	slow	slow	fast
Spontaneous aggregation	−	−	+ + +	−
Gm allotypes	a,z,f,x	n	b0,b1,b3, g,s,t, etc.	
Ga site reacting with rheumatoid factor*	+ + +	+ + +	−	+ + +
Combination with staphylococcal A protein	+ + +	+ + +	−	+ + +
Cross placenta	+ +	±	+ +	+ +
Complement fixation (Cı pathway)	+ + +	+ +	+ + + +	±
Binding to monocytes	+ + +	+	+ + +	±
Binding to heterologous skin	+ +	−	+ +	+ +
Blocking IgE binding	−	−	−	+
Antibody dominance	Anti-Rh	Anti-dextran Anti-levan	Anti-Rh	Anti-Factor VIII

Table 3.4. *Comparison of human IgG subclasses.*
* Other rheumatoid factors apparently react with Gm specific sites.

These give rise to differences in biological behaviour which are summarized in table 3.4.

Two subclasses of IgA have also been found, of which IgA1 constitutes 80–90% of the total. The IgA2 subclass is unusual in that it lacks interchain disulphide bonds between heavy and light chains. Class and subclass variation is not restricted to human immunoglobulins but is a feature of all the higher mammals so far studied: monkey, sheep, rabbit, guinea-pig, rat and mouse.

THE MAJOR HISTOCOMPATIBILITY COMPLEX (MHC)

Molecules within this complex were originally recognized through their ability to provoke vigorous rejection of grafts exchanged between different members of a species. In Chapter 2, brief mention was made of the necessity for cell-surface antigens to be associated with class I or class II MHC molecules in order that they may be recognized by T-lymphocytes. The intention now is to give more insight into the nature of these molecules.

Class I and class II molecules are membrane-bound heterodimers

Class I molecules consist of a heavy peptide chain of 43 kDa non-covalently linked to a smaller 11 kDa peptide called β_2-microglobulin. The largest part of the heavy chain is organized into three globular domains (α_1, α_2 and α_3; figure 3.18a) which protrude from the cell surface; a hydrophobic section anchors the molecule in the membrane and a short hydrophilic sequence carries the C-terminus into the cytoplasm.

X-ray analysis of crystals of a human class I molecule has provided an exciting leap forwards in our understanding of MHC function. Both β_2-microglobulin and the α_3 region resemble classical Ig domains in their folding pattern (cf. figure 3.10). However, the α_1 and α_2 domains which are most distal to the membrane, form an utterly surprising structure composed of two extended α-helices above a floor created by peptide strands held together in a β-pleated sheet, the whole forming an undeniable cavity (figure 3.18b and c). The appearance of these domains is so striking, I doubt whether the reader needs the help of gastronomic analogies such as 'two bananas on a plate' to prevent any class I structural amnesia. Delving into the unknown uncovered another curious feature. The cavity was occupied by a linear molecule, held by modern wisdom to be a linear peptide, which had co-crystallized with the class I protein. The significance of these unique findings for T-cell recognition of antigen will be revealed in the following chapter.

Class II MHC molecules are also transmembrane glycoproteins, in this case consisting of α and β polypeptide chains of molecular weight 34 kDa and 28 kDa respectively.

On the basis of considerable sequence homology with class I, a model has been proposed in which the α_2 and β_2 domains, the ones nearest to the cell membrane, assume the characteristic Ig fold, while the α_1 and β_1 domains mimic the class I α_1 and α_2 in forming a groove bounded by two α-helices and a β-pleated sheet floor (figure 3.18a and d).

Complement genes contribute to the remaining class III region of the MHC

A variety of other genes which congregate within the major histocompatibility complex chromosome region are grouped under the heading of class III. A notable cluster are the genes coding for two C4 isotypes and the two products, C2 and factor B, which each carry an active site for C3 convertase. Tumour necrosis factors (TNF) α and β are encoded under the class III umbrella as are two members of the human 70 kDa heat shock proteins.

Gene map of the major histocompatibility complex

The clusters of class I, II and III genes in the MHC of mouse and man are set out in figures 3.19 and 3.20. A number of silent or pseudo genes have been omitted from these gene maps in the interest of simplicity. The gap between class II and class I in the human can accommodate up to a 100 or so class III genes and new ones are constantly popping up.

The genes of the MHC display remarkable polymorphism

Unlike the immunoglobulin system where, as we shall see, variability is achieved in each individual

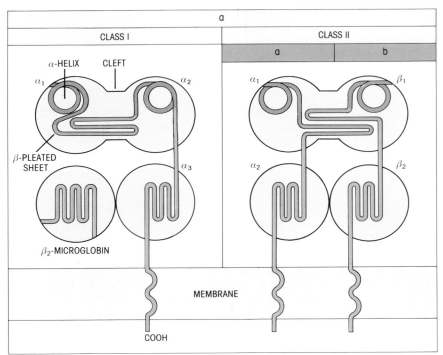

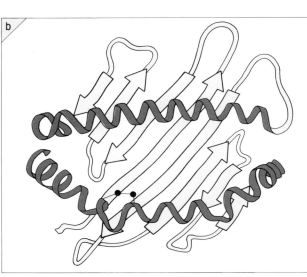

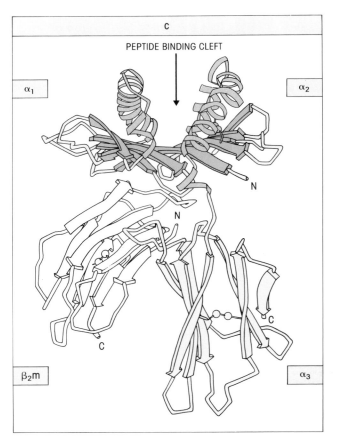

Figure 3.18. *Class I and class II major histocompatibility complex molecules. (a) Diagram showing domains and transmembrane segments; the α-helices and β-sheets are viewed end-on. (b) Schematic bird's eye representation of top surface of human class I molecule (HLA-A2) based on X-ray crystallographic structure. The strands making the β-pleated sheet are shown as thick grey arrows in the amino to carboxy direction, α-helices are represented as green helical ribbons. The inside facing surfaces of the two helices and the upper surface of the β-sheet form a cleft. The two black spheres represent an intrachain disulphide bond. (c) Side view of the same molecule clearly showing the anatomy of the cleft and the typical Ig folding of the α3 and β2-microglobulin domains (4 anti-parallel β-strands on one face and 3 on the other). (Reproduced from Bjorkman P.J. et al. (1987) **Nature**, 329, 506, with permission.)*

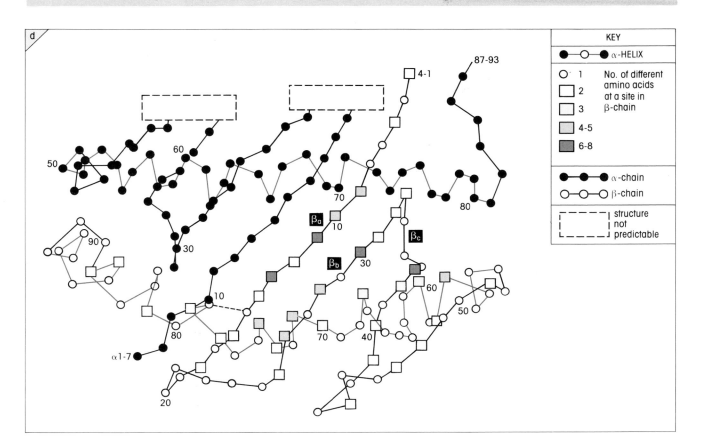

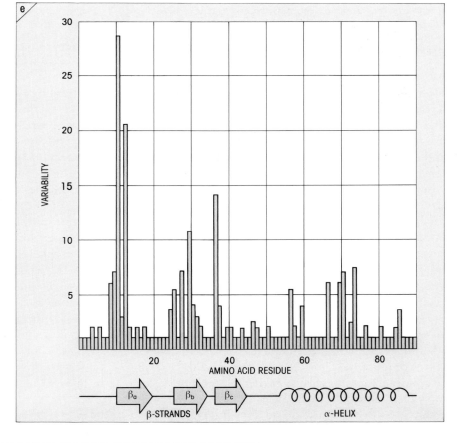

Figure 3.18. continued. (d) Model of the first domains of the a and β chains of HLA-DR (viewed from above as in (b)) showing the extent and location of the polymorphism (closely based on figure in March S.G.E. & Bodmer J.E. (1989) Immunology Today, 9, 305). DQ tends to have fewer amino acid substitutions at each polymorphic site, but unlike DR, they are distributed over both α-helices (e) Wu and Kabat type plot for the DRβ first domain (cf. figure 3.6) calculated from data of Marsh and Bodmer, ibid used for preceding figure (d), showing regions of amino acid variability. Individual β strands are picked out for comparison with (d).

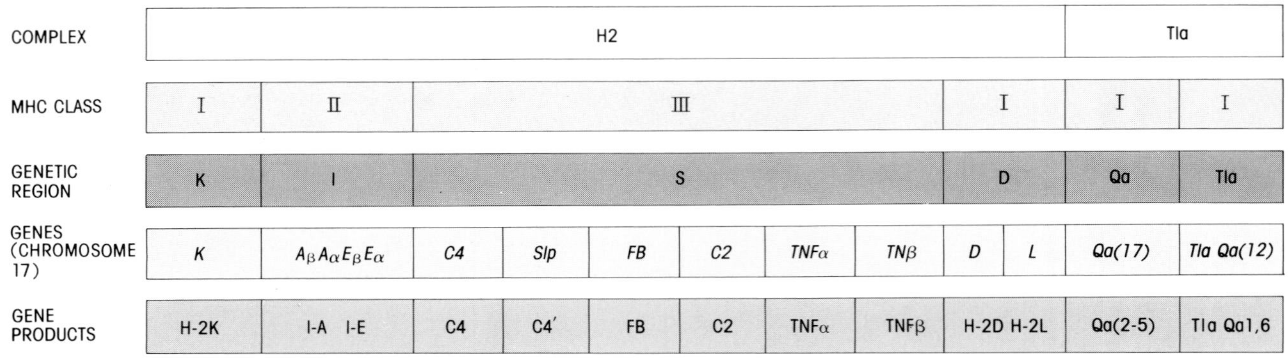

COMPLEX	H2									Tla	
MHC CLASS	I	II	III						I	I	I
GENETIC REGION	K	I	S						D	Qa	Tla
GENES (CHROMOSOME 17)	K	AβAαEβEα	C4	Slp	FB	C2	TNFα	TNβ	D L	Qa(17)	Tla Qa(12)
GENE PRODUCTS	H-2K	I-A I-E	C4	C4'	FB	C2	TNFα	TNFβ	H-2D H-2L	Qa(2-5)	Tla Qa1,6

Figure 3.19. *The genes in the major histocompatibility complex in the mouse. All class I molecules are associated with β₂-microglobulin. There are 17 Qa genes in the Qa region and 12 in the Tla region although most are silent. The class II molecules are αβ heterodimers. Slp (sex-limited protein) encodes a non-functional allele of C4, expressed under the influence of testosterone. The 21-hydroxylase B and A genes lie on either side of C4 as in the human.*

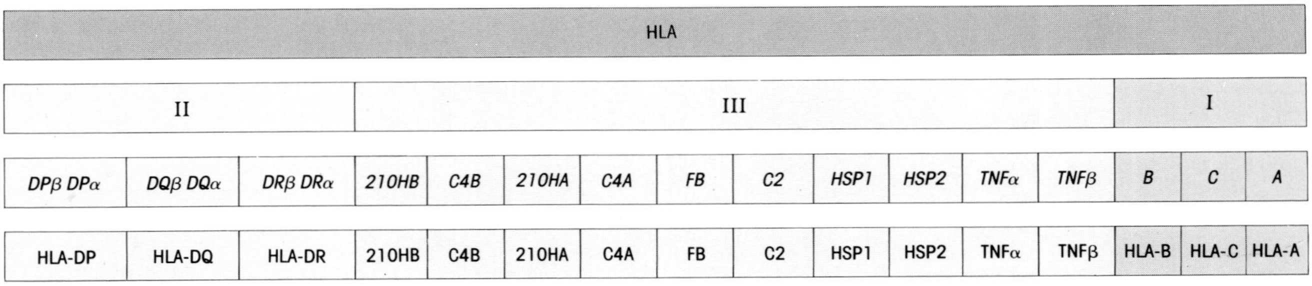

HLA															
II			III											I	
DPβ DPα	DQβ DQα	DRβ DRα	21OHB	C4B	21OHA	C4A	FB	C2	HSP1	HSP2	TNFα	TNFβ	B	C	A
HLA-DP	HLA-DQ	HLA-DR	21OHB	C4B	21OHA	C4A	FB	C2	HSP1	HSP2	TNFα	TNFβ	HLA-B	HLA-C	HLA-A

Figure 3.20. *The genes in the major histocompatibility complex of the human on chromosome 6. Three new class I genes which can direct the synthesis of class I proteins have been described: HLA-E, between HLA-B and -C, and HLA-F and -G, telomeric to HLA-A. They could be equivalent to murine Qa genes. The existence of many more silent class I genes is known (210HB, 21-hydroxylase; FB, complement factor B; HSP, 70 kDa heat shock protein; TNF, tumour necrosis factor).*

by a *multigenic* system, the MHC has evolved in terms of variability between individuals with a highly polymorphic system based on multiple alleles (i.e. alternative genes at each locus). Class I HLA-A and -B molecules are highly polymorphic, so are the class II peptides DQα, DQβ and DRβ, DPβ less so, while DRα and β2-microglobulin are invariant in structure. The amino acid changes responsible for this polymorphism are restricted to the α1 and α2 domains of class I and of the α₁ and β₁ domains of class II, and it is of considerable significance that they occur essentially in the β-sheet floor and the inner surfaces of the α-helices which line the central cavity (figure 3.18a) and also on the upper surface of the helices. I thought it would be more revealing to show the results of one such analysis in which the sequences of the first domains (β₁) of 41 DRβ alleles were compared for both the location and the extent of amino acid variability (figure 3.18d and e). Polymorphism affects both a-halices in DQ but the variability in individual amino acid substitution is lower.

Multiple allelic forms can be generated by a variety of mechanisms: point mutations, recombination, homologous but unequal crossing over, and gene conversion.

The latter mechanism has been identified as an important contributory factor in the formation of a series of spontaneous mutations in the *H-2K* region of C57BL mice. Most of the mutations contain clusters of multiple amino acid substitutions and seem to arise by transfer of stretches of up to 95 nucleotides from class I *Qa* genes to the α₁ and α₂ domains of *H-2K*. These intriguing findings have fostered the view that the large number of seemingly functionless *Qa* genes may represent a stockpile of genetic information for the generation of polymorphic diversity in the 'working' class I molecules. Evidence for gene conversion has also been obtained for the class II genes and an example is given in figure 3.21.

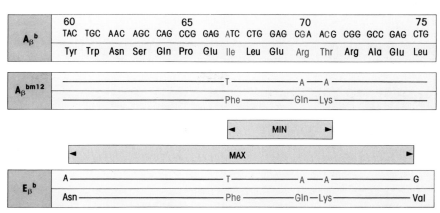

	60				65					70					75
A_β^b	TAC	TGC	AAC	AGC	CAG	CCG	GAG	ATC	CTG	GAG	CGA	ACG	CGG	GCC	GAG	CTG
	Tyr	Trp	Asn	Ser	Gln	Pro	Glu	Ile	Leu	Glu	Arg	Thr	Arg	Ala	Glu	Leu

A_β^{bm12} ————————————T————————A—A——————————
————————————Phe——————Gln—Lys——————————

◄ MIN ►

◄ MAX ►

E_β^b A————————————T————————A—A——————————G
Asn————————————Phe——————Gln—Lys——————————Val

Figure 3.21. *Evidence for gene conversion generating a class II mutant. A stretch of nucleotides from the parent strain E_β gene appears to have been transferred to A_β to produce the $A_\beta^{bm/2}$ mutant as shown by the comparison of DNA and amino acid sequences. The maximum and minimum possible sequences exchanged are indicated.*

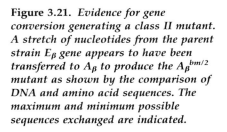

STRAIN	CBA	F₁ HYBRID	DBA/2
H-2 GENOTYPE	k/k	k×d ▼ k/d	d/d
	▼	▼	▼
LYMPHOCYTES (H-2 PHENOTYPE)	k ● k	k ● ◼ d	d ◼ ◼ d
ANTI H-2ᵏ	Killing	Killing	—
ANTI-H-2ᵈ	—	Killing	Killing

Figure 3.22. *Inheritance and co-dominant expression of MHC genes. The first familial generation (F1) obtained by crossing the pure parental strains CBA (H-2^k) and DBA/2 (H-2^d) has the H-2 genotype k/d. Since 100% of F1 lymphocytes are killed in the presence of complement by antibodies to H-2^k or to H-2^d (raised by injecting H-2^k lymphocytes into an H-2^d animal and vice versa), the MHC molecules encoded by both parental genes must be expressed on every lymphocyte. The same holds true for other tissues in the body.*

55

Nomenclature

Since much of the experimental work relating to the MHC is based on experiments in our little laboratory friend, the mouse, it may be helpful to explain the nomenclature used to describe the allelic genes and their products. If someone says to you in an obscure language, 'we are having free elections' you fail to understand, not because the idea is complicated but because you do not comprehend the language. It is much the same with the shorthand used to describe the H-2 system which looks unnecessarily frightening to the uninitiated. In order to identify and compare allelic genes within the H-2 complex in different strains, it is usual to start with certain pure inbred strains, obtained by successive brother–sister matings, to provide the prototypes. The collection of genes in the H-2 complex is called the haplotype and the haplotype of each prototypic

strain will be allotted a given superscript. For example, the DBA strain haplotype is designated $H-2^d$ and the genes constituting the complex are therefore $H-2K^d$, $I-A_\alpha^d$, $I-A_\beta^d$, $H-2D^d$ and so on; their products will be H-2K^d, I-A^d and H-2D^d and so forth. When new strains are derived from these by genetic recombination during breeding, they are assigned new haplotypes but the individual genes are designated by the haplotype of the prototype strain from which they were derived. Thus the A/J strain produced by genetic cross-over during interbreeding between ($H-2^k \times H-2^d$) F1 mice (cf. figure 3.22) is arbitrarily assigned the haplotype H-2^a, but table 3.5 shows that individual genes in the complex are identified by the haplotype symbol of the original parents.

If mixed haplotype heterodimers and inter-isotypic pairing (e.g. I-A$_\alpha^d$ E$_\beta^d$) could occur, this would increase the total range of MHC class II

Table 3.5. *The haplotypes of the H-2 complex of some commonly used mouse strains and recombinants derived from them.*

STRAIN	HAPLOTYPE	ORIGIN OF INDIVIDUAL REGIONS					
		K	A	(J)	E	S	D
C57BL	b	b	b	b	b	b	b
CBA	k	k	k	k	k	k	k
DBA/2	d	d	d	d	d	d	d
A/J	a	k	k	k	k*	d	d
B.10A(4R)	h4	k	k	b	b	b	b

A/J was derived by interbreeding (k × d) F1 mice, recombination occurring between E and S regions(*).

products dramatically, but the evidence for this is still controversial.

Inheritance of the MHC

Pure strain mice derived by prolonged brother—sister mating are homozygous for each pair of homologous chromosomes. Thus, in the present context, the haplotype of the MHC derived from the mother will be identical to that from the father and animals of the C57BL strain, for example, will each bear two chromosomes with the H-2^b haplotype (cf. table 3.5).

Let us see how the MHC behaves when we cross two pure strains of haplotypes H-2^k and H-2^d respectively. We find that the lymphocytes of the offspring (the F1 generation) all display *both* H-2^k and H-2^d molecules on their surface, i.e. there is co-dominant expression (figure 3.22). If we go further and breed F1s together, the progeny have the genotypes k, k/d and d in the proportions to be expected if the haplotype segregates as a single Mendelian trait. This happens because the H-2 complex spans 0.5 centimorgans, equivalent to a recombination frequency between the K and D ends of 0.5%, and the haplotype tends to be inherited *en bloc*. Only the relatively infrequent recombinations caused by meiotic cross-over events, as described for the A/J strain above, reveal the complexity of the system.

The tissue distribution of MHC molecules

Essentially, all nucleated cells carry class I molecules. These are abundantly expressed on lymphoid cells, less so on liver, lung and kidney and only sparsely on brain and skeletal muscle. In the human, the surface of the villous trophoblast does not display HLA-A, B or C components. Class II molecules are more restricted being especially associated with B-cells, antigen-presenting cells and macrophages; however, when activated by agents such as γ-interferon, capillary endothelia and many epithelial cells can be stained for surface class II and increased expression of class I.

MHC functions

Although originally discovered through transplantation reactions, the MHC molecules are utilized for vital biological functions by the host. Their function as cell surface markers to signal cytotoxic and helper T-cells will be explored in depth in subsequent chapters. Aside from the potential role of Qa genes in the generation of polymorphism, molecules encoded by the Tla complex are involved in differentiation events particularly in the embryo and possibly also in the placenta.

The MHC has been implicated in a variety of non-immunological phenomena such as body weight in mice, egg production in chickens and mating selection by body smells; many of these may have a hormonal basis and the evidence that class I molecules may also function as components of hormone receptors merits some consideration. For example, the Daudi tumour cell line which does not express surface class I because of a failure to synthesize β_2-microglobulin, lacks insulin receptors. If one strips class I, but not class II, from a cell surface by 'capping' with antibodies (see figure 2.6f), the binding of insulin is significantly diminished. Last, if a cell binds photoaffinity-labelled insulin, chemical links with H-2K but not H-2D may be seen. Associations with receptors for glucagon, epidermal growth factor and γ-endorphin have also been described. Of course, one of the lessons to be learned is that we should never look at immunological events as phenomena isolated from the biology of the whole individual—and beyond (figure 3.23).

THE T-CELL RECEPTOR

Receptors are transmembrane heterodimers

Like the B-lymphocyte, the T-cell has a specific receptor for antigen recognition on its surface. But whereas the B-cell receptor is a membrane-bound immunoglobulin M monomer, the T-cell receptor

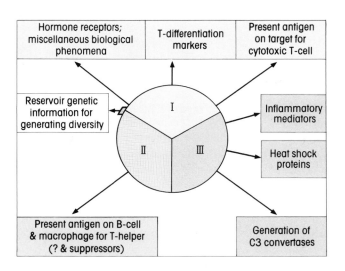

Figure 3.23. *The functions of MHC molecules.*

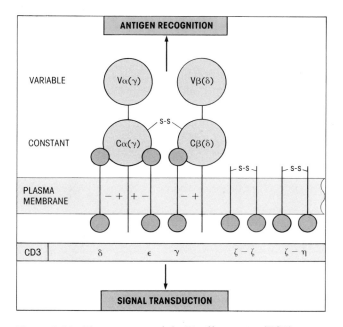

Figure 3.24. *The structure of the T-cell receptor (TCR). Antigen plus MHC is recognized by the α−β disulphide linked transmembrane heterodimer TCR2, or the alternative γ−δ TCR1. The receptor is intimately associated with the CD3 complex which transduces the signal produced by antigen recognition to the interior of the cell. (Based on Clevers H. et al. (1988) Ann. Rev. Immunol. 6, 629).*

(TCR) is a heterodimer composed of two chains, each of molecular weight 40−50 kDa, which are clearly not products of immunoglobulin genes (figure 3.24). There are two types of TCR each associated with a separate T-cell lineage. TCR1, composed of γ and δ chains, is the first to appear in ontogeny whereas TCR2 contains α and β chains and cells

bearing these receptors predominate in adult life, but not exclusively. Each chain folds into two domains, one having a relatively invariant structure homologous to the famous 'Ig fold', the other exhibiting a high degree of variability rather like an Ig Fab fragment. While it is safe to assume that the variable region has the job of binding to antigen plus MHC, we do not yet have the data to define the structural basis of that recognition process. The problem is that the T-cell receptor being membrane-bound, is insoluble and therefore cannot be crystallized and analysed by X-ray diffraction. A construct made by splicing variable domains of the receptor to Ig Fc genes would theoretically have been soluble but a functioning expression system could only be established with V_α (TCR). However, by expressing the TCR genes attached to a phosphatidyl inositol membrane anchor, soluble TCR heterodimers, apparently with antigen recognition ability, could be obtained by cleavage from the cell surface with a specific phospholipase. We must wait patiently for progress.

Both α and β chains are required for antigen specificity as shown by transfection of the T-receptor genes from a cytotoxic T-cell clone specific for fluorescein + H-2D^d to another clone of different specificity; when it expressed the new α and β genes, the transfected clone acquired the ability to lyse the fluoresceinated H-2D^d target cells. Another type of experiment utilized T-cell hybridomas formed by fusing single antigen-specific T-cells with T-cell tumours to achieve 'immortality'. A hybridoma recognizing chicken ovalbumin in association with I-A^d gave rise spontaneously to two variants, one of which lost the chromosome encoding the α chain, and the other, the β chain. Neither variant recognized antigen but when they were physically fused together, each supplied the complementary receptor chain and reactivity with antigen was restored.

In all immunocompetent T-cells, the antigen receptor is non-covalently but still intimately linked in a complex with CD3, a molecule composed of seven peptide chains (CD3-γ, -δ, -ε, ζ-ζ and ζ-η), which transduces the antigen recognition signal received by the α, β heterodimer to the inside of the cell. It really seems sensible to regard the complete receptor as a nine-peptide complex of the heterodimer with CD3 which can transiently associate with other membrane peptides such as CD3-p21 (figure 3.24) and possibly CD4 and CD8.

57

THE GENERATION OF DIVERSITY FOR ANTIGEN RECOGNITION

We know that the immune system has to be capable of recognizing virtually any pathogen that has arisen or might arise. The extravagant genetic solution to this problem of anticipating an unpredictable future involves the generation of millions of different specific antibodies, probably vastly more than the lifetime needs of the individual. Since this is probably more than the total number of genes in the body, there must be some clever ways to generate all this diversity. Before examining these mechanisms, we must first look at the genetic building blocks from which the final genes encoding antibody molecules and the T-cell receptor are constructed.

Multiple gene segments code for antibody

These fall into three clusters on three different chromosomes coding for κ, λ and heavy chains respectively. To simplify for the basis of discussion, we will assume that the most common variable region (*V*) gene utilized for the synthesis of mouse λ chains is the only one present and we will follow the genetic basis for the synthesis of this peptide (figure 3.25). In common with other eukaryotic proteins, the chain is encoded in multiple distinct gene segments separated by intervening nucleotide sequences, *introns*, which are removed either by DNA translocation or by excision of the corresponding mRNA sequence. There is a leader sequence required for passage of the peptide through the endoplasmic reticulum, a V_λ segment coding for amino acid residues 1 to 98, a joining segment (*J*—not to be confused with the J peptide in IgM and IgA) encoding the remaining 11 amino acids of the variable region, and a C_λ gene segment giving rise to the constant region. As a lymphocyte undergoes differentiation to become an immunocompetent cell capable of synthesizing λ chains, there is a rearrangement or translocation of the DNA bringing the *L*, V_λ and *J* segments together (figure 3.26) but still separated from the C_λ by an intron of 1250 nucleotides. Splicing of the transcribed RNA in the nucleus produces an mRNA which can now be used for the synthesis of a continuous λ chain peptide.

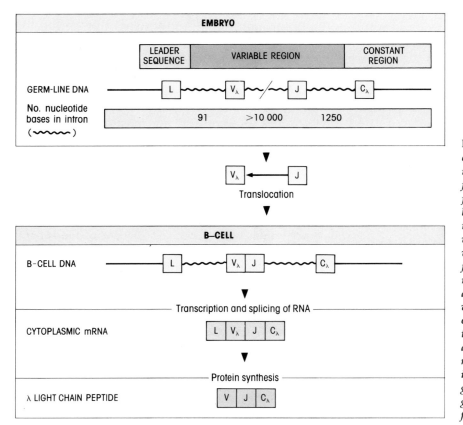

Figure 3.25. *Genetic basis for synthesis of mouse λ chain. As the cell becomes immunocompetent, the variable region is formed by the combination of V_λ with the joining segment J, a process facilitated by base sequences in the intron following the 3' end of the V_λ segment pairing up with sequences in the intron 5' to J. This variable region V_λ J segment is separate from the gene encoding the constant region as originally predicted by Dreyer and Bennett. The final joining occurs when the intervening sequence is spliced out of the RNA transcript. In practice there are a small number of further V_λ and C_λ genes in the region but the mechanism for generating the full mRNA is the same for each. In the human, the V_λ genes are more complex as is the case in general for V_κ and heavy chain genes (cf. figure 3.27).*

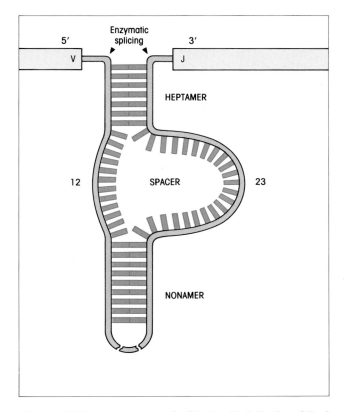

Figure 3.26. *Intron sequences facilitating V−J, V−D and D−J recombination. The characteristic sequences forming a base-paired (▦) heptamer, a spacer of 12 or 23 single bases (▦) and then a base-paired nonamer facilitate splicing and joining by enzymes. A protein binding to the J$_k$ recognition signal sequence containing the 23 base-pair spacer sequence has recently been purified and shown to have a 40-residue sequence related to the integrase motif of phages, bacteria and yeast, stongly suggesting that it could be a V-(D)-J recombinase.*

The same general principles apply to the arrangement of κ and heavy chain genes although they exist in far greater variety (figure 3.27). The 200 or so $V_κ$ genes occur as a series of five families or sets each containing closely related individual genes. Although the genes within a given set show some framework and hypervariable diversity, they resemble each other far more than they do $V_κ$ genes in other sets. There are five different *J* segments but just a single constant region gene.

The heavy chain constellation shows additional features: the subclass constant region genes form a single cluster and there is a group of 12 highly variable *D* segments inserted between the *V* and *J* regions. The *D* and *J* segments together encode almost the entire third hypervariable region, the first two being contributed by the *V* sequence.

A similar pattern of genes codes for the T-cell receptor

The gene segments encoding the T-cell receptor β chains follow a similar arrangement of *V, D, J* and constant segments to that described for the immunoglobulins (figure 3.28). Similarly, as an immunocompetent T-cell is formed, rearrangement of *V, D* and *J* genes occurs to form a continuous *VDJ* sequence and, as in the synthesis of antibody, the intron between *VDJ* and *C* is spliced out of the mRNA before translation.

The α chain gene pool lacks D segments but otherwise behaves in the same way. γ- and δ-genes forming the TCR1 obey similar rules.

The awkward location of the δ locus within the α gene cluster has been surprisingly informative with respect to the mechanism of translocation since T-cells which have undergone $V_α$−$J_α$ combination have no δ genes on the rearranged chromosome; in other words, the δ genes are completely excised.

59

The mechanisms which generate tremendous diversity from limited gene pools

Intrachain amplification of diversity

Simple VDJ combination joining increases diversity geometrically

During the rearrangement of germ-line genes to produce the immunocompetent cell, $V \rightarrow J$, $V \rightarrow D$ and $D \rightarrow J$ joining is random and will produce $V \times J$, or where appropriate, $V \times D \times J$ combinations (see table 3.6).

Variations on the combinatorial theme

Another ploy to squeeze more variation out of the germ-line repertoire involves variable boundary recombinations of *V, D* and *J* to produce different junctional sequences (figure 3.29).

Further diversity arises from the insertion of nucleotides at the N region of the D and J segments, a process associated with the expression of terminal deoxynucleotidyl transferase. This process greatly increases the repertoire of T-receptor γ genes which are otherwise rather limited in number.

Just to make sure that we are really impressed, it transpires that even after a V_HDJ_H rearrangement

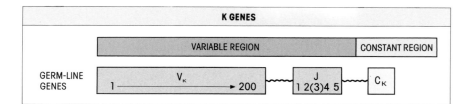

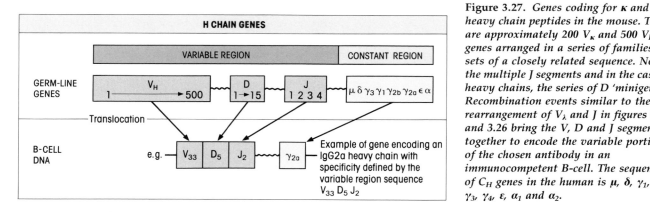

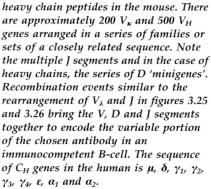

Figure 3.27. *Genes coding for κ and heavy chain peptides in the mouse. There are approximately 200 $V_κ$ and 500 V_H genes arranged in a series of families or sets of a closely related sequence. Note the multiple J segments and in the case of heavy chains, the series of D 'minigenes'. Recombination events similar to the rearrangement of $V_λ$ and J in figures 3.25 and 3.26 bring the V, D and J segments together to encode the variable portion of the chosen antibody in an immunocompetent B-cell. The sequence of C_H genes in the human is μ, δ, $γ_1$, $γ_2$, $γ_3$, $γ_4$, ε, $α_1$ and $α_2$.*

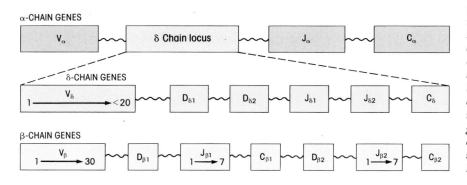

Figure 3.28. *Germ-line (unrearranged) sequence of genes encoding the α and β polypeptides of the murine T-cell receptor 2, and the δ-chain of the TCR1. In the committed cell, each chain is encoded by a recombination of one V, one D, one J and one constant region segment, e.g. $V_αD_αJ_αC_α$. Note the very large number of α-segments and the curious position of the δ genes in the midst of the TCRα locus. The γ-chain genes are arranged in 3 functional clusters, each containing V, J and C segments; like the α chains, there are no D regions.*

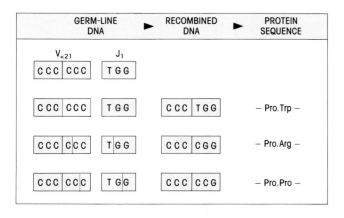

Figure 3.29. *Junctional diversity between two germ-line segments producing three variant protein sequences. The nucleotide triplet which is spliced out is coloured green.*

has occurred, an interchange with a quite different 5' V_H gene can still take place; since the process is not precise, bases can be lost and/or added at the region joining the new V_H to the N-terminal end of the D sequence. This V_H 'swapping' may prevent bias in the development of the heavy chain V-region repertoire because the earliest differentiating B-cells utilize the V_H segments most proximal to D with high frequency to form their V_HDJ_H rearrangements.

Yet additional mechanisms work on the D regions: in some cases the D segment can be read in three different reading frames and in others D–D combinations may be formed.

Since the third complementarity determining re-

	T-CELL RECEPTOR 2		IMMUNOGLOBULIN	
	ALPHA	BETA	HEAVY	KAPPA
V gene segments	100	30	500	200
D gene segments	—	2	15	—
J gene segments	50	6 + 6	4	4
D's in 3 reading frames	–	+	+	–
N region insertion	+	+ +	+ +	–
Junctional diversity	+ + +	+ + +	+ + +	+
Somatic hypermutation	–	–	+	+
Combinatorial joining (minimum)	$V \times J$ 100×50	$V \times D \times J$ $(30 \times 3 \times 12)$ $+(30 \times 3 \times 6)$	$V \times D \times J$ $500 \times 15 \times 4$	$V \times J$ 200×4
Total	5000	1620	3×10^4	800
	X		X	
Combinatorial association	8.1×10^6		2.4×10^7	

Table 3.6. *Combinatorial and somatic diversification of mouse V genes. The minimum number of specificities generated by straightforward combination of germ-line segments can be calculated. These will be increased by the further mechanisms listed, Indications are that great diversity can also be generated in TCR1 by the large number of δ gene segment and the tremendous junctional variation in γ chain resulting from N region nucleotide insertions. The calculation for the T-cell receptor β chain requires further explanation. The first of the two D segments, $D_{\beta1}$ can combine with 30 V genes, can be read in the 3 reading frames and can combine with all 12 $J_{\beta1}$ and $J_{\beta2}$ genes (30 × 3 × 12). $D_{\beta2}$ behaves similarly but can only combine with the 6 downstream $J_{\beta2}$ genes (30 × 3 × 6). Reproduced from Goverman J., Hunkappiller T. & Hood L. (1986) Cell 45, 475, with permission. Copyright 1986 by Cell Press.)*

gions (CDR3) in the various receptor chains are essentially composed of (D)J segments where junctional diversity mechanisms can introduce a very high degree of amino acid variability, one can see why it is that this hypervariable loop probably contributes the most flexibility in antigen binding specificity within these molecules.

Interchain amplification

The firmest evidence that B- and T-cells use similar recombination mechanisms comes from the SCID mouse which has a single autosomal recessive defect in its ability to link V, D and J segments successfully. Homozygous mutants fail to develop immunocompetent B- and T-cells and identical sequence defects in VDJ joint formation are seen in both pre-B and pre-T cell lines.

The immune system took an ingenious step forward when two different types of chain were utilized for the recognition molecules because the combinations produce new variability. Thus when one heavy chain is paired with different light chains the specificity of the final antibody is altered; for example, pairing of a heavy chain containing the T15 idiotype with three different light chains produced antibodies with different affinities for phosphorylcholine.

Random association between TCR1 γ and δ chains, TCR2 α and β chains, and Ig heavy and light chains yields a geometric increase in diversity. From table 3.6 it can be seen that approximately 200 TCR2 and 700 Ig germ-line segments can give rise to 8 million and 25 million different combinations respectively, by straightforward associations *without* taking into account all of the fancy additional D/J mechanisms described above. Hats off to evolution!

Somatic hypermutation

There is inescapable evidence that immunoglobulin V region genes can undergo significant somatic mutation. Analysis of 18 murine λ myelomas revealed 12 with identical structure, 4 showing just one amino acid change, 1 with 2 changes and 1 with 4 changes, all within the hypervariable regions and indicative of somatic mutation of the single mouse λ germ-line gene. In another study, following immunization with pneumococcal antigen, a single germ-line T15 V_H gene gave rise by mutation to several different V_H genes all encoding phosphorylcholine antibodies (figure 3.30).

A number of features of this somatic diversification phenomenon deserve mention. The mutations are the result of single nucleotide substitutions, they are restricted to the variable as distinct from the constant region and occur in both framework and hypervariable regions. The mutation rate calculated by dividing the substitutions by the nucleotide bases sequenced is remarkably high,

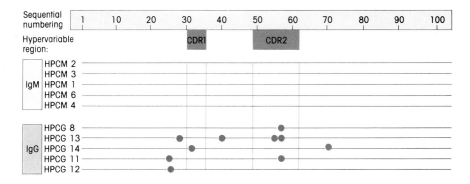

Figure 3.30. *Mutations in a germ-line gene. The amino acid sequences of the V_H regions of five IgM and five IgG monoclonal phosphorylcholine antibodies generated during an anti-pneumococcal response in a single mouse are compared with the primary structure of the T15 germ-line sequence. A line indicates identity with T15 prototype and a green circle a single amino acid difference. Mutations have only occurred in the IgG molecules and are seen in both hypervariable and framework segments (after Gearhart P.J. (1982)* **Immunol. Today 3, 107).**

between 2 and 4% for V_H genes as compared with a figure of less than 0.0001% for a non-immunological lymphocyte gene. In addition, the mutational mechanism is bound up in some way with class switch since mutations are more frequent in IgG and IgA than in IgM antibodies, affecting both heavy (figure 3.30) and light chains.

The perceived wisdom at the present time is that somatic mutation does not add to the repertoire available in the early phases of the primary response, but occurs during the generation of memory and is probably responsible for tuning the response towards higher affinity.

T-cell receptor genes, on the other hand, do not appear to undergo somatic mutation. Assuming this result is not biased by the selection of T-cell clones studied, it has been argued that this would be a useful safety measure since T-cells are so close to fully recognizing self, mutations could readily encourage the emergence of high affinity autoreactive receptors and autoimmunity.

One may ask how it is that this array of germ-line genes is protected from genetic drift. With a library of 800 or so *V* genes, selection would act only weakly on any single gene which had been functionally crippled by mutation and this implies that a major part of the library could be lost before evolutionary forces operated. One idea is that each subfamily of related *V* genes (legend, figure 3.27) contains a prototype coding for an antibody indispensable for protection against some common pathogen so that mutation in this gene would put the host at a disadvantage and would therefore be selected against. If any of the other closely related genes in its set become defective through mutation,

this indispensable gene could repair them by gene conversion, a mechanism in which it will be remembered that two genes interact in such a way that the nucleotide sequence of part or all of one becomes identical to that of the other. Although gene conversion was invoked earlier (figure 3.21) to account for the diversification of MHC genes, it can also act on families of genes to maintain a degree of sequence homogeneity.

SUMMARY

Immunoglobulins

Immunoglobulins (Ig) have a basic four-peptide structure of two identical heavy and two identical light chains joined by interchain disulphide links. Papain splits the molecule at the exposed flexible hinge region to give two identical univalent antigen binding fragments (Fab) and a further fragment (Fc). Pepsin proteolysis gives a divalent Ag binding fragment F(ab')$_2$ lacking the Fc.

There are perhaps 10^8 or more different Ig molecules in normal serum. Analysis of myeloma proteins which are homogeneous Ig produced by single clones of malignant plasma cells has shown the N-terminal region of heavy and light chains to have a variable amino acid structure and the remainder to be relatively constant in structure. Each chain is folded into globular domains. The variable region domains bind Ag, and three *hypervariable* loops on the heavy and three on the light chain form the Ag binding site. The constant region domains of the heavy chain (particularly the Fc) carry out a secondary biological function after the binding of Ag, e.g. complement fixation and macrophage binding.

In the human there are five major types of heavy chain giving five *classes* of Ig. IgG is the most abundant Ig particularly in the extravascular fluids where it neutralizes toxins and combats micro-organisms by fixing complement via the C1 pathway, and facilitating the binding to phagocytic cells by receptors for C3b and Fcγ. It crosses the placenta in late pregnancy and the intestine in the neonate. IgA exists mainly as a monomer (basic four-peptide unit) in plasma, but in the sero-mucous secretions where it is the major Ig concerned in the defence of the external body surfaces, it is present as dimer linked to a secretory component. IgM is a pentameric molecule, essentially intravascular, produced early in the immune response. Because of its high valency it is a very effective bacterial agglutinator and mediator of complement-dependent cytolysis and is therefore a powerful first-line defence against bacteraemia. IgD is largely present on the lymphocyte and probably functions as an Ag receptor. IgE binds firmly to mast cells and contact with antigen leads to local recruitment of anti-microbial agents through degranulation of the mast cells and release of inflammatory mediators. IgE is of importance in certain parasitic infections and is responsible for the symptoms of atopic allergy. Further diversity of function is possible through subdivision of classes into subclasses based on structural differences in heavy chains all present in each normal individual.

Allotypic structural variations are controlled by allelic genes and provide genetic markers. Idiotypic determinants unique to a given immunoglobulin are recognizable by anti-idiotypic antibodies and are associated with the hypervariable regions forming the Ag binding site.

Major histocompatibility complex (MHC)

Each vertebrate species has an MHC identified originally through its ability to evoke very powerful transplantation rejection. Each contains three classes of genes. Class I encode 44 kDa transmembrane peptides associated at the cell surface with β_2-microglobulin. Class II molecules are transmembrane heterodimers. Class III genes encode complement components linked to the formation of C3 convertases. The genes display remarkable polymorphism. A given MHC gene cluster is referred to as a 'haplotype' and is usually inherited *en*

bloc as a single Mendelian trait although its constituent genes have been revealed by cross-over recombination events.

Class I molecules are present on virtually all cells in the body except for the villous trophoblast in the human; class II are particularly associated with B-cells and macrophages but can be induced on capillary endothelial cells and epithelial cells by γ-interferon. Class I molecules associate with antigen on the surface of virally infected cells to signal cytotoxic T-cells. Class II signal T-helpers for B-cells and macrophages by a similar mechanism. Structural analysis indicates that the two domains distal to the cell membrane form a cavity bounded by two parallel α-helices sitting on a floor of β-sheet peptide strands; the walls and floor of the cavity and the upper surface of the helices are the sites of maximum polymorphic amino acid substitutions. Class I molecules may function as components of hormone receptors. Silent class I genes may increase polymorphism by gene conversion mechanisms.

T-cell receptor

Most T-cells bear a heterodimeric receptor (TCR2) consisting of transmembrane α and β chains, each with a variable and a constant region. Both chains are required for antigen recognition. A separate lineage (TCR1) bearing γδ receptors is transcribed strongly in early thymic ontogeny but is associated mainly with epithelial structures in the adult. The CD3 molecule forms an intimate part of the receptor and probably has a signal transducing role.

The generation of diversity for antigen recognition

Immunoglobulin heavy and light chains and T-cell receptor α and β chains generally are represented in the germ-line by between 30 and 500 variable region genes between 2 and 15 *D* segment minigenes (Ig heavy and TCR β only) and 4–50 short *J* segments. Constant region genes have single copies for each subclass. γ and δ chains are encoded by far fewer genes.

Random combination of any *V* with any *D* and then *J* in each gene cluster generates approximately 5000 T_α, 1600 T_β, 3×10^4 Ig heavy and 800 Ig light chains. Random association of T_α and T_β and Ig heavy and light chains produces the staggering total of 8×10^6 T-cell and 2.4×10^7 B-cell specificities. Further diversity can be developed by various $V \rightarrow D \rightarrow J$ junctional mechanisms which greatly increase the number of specificities which can be formed

63

from the relatively small γδ pool. In addition, after a primary response, B-cells but not T-cells undergo high-rate somatic mutation affecting the *V* regions and presumably helping to increase the affinity of the antibody response.

Further reading

Davie J.M. *et al.* (1986) Structural correlates of idiotopes. *Ann. Rev. Immunol.*, **4**, 147.

French M.A.H. (ed.) (1986) *Immunoglobulins in Health and Disease*. MTP Press, Lancaster, UK.

Hay F.C. (1989) *Immunology*. 2nd edn. I.M. Roitt, J. Brostoff & D.K. Male (eds). p. 6.1. Gower Medical Publishing, London. (On generation of diversity.)

Marsh S.G.E. & Bodmer J.G. (1989) HLA-DR and DQ epitopes and monoclonal antibody specificity. *Immunology Today*, **10**, 305.

Melchers F. *et al.* (eds) (1989) *Progress in Immunology*, **VII** (Proc. 7th Int. Congress Immunol; includes current description of effect of changes in MHC amino acids and most other aspects of immunology). Springer-Verlag, Berlin.

Raulet D.H. (1989) Structure and function of γ/δ T-cell receptor. *Ann. Rev. Immunol.* **7**, 175.

Unkeless J.C. (1989) Human Fcγ receptors. *Current Opinion in Immunol.* 2, 63.

CHAPTER 4

THE RECOGNITION OF ANTIGEN
I – Primary Interaction

What is an antigen?

A man cannot be a husband without a wife and a molecule cannot be an antigen without a corresponding antiserum or antibody — or T-cell receptor. The term 'antigen' is used in two senses, the first to describe a molecule which *gen*erates an immune response (also called an *immunogen*) and the second, a molecule which reacts with antibodies or primed T-cells irrespective of its ability to generate them. If this last situation sounds a trifle confusing, an example may help. A mouse injected with its own red cells, not too surprisingly, will not make any antibodies; if it is now given rat erythrocytes, antibodies are formed to both rat and *mouse* red cells and the latter bind to the animal's own cells *in vivo*, i.e. the mouse red cell acts as antigen in binding antibodies even though unable to evoke their formation. Similarly, *haptens*, which are small well-defined chemical groupings such as dinitrophenyl (DNP; cf. p. 35) or *m*-aminobenzene sulphonate, are not immunogenic on their own but will react with preformed antibodies induced by injection of the hapten linked to a 'carrier' molecule which is itself an immunogen (figure 4.1).

The part of the hypervariable regions on the antibody which contacts the antigen is termed the *paratope* and the part of the antigen which is in contact with the paratope is designated the *epitope*. To get some idea of size, if the antigen is a linear peptide or carbohydrate, the combining site can usually accommodate up to five or six amino acid residues or hexose units. With a globular protein as many as 16 or so amino acid side-chains may be in contact with an antibody (cf. figure 4.5).

Of epitopes and antigen determinants

Antibodies formed in response to immunization with a native globular protein (as distinct from a

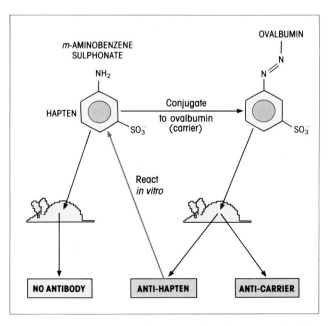

Figure 4.1. *The hapten on its own will not induce antibodies. However, it will react **in vitro** with antibodies formed to a conjugate with an immunogenic carrier.*

fibrillar protein) do not tend to react well with denatured preparations and this is consistent with the view that the majority recognize topographical (surface) structures (i.e. epitopes) which depend upon the conformation of the native molecule. For this reason, antibodies to native proteins do not usually react as strongly with peptides having the same primary sequence (figure 4.2). When individual epitopes are mapped using homogeneous monoclonal antibodies (cf. p. 136), they are frequently seen to involve amino acid residues far apart in the primary sequence, but brought together by the folding of the peptide chains in the native protein (figures 4.3 and 4.5). It seems reasonable to talk of *discontinuous* or assembled rather than *continuous* or sequential epitopes in these cases.

If one were to take each individual antibody within an antiserum raised to a protein antigen and plot the approximate centre of the corresponding epitope on the antigen surface, one would almost certainly finish up with a 'contour map' of epitope density indicating regions on the antigen surface of *dominant epitope clusters* (figure 4.4a). Each of these clusters is as near as I can get to defining an antigen *determinant*. It is important to be aware that each antigen usually bears several determinants on its surface, which may well be structurally distinct

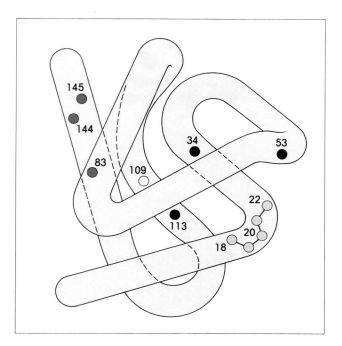

Figure 4.3. *Epitope residues on the folded peptide chain of sperm whale myoglobulin. Amino acid residues 34, 53, and 113 (●) contribute to the epitope recognized by one homogeneous monoclonal antibody, 83, 144 and 145 (●) to another. These are clearly* **discontinuous** *epitopes. Amino acids 18−22 ( ) are postulated to form part of a continuous epitope based on reactions with the isolated peptides. Much of the myoglobin chain is in the α-helical form. Residue 109 ( ) is critical for T-cell recognition and so far no antibodies reacting with this site have been demonstrated. (Based on Benjamin et al. (1986)* **Ann. Rev. Immunol. 2, 67.)**

from each other; thus a monoclonal antibody reacting with one determinant will usually not react with any other determinants on the same antigen unless the molecule has axes of symmetry (figure 4.4b).

Antigens and antibodies interact by spatial complementarity not by covalent bonding

Variation in hapten structure shows importance of shape

Once a method had been found for raising antibodies to small chemically defined haptens (figure 4.1), it then became possible to relate variations in the chemical structure of a hapten to its ability to bind to a given antibody. In one experiment, antibodies raised to *m*-aminobenzene sulphonate were

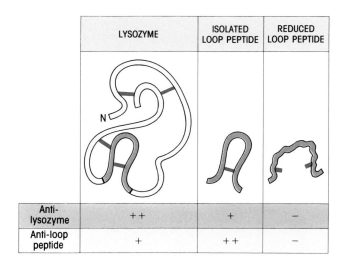

	LYSOZYME	ISOLATED LOOP PEPTIDE	REDUCED LOOP PEPTIDE
Anti-lysozyme	+ +	+	−
Anti-loop peptide	+	+ +	−

Figure 4.2. *Specificity and three-dimensional configuration in a globular protein, lysozyme. Antibodies to the whole molecule and to the isolated loop peptide do not react with the peptide after reduction of its disulphide bond, showing that the linear reduced peptide has lost the antigenic configuration it had when held as a loop even though the amino acid sequence was unchanged (from Maron E., Shiowa C., Arnon R. & Sela M. (1971)* **Biochemistry 10, 763).**

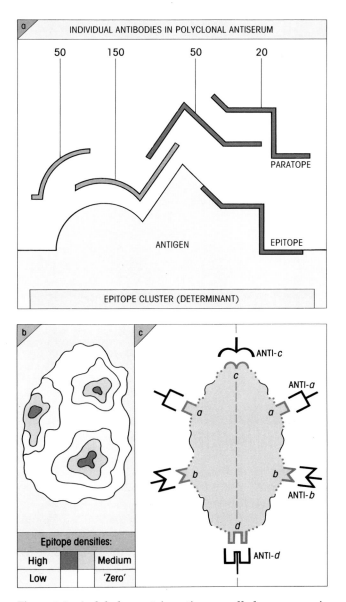

Figure 4.4. *A globular protein antigen usually bears a mosaic of determinants (dominant epitope clusters) on its surface, defined by the heterogenous population of antibody molecules in a given antiserum. (a) Highly idealized diagram showing individual antibodies in a polyclonal antiserum with different combining sites (paratopes) which react with overlapping epitopes forming a determinant on the surface of the antigen. The numbers refer to the relative frequency of each antibody specificity. (b) Hypothetical 'contour' map of surface showing how determinants represent regions of clustering but overlapping epitopes whose positions are plotted as the centre of the area making contact with antibody. The actual size of a single epitope may be gauged by looking at figure 4.5. (c) Cross-section of a theoretical antigen with an axis of symmetry displaying six determinants including two pairs which are identical. The clusters of overlapping antibodies to each determinant (one representative of each antibody cluster is shown) do not react with the other structurally unrelated determinants.*

Table 4.1. *Effect of variations in hapten structure on strength of binding to antibodies raised against* **m-aminobenzene sulphonate**.

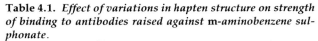
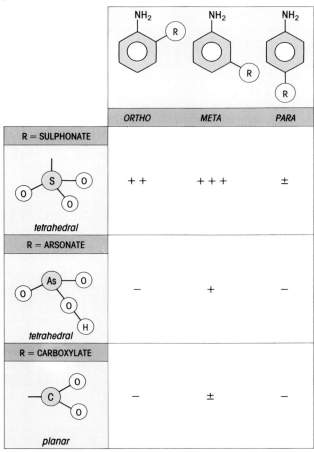

	ORTHO	META	PARA
R = SULPHONATE tetrahedral	+ +	+ + +	±
R = ARSONATE tetrahedral	−	+	−
R = CARBOXYLATE planar	−	±	−

(*From Landsteiner K. & van der Scheer J. (1936)* J. Exp. Med. 63, 325.)

67

tested for their ability to combine with *ortho, meta* and *para* isomers of the hapten and related molecules in which the sulphonate group was substituted by arsonate or carboxylate (table 4.1). The hapten with the sulphonate group in the *ortho* position combines somewhat less well with the antibody than the original *meta* isomer, but the *para*-substituted compound (chemically similar to the *ortho*) shows very poor reactivity. The substitution of arsonate for sulphonate leads to weaker combination with the antibody; both groups are negatively charged and have a tetrahedral structure but the arsonate group is larger in size and has an extra H atom. The amino benzoates in which the sulphonate is substituted by the negatively charged but planar carboxylate group show even less affinity for the antibody. It would appear that the overall *configuration* of the hapten is even more important than its *chemical* nature, i.e. the hapten is recognized by the overall three-dimensional shape of its outer electron cloud as distinct from its chemical reactivity. The production of antibodies against such strange moieties as benzene sulphonate and arsonate becomes more comprehensible if they are thought to be directed against a particular electron-cloud shape rather than a specific chemical structure.

Spatial complementarity of epitope and paratope can be demonstrated

It has proved possible, with not a little difficulty, to crystallize a complex of the Fab fragment of monoclonal anti-lysozyme with its antigen. X-ray analysis of these crystals was convincing; antigen and antibody fitted strongly together due to complementarity in shape over a wide area of contact (figure 4.5). Similar studies with three further monoclonal antibodies reacting with the same antigen confirmed the 'lock and key' type fit between paratope and epitope. It is important not to regard the 'lock and key' as inflexible entities like two pieces of rock since this might make it very difficult for an animal to produce an antibody with such a unique complementary surface. In fact, three of these four studies revealed significant changes in the polypeptide backbone of up to 2.5 Å and if one adds into the equation the possibility of rotational movement of the amino acid side chains and alterations in the angle of association of the variable domains of light and heavy chains (V_L/V_H) in the Fab, it would seem more correct to think of antigen and antibody as surfaces which are to some extent mutually deformable.

In each instance, the area of contact between epitope and paratope is quite large, of the order of 750 Å^2, and it transpires that this is of the order normally found for protein–protein interactions such as those between interacting Cγ3 domains in the immunoglobulin Fc region. None the less, calculation of the contributions of individual amino acid residues to the overall binding energy suggests that only a small number are actively involved (see e.g. the glutamine 121 in figure 4.5); the rest, although part of the epitope, may be passive. An important feature is that the majority of atoms concerned in this interaction are sufficiently close to exclude water and we will emphasize the significance of this later. The large area of contact also makes it likely that residues on more than one peptide chain will be implicated and indeed, in each case the epitopes are discontinuous.

Antigen–antibody bonds are readily reversible

If the link between epitope and paratope is entirely dependent on spatial complementarity and does not involve the formation of covalent chemical bonds, it should not be too difficult to pull them apart. This can easily be put to the test. If one puts a mixture of the hapten with antibody inside a dialysis bag, the hapten will be found to diffuse out into the surrounding fluid until an equilibrium is reached in which some hapten is bound to antibody and some is free; if this exterior fluid is continually renewed, all the hapten will be lost from the bag showing that it can be completely dissociated from the antibody (figure 4.6). With larger antigens, the complexes can be split by a change in pH which brings about alterations in protein conformation and destroys the complementarity of the two reactants. As will be seen subsequently (p. 92), this principle can be used for the purification of either antigens or antibodies by affinity chromatography.

The forces binding antigen to antibody become large as intermolecular distances become small

It should be stressed immediately that the forces which hold antigen and antibody together are in essence no different from the so-called 'non-specific' interactions which occur between any two unrelated proteins (or other macromolecules) as, for example, human serum albumin and human transferrin. These intermolecular forces may be classified under four headings:

(a) Electrostatic

These are due to the attraction between oppositely charged ionic groups on the two protein side-chains as, for example, an ionized amino group (NH_3^+) on a lysine of one protein and an ionized carboxyl group ($-COO^-$) of, say, glutamate on the other (figure 4.7a). The force of attraction (F) is inversely proportional to the square of the distance (d) between the charges, i.e.

$$F \propto 1/k_D d^2$$

where k_D is the dielectric constant. Thus as the charges come closer together, the attractive force increases considerably: if we halve the distance apart, we quadruple the attraction. Furthermore,

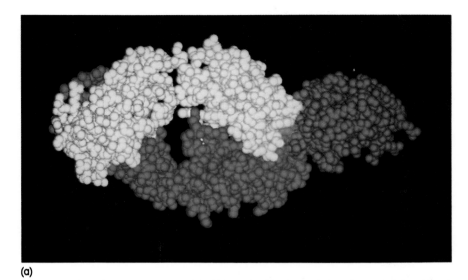
(a)

Figure 4.5. *The structure of the contact regions between a monoclonal Fab antilysozyme and lysozyme. (a) Space-filling model showing the Fab and lysozyme molecules fitting together snugly to form the complex. The antibody heavy chain is shown in blue, the light chain in yellow, lysozyme in green with its glutamine 121 in red. (b) Fab and lysozyme models pulled apart to show how the protuberances and depressions of each are complementary to each other. (c) End-on views of antibody combining site (left) and the antigenic region of lysozyme (right) obtained from (b) by rotating each molecule 90° about a vertical axis. Contact residues on both are shown in red except for Gln121 in light purple. The Gln121 fits into an antibody surface cavity surrounded by V_L and V_H residues 2, 5, 6, 7 and 16. The lysozyme epitope contact residues labelled 1—9 lie between residues 18 to 27 and labelled residues 10—16 are contributed by the peptide stretch from 117 to 128, i.e. this is clear evidence for a discontinuous epitope. All the hypervariable (complementarity determining) regions and two framework residues in the Fab make contact with the antigen. Most contacts are made by the heavy chain especially by the 3rd hypervariable region. It is not clear whether all the contacting residues contribute positively to the attractive forces between antigen and antibody; the striking influence of the Gln121 is revealed by the poor binding of lysozymes from other species in which the Gln121 is replaced by histidine. (Reproduced, with permission, from* Amit A. et al. (1986) Science **233,** 747—753. Copyright 1986 by the AAAS.)*

69

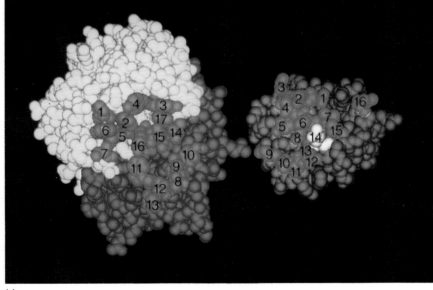
(b)

(c)

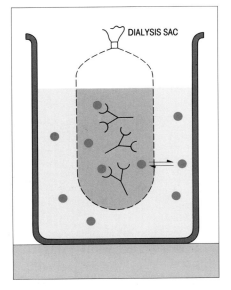

Figure 4.6. *Reversibility of the interaction between antibody (○—c) and hapten (●). Within the dialysis sac the hapten is partly in the free form and partly bound to antibody according to the affinity of the antibody. Only hapten can diffuse through the dialysis membrane and the external concentration then will equal the concentration of unbound hapten within the sac. Measurement of total hapten in the dialysis sac then enables the amount bound to antibody to be calculated. Constant renewal of the external buffer will lead to total dissociation and loss of hapten from inside the dialysis sac showing the reversible nature of the antigen—antibody bond.*

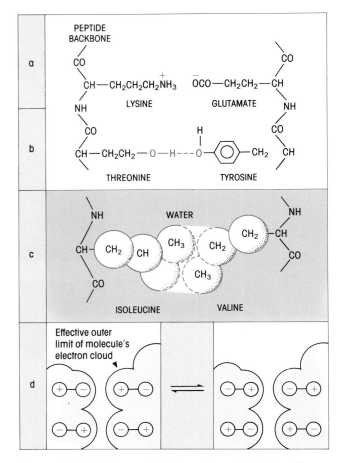

Figure 4.7. *Protein—protein interactions. (a) Coulombic attraction between oppositely charged ionic groupings. (b) Hydrogen bonding between two proteins. (c) Hydrophobic bonding: the region in which the water molecules are in contact with the hydrophobic groups (——) is considerably reduced when the hydrophobic groups on two proteins are in contact with each other (– – – –) and the lower free-energy of this system makes this a more probable state than separation of the hydrophobic groups. (d) Van der Waals force: the interaction between the electrons in the external orbitals of two different macromolecules may be envisaged (for simplicity!) as the attraction between induced oscillating dipoles in the two electron clouds.*

since the dielectric constant of water is extremely high, the exclusion of water molecules through the contiguity of the interacting residues to which we have already drawn attention, would greatly increase F.

Dipoles on antigen and antibody can also attract each other. In addition, electrostatic forces may be generated by charge transfer reactions between antibody and antigen; for example, an electron-donating protein residue such as tryptophan could part with an electron to a group such as dinitrophenyl which is electron accepting, thereby creating an effective +1 charge on the antibody and −1 on the antigen.

(b) Hydrogen bonding

The formation of reversible hydrogen bridges between hydrophilic groups such as ·OH, ·NH₂ and ·COOH depends very much upon the close approach of the two molecules carrying these groups (figure 4.7b). Although H-bonds are relatively weak, because they are essentially electrostatic in nature, exclusion of water between the reacting side-chains

would greatly enhance the binding energy through the gross reduction in dielectric constant.

(c) Hydrophobic

In the same way that oil droplets in water merge to form a single large drop, so non-polar, hydrophobic groups such as the side-chains of valine, leucine and phenylalanine tend to associate in an aqueous environment. The driving force for this hydrophobic bonding derives from the fact that water in contact with hydrophobic molecules, with which it cannot

H-bond, will associate with other water molecules but the number of configurations which allow H-bonds to form will not be as great as that occurring when they are surrounded completely by other water molecules, i.e. the entropy is lower. The greater the area of contact between water and hydrophobic surfaces, the lower the entropy and the higher the energy state. Thus if hydrophobic groups on two proteins come together so as to exclude water molecules between them, the net surface in contact with water is reduced (figure 4.7c) and the proteins take up a lower energy state than when they are separated (in other words, there is a force of attraction between them). It has been estimated that hydrophobic forces may contribute up to 50% of the total strength of the antigen−antibody bond.

(d) Van der Waals

These are the forces between molecules which depend upon interaction between the external 'electron clouds'. The deviation of gaseous molecules of say nitrogen or hydrogen from 'ideal' behaviour according to the kinetic theory is attributable to the Van der Waals attractions between them. The nature of this interaction is difficult to describe in non-mathematical terms but it has been likened to a temporary perturbation of electrons in one molecule effectively forming a dipole which induces a dipolar perturbation in the other molecule, the two dipoles then having a force of attraction between them; as the displaced electrons swing back through the equilibrium position and beyond, the dipoles oscillate (figure 4.7d). The force of attraction is inversely proportional to the seventh power of the distance, i.e.

$$F \propto 1/d^7$$

and as a result this rises very rapidly as the interacting molecules come closer together.

This last point underlines one essential feature common to all four types of force—they depend upon the close approach of both molecules before the forces become of significant magnitude, the more so if water molecules are excluded. And this is at the heart of the combination of antigen and antibody. The *complementary* electron-cloud shapes on the combining site of the antibody and the surface determinant of the antigen enable the two molecules to fit snugly together (cf. figure 4.5) so that the intermolecular distance becomes very small and the 'non-specific protein interaction forces' are considerably increased; the greater the areas of antigen and antibody which fit together, the greater the force of attraction, particularly if there is apposition of opposite charges and hydrophobic groupings.

By contrast, when the electron clouds of the two molecules effectively overlap, powerful repulsive forces are generated and energy must be expended in displacing the overlapping residues from their normal equilibrium positions.

The affinity or strength of binding of antigen and antibody

We saw from the electron microscope (E.M.) studies on the interaction between bifunctional dinitrophenyl (DNP) conjugates and antibody, that each DNP group fitted into one antibody combining site (figures 3.3 and 3.4). This means that small haptens by themselves are monovalent with respect to reaction with antibody. The experiment on mixing hapten with antibody in a dialysis bag (figure 4.6) showed that the combination with antibody was reversible and that the complex so formed could readily dissociate depending upon the strength of binding. This can be defined through the equilibrium constant (K) of the reaction:

$$Ab \quad + \quad H \quad \rightleftharpoons \quad AbH$$

given by the mass action equation,

$$K = \frac{[AbH]}{[Ab][H]}$$

where [Ab] is the concentration of free antibody combining sites and [H] the concentration of free hapten. If the antibody and hapten fit together very closely, the equilibrium will lie well over to the right; we refer to such antibodies which bind strongly to the hapten as *high affinity antibodies*. At a certain *free* hapten concentration $[H_c]$ where half of the antibody sites are bound,

$$[AbH] = [Ab] \text{ and } K = 1/[H_c]$$

i.e. the affinity constant K is equal to the reciprocal of the concentration of free hapten at the equilibrium point where half the antibody sites are in the bound form. In other words, when an antibody has a high affinity constant and binds hapten strongly, it only needs a low hapten concentration to half-saturate the antibody. It will be appreciated that an individual epitope on the surface of a complex antigen is also (by definition) monovalent and the strength of its combination with a univalent (Fab) antibody would also be defined by an affinity constant.

The value of K is determined by the difference in free energy (ΔG) between the antigen and antibody in the free state on the one hand and in the complexed form on the other, according to the equation

$$\Delta G = -RT \log_e K$$

where R is the universal gas constant and T the absolute temperature. Some energy may be required to alter the conformation of the antigen to allow strongly binding contact residues to interact either because displacement from the native position is required in order to make the contact, or because a residue has to be displaced on account of the steric repulsion forces which would be generated if it remained in its normal configuration (cf. figure 4.18).

One can study the interaction of hapten and antibody by the dialysis method described in figure 4.6 and use the data to calculate the affinity constant from the mass action equation. K values may sometimes be as high as 10^{11} l/mol.

Analysis of the binding at different hapten concentrations generally shows a heterogeneity (figure 4.8) which indicates that most antisera, even those raised against haptens with a simple structure, contain a variety of different antibodies with a range of binding affinities which depend upon the area of contact between the antibody and the hapten or epitope, the closeness of fit, conformation changes necessitated by electron-cloud overlap and the distribution of charged and hydrophobic groups.

The avidity of antiserum for antigen — the bonus effect of multivalency

While the term affinity describes the binding of antibody to a monovalent hapten or single antigen determinant, in most practical circumstances we are concerned with the interaction of an antiserum (i.e. the serum from an inmmunized individual) with a multivalent antigen. The term employed to express this binding,

$$nAb + mAg \rightleftharpoons Ab_nAg_m$$

(Ab = antibody; Ag = antigen) is *avidity*.

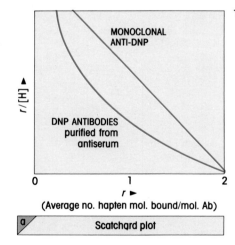

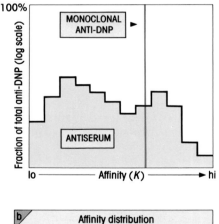

Figure 4.8. *Heterogeneity of IgG anti-hapten (dinitrophenyl: DNP) antibodies from the serum of an immunized animal contrasting with the homogeneity of a monoclonal IgG anti-DNP. (a) A Scatchard plot of hapten binding to antibodies purified from the serum. If r represents the average number of DNP molecules bound to each antibody molecule, of affinity constant k and number of binding sites n, in the presence of a free hapten concentration [H], then from the mass-action equation of equilibrium relationships (p.71) it can be shown that:*

r/[H] = nk − rk

Thus, a Scatchard plot of r/[H] against r for a single antibody species will be a straight line of slope k as seen for the monoclonal antibody; the deviation from a straight line given by anti-DNP from the antiserum clearly indicates the existence of antibodies with different affinities as may be confirmed by the binding of labelled DNP to many different bands after separation of the individual antibodies by isoelectric focusing of the serum. Extrapolation to r/[H] = o (at infinitely high concentration of antigen) gives the number of binding sites on each IgG molecule as 2 (cf. figure 3.4). For IgM antibodies the value would be 10. (b) Histogram showing a typical distribution of antibody affinities in the anti-DNP serum. Measurable affinities tend to range between 10^4 and 10^{10} or 10^{11} l/mol. and have skewed and not necessarily unimodal distributions. The monoclonal antibody of course gives a single affinity value.

The factors which contribute to avidity are complicated, including as they do the heterogeneity of antibodies in a given serum which are directed against each determinant on the antigen, and the heterogeneity of the determinants themselves (figures 4.4 and 4.8). But yet a further factor must be considered. The multivalence of most antigens leads to an interesting 'bonus' effect in which the binding of two antigen molecules by antibody is always greater, usually many-fold greater, than the arithmetic sum of the individual antibody links. This is illustrated in figure 4.9. The binding of the two antibodies to determinants 1 and 2 on the antigen can each be described by the individual change in free energy state on forming the epitope—paratope bond with its corresponding affinity constant, i.e.

$$\Delta G_1 = -RT \log_e k_1 \text{ and } \Delta G_2 = -RT \log_e k_2$$

For both antibodies operating in conjunction, the *overall* free energy change giving the avidity (K_{avid}) would be

$$\Delta G = \Delta G_1 + \Delta G_2 = -RT \log_e k_1 - RT \log_e k_2$$
$$= -RT(\log_e k_1 + \log_e k_2) = -RT(\log_e k_1 \times k_2)$$

Since $\Delta G = -RT \log_e K_{avid}$, $K_{avid} = k_1 \times k_2$.

The tremendous increase in equilibrium constant resulting from *multiplying* the contributing affinities (figure 4.9) is responsible for the bonus effect.

For those who prefer a more 'earthy' way of looking at molecular interactions, the mechanism of this effect may be interpreted by considering an analogy. Let us fabricate an unheard-of disease in which we cannot stop our hands opening and closing continuously. If we now try to hold an object in *one* hand it will fall the moment we open that hand. However, if we use *both* hands to hold the object, provided we open and close our hands at different times, there is much less chance of the object falling. The reversible combination of antigen and antibody is like the opening and closing of the hand; the more valencies holding the antigen the less likely it is to be lost when the complex dissociates at any one binding site (figure 4.10).

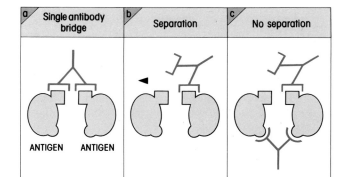

Figure 4.10. *The mechanism of the bonus effect. Each antigen—antibody bond is reversible and with a single antibody bridge between two antigen molecules (a), dissociation of either bond could enable an antigen molecule to 'escape' as in (b). If there are two antibody bridges, even when one dissociates the other prevents the antigen molecule from escaping and holds it in position ready to reform the broken bond. In effect, the orientation of the broken bond greatly increases the effective* combining concentration *of antibody and thereby speeds up the velocity of the association reaction:* $V_a = k_a[Ag] [Ab \uparrow]$.

The same considerations apply to the binding of antibody to a polymeric antigen with repeating determinants such as ovalbumin substituted by several DNP groups, or most bacterial polysaccharides or red cells with repeating blood-group determinants. As one moves from a univalent Fab fragment to a divalent IgG to a pentameric IgM, the bonus effect of multivalency produces striking increases in the strength of antigen—antibody complex formation.

Avidity being a measure of the functional affinity of an antiserum for the whole antigen is of obvious relevance to the reaction with antigen in the body. High avidity is superior to low for a wide variety of functions *in vivo*, immune elimination of antigen, virus neutralization, protective role against bacteria and so on.

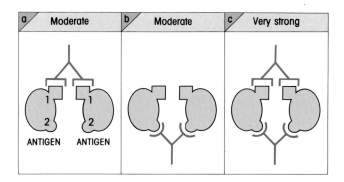

Figure 4.9. *The 'bonus' effect of multivalent attachment on binding strength. The force binding the two antigen molecules in (c) with two antibody bridges is many-fold greater than (a + b). If the affinity for determinant 1 is* k_1 *and for the second determinant* k_2, *the avidity of the mixture of antibodies for the antigen would be* $K_{avid} = k_1 \times k_2$. *To give a concrete example, if* k_1 *is* 10^4 *and* k_2 10^3, K_{avid} *would be* 10^7 *l/mol.*

ANTIGEN RECOGNITION — PRIMARY INTERACTION

The specificity of antigen recognition by antibody is not absolute

The ability of antibodies to discriminate between different antigens was well illustrated by the range of reactivity of an anti-hapten for a series of structurally related molecules as described in table 4.1. Since the strength of the reaction can be quantified by the affinity or avidity, we would relate the *specificity* of an antiserum to its relative avidity for the antigens which are being discriminated.

In so far as we recognize that an antiserum may have a relatively greater avidity for one antigen rather than another, by the same token we are saying that the antiserum is displaying relative rather than absolute specificity; in practice we speak of degrees of *cross-reactivity*. An antiserum raised against a given antigen can cross-react with a partially related antigen which bears one or more identical or similar determinants. In figure 4.11 it can be seen that an antiserum to antigen$_1$ (Ag$_1$) will react less strongly with Ag$_2$ which bears just one identical determinant because only certain of the antibodies in the serum can bind. Ag$_3$ which possesses a similar but not identical determinant will not fit as well with the antibody and the binding is even weaker. Ag$_4$, which has no structural similarity at all, will not react significantly with the antibody. Thus, based upon stereochemical considerations, we can see why the avidity of the antiserum for Ag$_2$ and Ag$_3$ is less than for the homologous antigen, while for the unrelated Ag$_4$ it is negligible. It would be customary to describe the antiserum as being highly specific for Ag$_1$ in relation to Ag$_4$ but cross-reacting with Ag$_2$ and Ag$_3$ to different extents.

By being directed towards single epitopes on the antigen, monoclonal antibodies frequently show high specificity in terms of their low cross-reactivity with other antigens. Occasionally, however, one sees quite unexpected binding to antigens which react poorly, if at all, with a specific antiserum. It is an instructive exercise to see how it is that a polyclonal antiserum containing a heterogeneous collection of antibodies can be more specific in discriminating between two antigens than a monoclonal antibody. The six hypervariable regions of an antibody encompass a relatively large molecular area composed of highly diverse amino acid side-chains and it is self-evident that a number of different epitopic structures could fit into different parts of this hypervariable 'terrain', albeit with a spectrum of combining affinities.

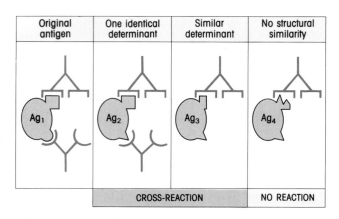

Figure 4.11. *Specificity and cross-reaction. The avidity of the serum antibodies (□——⊏ and ⊃——◯) for Ag$_1$ > Ag$_2$ > Ag$_3$ ≫ Ag$_4$.*

Thus, each antibody will react not only with the antigen which stimulated its production, but also with some possibly quite unrelated molecules. Figure 4.12 explains (I hope) how this may translate into a higher specificity for the polyclonal serum.

What the T-cell sees

We have on several occasions alluded to the fact that the T-cell receptor sees antigen on the surface of cells associated with an MHC class I or II molecule. Now is the time for us to go into the nuts and bolts of this relationship. (Warning! This represents one of the most active current areas of research in immunology and to follow what follows will require reasonable concentration. To those who feel this to be a trifle inconsiderate may I suggest reading the bold headings in this section and the text of the final subsection on p. 80)

Haplotype restriction reveals the need for MHC participation

Of dramatic significance has been the revelation that cytotoxic T-cells taken from an individual recovering from a viral infection will only kill virally infected cells which share an MHC haplotype. So important was this observation that it will pay us to look closely at the original experiments of Doherty and Zinkernagel. They found that cytotoxic T-cells from mice of the H-2^d haplotype infected with lymphocytic choriomeningitis virus could kill virally infected cells derived from any H-2^d strain but not cells of H-2^k or other H-2 haplotype. The

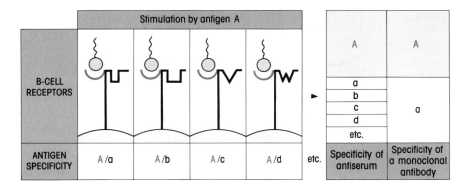

Figure 4.12. *Antigen A stimulates lymphocytes whose polyfunctional receptors bind A but could also bind other determinants as indicated (small letters). All antibodies in the resulting antiserum will have anti-A as a common specificity but the other specificities will be so diverse, none of them will reach appreciable concentrations to cross-react significantly with another antigen bearing a or b etc., i.e. the antiserum shows specificity for A. A monoclonal antibody on the other hand cannot dilute out its alternative specificity so in the example shown there would be strong cross-reaction with an unrelated antigen a. (With acknowledgement to Talmage D.W. (1959) Science 129, 1643.)*

reciprocal experiment with H-2^k mice shows that this is not just a special property associated with H-2^d (figure 4.13a). Studies with recombinant strains (cf. table 3.5) pin-pointed class I MHC as the restricting element and this was confirmed by showing that antibodies to class I MHC block this killing reaction. The same phenomenon has been repeatedly observed in the human. HLA-A2 individuals recovering from influenza have cytolytic T-cells which kill HLA-A2 target cells infected with influenza virus but not cells of a different HLA-A

tissue-type specificity (figure 4.13b). Note how cytotoxicity could be inhibited by antiserum specific for the donor HLA-A type but not by antisera to HLA-A1 or the HLA-DR framework.

In parallel, an entirely comparable series of experiments has established the role of MHC class II molecules in antigen presentation to helper T-cells. For example, a T-cell clone proliferating in response to ovalbumin on antigen-presenting cells with the I-A^b phenotype will fail to respond if antigen is presented in the context of I-A^k.

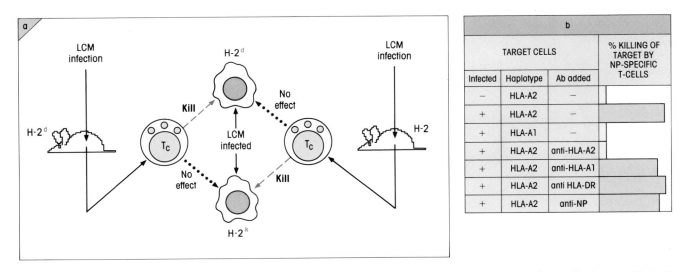

Figure 4.13. *T-cell killing is restricted by the MHC haplotype of the virus infected target cells. (a) Haplotype restricted killing of lymphocytic choriomeningitis (LCM) virus infected target cells by cytotoxic T-cells. Killer cells from H-2^d hosts only killed H-2^d infected targets, not those of H-2^k haplotype and vice versa. (b) Killing of influenza infected target cells by influenza nucleoprotein (NP)-specific T-cells from an HLA-A2 donor (cf. p. 284 for human MHC nomenclature). Killing was restricted to HLA-A2 targets and only inhibited by antibodies to A2, not to A1, nor to the class II HLA-DR framework or native NP antigen.*

Finally, transfection of the appropriate MHC genes endows cells of the wrong haplotype with the ability to present antigen to T-effector cells restricted to the haplotype of the transfected genes. Taken together, these findings unequivocally establish the participation of MHC molecules in T-cell recognition. What then of the antigen? For some time it was perplexing that in so many systems antibodies raised to the native antigen failed to block cytotoxicity (cf. figure 4.13b) despite consistent success with anti-MHC class I sera. We now think we know why.

T-cells see 'processed' antigen

It has long been known that denatured antigens tend to be better at eliciting T-cell-mediated skin reactions (delayed-type hypersensitivity) than native protein. There is now good evidence that exogenous soluble proteins need to be metabolically processed in some way by antigen-presenting cells before they can be recognized by T-helper cells. Consider the following experiment: if macrophages are pulsed with ovalbumin at 0°C, washed and then allowed to warm up to 37°C, they will induce a proliferative response in a T-cell clone specific for ovalbumin and the H-2 haplotype of the antigen-presenting macrophage. If the pulsed macrophages are fixed with glutaraldehyde within a few minutes

of reaching 37°C, they are unable to stimulate the T-cells, but if one waits for 1 hour at 37°C before fixation, a full-blooded T-cell proliferation can be induced (figure 4.14a). Clearly the antigen-presenting cell has to act on the ovalbumin in some way for it to be recognized by the T-cell and this processing takes around 1 hour. It is also blocked by chloroquine (figure 4.14b) which prevents the development of low pH in lysosomes and endosomes, and by cysteine proteinase inhibitors.

The current view is that exogenous soluble protein antigens are endocytosed by antigen presenting cells and, within the endosome, are subject to unfolding and limited proteolysis before fusion with a vesicle containing MHC class II molecules and return to the surface for presentation to T-cells.

What of the viral antigens recognized by cytolytic T-cells? The most obvious target would be the virally encoded proteins expressed on the surface of infected cells. But a molecule such as influenza nucleoprotein, which lacks a signal sequence or transmembrane region and so cannot be expressed on the cell surface, can none the less function as a target for cytotoxic T-cells and furthermore we have already noted that antibodies to native nucleoprotein have no influence on the killing reaction. It is unlikely that secreted nucleoprotein re-enters the cell by endocytosis and is processed by the pathway described for exogenous antigens since (i) chloro-

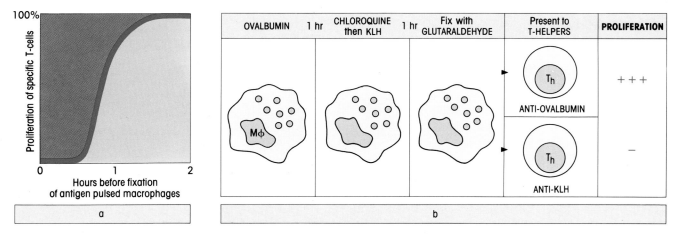

	OVALBUMIN	1 hr	CHLOROQUINE then KLH	1 hr	Fix with GLUTARALDEHYDE	Present to T-HELPERS	PROLIFERATION

a

b

Figure 4.14. *Evidence of processing of soluble protein by antigen-presenting cell. (a) Antigen-presenting macrophages are kept at 37°C after pulsing with antigen before fixation with glutaraldehyde; the ability to cause proliferation of specific T-cells does not appear until after 45 min. (b) Chloroquine, an agent which prevents low pH in lysosomes and endosomes blocks the processing of keyhole*

limpet haemocyanin (KLH) but has no effect on previously processed ovalbumin. Note that proteins with extended peptide chains such as fibrinogen, need minimal processing. (Based on Grey H.M. & Chesnut R. (1985) **Immunology Today** *6, 101; Ziegler K. & Unanue E. (1982)* **Proc. Nat. Acad. Sci. 79,** *175.)*

quine has no effect on killing and (ii) addition of nucleoprotein to uninfected cells does not make them targets for cytotoxic T-cells.

T-cells recognize a linear peptide sequence from the antigen

If we repeat the last experiment, but instead of using the whole nucleoprotein molecule, add a series of short peptides, each of about 16 amino acids, with sequences derived from the primary structure of the nucleoprotein, the uninfected cells now become susceptible to cytolytic T-cell attack (figure 4.15). This strongly supports the hypothesis that even protein antigens synthesized endogenously within the cell destined to become a cytotoxic target are first processed before presentation to T-cells. Note that only certain nucleoprotein peptides were recognized by the polyclonal T-cells in the donor population and these are to be regarded as T-cell epitopes. When clones of identical specificity are derived from these T-cells, each clone reacts with only one of the peptides; in other words, like B-cell clones, each clone is specific for one corresponding epitope.

Entirely analogous results are obtained when T-helper clones are stimulated by antigen presenting cells to which certain peptides derived from the original antigen had been added. Again, by synthesizing a series of such peptides, the T-cell epitope can be mapped with some precision.

Do MHC and peptide antigen interact positively to form a complex?

So far we have adduced evidence implicating a requirement for both MHC and peptide antigen in T-cell recognition. That they are all that is needed for reaction with the T-cell receptor is shown by experiments in which T-cell hybridomas (obtained by fusing a spontaneously dividing T-cell tumour with a normal T-cell of desired specificity; cf. B-cell hybridomas p. 136) are stimulated to produce lymphokines on contact with planar lipid membranes containing nothing more than the appropriate MHC and peptide. However, this does not tell us whether MHC and peptide actually complex together.

We are pretty convinced that they do: direct interaction between class II MHC and the corresponding peptides has been demonstrated by equilibrium dialysis, reaction with fluorescent peptide and covalent attachment of a radioactive peptide bearing a photoactivatable affinity label (cf. figure 3.12).

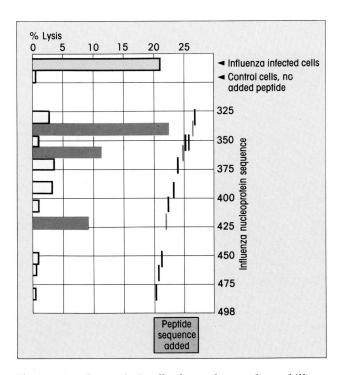

Figure 4.15. *Cytotoxic T-cells, from a human donor, kill uninfected target cells in the presence of short influenza nucleoprotein peptides. The peptides indicated were added to ^{51}Cr-labelled syngeneic (i.e. same as T-cell donor) mitogen-activated lymphoblasts and cytotoxicity assessed by ^{51}Cr release with a killer:target ratio of 50:1. The three peptides indicated in dark green induced good killing. Blasts infected with influenza virus of a different strain served as a positive control. (Reproduced from Townsend A.R.M. et al. (1986) Cell 44, 959, with permission. Copyright 1986 by Cell Press.)*

This latter system provides a convenient method for identifying which amino acids in the peptide are involved in binding to the MHC. Excess of the unlabelled peptide will block binding of the radioactive molecule; by replacing each individual amino acid in the peptide in turn with alternative amino acids to see when this blocking activity is lost, it is possible to define which residues are essential for the MHC interaction.

Although it can be done, it has proved to be more difficult to demonstrate direct binding to class I molecules, perhaps because their combining sites are already largely occupied by endogenous peptides (as suggested by existing X-ray crystallographic data (cf. p. 51)). The putative peptide strand lies within the groove formed by the two α-helices and the β-sheet floor and this cavity must be the obvious contender for the binding site for processed antigen peptide (figure 4.16). Physically, the groove provides a much greater opportunity for

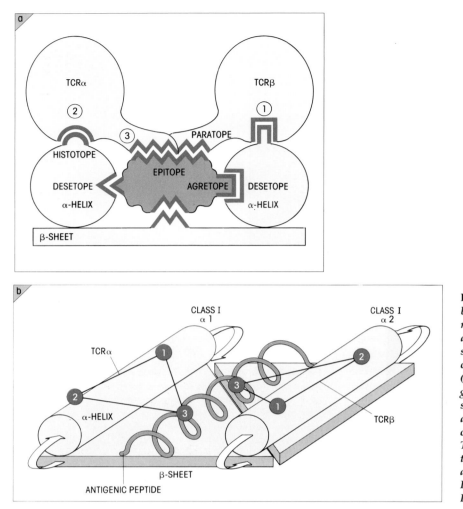

Figure 4.16. *Model of ternary complex between α and β chains of the T-cell receptor (TCR), MHC class I and antigenic peptide. (a) End on view showing the disposition of TCR complementarity determining regions (numbered) with peptide sitting in groove formed by α-helices and β-sheet floor. The various contact regions are defined. (b) Angled view of the complex showing CDR1 and 2 of each TCR chain in contact with α-helices and the two CDR3's interacting with the antigenic peptide (from Claverie J-M, Prochnicka-Chalufour A. & Bougueleret L. (1989)* **Immunology Today, 10, 10).**

building up forces of attraction with the peptide than would a flat surface. In addition, the location of many of the polymorphic amino acid residues on the floor and walls of the groove (cf. figure 3. 18d), could account for the variation in binding of a given peptide to different MHC alleles.

The recent rather remarkable observation that an antigenic peptide could act to some extent as a template and promote the folding of nascent class I heavy chain around itself, suggests that the full story of MHC-peptide interactions will have some surprises in store for us.

Polysaccharides are not degraded in the endosomes of antigen presenting cells, nor are they endowed with the physical properties to enable them to bind significantly to MHC molecules; accordingly, the reader will not be too surprised to be reminded that polysaccharides are unable to stimulate T-cells or to evoke T-cell mediated delayed-type hypersensitivity responses.

The T-cell receptor forms a ternary complex with MHC and antigenic peptide

Ignoring for the time being the role of accessory molecules in facilitating the interaction between T-cells and their antigen presenting target, at the molecular level it is difficult to contemplate the survival of any model which does not involve binding of the T-cell receptor to the MHC-peptide complex. Indirect evidence for contact between TCR and the other two components comes from studies in which amino acid residues on the peptide are systematically replaced by synthesis and those on the MHC by site directed mutagenesis. In accord with our previous deliberations, some of the changes in MHC residues lining the groove had profound effects on peptide binding whereas substitution of amino acids on the upper surface of the α-helices had no effect on the interaction with peptide but could influence T-cell recognition profoundly. Likewise, certain of the peptide side chains were also found to affect T-cell stimulation without changing its association with MHC.

Even while I am writing, I expect that in some laboratory, the binding of a soluble TCR construct to MHC-peptide complexes in planar artificial lipid membranes is being observed. It will take longer for us to have structural analysis of crystals of ternary complexes but meanwhile reasonable models of the predicted molecular interactions have been proposed. Of the three complementarity determinants assumed to be present in each TCR chain, CDR1 and CDR2 are much less variable than CDR3 which, like its immunoglobulin counterpart, has DJ sequences which result from a multiplicity of combinatorial and nucleotide insertion mechanisms (cf. p. 59). Since the MHC elements in a given individual are fixed and that great variability is expected in the antigenic peptide, a logical model would have CDR1 and CDR2 of each TCR chain contacting the α-helices, and the CDR3 concerned in binding to the peptide (figure 4.16). In accord with this view, two panels of T-cell clones recognizing two peptides differing only by one hydroxyl group (tyrosine for phenylalanine) and using the same MHC restriction element, differed only in the CDR3 hypervariable region.

Endogenous and exogenous antigens seem to be processed primarily by different pathways

Preprocessed antigenic peptides added exogenously to antigen-presenting cells appear to bind directly to unoccupied sites on surface MHC molecules, be they class I or class II, to form a complex able to stimulate T-cells. Whole protein antigens which have to undergo intracellular processing before association with MHC molecules are dealt with by two profoundly different mechanisms depending upon their route of entry. Exogenous antigens acquired by the antigen-presenting cells from the extracellular environment are processed via an endocytic pathway and normally become associated with class II molecules. By contrast, endogenous antigens such as viral proteins are degraded by a biosynthetic cytoplasmic pathway and usually, but not always, become complexed with class I MHC (see table 4.2).

Exogenous pathway

We have already discussed an outline of the fate of extracellular antigens taken up by endocytosis with

Table 4.2. *Pathways for presentation of exogenous and endogenous protein antigen (Ag)*

	Exogenous endocytic Ag	Endogenous cytoplasmic Ag	Exogenous peptide
Sensitive to:			
Chloroquine	+	−	−
Brefeldin A	− [a]	+	−
Cycloheximide	− [a]	+	−
MHC Presentation	Class II	Predominantly class I Sometimes class II	Class I and II

[a] Macrophages may require nascent synthesis of class II molecules

endosomes where they are cleaved at low pH by membrane-anchored-proteases before association with MHC class II (p. 76). It was noted that agents such as chloroquine which inhibit ATP driven proton pumps, block this process. In antigen-presenting cells such as interdigitating dendritic cells where the surface membrane actively recycles through the formation of cytoplasmic vesicles, the protease and MHC class II may be derived from molecules already on the surface. In macrophages where such cycling is relatively limited, vesicles containing newly-synthesized molecules may bud off from the Golgi system and fuse with the antigen-containing endosome before transport to the surface membrane (figure 4.17). Nascent MHC class II molecules contain a non-polymorphic 'invariant' peptide chain which is lost before the molecule reaches the surface; its function may be to control the endosome handling operation.

Endogenous pathway

The presentation of proteins synthesized within a cell to cytolytic T-cells is insensitive to chloroquine and is therefore independent of endosome mechanisms. It is likely that these cytoplasmic proteins are degraded by pH independent proteases linked to the 8.5 kDa ubiquitin molecule; they then fuse with newly synthesized class I molecules present within vesicles travelling to the cell surface after passage through the trans-Golgi apparatus (figure 4.17). The vital role of new class I synthesis in this pathway is highlighted by the failure to present endogenous antigens for T-cell cytotoxicity of cells treated with the protein synthesis inhibitor cycloheximide or with the fungal metabolite brefeldin-A which prevents proteins moving from the endoplasmic reticulum to the Golgi. Furthermore, transfection of cells with recombinant vaccinia virus containing

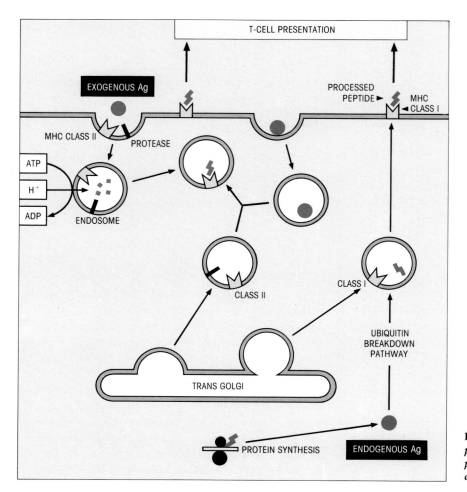

T-CELL PRESENTATION

EXOGENOUS Ag

PROCESSED
PEPTIDE ▶ ◀ MHC
CLASS I

MHC CLASS II PROTEASE

ATP

H⁺

ADP

ENDOSOME

CLASS II

CLASS I

UBIQUITIN
BREAKDOWN
PATHWAY

TRANS GOLGI

PROTEIN SYNTHESIS ENDOGENOUS Ag

Figure 4.17. *Distinct pathways for processing exogenous and endogenous protein antigens for presentation to T-cells.*

the gene encoding the adenovirus glycoprotein E19, profoundly inhibits the ability of vaccinia antigens to be presented to cytotoxic T-cells; the significance of this observation is that E19 specifically binds class I molecules in the endoplasmic reticulum and blocks intracellular transport.

Not all processed endogenous antigens are destined for class I presentation. For reasons which are not clear, but which may be related to the metabolic activity or particular cell type, some antigens finish up in association with class II. Examples are given by the chloroquine-insensitive susceptibility of measles and rabies infected cells to class II-restricted cytotoxic T-cells. We do not yet know how widespread is this phenomenon but it would be important to know whether presentation of cytoplasmic autoantigens by class II positive epithelial cells and processing of intracellular microbial antigens by macrophages for class II dependent T-cell recognition, proceed by this endogenous pathway.

The recognition of different forms of antigen by B- and T-cells is advantageous to the host

Antibodies combat microbes and their products in the extracellular body fluids where they exist essentially in their native form. Clearly it is to the host's advantage for the B-cell receptor to recognize epitopes on the native molecules.

T-cells, be they cytotoxic or lymphokine producers, have quite a different job; they have to seek out and bind to infected cells and carry out their effector function face to face with the target. First, the MHC molecules tell the effector T-lymphocyte that it is encountering a cell. Secondly, the T-cell does not want to attack an uninfected cell on whose surface a native microbial molecule is sitting adventitiously nor would it wish to have its antigenic target on the appropriate cell surface, blocked by an excess of circulating antibody. Thus it is of benefit for the infected cell to express the microbial antigen on its surface in a form distinct from that of the native molecule. As will now be more than abundantly clear, the solution was to make the T-cell recognize a processed peptide derived from the antigen and to hold it in a relatively restricted conformation (to improve binding affinities) by complexing it with the surface MHC molecules. The single T-cell receptor then recognizes both the MHC cell marker and the peptide infection marker in one operation.

Features associated with antigenicity

B-cell epitopes

This is a subject of particular interest to those wishing to make simple peptide substitutes for complex protein antigens. In general, large proteins, because they have more potential determinants, are better antigens than small ones. The more foreign an antigen, that is the less similar to self-configurations which induce tolerance, the more effective it is in provoking an immune response.

Parts of the peptide chains which protrude significantly from the globular surface tend to be sites of high epitope density. The least antigenic segments of the surface are associated with neighbouring concave regions containing water molecules which may be more difficult to displace, and we have noted earlier the importance attached to driving out the water molecules between antigen and antibody to achieve high binding forces. Much attention has been focused on the association between dominant antigenic regions and flexibility in the peptide chains as measured by the temperature factors derived from X-ray crystallography. If one considers the large area of potential contact between antigen and antibody, it is likely to be of value to have some flexibility in the shape of the antigen to allow it to take up a conformation which maximizes antibody

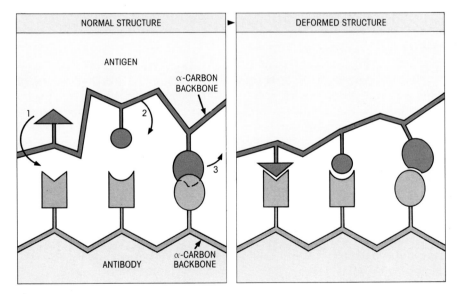

Figure 4.18. *Flexibility of antigen contributes to binding affinity. In the illustration we show three types of energy consuming reactions required to deform the antigen thereby allowing positive interaction between residues in the paratope and epitope: 1) bond rotation exposing a hydrophobic side chain normally buried within the interior of the protein antigen, 2) flexing of the α-carbon backbone to bring interacting residues close together, and 3) lateral displacement of a residue whose electron clouds would overlap with those on the antibody. Provided the total deformation energy is less than the energy of attraction of antibody for deformed antigen, complex formation will be favoured. Expressed mathematically:*

$$\text{Energy required to deform antigen} = (\Delta G1 + \Delta G2 + \Delta G3)$$
$$= \Delta G_{def}$$

Energy of association of deformed antigen + antibody =
$$\Sigma \text{ (individual binding energies)} = \Delta G_{binding}$$
(attractive force gives negative ΔG).
Overall energy change for complex formation
$$= \Delta G_{def} + \Delta G_{binding} = -RT\log_e K$$
Provided $-\Delta G_{binding} > \Delta G_{def}$, antigen and antibody will associate at equilibrium with a reasonable affinity constant K.

If the antigen were completely rigid, it would be unable to approach close enough to the antibody to generate significant binding energy. Clearly, the same considerations could apply to structural changes in the antibody molecule.

ANTIGEN RECOGNITION — PRIMARY INTERACTION

contact; the assumption is that the energy expended in inducing this conformational change is more than compensated by the intrinsic free energy change associated with formation of the new binding sites. This input of energy to produce conformational change leading to strong binding appears to be the factor behind the occurrence of normally 'buried' hydrophobic side-chains as contact residues for antibody (figure 4.18).

T-cell epitopes

T-cell epitopes can be identified fairly closely by making linear synthetic peptides but the exact form of the naturally processed peptide is not easy to predict. In different systems, maximal T-cell stimulation has occurred with anything between 9-mer and 16-mer peptides and some response was reported with a 5-mer. It has been calculated that the MHC class I and II groove can accommodate an elongated peptide of 8 amino acids but one of about 20 residues if present in the form of a contracted α-helix. In one study, naturally processed hen egg white lysozyme peptides were isolated from complexes with the I-E murine class II molecule formed in antigen-presenting cells. The peptides were heterogeneous but tended to be between 15 and 20 residues in length. This was the material with antigenic activity as could be demonstrated by re-insertion into purified I-E to produce a stimulatory complex for T-cell hybridomas.

We have come a long way in pinning down the molecular immunology of T-cell recognition, but we still have difficulty in predicting potential T-cell epitopes with complete confidence. The Berzofsky model looks for amphipathic sequences forming a helix with hydrophilic residues on one surface contacting the T-cell receptor and hydrophobic residues on the other, interacting with MHC groove. The other predictive 'motif' developed by Rothbard identifies a consensus sequence starting with a charged residue or glycine, followed by two or three consecutive hydrophobic residues and terminating in a polar amino acid. So far, neither 'motif' seems to win all the time but their success rates are not bad.

Because B-cells tend to react with the natively folded protein antigen while T-cells recognize unfolded peptide chains, linear peptides mimic the potency of the parent antigen for stimulation of T-cells much more readily than they do for reaction with antibody.

SUMMARY

An antigen is defined by its antibody. The contact area with an antibody is called an *epitope* and the corresponding area on an antibody, a *paratope*. Antisera recognize a series of dominant epitope clusters on the surface of an antigen; each cluster is called a determinant. Antigens and antibodies interact by spatial complementarity, not by covalent binding, and the forces of interaction include electrostatic, hydrogen-bonding, hydrophobic and Van der Waals; the forces become large as separation of antigen and antibody diminishes, especially when water molecules are excluded.

The strength of binding to a single antibody combining site is measured by the affinity. The reaction of multivalent antigens with the heterogeneous mixture of antibodies in an antiserum is defined by avidity and is usually much greater than affinity due to the 'bonus effect of multivalency'.

Specificity of antibodies is not absolute and they may cross-react with other antigens to different extents measured by their relative avidities.

T-cells see antigen in association with MHC molecules. They are restricted to the haplotype of the cell which first primed the T-cell. Protein antigens are processed by antigen-presenting cells to form peptides which associate with the MHC molecules binding to their central groove. Recognition by the T-cell receptor leads to formation of a ternary complex in which it is envisaged that the first and second hypervariable regions (CDR1 and CDR2) of each TCR chain contact the MHC α-helices while the CDR3s, having the greatest variability, interact with the antigenic peptide. Exogenous antigens are taken up by endocytosis, the endosome acidified in a chloroquine sensitive step, and the antigen subjected to proteolytic degradation before returning to the surface in association with class II MHC. Endogenous antigens such as viral proteins are cleaved by ubiquitin-dependent proteolysis and the peptides so-formed enter vesicles containing newly-synthesized class I MHC; the peptide-MHC complex is then transported to the surface for presentation to cytotoxic T-cells. In some incompletely defined circumstances, the endogenous peptides complex with class II MHC.

B-cells recognize epitopes on the native antigen; this is important because antibodies react with native antigen in the extracellular fluid. T-cells must contact infected cells and to avoid confusion between the two systems, the infected cell signals itself to the T-cell by the combination of MHC and degraded antigen.

The larger and more foreign a protein, the more likely it is to provoke antibody production; the protruding regions and probably the 'flexible' segments of globular proteins tend to be associated with higher epitope densities. If energy expended in distorting the antigen structure from its equilibrium state to enable it to combine more effectively with the complementary shape of the antibody surface is less than the energy of interaction of the 'distorted' antigen with its antibody, a complex will be formed.

T-cell epitopes are linear peptides usually about 9−15 amino acids long. The two major algorithms for predicting T-cell epitopes from a given structure are the Berzovsky amphipathic helix and the Rothbard 5-amino acid 'motif' but neither is yet 100% reliable.

Further reading

Austyn J.M. (1989) Antigen-presenting cells. *In Focus* series (Rickwood D. & Male D. Eds) IRL Press, Oxford.

Getzoff E.D., Tainer, J.A., Lerner R.A. & Geysen H.M. (1988) The chemistry and mechanism of antibody binding to protein antigens. *Adv. Immunol.*, **43**, 1.

Karush F. (1976) Multivalent binding and functional affinity. In *Contemporary Topics in Molecular Immunology.* F.P. Inman (ed.). Vol. 5, p. 217. Plenum Press, New York. (Bonus effect of multivalency.)

Kindt T.J., Long E.O. & Rothbard J.B. (Eds). (1989/90) *Current Opinion in Immunology.* Current Science, London. (Excellent pithy reviews on recognition of antigens by antibodies and T-cells.)

Melchers, F. *et al.* (Eds) (1989) *Progress in Immunol.*, **VII**, Springer Verlag, Berlin. (Articles on TCR-MHC-peptide interactions and relation Ig structure to Ag binding by top people.)

Nisonoff A. & Pressman D. (1957) Closeness of fit and forces involved in the reactions of antibody homologous to the p-(p'azophenylazo)-benzoate ion group. *J. Amer. Chem. Soc.*, **79**, 1616.

Townsend A.R.M. & Bodmer B. (1989) Antigen recognition by class I restricted T-lymphocytes. *Ann. Rev. Immunol.*, **7**, 601.

Novotny J., Bruccoleri R.E. & Saul F.A. (1989) On the attribution of binding energy in antigen−antibody complexes. *Biochemistry*, **28**, 4735. (View that only certain residues in epitope actively involved, others passive.)

CHAPTER 5

THE RECOGNITION OF ANTIGEN
II – Detection and Application

After exploring the intimacy of antigen–antibody interactions at the molecular level, this chapter will be more concerned with the practical aspects of methods used to detect and exploit antigen recognition.

Precipitation

The classical precipitin reaction

When an antigen solution is mixed in correct proportions with a potent antiserum, a precipitate is formed. Quantitative analysis of this interaction by the method shown in figure 5.1 gives both the antibody content of the immune serum and also an indication of the valency of the antigen, i.e. the effective number of dominant combining sites (determinants). This can vary enormously depending on the antigen, its size, and the species making the antibody. With hyperimmune rabbit antisera containing predominantly IgG antibodies, ovalbumin may have a valency of 10 and human thyroglobulin as many as 40 determinants on its surface.

It will be noted from the precipitin curve in figure 5.1 that as more and more antigen is added, an optimum is reached after which consistently less precipitate is formed. At this stage the supernatant can be shown to contain soluble complexes of antigen (Ag) and antibody (Ab), many of composition Ag_4Ab_3, Ag_3Ab_2 and Ag_2Ab (figure 5.2). In

extreme antigen excess (AgXS; figure 5.1) ultracentrifugal analysis reveals the complexes to be mainly of the form Ag_2Ab, a result directly attributable to the two combining sites or divalence of the IgG antibody molecule (cf. E.M. study, figure 3.3 and Scatchard analysis, figure 4.8). Between these extremes the cross-linking of antigen and antibody will generally give rise to three-dimensional lattice structures, as suggested by Marrack, which coalesce, largely through Fc–Fc interaction, to form large precipitating aggregates. Sera frequently contain up to 10% of non-precipitating antibodies which are effectively univalent because of the asymmetric presence of a sugar on one Fd region which stereochemically blocks the adjacent combining site.

Quantification by nephelometry

The small aggregates formed when dilute solutions of antigen and antibody are mixed creates a cloudiness or turbidity which can be measured by the scattering of an incident light source (nephelometry). Greater sensitivity can be obtained by using monochromatic light from a laser and by adding polyethylene glycol to the solution so that aggregate size is increased. In favoured laboratories which can sport the appropriate equipment, this method is replacing single radial immunodiffusion for the estimation of immunoglobulins, C3, C-reactive protein, etc.

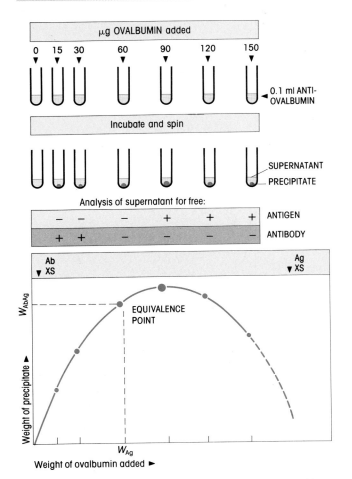

Figure 5.1. *Quantitative precipitin reaction between rabbit anti-ovalbumin and ovalbumin (the classical method of Heidelberger & Kendall which goes back as far as 1935). The antibodies are predominantly IgG. Increasing amounts of ovalbumin are added to a constant volume of the antiserum placed in a number of tubes. After incubation the precipitates formed are spun down and weighed. Each supernatant is split into two halves: by adding antigen to one and antibody to the other, the presence of reactive antibody or antigen respectively can be demonstrated. The antibody content of the serum can be calculated from the equivalent point where virtually no antigen or antibody is present in the supernatant. All the antigen added is therefore complexed in the precipitate with all the antibody available and the antibody content in 0.1 ml of serum would therefore be given by $(W_{AgAb} - W_{Ag})$. Analysis of the precipitate formed in antibody excess (AbXS), where the antigen-combining sites are largely saturated, gives a measure of the molar ratio of antibody to antigen in the complex and hence an estimate of the effective antigen valency.*

Visualization of the precipitation reaction in gels

Ouchterlony double diffusion

In this method, antigen and antibody placed in wells cut in agar gel diffuse towards each other and

precipitate to form an opaque line in the region where they meet in optimal proportions. A preparation containing several antigens will give rise to multiple lines. The immunological relationship between two antigens can be assessed by setting up the precipitation reactions in adjacent wells; the lines formed by each antigen may be completely confluent indicating immunological identity, they may show a 'spur' as in the case of partially related antigens, or they may cross, indicative of unrelated antigens (figure 5.3). The origins of these patterns are explained in figure 5.4. It should be emphasized that even in the case of confluent lines this can only indicate immunological identity in terms of the antiserum used, not necessarily molecular identity. For example, purified antibodies to the dinitrobenzene hapten would give a line of confluence when set up against dinitrophenyl (DNP)—ovalbumin and DNP—serum albumin conjugates placed in adjacent wells.

Where reagents are present in balanced proportions, the line formed will generally be concave to the well containing the reactant of higher molecular weight, be it antigen or antibody. This is a consequence of the usually slower diffusion rate of larger sized molecules.

The gel precipitation method can be made more sensitive by incorporating the antiserum in agar and allowing the antigen to diffuse into it (Feinberg). This method of single radial immunodiffusion is used for the quantitative estimation of antigens.

Single radial immunodiffusion (SRID)

When antigen diffuses from a well into agar containing suitably diluted antiserum, initially it is present in a relatively high concentration and forms soluble complexes; as the antigen diffuses further the concentration continuously falls until the point is reached at which the reactants are nearer optimal proportions and a ring of precipitate is formed. The higher the concentration of antigen, the greater the diameter of this ring (figure 5.5). By incorporating, say, three standards of known antigen concentration in the plate, a calibration curve can be obtained and used to determine the amount of antigen in the unknown samples tested (figure 5.6). The method is used routinely in clinical immunology, particularly for immunoglobulin determinations, and also for substances such as the third component of complement, transferrin, C-reactive protein and the embryonic protein, α-fetoprotein, which is associated with certain liver tumours.

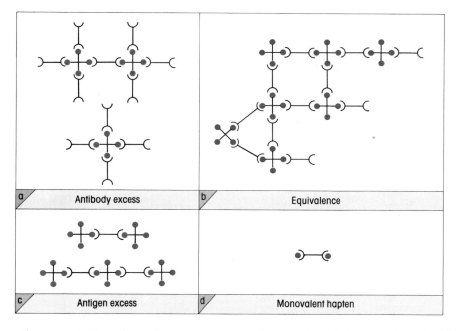

a	Antibody excess
b	Equivalence
c	Antigen excess
d	Monovalent hapten

Figure 5.2. *Diagrammatic representation of complexes formed between a hypothetical tetravalent antigen (•⫞•) and bivalent antibody (◯—◯) mixed in different proportions. In practice, the antigen valencies are unlikely to lie in the same plane or to be formed by identical determinants as suggested in the figure. (a) In extreme antibody excess, the antigen valencies are saturated and the molar ratio Ab:Ag approximates to the valency of the antigen. (b) At equivalence, large lattices are formed which aggregate to form a typical immune precipitate. This secondary aggregation, and hence precipitation tends to be inhibited by high salt concentration. (c) In extreme antigen excess where the two valencies of each antibody molecule become rapidly saturated, the complex Ag_2Ab tends to predominate. (d) A monovalent hapten binds but is unable to cross-link antibody molecules.*

87

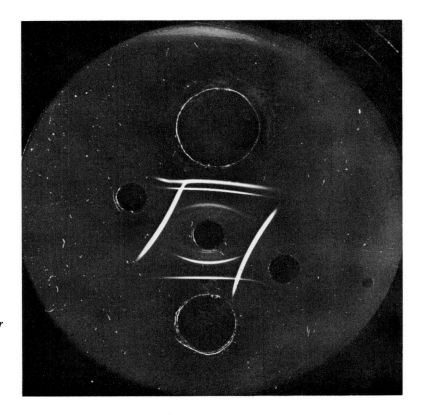

Figure 5.3. *Multiple lines formed in the Ouchterlony test (double-diffusion precipitation) when rabbit antiserum (centre well) reacts in agar gel with four different antigen preparations (peripheral wells). Non-identity and partial identity of antigens are shown respectively by crossing over and spur formation between precipitin lines.*

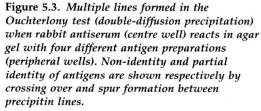

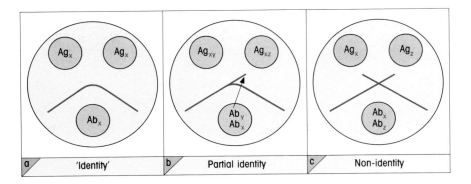

Figure 5.4. *(a) Line of confluence obtained with two antigens which cannot be distinguished by the antiserum used. (b) Spur formation by partially related antigens having a common determinant x but individual determinants y and z reacting with a mixture of antibodies directed against x and y. The antigen with determinants x and z can only precipitate antibodies directed to x. The remaining antibodies (Ab_y) cross the precipitin line to react with the antigen from the adjacent well which has determinant y giving rise to a 'spur' over the precipitin line. (c) Crossing over of lines formed with unrelated antigens.*

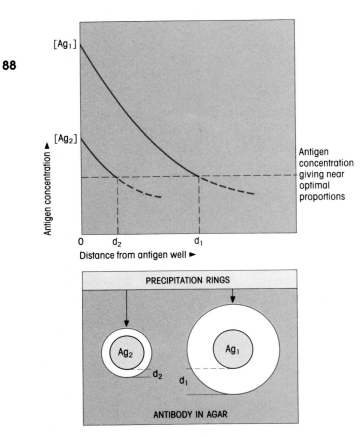

Figure 5.5. *Single radial immunodiffusion: relation of antigen concentration to size of precipitation ring formed. Antigen at the higher concentration [Ag_1] diffuses further from the well before it falls to the level giving precipitation with antibody near optimal proportions.*

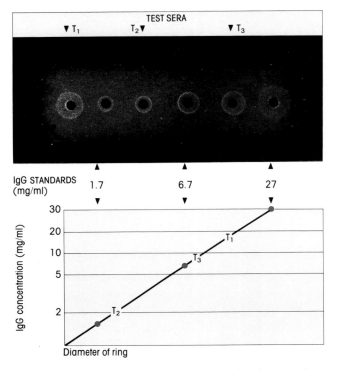

Figure 5.6. *Measurement of IgG concentration in serum by single radial immunodiffusion. The diameter of the standards (●) enables a calibration curve to be drawn and the concentration of IgG in the sera under test can be read off:*
T_1—serum from patient with IgG myeloma; 15 mg/ml
T_2—serum from patient with hypogammaglobulinaemia; 2.6 mg/ml
T_3—normal serum; 9.6 mg/ml.
(Courtesy of Dr F.C. Hay.)

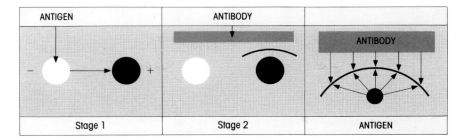

ANTIGEN	ANTIBODY	
		ANTIBODY
Stage 1	Stage 2	ANTIGEN

Figure 5.7. *The principle of immunoelectrophoresis.* **Stage I:** *Electrophoresis of antigen in agar gel. Antigen migrates to hypothetical position shown.* **Stage 2:** *Current stopped. Trough cut in agar and filled with antibody. Precipitin arc formed. Because antigen theoretically at a point source diffuses radially and antibody from the trough diffuses with a plane front, they meet in optimal proportions for precipitation along an arc. The arc is closest to the trough at the point where antigen is in highest concentration.*

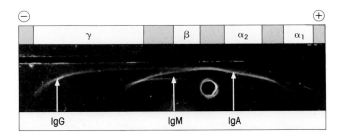

Figure 5.8. *Major human immunoglobulin classes demonstrated by immunoelectrophoretic analysis of human serum using a rabbit antiserum in the trough. The position of the main electrophoretic globulin fractions is indicated. Three of the five major immunoglobulin classes can be recognized: immunoglobulin G (IgG), immunoglobulin A (IgA) and immunoglobulin M (IgM). The IgG precipitin arc extends from the γ region well into the α_2-globulin mobility range reflecting the tremendous heterogeneity of the antibody population with respect to amino acid composition and net charge.*

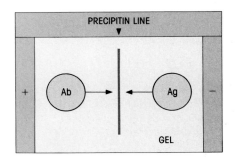

Figure 5.9. *Countercurrent immunoelectrophoresis. Antibody moves 'backwards' in the gel on electrophoresis due to endosmosis; an antigen which is negatively charged at the pH employed will move towards the positive pole and precipitate on contact with antibody.*

89

Immunoelectrophoresis

The principle of this is described in figure 5.7. The method is of value for the identification of antigens by their electrophoretic mobility, particularly when other antigens are also present. In clinical immunology, semi-quantitative information regarding immunoglobulin concentrations and identification of myeloma proteins is provided by this technique (figure 5.8).

There have been some felicitous developments of the principle combining electrophoresis with immunoprecipitation in which movement in an electric field drives the antigen directly into contact with antibody. *Countercurrent immunoelectrophoresis* may be applied to antigens which migrate towards the positive pole in agar (see figure 5.9). This qualitative technique is much faster and considerably more sensitive than double diffusion (Ouchterlony) and is used for the detection of hepatitis B antigen or antibody, DNA antibodies in SLE (p. 307), autoantibodies to soluble nuclear antigens in mixed connective tissue disease, and *Aspergillus* precipitins in cases with allergic bronchopulmonary aspergillosis. *Rocket electrophoresis* is a quantitative method which involves electrophoresis of antigen into a gel containing antibody. The precipitation arc has the appearance of a rocket, the length of which is related to antigen concentration (figure 5.10). Like countercurrent electrophoresis this is a rapid method but again the antigen must move to the positive pole on electrophoresis; it is therefore suitable for proteins such as albumin, transferrin and caeruloplasmin but immunoglobulins are more conveniently quantitated by single radial immunodiffusion. One powerful variant of the rocket system, Laurell's *two-dimensional* or *crossed immunoelectrophoresis*, involves a preliminary electrophoretic separation of an antigen mixture in a direction perpendicular to that of the final 'rocket-stage' (figure 5.11). In this way one can quantitate each of several antigens in a mixture. One straight-

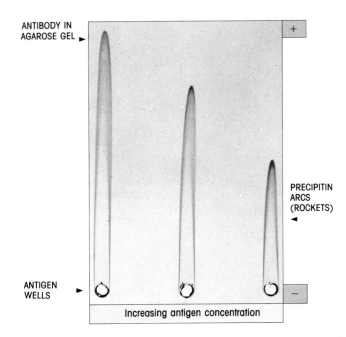

Figure 5.10. *Rocket electrophoresis. Antigen, in this case human serum albumin, is electrophoresed into gel containing antibody. The distance from the starting well to the front of the rocket-shaped arc is related to antigen concentration. In the example shown, human serum albumin is present at relative concentrations from left to right: 3, 2 and 1. (Reproduced from Weir* et al. *(eds) (1986)* Handbook of Experimental Immunology 1, *figure 32.42, with permission.)*

forward example is the estimation of the degree of conversion of the third component of complement (C3) to the inactive form C3c (cf. figure 1.10) which may occur in the serum of patients with active SLE or the synovial fluid of affected joints in active rheumatoid arthritis, to give but two examples (figure 5.11b). The remarkable ability of the technique to resolve a highly complex mixture of antigens is clearly seen in figure 5.11c.

Indirect precipitation of complexes

For a variety of reasons, addition of antibody to an antigen may give rise to a soluble complex. If one wishes to analyse the complex for its antibody content or to identify the antigens within it, the complex can be brought out of solution either by changing its solubility or by adding an anti-immunoglobulin precipitating reagent as in figure 5.12. An example of how this technique was used to characterize the main chain of human class I MHC molecules is given in figure 5.13.

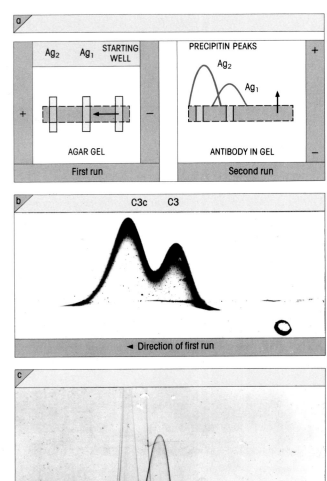

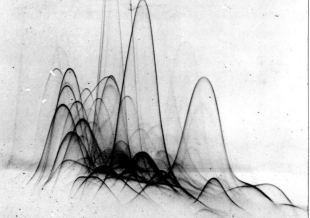

Figure 5.11. *Crossed immunoelectrophoresis. (a) Antigens are separated on the basis of electrophoretic mobility in agar. A strip (dotted) containing the separated antigens is cut out as shown, laid over another gel which contains antiserum, and electrophoresis carried out in a direction at right angles to the first to drive the antigens through the antiserum to form precipitin peaks; the area under the peak is related to the concentration of antigen. (b) Actual run showing C3 conversion (C3→C3c) in serum (stained gel). In this case the arcs interact because of common antigenic determinants. (Courtesy of Dr C. Loveday.) (c) 'Himalayan fantasy' showing a highly complex mixture of antigens from* Mycobacterium intracellulare. *(Reproduced from Weir* et al. *(eds) (1986)* Handbook of Experimental Immunology 1, *figure 32.44, with permission.)*

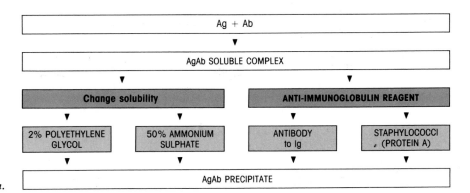

Figure 5.12. *Precipitation of soluble complexes either (i) by changing the solubility so that the complexes are precipitated while the uncombined Ag and Ab remain in solution, or (ii) by adding a precipitating anti-immunoglobulin antibody or staphylococcal organisms which bind immunoglobulin Fc to the protein A on their surface and can then be spun down.*

Ag + Ab

AgAb SOLUBLE COMPLEX

Change solubility

ANTI-IMMUNOGLOBULIN REAGENT

2% POLYETHYLENE GLYCOL

50% AMMONIUM SULPHATE

ANTIBODY to Ig

STAPHYLOCOCCI (PROTEIN A)

AgAb PRECIPITATE

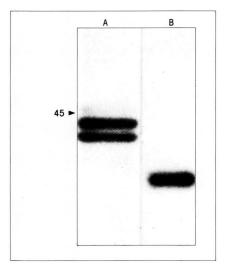

Figure 5.13. *Analysis of membrane-bound class I MHC antigens (cf. p. 51). The membranes from human cells pulsed with ^{35}S-methionine were solubilized in a detergent, mixed with a monoclonal antibody to HLA-A and B molecules and immunoprecipitated with staphylococci. An autoradiograph (A) of the precipitate run in SDS-polyacrylamide gel electrophoresis shows the HLA-A and B chains as a 43 000 molecular weight doublet (the position of a 45 000 marker is arrowed). If membrane vesicles were first digested with Proteinase K before solubilization, a labelled band of molecular weight 39 000 can be detected (B) consistent with a transmembrane orientation of the HLA chain: the 4000 hydrophilic C-terminal fragment extends into the cytoplasm and the major portion, recognized by the monoclonal antibody and by tissue typing reagents, is present on the cell surface (cf. figure 3.18). (From data and autoradiographs kindly supplied by Dr M.J. Owen.)*

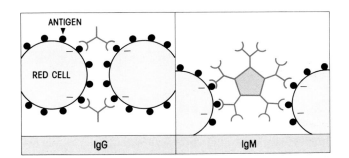

Figure 5.14. *Mechanism of agglutination of antigen-coated particles by antibody cross-linking to form large macroscopic aggregates. If red cells are used, several cross-links are needed to overcome the electrical charge at the cell surface. IgM is superior to IgG as an agglutinator because of its multivalent binding and because the charged cells are further apart.*

91

Agglutination by antibody

Whereas the cross-linking of multivalent protein antigens by antibody leads to precipitation, cross-linking of cells or large particles by antibody directed against surface antigens leads to agglutination. Since most cells are electrically charged, a reasonable number of antibody links between two cells is required before the mutual repulsion is overcome. Thus agglutination of cells bearing only a small number of determinants may be difficult to achieve unless special methods such as further treatment with an antiglobulin reagent are used. Similarly, the higher avidity of multivalent IgM antibody relative to IgG (cf. p. 73) makes the former more effective as an agglutinating agent, molecule for molecule (figure 5.14).

Agglutination reactions are used to identify bacteria and to type red cells; they have been observed with leucocytes and platelets and even with spermatozoa in certain cases of male infertility due to sperm agglutinins. Because of its sensitivity and convenience, the test has been extended to the identification of antibodies to soluble antigens which have been artificially coated on to various types of particle. Red cells have been popular and they can be coated with proteins after first modifying their surface with tannic acid or chromium chloride, or by direct use of bifunctional cross-linking agents such as bisdiazobenzidine. The large, rapidly sedimenting red cells of the turkey are finding increasing favour for this purpose. The tests are usually carried out in the wells of plastic agglutination trays where the settling pattern of the cells on the bottom of the cup may be observed (figure 5.15); this provides a more sensitive indicator than macroscopic clumping. Inert particles such as bentonite and polystyrene latex have also been coated with antigens for agglutination reactions, particularly those used to detect the rheumatoid factors (figure 5.16).

Purification of antigens and antibodies by affinity chromatography

The principle is simple and *very* widely applied. Antigen or antibody is bound through its free amino groups to cyanogen-bromide-activated Sepharose particles. Insolubilized antibody, for example, can be used to pull the corresponding antigen out of solution in which it is present as one component of a complex mixture, by absorption to its surface. The uninteresting garbage is washed away and the required ligand released from the affinity absorbent by disruption of the antigen−antibody bonds by changing the pH or adding chaotropic ions such as thiocyanate (figure 5.17). Likewise, an antigen immunosorbent can be used to absorb out an antibody from a mixture whence it can be purified by elution. The potentially damaging effect of the eluting agent can be avoided by running the antiserum down an affinity column so prepared as to have relatively weak binding for the antibody being purified; under these circumstances, the antibody is retarded in flow rate rather than being firmly bound. If a protein mixture is separated by iso-

electric focusing into discrete bands, an individual band can be used to affinity purify specific antibodies from a polyclonal antiserum; quite useful when supplies of antigen are painfully limited.

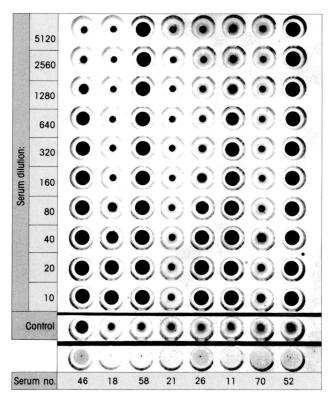

Figure 5.15. *Tanned red cell haemagglutination test for thyroglobulin autoantibodies. Thyroglobulin-coated cells were added to dilutions of patients' sera. Uncoated cells were added to a 1:10 dilution of serum as a control. In a positive reaction, the cells settle as a carpet over the bottom of the cup. Because of the 'V'-shaped cross-section of these cups, in negative reactions the cells fall into the base of the 'V' forming a small easily recognizable button. The reciprocal of the highest serum dilution giving an unequivocally positive reaction is termed the* **titre**. *The titres reading from left to right are: 640, 20, >5120, neg, 40, 320, neg, >5120. The control for serum No. 46 was slightly positive and this serum should be tested again after absorption with uncoated cells.*

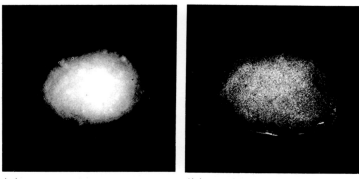

(a)   (b)

Figure 5.16. *Macroscopic agglutination of latex coated with human IgG by serum from a patient with rheumatoid arthritis. This contains rheumatoid factor, an autoantibody directed against determinants on IgG. (a) Normal serum, (b) patient's serum.*

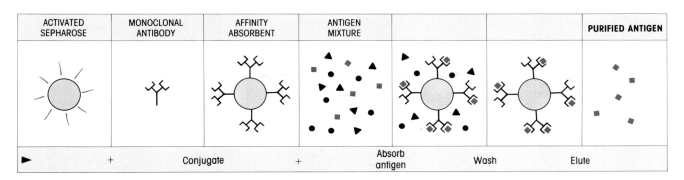

ACTIVATED SEPHAROSE	MONOCLONAL ANTIBODY	AFFINITY ABSORBENT	ANTIGEN MIXTURE			PURIFIED ANTIGEN
►	+	Conjugate	+	Absorb antigen	Wash	Elute

Figure 5.17. *Affinity chromatography. A column is filled with Sepharose-linked antibody. The antigen mixture is poured down the column. Only the antigen binds and is released by change in pH for example. An antigen-linked affinity column will purify antibody obviously.*

Immunoassay of antigen and antibody with labelled reagents

Antigen and antibody can be used for the detection of each other and an ingenious plethora of immunoassay techniques have been developed in which the final read-out of the reaction involves a reagent conjugated with an appropriate label. Radiolabelling with ^{131}I, or now more usually ^{125}I, is a tried and trusted technique with a very long history and we will describe the principles of various immunoassay techniques using this as a label.

Soluble phase immunoassays

For antibody

If a reasonable excess of labelled antigen is added to an antiserum, most of the antibodies of moderate affinity will be complexed and precipitation of the complexes followed by measurement of the label will give an estimate of the antigen binding capacity of the serum (figure 5.18). By using antibodies to different immunoglobulin classes and subclasses as the antiglobulin reagent, it is possible to determine the distribution of antibody activity among the classes. For example, addition of a radioactive antigen to human serum followed by a precipitating rabbit anti-human IgA would indicate how much antigen had been bound to the serum IgA.

Classical radioimmunoassay (RIA) for antigen

The binding of radioactively labelled antigen to a limited fixed amount of antibody can be partially inhibited by addition of unlabelled antigen and the extent of this inhibition can be used as a measure of the unlabelled material added. The principle of this form of saturation analysis is explained in figure 5.19. Methods vary in the means used to separate free antigen from that bound to antibody and we have discussed the main ones already.

With the development of methods for labelling antigens to a high specific activity, very low concentrations down to the 10^{-12} g/ml level can be detected and most of the protein hormones can now be assayed with this technique. One disadvantage is that these methods cannot distinguish active

93

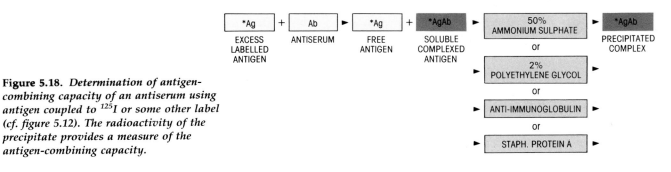

Figure 5.18. *Determination of antigen-combining capacity of an antiserum using antigen coupled to ^{125}I or some other label (cf. figure 5.12). The radioactivity of the precipitate provides a measure of the antigen-combining capacity.*

*Ag + Ab ► *Ag + *AgAb ►
EXCESS LABELLED ANTIGEN — ANTISERUM — FREE ANTIGEN — SOLUBLE COMPLEXED ANTIGEN

50% AMMONIUM SULPHATE
or
2% POLYETHYLENE GLYCOL
or
ANTI-IMMUNOGLOBULIN
or
STAPH. PROTEIN A

► *AgAb
PRECIPITATED COMPLEX

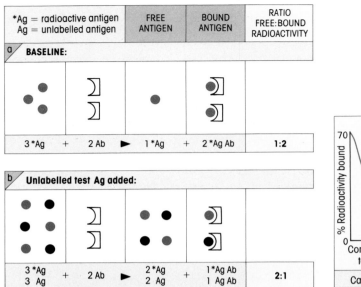

*Ag = radioactive antigen Ag = unlabelled antigen	FREE ANTIGEN	BOUND ANTIGEN	RATIO FREE:BOUND RADIOACTIVITY
a BASELINE:			
3 *Ag + 2 Ab ► 1 *Ag + 2 *Ag Ab	1:2		
b Unlabelled test Ag added:			
3 *Ag 3 Ag + 2 Ab ► 2 *Ag 2 Ag + 1 *Ag Ab 1 Ag Ab	2:1		

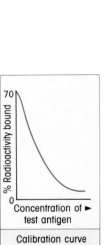

Calibration curve

Figure 5.19. *Principle of radioimmunoassay (simplified by assuming a very highly avid antibody and one combining site per antibody molecule). (a) If we add 3 mol of radio-labelled Ag (●) to 2 mol of Ab, 1 mol of Ag will be free and 2 bound to Ab. The ratio of the counts of free to bound will be 1:2. (b) If we now add 3 mol of unlabelled Ag (●) plus 3 mol radio Ag to the Ab, again only 2 mol of total Ag will be bound, but since the Ab cannot distinguish labelled from unlabelled Ag, half will be radioactive. The remaining antigen will be free and the ratio free: bound radioactivity changes to 2:1. This ratio will vary with the amount of unlabelled Ag added and this enables a calibration curve to be constructed.*

94

protein molecules from biologically inactive fragments which still retain antigenic determinants. Other applications include the assay of carcino-embryonic antigen, hepatitis B (Australia) antigen and smaller molecules such as steroids, prostaglandins and morphine-related drugs (appropriate antibodies are raised by coupling to an immunogenic carrier).

Solid phase immunoassays

For antibody

The antibody content of a serum can be assessed by the ability to bind to antigen which has been insolubilized by physical adsorption to a plastic tube or micro-agglutination tray with multiple wells; the bound immunoglobulin may then be estimated by addition of a labelled anti-Ig raised in another species (figure 5.20). Consider, for example, the

determination of DNA autoantibodies in systemic lupus erythematosus (cf. p. 307). When a patient's serum is added to a microwell coated with antigen (in this case DNA), the autoantibodies will bind to the plastic and remaining serum proteins can be readily washed away. Bound antibody can now be estimated by addition of ^{125}I-labelled purified rabbit anti-human IgG; after rinsing out excess unbound reagent, the radioactivity of the tube will clearly be a measure of the autoantibody content of the patient's serum. The distribution of antibody in different classes can obviously be determined by using specific antisera. Take the radioallergosorbent test (RAST) for IgE antibodies in allergic patients. The allergen (e.g. pollen extract) is covalently coupled to an immunoabsorbent, in this case a paper disc, which is then treated with patient's serum. The amount of specific IgE bound to the paper can now be estimated by addition of labelled anti-IgE.

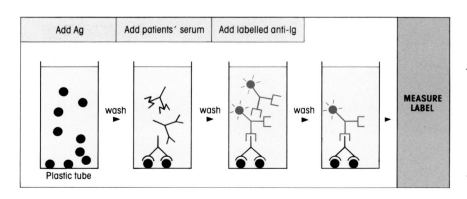

Add Ag	Add patients´ serum	Add labelled anti-Ig	MEASURE LABEL
Plastic tube			

Figure 5.20. *Solid phase immunoassay for antibody. By attaching antibody to the solid phase, the system can be used to assay antigen (cf. sandwich two-site assay below). To reduce non-specific binding of IgG to the solid phase after adsorption of the first reagent, it is usual to add an irrelevant protein such as gelatin, or more recently α_1-glycoprotein, to block any free sites on the plastic.*

Immunoradiometric assay for antigen

This differs from radioimmunoassay in the sense that the labelled reagent is used in excess. For the estimation of antigen, antibodies are coated on to a solid surface such as plastic and the test antigen solution added; after washing, the amount of antigen bound to the plastic can be estimated by adding an excess of radio-labelled antibody. The specificity of the method can be improved by the sandwich assay which uses solid phase and labelled antibodies with specificities for different parts of the antigen:

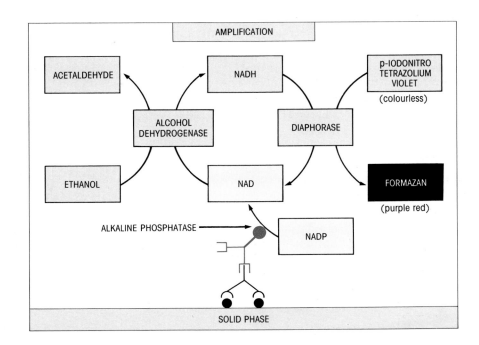

One widely used application is the radioimmunosorbent test (RIST) for IgE. Rabbit anti-IgE is coupled by cyanogen bromide to microcrystalline cellulose and reacted with dilutions of an IgE-containing standard serum or the patient's serum under test. Bound IgE is then measured by addition of labelled anti-IgE.

A wide variety of labels is available

Because of health hazards and the deterioration of reagents through radiation damage, types of label other than radioisotopes have been sought.

ELISA (enzyme-linked immunosorbent assay)

Perhaps the most widespread alternative has been the use of enzymes which give a coloured reaction product, usually in solid phase assays. Enzymes such as horse radish peroxidase and phosphatase have been widely employed. One clever ploy for amplifying the phosphatase reaction is to use NADP as a substrate to generate NAD which now acts as a coenzyme for a second enzyme system (figure 5.21). Pyrophosphatase from *E. coli* provides a good conjugate because the enzyme is not present in tissues, is stable and gives a good reaction colour. Chemiluminescent systems based on enzymes such as luciferase can also be applied.

Other labels

Conjugation with the vitamin biotin is frequently used since this can readily be detected by its reaction with enzyme-linked avidin (or even better, streptavidin) to which it binds with ferocious specificity and affinity ($K = 10^{15} \text{ M}^{-1}$).

Fluorescent labels have an important role to play in lowering the limits of detection of immunoassay methods and special mention should be made of time resolved fluorescence assay based upon chelates of rare earths such as Europium 3^+ (figure 5.22).

Figure 5.21. *Coenzyme-geared amplification of the phosphatase reaction to reveal solid phase anti-immunoglobulin label.*

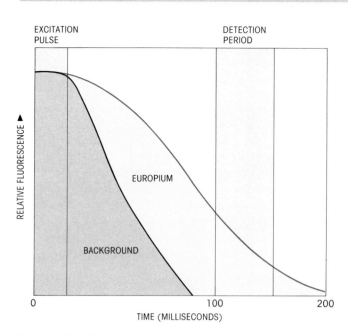

Figure 5.22. *The principle of time-resolved fluorescence assay. The problem with conventional methods of detection of low fluorescent signals is interference from reflection of incident light and background instrument fluorescence. By using just a short excitation pulse and measuring the signal after background has fallen to zero but before the Europium with its long fluorescence half-life has decayed completely, good discrimination between a weak signal and background becomes possible.*

The ambient analyte principle

The advent of highly sensitive fluorescence probes will allow the wide exploitation of the ambient analyte principle which states that the percentage occupancy of combining sites for a given antibody is dependent upon the concentration of antigen (analyte) in the solution but is independent of the amount of antibody, provided this is relatively small compared with the analyte (Ekins). The same is true for any binding system with ligand specificity.

Thus, in an assay for a hormone, for example, it is possible to use a microspot of the first (or capture antibody) labelled with one fluorescent reagent to bind the hormone from a test solution, and then to obtain a measure of occupied antibody sites by using a second antibody to the hormone (cf. 'sandwich assay', p. 95) labelled with a second distinct flourescent label. The ratio of the two labels will be a measure of the original hormone concentration. By using a number of microspots with capture antibodies of differing specificities on the same support, one can envisage the exciting possibility of being able to screen a single sample for multiple analytes in one test.

Immunoblotting (Western blots)

After separation from a complex mixture by electrophoresis in a solid phase such as polyacrylamide or agar gel, antigens can be 'blotted' by transverse electrophoresis on to nitrocellulose sheets where they bind non-specifically and can be identified by staining with appropriately labelled antibodies. This technique has been used widely, as for example in the identification of components of neurofilaments which have been separated in sodium dodecyl sulphate (SDS)-polyacrylamide gels. Obviously, such a procedure will not work with antigens which are irreversibly denatured by this detergent and it is best to use polyclonal antisera for blotting to increase the chance of having antibodies to whichever epitopes do survive the denaturation procedure; a surprising number do (figure 5.23). Conversely, the spectrotype of an antiserum can be revealed by isoelectric focusing, blotting and then staining with labelled antigen.

Immunohistochemistry — localization of antigens in cells and tissues

Immunofluorescence

Because fluorescent dyes such as fluorescein and rhodamine can be coupled to antibodies without destroying their specificity, the conjugates can combine with antigen present in a tissue section and be visualized in the fluorescence microscope. In this way the distribution of antigen throughout a tissue and within cells can be demonstrated. Looked at another way, the method can also be used for the detection of antibodies directed against antigens already known to be present in a given tissue section or cell preparation. There are three general ways in which the test is carried out.

1. Direct test

The antibody to the tissue substrate is itself conjugated with the fluorochrome and applied directly (figure 5.24a). For example, suppose we wished to show the tissue distribution of a gastric autoantigen reacting with the autoantibodies present in the serum of a patient with pernicious anaemia. We would isolate IgG from the patient's serum, conjugate it with fluorescein, and apply it to a section of human gastric mucosa on a slide. When viewed in

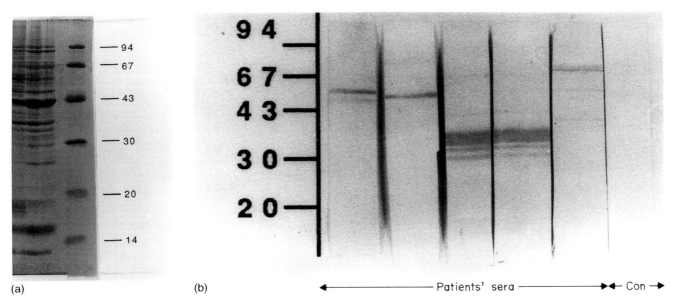

(a)   (b)   ◄——————— Patients' sera ———————►◄— Con —►

Figure 5.23. *Western blot analysis of human polymorph primary granules with sera from patients with systemic vasculitis. Human polymorph post-nuclear supernatant was run on SDS-PAGE. (a) Gel stained for protein with Coomassie Blue. Numbers refer to molecular weight markers (kDa). (b) Blots from gel stained with sera from five patients and one control (RHS) and visualized with alkaline phosphatase-conjugated goat anti-human IgG. Three different patterns of autoantibody reaction are evident. (Kindly supplied by Drs J. Cambridge & B. Leaker.) The antibodies used for immunoblotting are usually labelled with enzymes or biotin (followed by labelled avidin) but in many* laboratories, *colloidal gold conjugates are becoming the method of choice. Often IgG antibodies are picked up by labelled staphylococcal protein A although this may well be superseded by streptococcal protein G which reacts with all IgG subclasses and with IgG from a wide variety of species. One method for relating the position of a peptide in a Western blot is to use colloidal gold for staining total protein red, and peroxidase labelled antibody to stain the immunoreactive band blue; the two colours can be differentiated by photography with appropriate filters.*

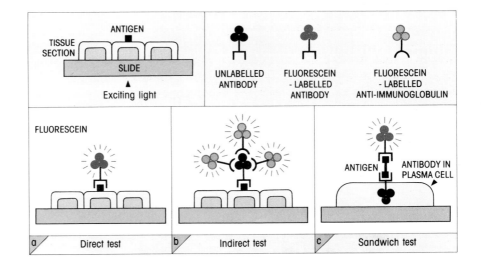

Figure 5.24. *The basis of fluorescence antibody tests for identification of tissue antigens or their antibodies.* ● = *fluorescein labelled.*

the fluorescence microscope we would see that the cytoplasm of the parietal cells was brightly stained. By using antisera conjugated to dyes which emit fluorescence at different wavelengths, two different antigens can be identified simultaneously in the same preparation. In figure 2.6h (p. 21), direct staining of fixed plasma cells with a mixture of rhodamine-labelled anti-IgG and fluorescein-conjugated anti-IgM craftily demonstrates that these two classes of antibody are produced by different cells. The technique of coupling biotin to the anti-serum and then finally staining with fluorescent avidin is finding increasing favour.

ANTIGEN RECOGNITION — DETECTION AND APPLICATION

2. Indirect test

In this double-layer technique, the unlabelled antibody is applied directly to the tissue substrate and visualized by treatment with a fluorochrome-conjugated anti-immunoglobulin serum (figure 5.24b). In this case, in order to find out whether or not the serum of a patient has antibodies to gastric parietal cells, we would first treat a gastric section with the serum, wash well and then apply a fluorescein-labelled rabbit anti-human immunoglobulin; if antibodies were present, there would be staining of the parietal cells (figure 5.25).

This technique has several advantages. In the first place the fluorescence is brighter than with the direct test since several fluorescent anti-immunoglobulins bind on to each of the antibody molecules present in the first layer (figure 5.24b). Secondly, since the conjugation process is lengthy, much time can be saved when many sera have to be screened for antibody because it is only necessary to prepare a single labelled reagent, viz. the anti-immunoglobulin. Furthermore, the method has great flexibility. For example, by using conjugates of antisera to individual immunoglobulin heavy chains, the distribution of antibodies among the various classes and subclasses can be assessed at least semi-quantitatively. One can also test for complement fixation on the tissue section by adding a mixture of the first antibody plus a source of complement, followed by a fluorescent anti-complement reagent as the second layer. Even greater sensitivity can be attained by using a third layer. Thus, in the example quoted of antibodies to parietal cells, we could treat the stomach section sequentially with the following: patient's serum containing antibodies to parietal cells, then a rabbit anti-human IgG, and finally a fluorescein-conjugated goat anti-rabbit IgG. However, as with most immunological techniques as *sensitivity* is increased, *specificity* becomes progressively reduced and careful controls are essential.

Applications of the indirect test may be seen in figure 5.25a and in Chapter 14 (e.g. figure, 14.2, p. 307).

3. Sandwich test

This is a double-layer procedure designed to visualize specific antibody. If, for example, we wished to see how many cells in a preparation of lymphoid tissue were synthesizing antibody to pneumococcus polysaccharide, we would first fix the cells with ethanol to prevent the antibody being washed away during the test, and then treat with a solution of the polysaccharide antigen. After washing, a fluorescein-labelled antibody to the polysaccharide would then be added to locate those cells which had specifically bound the antigen (figure 5.24c). The name of the test derives from the fact that antigen is sandwiched between the antibody present in the cell substrate and that added as the second layer.

Reaction with cell surface antigens

Surface antigens can be detected and localized by the use of labelled antibodies. Because antibodies cannot readily penetrate living cells except by endocytosis, treatment of cells with labelled antibody in

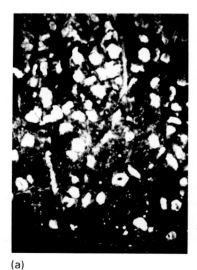
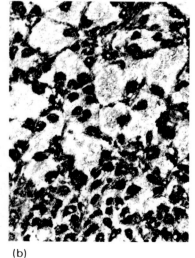

(a)　　　　　　　　　　(b)

Figure 5.25. *Staining of gastric parietal cells by (a) fluorescein and (b) peroxidase-linked antibody. The sections were sequentially treated with human parietal cell autoantibodies and then with the conjugated rabbit anti-human IgG. The enzyme was visualized by the peroxidase reaction. (Courtesy of Miss V. Petts.)*

the cold (to minimize endocytosis) leads to staining only of antigens on the surface. We have previously seen the example of fluorescent staining of the surface of B-lymphocytes with anti-immunoglobulin, and figure 2.6f in Chapter 2 shows the distribution of antigens on the surface of viable human thyroid cells demonstrated with thyroid autoantibodies by the indirect test.

A close look at these examples reveals the patchy distribution of these surface antigens seen when they are visualized with conventional divalent antibodies. However, when B-cells are stained directly with a fluorescein-tagged *uni*valent Fab anti-immunoglobulin, the resulting fluorescence is seen as a smooth ring. This implies that the patchy fluorescence is the result of micro-agglutination through cross-linking of the antigens and, further, that the antigens are freely mobile in the plane of the surface membrane; this becomes quite striking as the cells are warmed up to 37°C when the patches coalesce into caps at one pole of the cell (figure 2.6f) before being taken into the cytoplasm by endocytosis. In fact, after combination with antibody, many antigens are removed from the cell surface either through capping and endocytosis, or shedding into the extracellular medium as complexes. This 'stripping' process may have deleterious consequences for the host if it makes virally infected cells or tumours refractory to immunological attack.

Measurement of cell surface fluorescence by flow cytofluorography

The amount of fluorescent antibody bound to each cell can be quantified by a technique known as flow cytofluorography. Suppose we have stained a subpopulation of lymphocytes with a specific antibody; it is now possible to make the cells flow obediently in a single stream past a laser beam. A light detector at right angles to the beam can be used to record the strength of the fluorescent signal while another detector gives information about cell size by forward light scatter (figure 5.26). An example of the quantitative data which can be generated by these machines is given in figure 5.27.

In a recent extension of this technique, cells lightly fixed with glutaraldehyde become permeable to antibody so that intracellular antigens can be picked out by fluorescent antibodies. With the advent of 3-colour fluorescence, a combination of three different cell surface and/or intracellular antigens can now be looked at in each individual cell.

Other labelled antibody methods

In place of fluorescent markers, other workers have evolved methods in which enzymes such as peroxidase or phosphatase are coupled to antibodies and these can be visualized by conventional histo-

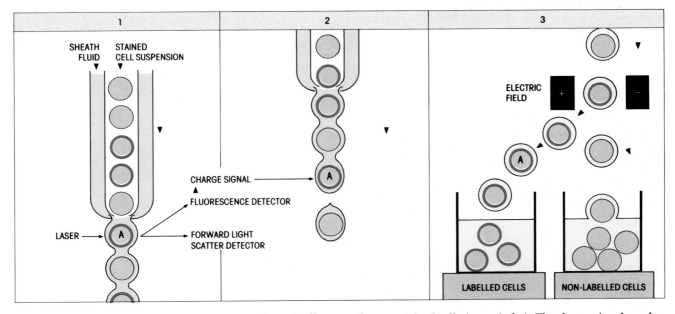

Figure 5.26. *The principle of the fluorescence activated cell sorter (FACS), designed by the Herzenbergs and colleagues, for flow cytofluorographic measurement of the fluorescence on stained cells (green rimmed circles) and physical separation from unstained cells (grey circles). The charge signal can be activated to separate cells of high from low fluorescence or of large from small size.*

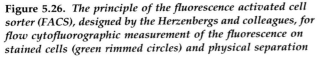

ANTIGEN RECOGNITION — DETECTION AND APPLICATION

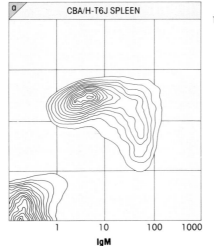

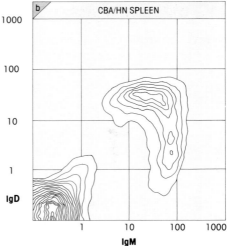

Figure 5.27. *Flow cytofluorographic analysis in a fluorescence activated cell sorter (FACS) of spleen cells from (a) CBA/J and (b) CBA/N mice stained with both fluorescein-labelled anti-IgM and Texas Red conjugated anti-IgD. The axes represent relative fluorescence while the contours give an indication of cell numbers. The CBA/N strain which is defective in its response to type II thymus independent antigens like pneumococcus polysaccharide (cf. p. 120) lacks the population with low surface IgM and high IgD seen in the normally responding strain CBA/J (Parks D.R., Hardy R.R. & Herzenberg L.A. (1983) Immunol. Today 4, 145). Since Texas*

Red is excited at a different wavelength from fluorescein, the FACS had to be fitted with two lasers to acquire this data; with the advent of newer dyes such as the algal photosynthetic pigment, phycoerythrin, which have fluorescence emission peaks well separated from fluorescein yet can be excited at the same wavelength, comparable results can be obtained with a single laser. Light scatter measurements in the FACS also provide information on cell size and viability which allows discrimination against dead cells and analysis of fluorescence in relation to cell size.

chemical methods at both light microscope (figure 5.25b) and electron microscope (figure 5.28) level.

Ferritin antibody conjugates and colloidal gold bound to antibody (figure 5.29) have been widely used as electron-dense immunolabels by electron-microscopists. A new ultra small probe consisting of Fab' fragments linked to undecagold clusters allows more accurate spatial localization of antigens

and its small size enables it to mark sites which are inaccessible to the larger immunolabels. However, clear visualization requires a high resolution scanning transmission E.M.

Localization in tissues of a gene product

To get more feel for the way immunology interacts

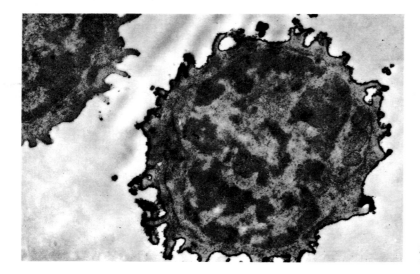

Figure 5.28. *Electron microscopic visualization of human IgG on the surface of a B-lymphocyte by treatment of viable cell suspensions with peroxidase-coupled anti-IgG. Note the adjacent unstained lymphocyte. (Courtesy of Miss V. Petts.)*

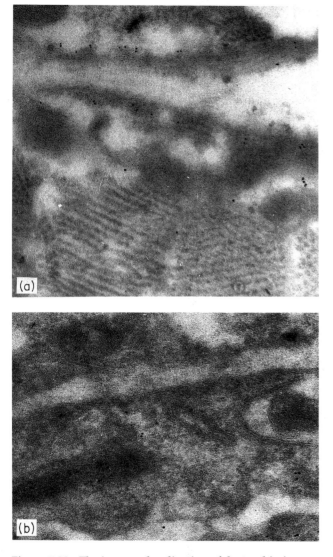

with other disciplines, it is instructive to follow the trail leading from the identification of a gene defect in Duchenne muscular dystrophy to the localization of the gene product within muscle tissue. The normal gene, which encodes the protein dystrophin, was sequenced and using either a peptide corre-

sponding with part of this sequence, or a fusion protein produced when this gene was expressed in bacteria, rabbit antisera were raised and purified. Immunofluorescence showed binding of the antibodies to the surface membrane of intact human and mouse skeletal muscle. Excellent controls were provided by muscle from Duchenne patients and *mdx* mice (a model for Duchenne), neither of which express dystrophin. E.M. studies with immunogold pin-pointed the anatomical location of the antigen even more closely and showed convincingly that the major distribution of dystrophin was on the cytoplasmic face of the plasma membrane of muscle fibres (figure 5.29).

Cell separation techniques

Certain useful gross separations of immunological cells can be achieved by physical means. Adherence to plastic surfaces largely removes phagocytic cells while passage down nylon-wool columns greatly enriches lymphocyte populations for T- at the expense of B-cells. Lymphocyte preparations are customarily made by centrifugation over a Ficoll density step which separates them from other peripheral blood white cells of higher buoyant density.

However, the development of a wide range of monoclonal antibodies directed to specific differentiation antigens on the surface of different cellular subpopulations can be exploited by a variety of techniques to achieve more effective fractionation (summarized in figure 5.30).

We have already looked at the manner in which cells stained by fluorescent antibodies can be analysed one at a time in a flow cytofluorimeter. After flowing past the laser, the liquid stream is broken up into droplets each containing a single cell and if one wishes to separate the stained cell population, the droplet containing a cell giving a fluorescent signal is charged and deviated from the stream by an electric field into a suitable collector—hence the name *fluorescence activated cell sorter* (FACS; cf. figure 5.26). An experiment in which cells were sorted on the basis of surface immunoglobulin in one of these elegant but expensive machines is documented in figure 5.31.

Cells bearing antibody can also be selected by *panning* to dishes coated with an anti-immunoglobulin (figure 5.30). Alternatively, they can form *rosettes* with anti-immunoglobulin-coated erythrocytes and these can readily be separated from unrosetted cells by centrifugation. Antibody-coated

Figure 5.29. *The immuno-localization of dystrophin in normal and* **mdx** *mouse skeletal muscle.* **mdx** *mice are a model for human Duchene muscular dystrophy and both have a defective gene encoding dystrophin. Gold particles (5 nm) indicating the location of dystrophin immune complexes are seen along the plasma membrane (open arrows) of the normal mouse myofibres (a), but not the* **mdx** *plasma membrane (b). MF, myofibre; END, endothelial cell. (Reproduced from Watkins S.C., Hoffman E.P., Slayter H.S. & Kunkel L.M. (1988)* **Nature**, *333, 863, with kind permission of the authors and* **Nature**.)

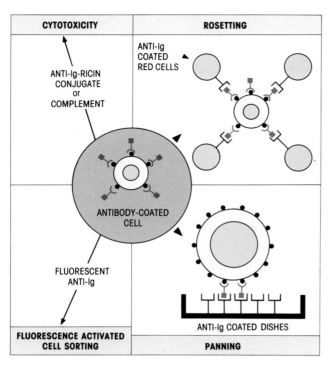

Figure 5.30. *Major methods for separating cells coated with a specific antibody.*

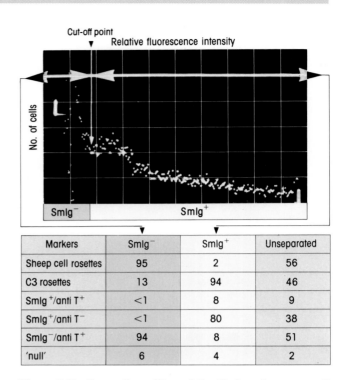

Markers	SmIg$^-$	SmIg$^+$	Unseparated
Sheep cell rosettes	95	2	56
C3 rosettes	13	94	46
SmIg$^+$/anti T$^+$	<1	8	9
SmIg$^+$/anti T$^-$	<1	80	38
SmIg$^-$/anti T$^+$	94	8	51
'null'	6	4	2

Figure 5.31. *Separation of B- and T-cells from human tonsil lymphocytes by the fluorescence activated cell sorter. After staining with fluorescein-conjugated anti-Ig, the viable cells were analysed by flow cytofluorimetry to give the histogram shown. The lymphocytes were separated into a surface membrane Ig positive (SmIg$^+$) and a negative (SmIg$^-$) population depending upon the fluorescence intensity being either above or below the arbitrary cut-off point. Analysis of the % of cells positive for each marker is shown. 'Null' cells were negative with both anti-Ig and anti-T reagents. (Data kindly provided by Dr M.F. Greaves.)*

cells can also readily be separated by cluster formation with anti-immunoglobulin bearing magnetic particles. Such techniques have frequently been employed to fractionate CD4 (helper) from CD8 (cytotoxic/suppressor) human lymphocytes (cf. table 6.3) or the corresponding L3T4 and Ly2 mouse populations.

Sometimes one wishes to deplete certain populations such as mature T-lymphocytes in bone marrow cell suspension to limit graft-versus-host reactions (cf. p. 279). For this, cells labelled with anti-T can be killed by addition of complement or of an antibody conjugated to a highly toxic molecule such as ricin-A chain (figure 5.30).

Neutralization of biological activity

To continue our discussion on the interaction of antigen and antibody we may focus attention on a number of biological reactions which can be inhibited by addition of specific antibody. Thus the agglutination of red cells by interaction of influenza virus with receptors on the erythrocyte surface can be blocked by anti-viral antibodies and this forms the basis for their serological detection. Neutralization of the growth of hapten-conjugated bacterio-

phage provides an exquisitely sensitive assay for anti-hapten antibodies. A test for antibodies to salmonella H antigen present on the flagella depends upon their ability to inhibit the motility of the bacteria *in vitro*. Likewise, mycoplasma antibodies can be demonstrated by their inhibitory effect on the metabolism of the organisms in culture. The successful treatment of cases of drug overdose with the Fab fragment of specific antibodies has been described and may become a practical proposition if a range of hybridomas can be assembled. Antibodies to hormones such as insulin and thyroid stimulating hormone (TSH), or to cytokines, can be used to probe the specificity of biological reactions *in vitro*; for example, the specificity of the insulin-like activity of a serum sample on rat epididymal fat pad can be checked by the neutralizing effect of an antiserum. Such antibodies can be effective *in vivo* and, as part of the world-wide effort to prevent disastrous over-population, attempts are in progress to immunize against chorionic gonadotropin using fragments of the β chain coupled to appropriate carriers, since this hormone is needed to sustain the implanted ovum.

SUMMARY

The formation of single bands of precipitate when antigen and antibody react in gels can be used qualitatively to study the number of reacting components and the immunological relationship between different antigens (Ouchterlony double-diffusion system) and the electrophoretic mobility of the antigens (immunoelectrophoresis). Quantitative measurement of antigen concentration is made by single radial immunodiffusion, 'rocket' electrophoresis and two-dimensional electrophoresis. Laser nephelometry provides a sensitive method for the quantification of antigens in solution.

Antibodies can also be detected by macroscopic agglutination of particles coated with antigen. Insoluble immunoabsorbents prepared by coupling antibody to Sepharose can be used to affinity-purify antigens from complex mixtures and reciprocally to purify antibodies.

Many immunoassay techniques which exploit the mutual interaction of antigens and antibodies using labelled reagents have been devised. Labels include radioactivity, enzymes and fluorescent probes. In soluble phase systems, antibody can be estimated by addition of excess labelled antigen followed by precipitation of the complex. Radioimmunoassay of antigen is a form of saturation analysis in which the test material competes with labelled antigen for a limited amount of antibody, the amount of label displaced being a measure of the antigen in the test sample. Immunoradiometric tests involve the binding of antigen to solid phase antibody and of antibody to solid phase antigen followed by estimation of ligand by excess of an appropriate labelled antibody. The 'ambient analyte' principle allows assays to be carried out on microspots of the captive reagent. Antigens in mixtures can be identified by 'immunoblotting'.

The localization of antigens in tissues, within cells or on the cell surface can be achieved microscopically using antibodies tagged with fluorescent dyes or enzymes such as peroxidase whose reaction product can be readily visualized. In the direct test, the labelled antibody is applied directly to the tissue; in the indirect test the label is conjugated to an anti-Ig used as a second amplifying antibody. Fluorescent antibody bound to the surface of single cells, e.g. lymphocytes, can be quantified by flow cytofluorography. For ultrastructural studies, antibodies may be tagged with peroxidase or colloidal gold.

Cells labelled on their surface by a specific antibody can be selectively fractionated by the fluorescence activated cell sorter, by panning or rosette formation, or killed by complement-mediated cytotoxicity or by an anti-immunoglobulin conjugated to a toxin.

Antigens with biological activity, e.g. bacterial toxins or hormones such as human chorionic gonadotropin, may be neutralized *in vivo* by antibody.

103

Further reading

Beverley P.C.L. (ed.) (1986) Monoclonal antibodies. *Methods in Hematology*, **13**. Churchill Livingstone, Edinburgh, UK.

Edwards R. (1985) *Immunoassay: an Introduction*. Heinemann Medical Books, London.

Harlo E. & Lane D. (eds) (1988) *Antibodies: a laboratory manual*. Cold Spring Harbor Laboratory. (An excellent laboratory manual on how to make and use antibodies.)

Hudson L. & Hay, F.C. (1989) *Practical Immunology*, 3rd edn. Blackwell Scientific Publications, Oxford. (Extremely valuable for those carrying out immunological techniques.)

Johnstone A. (ed.) (1989) Immunological techniques. *Current Opinion in Immunology*, **1**, 927.

Larsson L-I. (1988) *Immunochemistry: theory and practice*. C.R.C. Press. (A detailed practical manual not necessarily suitable for beginners but rather expensive.)

De Lellis R.A. (ed.) (1989) *Advances in immunohistochemistry*. Raven Press. (A well-written multi-author volume.)

Pretlow II T.G. & Pretlow T.P. (1987) *Cell separation: methods and selected applications*, **5**. Academic Press.

Weir D.M. (ed.) (1986) *Handbook of Experimental Immunology*, **1—4**, 4th edn. Blackwell Scientific Publications, Oxford.

THE ACQUIRED IMMUNE RESPONSE

I – Consequences of Antigen Recognition

WHERE DOES IT ALL HAPPEN? — THE ANATOMY OF THE IMMUNE RESPONSE

For an effective immune response an intricate series of cellular events must occur. Antigen must bind and if necessary be processed by antigen-presenting cells which must then make contact with and activate T- and B-cells; T-helpers must assist certain B-cells and cytotoxic T-cell precursors and there have to be mechanisms which amplify the numbers of potential effector cells by proliferation and then bring about differentiation to generate the mediators of humoral and cellular immunity. In addition, memory cells for secondary responses must be formed and the whole response controlled so that it is adequate but not excessive and is appropriate to the type of infection being dealt with. By working hard, we can isolate component cells of the immune system and persuade them to carry out a number of responses to antigen in the test tube, but compared with the efficacy of the overall development of immunity in the body, our efforts still leave much to be desired. *In vivo* the integration of the complex cellular interactions which form the basis of the immune response takes place within the organized architecture of peripheral, or secondary, lymphoid tissue which includes the lymph glands, spleen and unencapsulated tissue lining the respiratory, alimentary and genito-urinary tracts.

These tissues become populated by cells of reticular origin and by macrophages and lymphocytes derived from bone marrow stem cells, the T-cells first differentiating into immunocompetent cells by a high pressure training period in the thymus, the B-cells undergoing their education in the bone marrow itself (figure 6.1). In essence, the lymph nodes filter off and if necessary respond to foreign material draining body tissues, the spleen monitors the blood and the unencapsulated lymphoid tissue is strategically integrated into mucosal surfaces of the body as a forward defensive system based on IgA secretion.

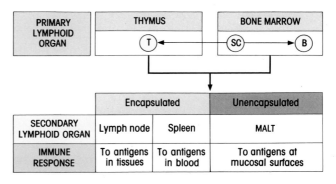

Figure 6.1. *The functional organization of lymphoid tissue. Stem cells (SC) arising in the bone marrow differentiate into immunocompetent T- and B-cells in the primary lymphoid organs and then colonize the secondary lymphoid tissues where immune responses are organized. The mucosal-associated lymphoid tissue which produces the antibodies for mucosal secretions is often referred to as the MALT system.*

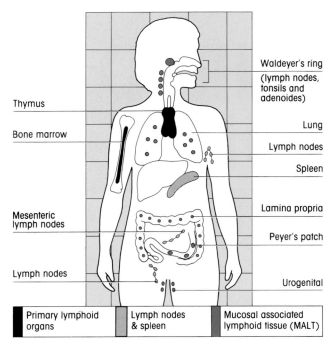

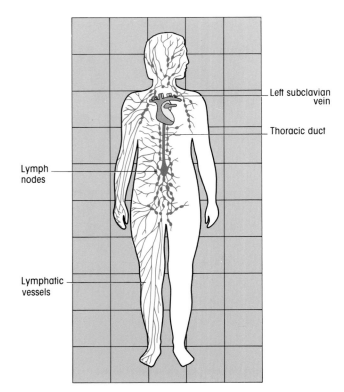

Thymus

Bone marrow

Mesenteric
lymph nodes

Lymph nodes

Waldeyer's ring
(lymph nodes,
tonsils and
adenoides)

Lung

Lymph nodes

Spleen

Lamina propria

Peyer's patch

Urogenital

| Primary lymphoid organs | Lymph nodes & spleen | Mucosal associated lymphoid tissue (MALT) |

Fig. 6.2. *The distribution of major lymphoid organs and tissues throughout the body.*

Left subclavian vein

Thoracic duct

Lymph nodes

Lymphatic vessels

Fig. 6.3. *The network of lymph nodes and lymphatics. Lymph nodes occur at junctions of the draining lymphatics. The lymph finally collects in the thoracic duct and thence returns to the bloodstream via the left subclavian vein.*

The anatomical disposition of these lymphoid tissues is illustrated in figure 6.2. The lymphatics and associated lymph nodes form an impressive network draining the viscera and the more superficial body structures before returning to the blood by way of the thoracic duct (figure 6.3).

Communication between these tissues and the rest of the body is maintained by a pool of recirculating lymphocytes which pass from the blood into the lymph nodes, spleen and other tissues and back to the blood by the major lymphatic channels such as the thoracic duct (figures 6.4 and 6.8).

Lymphocytes traffic between lymphoid tissues

This traffic of lymphocytes between the tissues, the bloodstream and the lymph glands enables antigen-sensitive cells to seek the antigen and to be recruited to sites at which a response is occurring, while the dissemination of memory cells and their progeny enables a more widespread response to be organized throughout the lymphoid system. Thus, antigen-reactive cells are depleted from the circulating pool of lymphocytes within 24 hours of antigen first localizing in the lymph nodes or spleen; several days later, after proliferation at the site of antigen

localization, a peak of activated cells appears in the thoracic duct. When antigen reaches a node in a primed animal, there is a dramatic fall in the output of cells in the efferent lymphatics, a phenomenon described variously as 'cell shutdown' or 'lymphocyte trapping' and which probably results from the antigen-induced release of a T-cell soluble factor (cf. the lymphokines, p. 28); this is followed by an output of activated blast cells which peaks at around 80 hours.

Lymphocytes enter a lymph node through the afferent lymphatics and by passage across the specialized high-walled endothelium of the post-capillary venules (HEV) (cf. figure 6.4). They are guided to the HEV by interaction between their homing receptors and complementary binding proteins, known as vascular addressins, on the surface of the endothelial cells (figure 6.4b). The lymphocyte homing receptor, recognized by the monoclonal antibody (MEL-14 in the mouse and Leu-8 in the human), is polyubiquitinated and has a characteristic 'mongrel' structure indicative of a mixed ancestry; adjacent to the cytoplasm are repeating

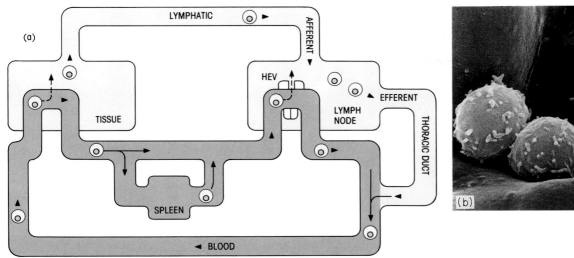

Figure 6.4. *Traffic and recirculation of lymphocytes through encapsulated lymphoid tissue. (a) Blood-borne lymphocytes enter the tissues and lymph nodes passing through the high-walled endothelium of the post-capillary venules (HEV) and leave via the draining lymphatics. The efferent lymphatics finally emerging from the last node in each chain join to form the thoracic duct which returns the lymphocytes to the bloodstream. In the spleen, lymphocytes enter the lymphoid area (white pulp) from the arterioles, pass to the sinusoids of the erythroid area (red pulp) and leave by the splenic vein. (b) Lymphocytes adhering to HEV (scanning electron micrograph kindly provided by Dr W. van Ewijk).*

structures homologous with complement-binding proteins (cf. p. 18), next there is a sequence similar to that of epidermal growth factor, and finally the N terminal portion has a lectin-like configuration capable of binding firmly to a phosphomannosyl oligosaccharide grouping within the HEV addressin. As a consequence of this binding to the HEV, the lymphocyte elbows its way either between or through the endothelial cells, across the basement membrane and into the substance of the lymph node itself.

This homing interaction can be recreated *in vitro* by the adherence of lymphocytes to the HEV of thin lymph node sections or to supported artificial membranes incorporating purified vascular addressin molecules. This technical breakthrough has made it possible to make much faster progress in the analysis of the homing phenomenon. Thus adherence of lymphocytes to HEV can be blocked by the monoclonal MEL-14, or by addition of a mannose-6-phosphate rich polysaccharide, or by hydrolysis of terminal sialic acid residues on the HEV. Of considerable physiological significance is the finding of a quite distinct vascular addressin on Peyer's patch HEV and on other elements of the mucosal associated lymphoid tissue (MALT). This MALT-specific binding molecule encourages lymphocytes with the MALT homing receptor (CDw 44; table 6.1, p. 116) to circulate within and between the

collections of lymphoid tissue guarding the external body surfaces; thus lymphocytes, such as those programmed to manufacture dimeric IgA destined for secretion, will not waste time cooling their heels in encapsulated peripheral lymph nodes which play no role in mucosal protection.

Further homing systems allow leucocytes to localize at sites of inflammation, undoubtedly a useful activity. The reader will recall the upregulation of the neutrophil binding molecule ELAM-1 on endothelial cells by the cytokines TNF and IL-1 (p. 142) while vascular addressins for lymphocytes make an appearance under the influence of T-cell lymphokines like IFNγ. LFA-1/ICAM-1 interactions (cf. p. 119) only add some intercellular stickiness without providing the specificity of the homing receptors which shunt the circulating lymphocytes into their 'correct' compartment. Rumour has it that we may expect the future to reveal there to be a family of these homing molecules to guide lymphocytes through the labyrinth of organized lymphoid tissue.

Lymph node

The encapsulated tissue of the lymph node contains a meshwork of reticular cells and their fibres organized into sinuses. These act as a filter for lymph draining the body tissues and possibly bearing

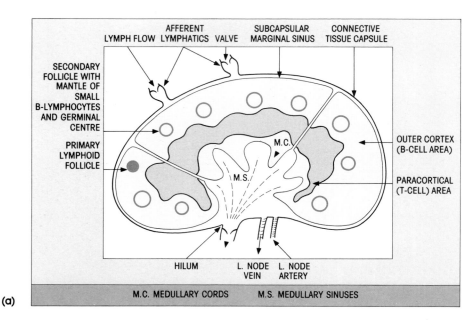

AFFERENT
LYMPH FLOW LYMPHATICS VALVE   SUBCAPSULAR   CONNECTIVE
MARGINAL SINUS   TISSUE CAPSULE

SECONDARY
FOLLICLE WITH
MANTLE OF
SMALL
B-LYMPHOCYTES
AND GERMINAL
CENTRE

PRIMARY
LYMPHOID
FOLLICLE

M.C.

OUTER CORTEX
(B-CELL AREA)

M.S.

PARACORTICAL
(T-CELL) AREA

HILUM   L. NODE   L. NODE
VEIN   ARTERY

(a)

M.C. MEDULLARY CORDS   M.S. MEDULLARY SINUSES

Figure 6.5. Above and facing page. *Lymph node.*
(a) Diagrammatic representation. (b) Human lymph node, low
power view. (c) Secondary lymphoid follicle showing
germinal centre surrounded by a mantle of small
B-lymphocytes stained by anti-human IgD labelled with
horse-radish peroxidase (brown colour). There are few IgD
positive cells in the centre but both areas contain IgM
positive B-lymphocytes. (d) Medulla stained with methyl
green pyronin to show the basophilic (pink) cytoplasm of the
plasma cells with their abundant ribosomes. (e) Medullary
sinus of lymph node draining site of lithium carmine injection
showing macrophages which have phagocytosed the colloidal
dye. (f) Node from mouse immunized with the thymus-
independent antigen, pneumococcus polysaccharide SIII,
revealing prominent stimulation of secondary follicles with
germinal centres. (g) Methyl green pyronin stain of lymph

node draining site of skin painted with the contact sensitizer
oxazolone, highlighting the generalized expansion and
activation of the paracortical (T-cell), the T-blasts being
strongly basophilic. (h) The same study in a neonatally
thymectomized mouse shows a lonely primary nodule
(follicle) with complete lack of cellular response in the
paracortical area.

SS, subcapsular sinus; PN, primary nodule; SF, secondary
follicle; LM, lymphocyte mantle of SF; GC, germinal centre;
PA, paracortical area; MC, medullary cords; MS, medullary
sinus; PC, plasma cell; SM, sinusoidal macrophage. ((b)
photographed by Dr P.M. Lydyard, (c) and (d) photographed
by Dr K.A. MacLennan, (e) courtesy of Anatomy Dept.,
Middlesex Hospital Medical School, (f), (g) and (h) courtesy
of Dr M. de Sousa and Prof. D.M.V. Parrott.)

foreign antigens which enters the subcapsular sinus by the afferent vessels and diffuses past the lymphocytes in the cortex to reach the macrophages of the medullary sinuses (figure 6.5) and thence the efferent lymphatics (figures 6.4 and 6.5). What is so striking about the organization of the lymph node is that the T- and B-lymphocytes are very largely separated into different anatomical compartments.

B-cell areas

The follicular aggregations of B-lymphocytes are a prominent feature of the outer cortex. In the unstimulated node they are present as spherical collections of cells termed *primary nodules* (figure 6.5h) but after antigenic challenge they form *secondary follicles* (figure 6.5c) which consist of a corona or mantle of concentrically packed, resting small B-

lymphocytes possessing both IgM and IgD on their surface surrounding a pale-staining *germinal centre*. This contains large, usually proliferating, B-blasts, a minority of T-cells, scattered conventional reticular macrophages containing 'tingible bodies' of phago-cytosed lymphocytes, and a tight network of specialized follicular dendritic cells with elongated cytoplasmic processes and few, if any, lysosomes. Germinal centres are greatly enlarged in secondary antibody responses and they are regarded as important sites of B-cell maturation and the generation of B-cell memory. Following antigenic stimulation, the B-cells divide with a short cycle time, many die and are taken up by macrophages. Differentiating plasmablasts appear and migrate to become plasma cells in the medullary cords of lymphoid cells which project between the medullary sinuses (figure 6.5d). This maturation of antibody-forming cells at a site

108

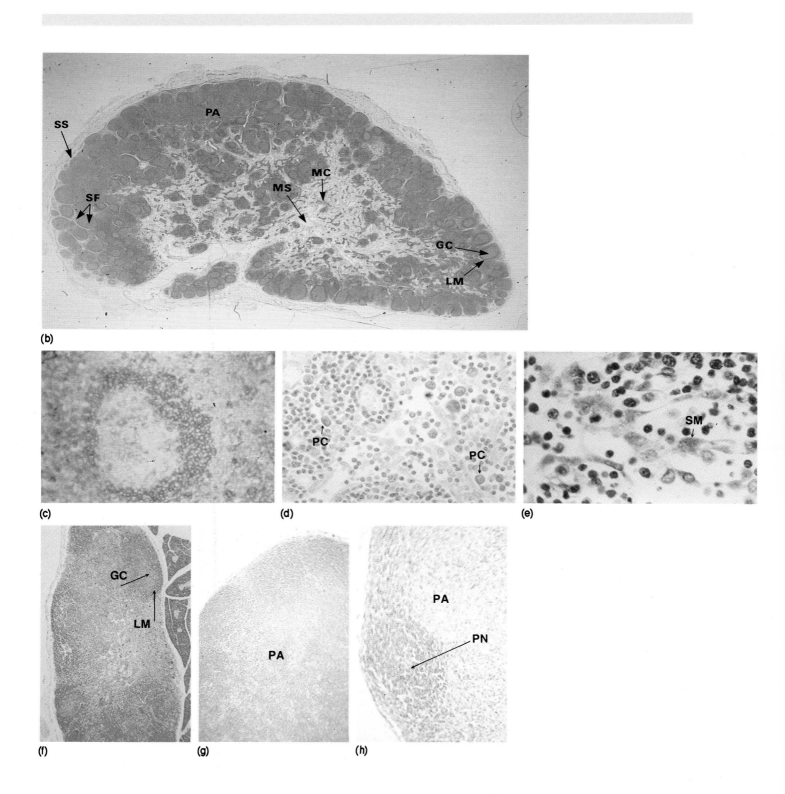

(b)

(c)

(d)

(e)

(f)

(g)

(h)

distant from that at which antigen triggering has occurred is also seen in the spleen where plasma cells are found predominantly in the marginal zone. My guess is that this movement of cells acts to prevent the generation of high local concentrations of antibody within the germinal centre so avoiding neutralization of the antigen on the follicular dendritic cells and premature shutting off of the immune response.

The remainder of the outer cortex is also essentially a B-cell area with scattered T-cells.

T-cell areas

T-cells are mainly confined to a region referred to as the paracortical (or thymus-dependent) area (figure 6.5a); in nodes taken from children with selective T-cell deficiency (figure 11.14) or neonatally thymectomized mice (figure 6.5h), the paracortical region is seen to be virtually devoid of lymphocytes. Furthermore, when a T-cell mediated response is elicited in a normal animal, say by a skin graft or by painting chemicals such as picryl chloride on the skin to induce contact hypersensitivity, there is a marked proliferation of cells in the thymus-dependent area and typical lymphoblasts are evident (figure 6.5g). In contrast, stimulation of antibody formation by the thymus-independent antigen, pneumococcus polysaccharide SIII, leads to proliferation in the cortical lymphoid follicles with development of germinal centres while the paracortical region remains inactive, reflecting the inability to develop cellular hypersensitivity to the polysaccharide (figure 6.5f). As expected, nodes taken from children with congenital hypogamma-globulinaemia associated with failure of B-cell development conspicuously lack primary and secondary follicules.

Spleen

On a fresh section of spleen, the lymphoid tissue forming the white pulp is seen as circular or elongated grey areas within the erythrocyte-filled red pulp consisting of splenic cords lined with macrophages and venous sinusoids. As in the lymph node, T- and B-cell areas are segregated (figure 6.6). The spleen is a very effective blood filter removing effete red and white cells and responding actively to blood-borne antigens, the more so if particulate. Plasmablasts and mature plasma cells are present in the marginal zone extending into the red pulp.

Mucosal-associated lymphoid tissue

The respiratory, alimentary and genito-urinary tracts are guarded immunologically by subepithelial accumulations of lymphoid tissue which are not constrained by a connective tissue capsule (figure 6.7). These may occur as diffuse collections of lymphocytes, plasma cells and phagocytes throughout the lung and the lamina propria of the intestinal wall (figure 6.7a and b) or as more clearly organized tissue with well-formed follicles. In man, the latter includes the lingual, palatine and pharyngeal tonsils (figure 6.7c) the small intestinal Peyer's patches (figure 6.7d) and the appendix. It is generally agreed that this mucosal-associated lymphoid tissue (MALT) forms a separate interconnected secretory system within which cells committed to IgA or IgE synthesis may circulate.

In the gut, antigen enters the Peyer's patches (figure 6.7d) across specialized epithelial cells and stimulates the antigen-sensitive lymphocytes; after activation these drain into the lymph and after a journey through the mesenteric lymph nodes and the thoracic duct, they pass from the bloodstream

Facing page

Figure 6.6. *Spleen. (a) Diagrammatic representation. (b) Low power view showing lymphoid white pulp (WP) and red pulp (RP). (c) High power view of secondary follicle (SF) with germinal centre (GC) surrounded by periarteriolar (T-cell) lymphoid tissue, showing arteriole (A), marginal zone (MZ) and red pulp (RP). (d) Localization of the thymus-independent antigen, ficoll, on the marginal zone macrophages. The ficoll is* visualized by labelling with the red flourescent dye tetramethyl-rhodamine. (e) Preferential localization of a thymus-dependent antigen (conjugated to green fluorescein) on the follicular dendritic cells (ignore orange fluorescence). ((b) photographed by Dr P.M. Lydyard, (c) by Dr K.A. MacLennan, (d) and (e) kindly provided by Prof. J.H. Humphrey.)*

110

CHAPTER 6

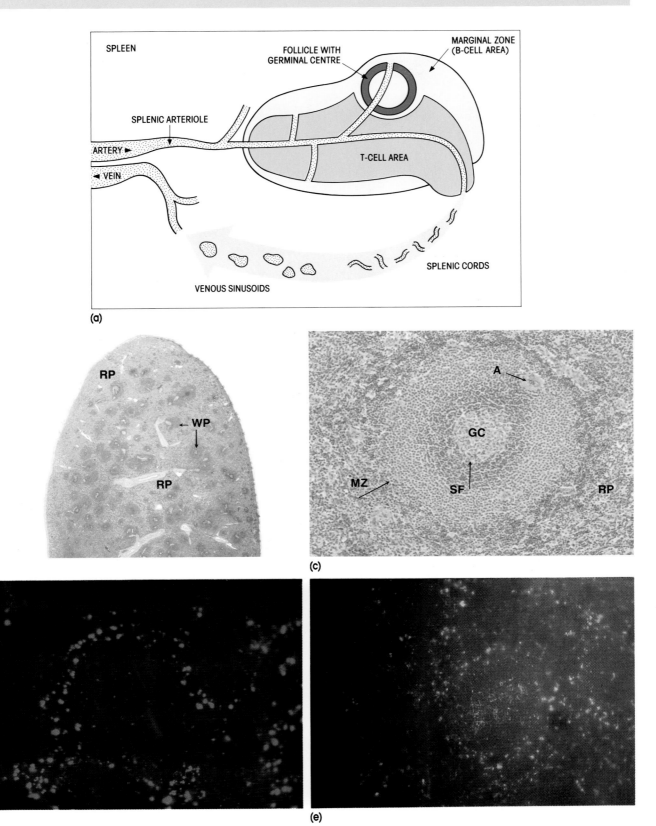

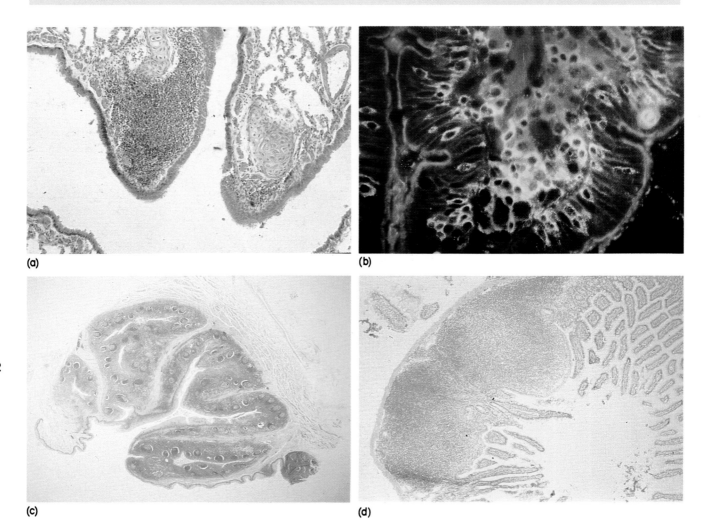

(a)

(b)

(c)

(d)

Figure 6.7. *The IgA secretory immune system (MALT). (a) Section of lung showing a diffuse accumulation of lymphocytes (Ly) in the bronchial wall. (b) Section of human jejunum showing lymphoid cells (Ly) stained green by a fluorescent anti-leucocyte monoclonal antibody, in the mucosal epithelium (ME) and in the lamina propria (LP). A red flourescent anti-IgA conjugate stains the cytoplasm of plasma cells (PC) in the lamina propria and detects IgA in the surface mucus, altogether a super picture! (c) Low power view of human tonsil showing the MALT with numerous secondary follicles (SF) containing germinal centres. (d) Peyer's patches (PP) in mouse ileum. The T-cell areas are stained brown by a peroxidase-labelled monoclonal antibody to Thy 1. ((a) was kindly provided by Dr P. Lydyard, (b) by Prof. G. Jannosy, (c) by Mr C. Symes and (d) by courtesy of Dr E. Andrew.)*

into the lamina propria (figure 6.8) where they become IgA-forming cells which, because they are now widely distributed, protect a wide area of the bowel with protective antibody. The cells also appear in the lymphoid tissue of the lung and in other mucosal sites presumably guided by the interactions of specific homing receptors with appropriate HEV addressins as discussed earlier.

In the mouse, but apparently not so in man, intra-epithelial lymphocytes are predominantly T-cells with the γδ (TCR1) receptor. Since a number of cloned γδ-T-cells have been found to have specificity for heat shock proteins, which are widely distributed in nature and usually highly immunogenic, it has been postulated that they act as a relatively primitive first line of defence at the outer surfaces of the body.

Bone marrow can be a major site of antibody synthesis

A few days after a secondary response, activated memory B-cells can be shown to migrate to the

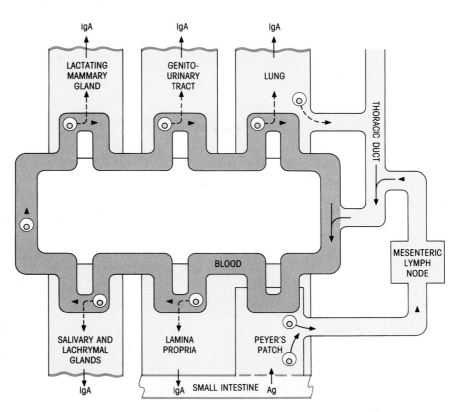

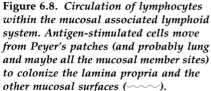

Figure 6.8. *Circulation of lymphocytes within the mucosal associated lymphoid system. Antigen-stimulated cells move from Peyer's patches (and probably lung and maybe all the mucosal member sites) to colonize the lamina propria and the other mucosal surfaces (*〜〜〜*).*

bone marrow where they mature into plasma cells. Bone marrow is a much neglected site of antibody synthesis which proves to be a major source of serum Ig, contributing up to 80% of the total Ig-secreting cells in the 100-week-old mouse. The peripheral lymphoid tissue responds rapidly to antigen, but only for a relatively short time, whereas bone marrow starts slowly and gives a long-lasting massive production of antibody to antigens which repeatedly challenge the host.

The handling of antigen

Where does antigen go when it enters the body? If it penetrates the tissues it will tend to finish up in the draining lymph nodes. Antigens which are encountered in the upper respiratory tract or intestine are trapped by local mucosal-associated lymphoid tissue, whereas antigen in the blood provokes a reaction in the spleen. Macrophages in the liver and lung will filter blood-borne antigens and degrade them without producing an immune response since they are not strategically placed with respect to lymphoid tissue.

Macrophages are general antigen-presenting cells

'Classically', it has always been recognized that antigens draining into lymphoid tissue are taken up by macrophages. They are then partially, if not completely, broken down in the lysosomes; some may escape from the cell in a soluble form to be taken up by other antigen-presenting cells and a fraction may reappear at the surface either as a large fragment or as a processed peptide associated with class II major histocompatibility molecules. Although resting resident macrophages do not express MHC class II, antigens are usually encountered in the context of a microbial infectious agent which can induce the expression of class II by its adjuvant-like properties expressed through molecules such as bacterial lipopolysaccharide (LPS). There is general agreement that the antigen-presenting cell must bear antigen on its surface for effective activation of lymphocytes and we have ample evidence that antigen-pulsed macrophages can stimulate specific T- and B-cells both *in vitro* (e.g. figure 4.14, p. 76) and when injected back *in vivo*. Some antigens, such as polymeric carbohydrates like ficoll, cannot be degraded because the macrophages lack the enzymes required; in these instances, specialized macrophages in the marginal zone of the spleen or the lymph node subcapsular sinus, trap and present the antigen to B-cells directly, apparently without any processing or intervention from T-cells (figure 6.6d).

Follicular dendritic cells stimulate B-cells in germinal centres

Secondary antibody responses can be boosted by quite small amounts of immunogen which complex with circulating antibody and fix C3 so that they localize very effectively on the surface of the follicular dendritic cells within the germinal centres of secondary follicles (figure 6.6e). These cells have very elongated processes which can make contact with numerous lymphocytes and their surface receptors for IgG Fc, and iC3b enable them to trap the complexed antigen very efficiently and hold the antigen on their surface for extended periods, in keeping with the memory function of secondary follicles. Evidence for this notion may be derived from animals effectively depleted of complement by injection of cobra venom factor which contains the reptilian equivalent of C3b. This fires the alternative pathway by forming a complex with factor B but because of its insensitivity to the mammalian C3b inactivator, it persists long enough to discharge the feedback loop to exhaustion and deplete C3 completely. Such mice can neither localize antigen—antibody complexes on their follicular dendritic cells, nor generate B-memory cells in response to T-dependent antigens (see p. 120).

One to three days after secondary challenge, the filamentous dendrites on the follicular cells to which the immune complexes are bound, form into beads (figure 6.9) which break off as 'immune-complex coated bodies'. These bind to and are processed by germinal centre B-cells so that the antigen is now in a form in association with B-cell MHC class II, that can stimulate T-helper cells and kick off the secondary response. Even by day 14, antigen can still be detected on the surface of filiform follicular dendritic cells which may now be devoted to the generation of B-memory cells.

Interdigitating dendritic cells present antigen to T-lymphocytes

We have already described experiments in which macrophages can present antigen to T-cells and have just hinted that B-cells can do the same. However, in the paracortical region of the lymph node,

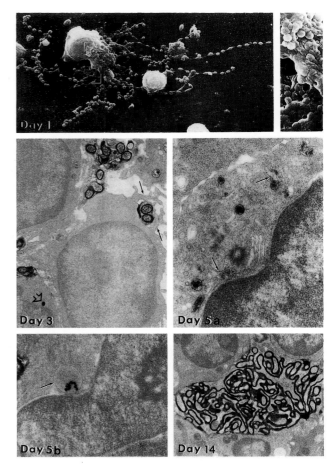

Figure 6.9. *Association of antigen (horseradish peroxidase, HRP) with follicular dendritic cells (FDC) after injection into immunized mice. Day 1: isolated FDC with 'beaded' dendrites (× 1700); right: high magnification of beads (× 4843). Day 3: bead dispersion among germinal centre B-cells (note attached beads surrounded by microvilli (arrows), × 5873). Day 5a: germinal centre B-cell with HRP (black) in endocytic vesicles, apparently being degraded (arrows) (note association with Golgi, × 13601); Day 5b: gold conjugated antigen in germinal centre B-cell endocytic vesicle (× 13601). Day 14: tightly convoluted HRP positive filiform FDC dendrites (× 4431). Kindly provided by Drs J.G. Tew, M.H. Kosco & A.K. Szakal from an article in* **Immunology Today** *(1989), 10, 231, and reproduced with permission from Elsevier Trends Journals, Cambridge.*

which is essentially T-cell country, there is another type of antigen-presenting cell, the interdigitating dendritic cell, which is dedicated exclusively to the potent stimulation of antigen-specific T-cells.

Figure 6.10a shows the large area of close contact of one of these cells with the membranes of surrounding T-lymphocytes rather well. These dendritic cells lack receptors for Ig and C3 but constitutively express high levels of surface MHC class I and II, are positive for the leucocyte common antigen (giving away their bone marrow origin) and bear the β-integrin adhesion molecule p150,95. Unlike the macrophages which in a sense are 'brutal microbe crunchers', the dendritic cells are not phagocytic although the interdigitating cells must have just whatever limited powers of degradation are required for the processing of antigen for T-cell recognition.

There is much evidence that dendritic cells such as the Langerhans' cells of the skin (cf. figure 2.6i), can pick up and process antigen in the periphery, then travel as 'veiled' cells in the lymph (figure 6.10b) to deliver the antigen for effective presentation to paracortical T-cells in the draining node. For example, dendritic cells from nodes draining the skin site of contact sensitization to picryl chloride can transfer sensitivity to a naïve animal. It has also been shown that veiled cells isolated from gut lymphatics of appropriately infected rats were associated with salmonella antigens. Sites of chronic T-cell inflammation seem to attract these cells since abnormally high numbers are found closely adhering to activated T-lymphocytes in synovial tissue from patients with ongoing rheumatoid arthritis and in the glands of subjects with chronic autoimmune thyroiditis lesions.

THE ACTIVATION OF T-CELLS

The surface markers of cells in the immune system

In order to discuss the events which occur in lymphocyte activation, and indeed in the operation of the immune system as a whole, it is imperative to establish a nomenclature which identifies the surface markers on the cells involved since these are used for communication and are usually functional molecules reflecting the state of cellular differentiation. The nomenclature system is established as follows. Immunologists from the far corners of the world who have produced monoclonal antibodies directed to surface molecules on B- and T-cells, macrophages, neutrophils and NK cells, get together every so often to compare the specificities of their reagents, in international workshops whose spirit of co-operation should be a lesson to most politicians. Where a cluster of monoclonals are found to react with the same polypeptide, they clearly represent a series of reagents defining a given marker and we label it with a CD (cluster determinant) number. The number of CD specificities on leuco-

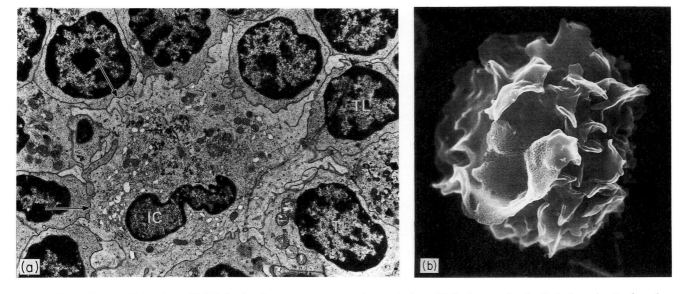

Figure 6.10. *(a) Interdigitating cell (IC) in the thymus-dependent area of the rat lymph node. This is thought to be an antigen-presenting cell derived from the Langerhans' cell in the skin which travels to the node in the afferent lymph as a 'veiled' cell bearing antigen on its profuse surface processes. Intimate contacts are made with the surface membranes (arrows) of the surrounding T-lymphocytes (TL). The cytoplasm of the IC contains relatively few organelles and* *does not show Birbeck granules (racket-shaped cytoplasmic organelles, characteristic of the Langerhans' cell), but these granules appear after antigenic stimulation (× 2000). (From Kamperdijk E.W.A., Hoefsmit E.Ch.H., Drexhage H.A. & Balfour B.H. (1980). In Mononuclear Phagocytes, 3rd edn. Van Furth R. (ed.). Rijhoff Publishers, The Hague. Courtesy of authors and publishers.) (b) Scanning electron micrograph of veiled cell (courtesy of Dr G.G. MacPherson).*

cytes is coming up into the 80s(!) at the time of writing but I have selected just some of them in table 6.1 which are the ones most likely to be relevant to our discussions. This can be used for reference but I regret to have to tell the reader that familiarity with the numbers can be a great help.

Immunocompetent T- and B-cells differ in many respects

We should now focus on the main surface markers which help us to differentiate T- and B-cells. The main relevant characteristics of human lymphocytes are set out in table 6.2.

The most clear-cut difference is established by reagents which recognize the antigen receptors, anti-CD3 for T-cells and anti-immunoglobulin for B-cells, and in laboratory practice these are the markers most often used to enumerate the two lymphocyte populations. Quite often, the adventitious formation of rosettes through the binding of sheep erythrocytes to CD2 (figure 2.6e) is used for the detection and separation of T-cells.

Attention should also be drawn to the so-called 'non-specific mitogens' which activate populations and sometimes subpopulations of T- or B-cells in a way which is unrelated to the antigen specificity of the lymphocyte receptors because they react with constant, as distinct from highly variable, structures on the cell surface. For this reason, they are often termed polyclonal B- or T-cell activators. Of notable interest have been the recent observations that a proportion of the T-cell population in mice is stimulated by staphylococcal enterotoxins, which cause food poisoning in humans, and by the pyro-

CD	Main cellular association	Membrane component
CD2	T	Receptor for LFA-3 and sheep r.b.c.
CD2R	act. T	Abs activate through these epitopes
CD3	T	Transducing elements of T-cell receptor
CD4	T subset	MHC class II, HIV receptor
CD5	T, B subset	Ab increases 2nd messenger pool
CD8	T subset	MHC class I receptor
CD10	CALL, germinal centre B,G	Neutral endopeptidase, CALLA
CD11a	Leucocytes	LFA-1 α chain
CD11b	M, G, NK	CR3, iC3b receptor α chain
CD11c	M, G, NK, B subset	α chain of gp 150/95 adhesion mol.
CD16	NK, G, macrophages	Fcγ RIII
CD18	Leucocytes	β chain to CD11a, b, c
CD19	B	Pan B-cell marker
CD20	B	? part of regulated Ca^{2+} channel
CD21	B subset	CR2, C3d/EBV receptor
CD23	B subset, act M, Eo	Fcε RII
CD25	act T, B, M	IL-2R β chain
CD29	Leucocytes	VLA β, integrin β1-chain
CD30	act T, B, Reed–Sternberg	
CDw32	M, G, B	Fcγ RII
CD35	G, M. B	CR1, receptor for C3b and C4b
CD45	Leucocytes	Leucocyte common antigen, T200
CD45 RA	T subset, B, G, M	Restricted T200, gp 220
CD45 RB	''	Restricted T200
CD45 RO	''	Restricted T200, gp 180
CD46	Leucocytes	Membrane cofactor protein (C3b breakdown)
CDw49b	Plt, cultured T	VLA-α2 chain, collagen receptor
CDw49d	M, T, B, LHC	VLA-α4 chain, Peyer's patch homing R
CDw49f	Plt	VLA-α6 chain, laminin receptor
CDw52	Leucocytes	Campath-1, therapeutic anti-lymphocyte
CD54	Broad	ICAM-1, rhinovirus receptor
CD55	Broad	Decay accelerating factor (C3b breakdown)
CD56	NK, act lymphocytes	Pan NK marker (? isoform of NCAM)
CD57	NK, T, B subset,	HNK1, carbohydrate of NK cells
CD58	Leucocytes, epithelial cells	LFA-3
CD64	M	High affinity Fcγ RI
CD68	Macrophages	Best macrophage marker available
CD69	act B, T	Small germinal-centre T-cells
CDw70	act B, T, Reed–Sternberg	Strong selectivity for Hodgkin Reed–Sternberg cells
CD71	Proliferating cells, macrophages	Transferrin receptor
CD72	B	Pan B-cell marker
CD73	B subset, T subset	Ecto-5'-nucleotidase, glycosyl P1 anchor
CDw75	Mature B (T subset)	Germinal centre B-cells
CD76	''	Mantle zone in 2° follicles
CD77	Resting B	Germinal centre B-cells, Burkitt centrocytic & centroblastic lymphomas

Table 6.1. *Cluster determinants (CD) on human cells. M=macrophage; G= granulocyte; NK=natural killer cell; Eo= eosinophil; Plt=platelet; CALL= common acute lymphoblastic leukaemia.*

Table 6.2. *Comparison of human T- and B-cells.*

	T	B
% in peripheral blood	65–80	8–15
ANTIGEN RECEPTOR MARKERS:		
Surface Ig	−	++
*CD3(T3)	++	−
OTHER RECEPTORS:		
Sheep cell rosettes (CD2)	++	−
Fcγ receptors	+ (some)	++
C3b receptors (CR1, CR2)	±	++
EBV receptors (= CR2)	−	++
Measles receptors	++	−
MHC:		
Class I	++	++
Class II	only activated cells	++
POLYCLONAL ACTIVATION:	anti-CD3 concanavalin A phytohaemagglutinin (PHA) pokeweed mitogen (PWM) enterotoxin superantigen	anti-Ig *Staph. aureus* (str. Cowan 1) EBV pokeweed mitogen (PWM)

* CD3 was best known by one of the monoclonals which first defined it, viz. T3.

Table 6.3. *T-cell subsets in man and mouse.*

	HUMAN	MOUSE
Pan T markers	CD3 CD2	Thy1
T-helper/T-delayed hypersensitivity	CD4	L3T4
	CD5	Ly1
T-cytotoxic/suppressor	CD8	Ly2

genic exotoxin A, the 'scarlet' toxin, of group A streptococci. Staphylococcal enterotoxin B, for example, is extraordinarily mitogenic for T-cells carrying the T-cell receptor variable gene families Vβ3 and Vβ8 irrespective of their specificity for antigen. It therefore behaves as a polyclonal activator of particular subpopulations of T-cells and the term 'superantigen' has evolved as a label to describe this class of stimulator. We will see in subsequent chapters that the minor lymphocyte stimulating (Mls) gene products on allogeneic lymphocytes which can activate up to 20% of murine T-cells through recognition of invariable segments of certain Vβ families, must be put in the same category.

Monoclonal antibodies also help to define specialized T-cell subsets of which the most prominent are shown in table 6.3 with their murine counterparts. CD4 and L3T4 are markers of helper T-cell populations which promote activation and maturation of B-cells and cytotoxic T-cells, and control antigen-specific chronic inflammatory reactions through stimulation of macrophages. CD4 molecules form subsidiary links with class II MHC on the cell presenting antigen. Similarly, the CD8 and Ly2 molecules on cytolytic T-cells connect with MHC class I (figure 6.13).

The activation of T-cells requires two signals

Antibodies to the T-cell receptor, either anti-idiotype or anti-T3, when insolubilized by coupling to Sepharose, will not activate resting T-cells on their own. Addition of interleukin-1 (IL-1) now readily induces RNA and protein synthesis, the cell enlarges to a blast-like appearance, interleukin-2 (IL-2) synthesis begins and the cell moves from G_0 into the G_1 phase of the mitotic cycle. Thus, two signals are required for the activation of a resting T-cell (figure 6.11). Antigen in association with MHC class II on the surface of antigen-presenting cells is clearly capable of fulfilling these requirements. Ternary complex formation between the T-cell receptor, antigen and MHC provides signal 1 through the receptor/CD3 complex and exposes the T-cell to a costimulatory signal 2 from the antigen-presenting cell, presumably IL-1 in high local concentrations or in a membrane-bound form. We shall see in a subsequent chapter that delivery of signal 1 to a resting T-cell in the absence of signal 2 leads to unresponsiveness or tolerance; thus, through its provision of signal 2, the antigen-presenting cell confers immunogenicity on the antigen. Things are not the same with T-cells which have already been activated; they are happy to be stimulated by just signal 1 alone.

The biochemical repercussions of these activation signals are complicated, but figure 6.12 makes some attempt to set out a minimally accepted overall scheme leading to synthesis of RNA and protein, including IL-2. The very earliest detectable events involve increased turnover of phosphatidyl inositol compounds and a rapid increase in cytoplasmic calcium concentration either through the opening of a Ca^{2+} channel in the plasma membrane or more probably by mobilization of intracellular stores under the influence of inositol triphosphate, itself

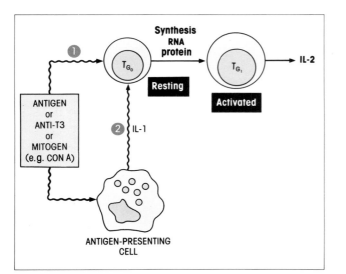

Figure 6.11. *Activation of resting T-cells requires two signals.*

dependent protein kinase C linked to the formation of IL-2. Further breakdown of diacyglycerol to arachidonic acid leads through mediators of the 5-lipoxygenase pathway to increased cyclic-GMP formation and this greatly enhances the activity of cGMP-dependent protein kinase(s) responsible for phosphorylation of a number of substrates, including non-histone acidic nuclear proteins critical for gene expression. cGMP has also been implicated in the activation of DNA-dependent RNA polymerases and the initiation of ribosomal and other RNA synthesis.

Accessory molecules play a role in T-cell activation

The avidity of binding of a naive T-cell to an appropriate presenting cell mediated solely through TCR recognition of a specific antigen/MHC complex is insufficient to allow more than a transient embrace. However, the interaction is greatly enhanced by the presence of complementary pairs of molecules on

118   derived by the action of an activated phospholipase on phosphatidyl inositol diphosphate. The other cleavage product, diacylglycerol, activates a calcium-

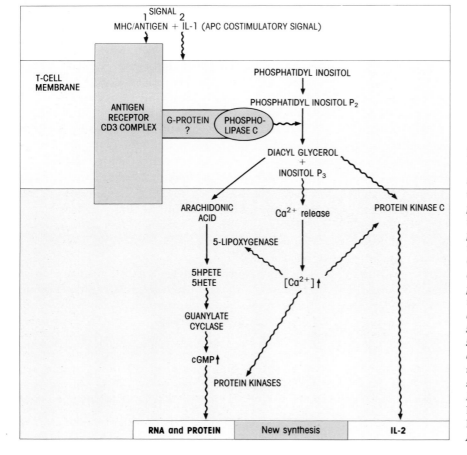

Figure 6.12. *Biochemical pathways of T-cell activation. A crucial event stimulated by antigen plus interleukin-1 would seem to be activation of the phospholipase which splits phosphatidyl inositol diphosphate to the reactive products diacylglycerol and inositol triphosphate. The increased intracellular Ca^{2+} concentration activates a number of different enzyme systems, including protein kinases, which lead finally to new synthesis of RNA, protein and interleukin-2 (5HPETE, 5-hydroperoxyeicosatetraenoic acid; 5HETE, 5-hydroxyeicosatetraenoic acid; cGMP, cyclic 3', 5'-guanosine monophosphate). (The arachidonic acid sequence is distilled from a review by Hadden J.W. (1987). In* **Mechanisms of Lymphocyte Activation and Immune Regulation.** *Gupta S., Paul W. and Fauci A. (eds), p.69. Plenum Press, N.Y.)*

the two cells (figure 6.13) which increase adhesion and permit signalling through the TCR to occur.

Without in any way questioning the importance of these molecules for cellular contact, which is now well established, LFA-1, CD2 and CD4/8 are seen to play a role in the regulation of the T-cell signal. It is instructive to take on board and ponder some of the evidence.

1 The ability of IL-1 plus insolubilized anti-CD3 coupled to Sepharose to stimulate T-cells is inhibited by anti-CD4 even though no CD4-MHC II attachment is involved.

2 Anti-CD3 also activates T-cells from patients who fail to express LFA-1 showing that adherence through LFA-1 is not essential for signalling; none the less, anti-LFA-1 inhibited activation of *normal* lymphocytes by anti-CD3.

3 CD2 is physically associated with the CD3−TCR complex, and monoclonal antibodies to two different epitopes on CD2 will activate T-cells through

an antigen-independent but TCR-mediated pathway in the presence of LFA-3 positive cells.

Lest the reader, if still awake(!), should by now have lost sight of the relevance of adhesion forces, let me quote one further rather fancy experimental result. Transfection of a murine antigen-presenting cell with human LFA-3 resulted in a 400% enhancement of the antigen-specific response of a T-cell hybridoma expressing a truncated human CD2 molecule which retained LFA-3 binding activity but had lost its signal-transducing cytoplasmic tail, i.e. it could adhere but not signal.

As a further twist to the story, antigen receptor cross-linking increases the avidity of LFA-1 for ICAM-1 through some intracellular signal. This increase in avidity is both rapid and transient, so providing a dynamic mechanism for antigen-specific regulation of lymphocyte adhesion and separation.

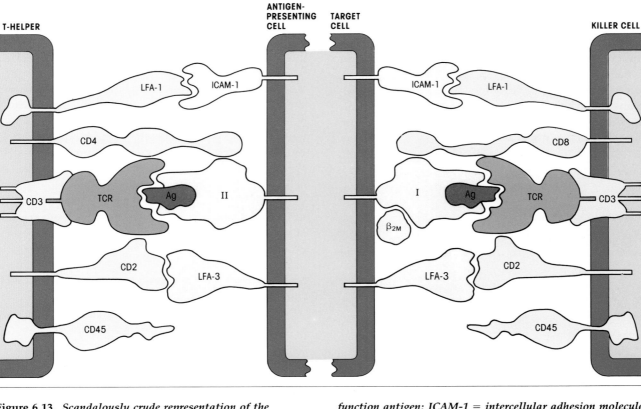

Figure 6.13. *Scandalously crude representation of the molecules involved in T-cell activation. There are multiple interactions between T-helpers and T-killers on the one hand and their antigen-presenting and target cells on the other. TCR = T-cell antigen-specific receptor; I and II refer to MHC class; CD45 = leucocyte common antigen; LFA = lymphocyte function antigen; ICAM-1 = intercellular adhesion molecule; CD2 = receptor for LFA-3-like molecule on sheep erythrocytes; LFA-1 is a member of the integrin family which includes the Mac-1 iC3b receptor; the others are members of the Ig super-family. Murine equivalents of CD4 and CD8 are L3T4 and Ly2 respectively.*

CONSEQUENCES OF ANTIGEN RECOGNITION

Last, one should mention the leucocyte common antigen CD45 which exists in several isoforms by discreet shuffling of its three N terminal exons. CD45 is a potent regulator of signal transduction, and proliferation induced through T- (or B-) surface molecules is inhibited by anti-CD45.

T-cell signalling is regulated by protein tyrosine phosphorylation

At least this is the way current thinking is moving. The conversion of phosphorylase *b* to the active *a* form originally drew attention to the importance of protein phosphorylation for the regulation of cellular processes and we now know that transforming proteins of certain oncogenic retroviruses and receptors for a number of growth factors or hormones have protein tyrosine kinase activity. T-cells have such an enzyme, p56^{lck}, bound to the internal side of the plasma membrane and physically associated with CD4 (or with CD8). After cell activation, p56^{lck} is modulated and the zeta (ζ) chains of the CD3 complex become phosphorylated. Just how this is related to the early events involving phosphatidylinositol diphosphate turnover, changes in intracellular Ca^{2+} and protein kinase C activation, has yet to be disentangled. The realization that the cytoplasmic domains of CD45 show considerable homology with known protein tyrosine phosphatases makes the idea that its potent downregulating ability may be related to dephosphorylation of CD3 zeta chains quite attractive (figure 6.14).

THE ACTIVATION OF B-CELLS

B-cells respond to three different types of antigen

1. Type 1 thymus-independent antigens

Certain antigens such as bacterial lipopolysaccharides, at a high enough concentration, have the ability to activate a substantial proportion of the B-cell pool polyclonally, i.e. without reference to the antigen specificity of the surface receptor hypervariable regions. At low concentrations, which do not cause polyclonal activation, those

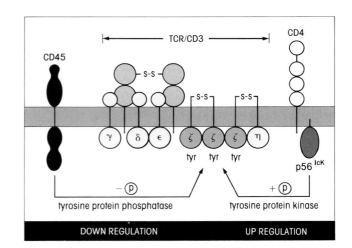

Figure 6.14. *Speculative model of regulation of T-cell signalling through the TCR/CD3 complex by phosphorylation of zeta chain tyrosines. (Note CD4 is probably physically associated with the TCR/CD3 complex during upregulation.)*

B-cells with Ig receptors *specific* for these antigens will focus them passively on their surface and be stimulated by their inherent mitogenic power (figure 6.18a).

2. Type 2 thymus-independent antigens

Certain linear antigens which are not readily degraded in the body and which have an appropriately spaced, highly repeating determinant — pneumococcus polysaccharide, ficoll, D-amino acid polymers and polyvinylpyrrolidone, for example — are also thymus-independent in their ability to stimulate B-cells directly without the need for T-cell involvement. They persist for long periods on the surface of specialized macrophages located at the subcapsular sinus of the lymph nodes and the splenic marginal zone (figure 6.6d), and can bind to antigen-specific B-cells with great avidity through their multivalent attachment to the complementary Ig receptors which they cross-link (figure 6.18b).

In general, the thymus-independent antigens give rise to predominantly IgM responses, some IgG3 in the mouse, and relatively poor, if any, memory.

3. Thymus-dependent antigens — the need for collaboration with T-helper cells

Many antigens are thymus-dependent in that they provoke little or no antibody response in animals which have been thymectomized at birth and have few T-cells. In general, antigens cannot fulfil the molecular requirements for direct stimulation; they may be univalent with respect to the specificity of each determinant, they may be readily degraded by phagocytic cells and they may lack mitogenicity. If they bind to B-cell receptors they will sit on the surface just like a hapten and not trigger the B-cell (figure 6.15). Cast your mind back to the definition of a hapten—a small molecule like dinitrophenyl (DNP) which binds to preformed antibody (e.g. the surface receptor of a specific B-cell) but fails to stimulate antibody production (i.e. stimulate the B-cell). Remember also that haptens become immunogenic when coupled to an appropriate carrier protein (p. 65). We now know that the carrier functions to stimulate T-helper cells which cooperate with B-cells to enable them to respond to the hapten by providing some accessory signals (figure 6.15). It should also be evident from figure 6.15 that while one determinant on an antigen is behaving as a hapten in binding to the B-cell, the other determinants subserve a carrier function in recruiting T-helper cells.

It is worthwhile examining the evidence on which these assertions are based. The first experiment in figure 6.16 shows that boosting with a hapten-carrier conjugate produces a secondary antibody response (not altogether surprising). The second shows that boosting with the hapten on a different carrier is ineffective unless the animal had already been separately primed to the second carrier (experiment 3). The last experiment shows that if the hapten and carrier are not physically linked together, they are not able to induce a secondary response. The roles of cooperating carrier-primed T-cells in the secondary response to carrier-hapten conjugates are revealed by the adoptive transfer experiments in figure 6.17.

Antigen processing by B-cells

The need for physical linkage of hapten and carrier strongly suggests that T-helpers must recognize the carrier determinants on the responding B-cell in order to provide the relevant accessory stimulatory signals. However, since T-cells only recognize processed membrane-bound antigen in association with MHC molecules, the T-helpers cannot recognize native antigen bound simply to the Ig-receptors of the B-cell as naïvely depicted in figure 6.15. All is not lost, however, since primed B-cells can present antigen to T-helper cells—in fact, they work at much lower antigen concentrations than conven-

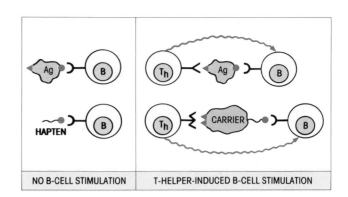

Figure 6.15. *T-helper cells cooperate through carrier determinants to help B-cells respond to hapten or equivalent determinants on antigens by providing accessory signals. (For simplicity we are ignoring the MHC component and epitope processing in T-cell recognition, but we won't forget it.)*

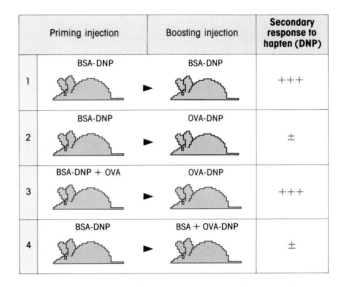

Figure 6.16. *The role of carrier priming in the secondary response to hapten. The boosting injection only produces a secondary hapten response when the hapten is physically linked to a carrier to which the animal is already primed (after Rajewsky): BSA, bovine serum albumin; DNP, dinitrophenyl; Ova, chicken ovalbumin.*

121

tional presenting cells because they can focus antigen through their surface receptors. They must therefore be capable of 'processing' the antigen and the current view is that antigen bound to surface Ig is internalized in endosomes which then fuse with vesicles containing MHC class II molecules with their invariant chain, and membrane-bound cathepsins B and D. Processing of the protein antigen presumably begins with the action of cathepsin B which is a neutral protease and is continued, as the vesicle is slowly acidified, by cathepsin D. The

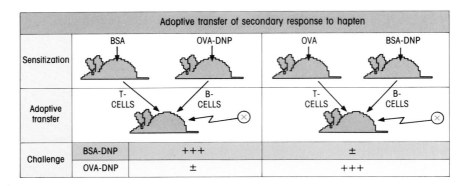

Adoptive transfer of secondary response to hapten					
Sensitization	BSA	OVA-DNP		OVA	BSA-DNP
Adoptive transfer	T-CELLS	B-CELLS		T-CELLS	B-CELLS
Challenge	BSA-DNP	+++		±	
	OVA-DNP	±		+++	

Figure 6.17. *The secondary response of B-cells primed to dinitrophenyl (DNP) depends upon help from T-cells sensitized to carrier determinants. Spleen cells from primed mice were fractionated into T-cells by nylon wool filtration or panning off B-cells with anti-Ig plates; B-cell fractions were obtained by killing T-cells with anti-Thy 1 plus complement. Appropriate mixtures of T- and B-cells were transferred to irradiated hosts of the same strain and then challenged with either of the two hapten-carrier conjugates. BSA, bovine serum albumin; OVA, ovalbumin.*

resulting antigenic peptide is then recycled to the surface in association with the class II molecules where it is available for recognition by specific T-helpers (figures 6.18c and 6.19). The need for the physical union of hapten and carrier is now revealed; the hapten leads the carrier to be processed into the cell which is programmed to make anti-hapten antibody and, following stimulus by the T-helper recognizing processed carrier, it will carry out its programme and ultimately produce antibodies which react with the hapten (is there no end to the wiliness of nature?!).

The nature of B-cell activation

Cross-linking of B-cell surface receptors, for example by anti-IgM conjugated to insoluble Sepharose particles, induces the early activation events. The involvement of antigen-presenting cells in the activation process is still not clearly defined. The polymeric type-2 thymus-independent antigens with repeating determinants firmly cross-link Ig receptors to form a stable matrix, but they are normally presented on specialized macrophages which produce an assortment of possible accessory factors like IL-1 and C3. The latter is of interest since antibodies to the CR2 receptor for C3b are mitogenic for B-cells and, furthermore, the polyclonal activator Epstein Barr (EB) virus is known to bind to this receptor.

Be that as it may, Ig receptor cross-linking leads to a series of changes which probably closely parallel those seen in T-cell activation, GTP-dependent hydrolysis of phosphatidyl inositol diphosphate by phospholipase C, formation of inositol triphosphate with mobilization of intracellular Ca^{2+}, and of diacylglycerol and activation of protein kinase C (cf. figure 6.12). The kappa-gene enhancer binding protein NFκB, which exists as a dimer bound to an inhibitor in the cytoplasm, releases the inhibitor on activation of the protein kinase and moves into the nucleus where its appearance is associated with κ-gene transcription. Not surprisingly, like the T-cell receptor, it turns out that the surface IgM receptor is associated with a complex of two or even three membrane proteins which may also undergo phosphorylation in relationship to B-cell signalling. Note that $F(ab')_2$ anti-μ is far more mitogenic for B-cells than is the intact immunoglobulin, and this raises the possibility that simultaneous engagement of both the IgM antigen-receptor and the Fcγ receptor by IgG anti-μ or by immune complexes containing IgG could downregulate the cell, possibly through the adenyl cyclase–protein kinase A pathway.

This cross-linking model seems appropriate for an understanding of stimulation by type 2 thymus-independent antigens, and like the T-cell polyclonal activators, the type I T-independent antigens probably bypass the specific receptor and act directly on downstream molecules such as diacylglycerol and protein kinase C. T-dependent antigens pose a different problem. These are usually univalent with respect to B-cell receptors, and it is not easy to see how Ig receptors can be cross-linked unless this was to occur weakly through some type of linked array of native antigen on an initial antigen-presenting cell prior to B-cell processing (cf. figure 6.18c). Of course, it is also possible that Ig receptors undergo spontaneous endosome recycling and that no stimulus is received by the B-cell until a helper T-cell reacts with the processed antigen and class II

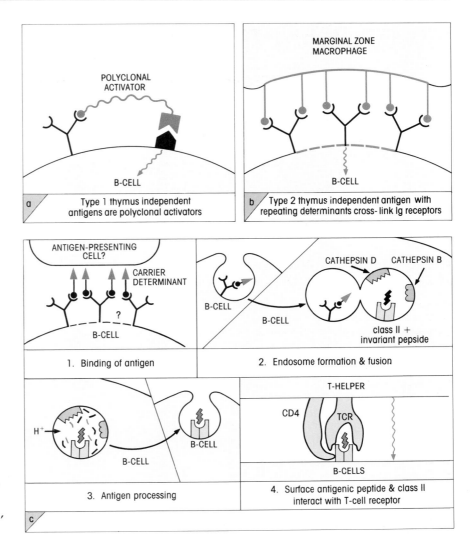

Figure 6.18. *B-cell recognition of three types of antigen.* ∿∿→ *, activation signal;* Υ *, surface Ig receptor;* – – – , *cross-linking of receptors.*

MHC on its surface. The nature of the T-cell activating signal is not entirely clear but interleukin-4 (IL-4), a soluble T-cell product previously known as B-cell stimulatory factor-1, plays a major role. Resting B-cells bear IL-4 receptors, the engagement of which leads to an abrupt increase in density of surface MHC class II and conditions the cell for a costimulatory signal from the T-cell (CD4?) which pushes it into the G1 phase of the mitotic cycle.

Like the activated T-cell, the stimulated B-lymphocyte also acquires a number of surface receptors for growth factors derived from T-helpers and the stage is now set for the proliferation which characterizes the next phase in the immune response.

Clonal expansion is achieved by T-cell soluble factors

Thymus-independent polyclonal activators drive B-cells into division independently of Ig receptors through their innate mitogenic potential, while Ig receptor cross-linking together with macrophage accessory factors are probably sufficient to enable type-2 thymus-independent antigens to get the B-cells cycling. Our discussion will focus on the T-dependent responses which actually have much greater flexibility in terms of antibody class, affinity, memory and probably clone size.

The first expansion occurs in the activated helper-T population which express surface receptors of high affinity for interleukin-2 (IL-2) and proliferate in response to IL-2 produced either by themselves or by another subpopulation (figure 6.20).

CONSEQUENCES OF ANTIGEN RECOGNITION

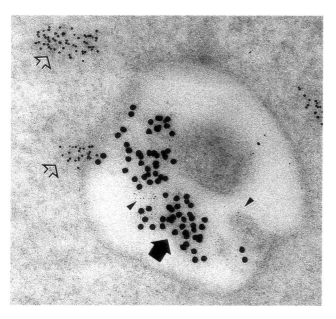

Figure 6.19. *Demonstration that endocytosed B-cell surface Ig receptors enter cytoplasmic vesicles geared for antigen processing. Surface IgG was cross-linked with goat anti-human Ig and rabbit anti-goat Ig conjugated to 15-nm gold beads (large dark arrow). After 2 min the cell sections were prepared and stained with anti-HLA-DR invariant chain (2-nm gold; arrowhead) and anti-cathepsin B (5-nm gold; clear arrow). Thus the internalized IgG is exposed to proteolysis in a vesicle containing class II molecules. The presence of invariant chain shows that the class II molecules derive from the endoplasmic reticulum and golgi, not from the cell surface. Note the clever use of different-sized gold particles to distinguish the antibodies used for localizing the various intravesicular proteins, etc. Photograph reprinted by permission from the authors, L.E. Guagliardi and colleagues, and from* **Nature** *343, 133. Copyright © 1990 Macmillan Magazines Ltd.*

124

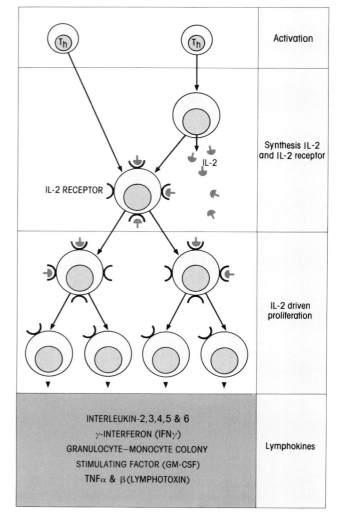

Figure 6.20. *Activated T-blasts expressing surface receptors for interleukin-2 proliferate in response to IL-2 produced by itself or by another T-cell subset. Expansion is controlled through down-regulation of the IL-2 receptor by IL-2 itself. The expanded population secretes a wide variety of biologically active lymphokines of which IL-4 also enhances T-cell proliferation.*

The T-cell blasts also produce an impressive array of other soluble factors (lymphokines), one of which, IL-4, is also a T-cell growth factor. They can induce changes in the status of many other cell types, B-cells, cytotoxic T-cell precursors, macrophages, endothelial cells and so on and for this reason they are often referred to as *inducer* cells. However, in the present context we will restrict ourselves to the expansion of newly activated B-cells.

The secretion of interleukins is polarized to the region of T–B surface contact so that the B-cell is exposed to very high local concentrations of the growth factors. This was rather elegantly demonstrated by the following experiment. Cytoplasmic processes of a T-helper clone were forced into the 3-micron pores of a nucleopore membrane on the far side of which had been placed a T-cell stimulating anti-receptor idiotype. Judicious controls showed that IL-4 was preferentially released at the pole of the cell being stimulated.

IL-4 not only activates resting B-cells, but also acts as a potent growth factor for cells in G1. IL-5, previously known as B-cell growth factor II or T-cell replacing factor, also promotes clonal expansion. IL-2 may do so only at very high concentrations.

Further T-cell factors bring about maturation of effector cells

After clonal expansion of the activated B-blasts,

maturation to cells with effector function occurs. The factors which control these changes have not been fully worked out but we have some idea of the influence of certain lymphokines, alone or in concert, on the switch from IgM to production of other isotypes (see figure 6.21). IL-6, appearing as B-cell stimulating factor 2, B-cell differentiation factor or IFNβ₂ in previous incarnations, not only influences the switch to IgG, but is an important growth factor.

What is going on in the germinal centre?

The secondary follicle with its corona or mantle of small lymphocytes surrounding the pale germinal centre is a striking and unique cellular structure, often picked out proudly by immunologists with a rather untutored histological background (like myself) to bolster their otherwise shaky morphological prowess. None the less, until recently, the nature of the events occurring within it were shrouded in mystery, as if it were yet another 'black box'. First, let us recall what we are looking at.

Germinal centres do not normally occur in the embryo; only small lymphocytes aggregated into primary follicles are first seen. About 4 days after antigen is given, dividing centroblasts appear within the primary follicles and 24 hours later tingible body macrophages are observed. The division into a dark zone containing centroblasts and a light zone with centrocytes appears only after 1−3 weeks. Follicular dendritic cells are attracted to or develop at this site and, to complete the picture, T-cells making up approximately 5% of the local population are present. In the primary response, nearly 70% of B-cells have surface IgM and only 10% IgG; however, after secondary challenge, the proportions are reversed, 30% M and 70% G, although it is significant that germinal centre B-cells in Peyer's patches are predominantly IgA. Note the contrast with the mantle lymphocytes which express IgM and IgD simultaneously and are probably naive cells.

Secondary challenge with antigen or immune complexes induces enlargement of germinal centres, formation of new ones, appearance of B-memory cells and development of Ig producing cells of higher affinity. B-cells entering the germinal centre become centroblasts which divide with a very short cycle time of 6 hours, temporarily lose their surface

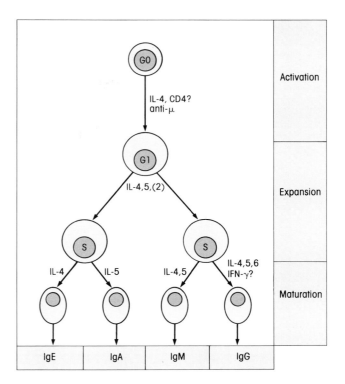

Figure 6.21. *Clonal expansion and maturation of activated B-cells under the influence of T-cell derived soluble factors. c-Myc expression, which is maximal 2 h after antigen or anti-μ stimulation, parallels sensitivity to growth factors; transfection with c-myc substitutes for anti-μ. The nature of the signals for memory cell differentiation is unknown.*

Ig and FcεII receptor (CD23), and have a high spontaneous death rate. Later, the B-cells express a single Ig isotype on their surface and are potent presenters of antigen to T-cells. As the centrocytes mature, they differentiate either into immunoblast plasma cell precursors which secrete Ig in the absence of antigen or memory B-cells.

How has this all been pieced together in the current, admittedly still speculative, scenarios? Following secondary antigen challenge, primed B-cells may be activated by paracortical T-helper cells in association with interdigitating dendritic cells or macrophages, and migrate to the germinal centre. Activation can also occur by complexes on follicular dendritic cells (cf. p. 114) with perhaps a further proliferative stimulus from cleaved CD23 derived from the surface of the dendritic cells and stimulated B-cells, and at some stage from T-cell lymphokines released in response to antigen-presenting B-cells. During this particularly frenetic bout of cell division, it is postulated that somatic mutation of B-cell Ig genes occurs with high frequency probably under the influence of T-cell interleukins. At this stage the

B-cells are vulnerable and die readily whence they are taken up as the 'tingible bodies' by macrophages, unless rescued by association with antigen on a follicular dendritic cell. This will only occur if the mutated surface Ig receptor still binds antigen, and as the concentration of antigen gradually falls, only if the receptor is of high affinity will the association with follicular dendritic cell occur. This clearly would provide a mechanism for the maturation of affinity during the T-dependent immune response. The cells either migrate to the sites of plasma cell activity (e.g. lymph node medulla) or go to expand the memory B-cell pool depending upon the differentiating signals received from T-cells and follicular dendritic cells (figure 6.22). Obscurity still surrounds the signals which guide cells along the pathway to memory and encourage the abnormally high mutation rate in the Ig variable region genes which precedes this within the secondary follicle germinal centre.

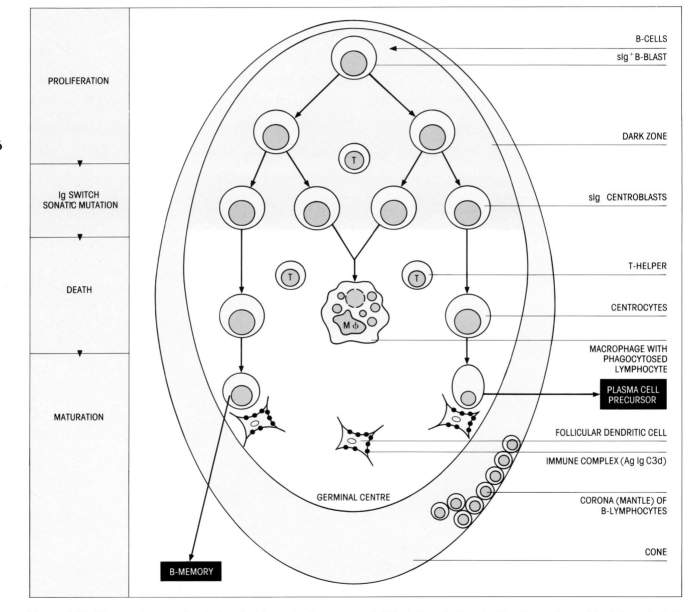

Figure 6.22. *The events occurring in lymphoid germinal centres. Expression of LFA-1 and ICAM-1 on B-cells and follicular dendritic cells in the germinal centre makes them 'sticky'. Germinal centre B-cells can be enriched through their affinity for the peanut agglutinin lectin. The T-helper cells bear the unusual CD57 marker.*

SUMMARY

Lymphocytes mediate acquired immune responses which involve a first phase of induction or activation, a second phase of clonal proliferation and a final phase in which a proportion of the lymphocytes become effector cells and the remainder an expanded population of memory cells able to provide secondary responses.

The immune response occurs most effectively in structured secondary lymphoid tissue. The lymph nodes filter and screen lymph flowing from the body tissues while spleen filters the blood. B- and T-cell areas are separated. B-cell structures appear in the lymph node cortex as primary follicles or secondary follicles with germinal centres after antigen stimulation; T-cells occupy the paracortical area; plasma cells synthesizing antibody appear in medullary cords which penetrate the macrophage-lined medullary sinuses. Lymphoid tissue guarding the gastro-intestinal tract is unencapsulated and somewhat structured (tonsils, Peyer's patches, appendix) or present as diffuse cellular collections in the lamina propria. Together with the subepithelial accumulations of cells lining the mucosal surfaces of the respiratory and genito-urinary tracts, they form the 'secretory immune system' which bathes the surface with protective IgA antibodies. Bone marrow is a major site of antibody production. Lymphocyte recirculation between the blood and lymphoid tissues is guided by specialized homing receptors on the surface of the high-walled endothelium of the postcapillary venules.

Antigen is presented to lymphocytes by macrophages and by specialized antigen-presenting cells in T- and B-cell areas. Dendritic cells in secondary follicles bind immune complexes firmly and persistently and are linked with B-cell memory.

Cells of the haematopoietic system are characterized by their surface differentiation molecules which are defined by possession of antigen determinants recognized by a cluster (3 or more) of monoclonal antibodies through which they are assigned a CD (cluster determinant) number.

T- and B-cells are readily distinguished by surface markers, CD3 on T-cells and surface Ig on B-cells. T-cells also form spontaneous rosettes with sheep erythrocytes through their CD2 molecules.

Activation of T-cells requires two signals, one through the T-cell CD3 complex, the other a costimulatory signal from antigen-presenting cells, probably IL-1. Cleavage of phosphatidyl inositol diphosphate leads to mobilization of intracellular Ca^{2+}, activation of protein kinases and subsequent synthesis of RNA and protein including interleukin-2 (IL-2).

Accessory molecules such as LFA-1, CD2 and CD4 (or 8) enhance cellular adhesiveness to the cell presenting antigen and play a role in regulating the activation signal. CD45 (leucocyte common antigen) is a phosphatase which may downregulate activation by dephosphorylating the phosphate group introduced into the CD3 complex by a tyrosine phosphorylase associated with T-cell stimulation. B-cells respond to three different types of antigen, thymus-independent type-1 (polyclonal activators), thymus-independent type-2 (polymeric nondegradable) and thymus-dependent which require T-helper recognition of one determinant on the antigen (carrier) to help a B-cell respond to another determinant (hapten) on the same molecule. B-cells process antigen which binds to their Ig receptors and re-express it on their surface with class II MHC. B-cells are activated either by non-specific polyclonal activation, or Ig receptor cross-linking associated with a macrophage signal, or by a signal from helper T-cells recognizing peptide antigen in association with class II MHC. A strong candidate for this signal is known to be capable of activating resting G_0 B-cells. These events lead to phosphatidyl inositol diphosphate breakdown and comparable cascade reactions to those seen in activation of T-cells.

Activated T-cells secrete IL-2 which drives division in cells expressing IL-2 receptors. The T-cells produce a series of lymphokines which clonally expand activated B-cells, cause their maturation into antibody synthesizing cells and class-switching to IgG and other isotypes. In germinal centres, activated B-cells undergo frenetic division, Ig somatic mutation and selection for high affinity on follicular dendritic cells bearing IgG antibody complexes before leaving as progenitors of plasma cells and B-memory cells.

Further reading

Feldmann M., Maini R.N. & Woody J.N. (eds) (1989) *T-cell Activation in Health and Disease*. Academic Press, London.

Gupta S., Paul W. & Fauci A. (eds) (1987) *Mechanisms of Lymphocyte Activation and Immune Regulation*. Plenum Press, New York.

Hamaoka T. & Ono S. (1986) Regulation of B-cell differentiation. *Ann. Rev. Immunol.*, **4**, 167.

Henry K. & Farrer-Brown G. (1981) *Colour Atlas of Thymus and Lymph Node Histology with Ultrastructure.* Wolfe Medical Publications, London.

Melchers F. & Andersson J. (1986) Factors controlling the B-cell cycle. *Ann. Rev. Immunol.*, **4**, 13.

128

THE ACQUIRED IMMUNE RESPONSE
II – Production of Effectors

THE SYNTHESIS OF HUMORAL ANTIBODY

Detection and enumeration of antibody-forming cells

Immunofluorescence

Cells containing antibody within their cytoplasm can be identified by the 'sandwich' technique (see figure 5.24). For example, a cell making antibodies to tetanus toxoid if treated first with the antigen will subsequently bind a fluorescein-labelled anti-tetanus antibody and can then be visualized in the fluorescence microscope.

Plaque techniques

Antibody-secreting cells can be counted by diluting them in an environment in which the antibody formed by each individual cell produces a readily observable effect. In one of the most widely used techniques, developed from the original method of Jerne and Nordin, the cells from an animal immunized with sheep erythrocytes are suspended together with an excess of sheep red cells and complement within a shallow chamber formed between two microscope sides. On incubation the antibody-forming cells release their immunoglobulin which coats the surrounding erythrocytes. The comple-

ment will then cause lysis of the coated cells and a plaque clear of red cells will be seen around each antibody-forming cell (figure 7.1). Direct plaques obtained in this way largely reveal IgM producers since this antibody has a high haemolytic efficiency. To demonstrate IgG synthesizing cells it is necessary to increase the complement binding of the erythrocyte—IgG antibody complex by adding a rabbit anti-IgG serum; thus develops the 'indirect plaques' and can be used to enumerate cells making antibodies in different immunoglobulin subclasses, provided the appropriate rabbit antisera are available. The method can be extended by coating an antigen such as pneumococcus polysaccharide on to the red cell, or by coupling hapten groups to the erythrocyte surface.

In the 'Elispot' modification, the antibody-forming cell suspension is incubated on a dish of immobilized antigen. The secreted antibody is captured locally and is visualized after removal of the cells, by treatment with peroxidase-labelled anti-Ig, and development of the colour reaction by incorporating the substrate in a gel which is poured over the floor of the dish. Limited diffusion of the coloured reaction product in the gel provides a series of macroscopic spots which can be readily enumerated (figure 7.2).

Protein synthesis

In the normal antibody-forming cell there is a rapid turnover of light chains which are present in slight

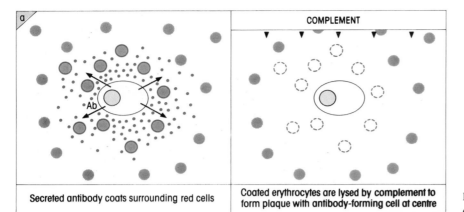

	COMPLEMENT
Secreted antibody coats surrounding red cells	Coated erythrocytes are lysed by complement to form plaque with antibody-forming cell at centre

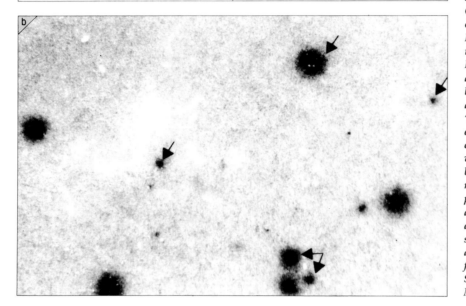

Figure 7.1. *Jerne plaque technique for enumerating antibody-forming cells (Cunningham modification). (a)* **The** *direct technique for cells synthesizing IgM haemolysin is shown. The* **indirect** *technique for visualizing cells producing IgG haemolysins requires the addition of anti-IgG to the system. The difference between the plaques obtained by direct and indirect methods gives the number of 'IgG' plaques. The* **reverse plaque** *assay enumerates total Ig producing cells by capturing secreted Ig on red cells coated with anti-Ig. Multiple plaque assays can be carried out by a modification using microtitre plates. (b) Photograph of plaques which show as circular dark areas (some of which are arrowed) under dark-ground illumination. They vary in size depending upon the antibody affinity and the rate of secretion by the antibody-forming cell. (Courtesy of Mr C. Shapland, Ms P. Hutchings & Dr D. Male.)*

excess. Defective control occurs in many myeloma cells and one may see excessive production of light chains or complete suppression of heavy chain synthesis. Interchain disulphide bridges may form while the heavy chains are still attached to the ribosomes (figure 7.3) but the sequence in which the intermediates arise varies with the nature of the immunoglobulin. Using 'pulse and chase' techniques with radioactive amino acids it was found that the build-up of both light and heavy chains proceeds continuously starting from the N-terminal end. Furthermore, isolation of the mRNA for each type of chain has shown them to be of appropriate size to allow synthesis of the complete peptides. The evidence therefore confirms the present view that the messenger regions for variable and constant regions are spliced together before leaving the nucleus.

Differential splicing mechanisms also provide a rational explanation for the co-expression of surface IgM and IgD with identical V regions on a single cell (figure 7.4), and for the switch from production of membrane-bound IgM receptor to secretory IgM in the antibody-forming cell (figure 7.5).

Class switching occurs in individual B-cells

The synthesis of antibodies belonging to the various immunoglobulin classes proceeds at different rates. Usually there is an early IgM response which tends to fall off rapidly. IgG antibody synthesis builds up to its maximum over a longer time period. On secondary challenge with antigen, the time course of the IgM response resembles that seen in the primary. By contrast, the synthesis of IgG antibodies rapidly accelerates to a much higher titre and there is a relatively slow fall-off in serum anti-

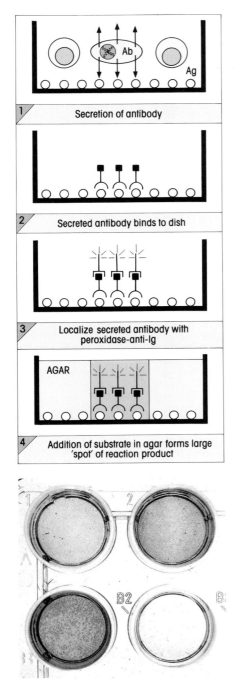

Figure 7.2. *'Elispot' (from ELISA technique) system for enumerating antibody-forming cells. The picture shows spots formed by hybridoma cells making autoantibodies to thyroglobulin revealed by alkaline phosphatase-linked anti-Ig (courtesy of P. Hutchings). Increasing numbers of hybridoma cells were added to the top two and bottom left-hand wells which show corresponding increases in the number of 'Elispots'. The bottom right-hand well is a control using a hybridoma of irrelevant specificity.*

body levels (figure 7.6). The same probably holds for IgA and in a sense both these immunoglobulin classes provide the main *immediate* defence against future penetration by foreign antigens.

There is evidence that individual cells can switch over from IgM to IgG production. Several days after immunization with salmonella flagella, isolated cells taken into micro-drop cultures were shown to produce both IgM and IgG immobilizing antibodies. In another study it was shown that antigen challenge of irradiated recipients receiving relatively small numbers of lymphoid cells, produced splenic foci of cells, each synthesizing antibodies of different heavy chain class bearing a single idiotype; the common idiotype suggests that each focus is derived from a single precursor cell whose progeny can form antibodies of different class.

Antibody synthesis in most classes shows considerable dependence upon T-cooperation in that the responses in T-deprived animals are strikingly deficient; such is true of mouse IgG1, IgG2a, IgA, IgE and part of the IgM antibody responses. T-independent antigens such as the polyclonal activator, LPS endotoxin, induce synthesis of IgM with some IgG2b and IgG3. Immunopotentiation by complete Freund's adjuvant, a water-in-oil emulsion containing antigen in the aqueous phase and a suspension of killed tubercle bacilli in the oily phase (p. 238), seems to occur, at least in part, through the activation of helper T-cells which stimulate antibody production in T-dependent classes. The prediction from this that the response to T-independent antigens (e.g. pneumococcus polysaccharide, p. 120) should not be potentiated by Freund's adjuvant is borne out in practice; furthermore, as mentioned previously, these antigens evoke primarily IgM antibodies and poorly defined immunological memory as do T-dependent antigens injected into T-cell deficient neonatally thymectomized hosts.

Thus, in rodents at least, the switch from IgM to IgG and other classes appears to be largely under T-cell control presumably mediated by soluble factors as suggested earlier (p. 125), although it is often difficult to establish whether a given agent is itself causing the switch or is a particularly good growth promoter for the Ig class resulting from the switch. Let us take another look at the stimulation of small surface IgM positive B-cells by LPS; as we noted, on its own the non-specific mitogen evokes the synthesis of IgM, IgG3 and some IgG2b. Following addition of interleukin-4 (IL-4) to the system, there is heightened production of IgE and IgG1 whereas interferon-γ (IFNγ) stimulates IgG2a secretion at

131

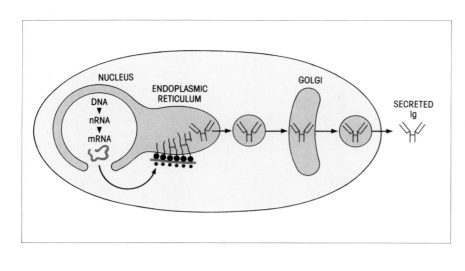

Figure 7.3. *Synthesis of mouse IgG2a immunoglobulin. As the H-chains near completion, adjacent peptide chains can spontaneously cross-link through their constant regions. It is thought that the light chains may aid release of the terminal chains from the ribosome by forming the L—H—H molecule. Combination with a further light chain would yield the full immunoglobulin L—H—H—L (based on Askonas B.A. & Williamson A.R. (1986)* **Biochem. J.** *109, 637). The order in which the interchain disulphide bridges are formed varies in different immunoglobulins depending on the relative strengths of the bonds as assessed by susceptibility to reduction. Surface receptor Ig would be inserted by its hydrophobic sequences into the membrane of the endoplasmic reticulum as it was synthesized.*

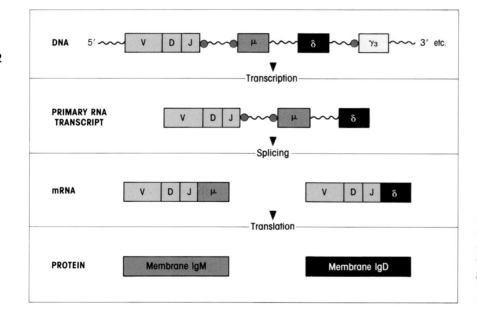

Figure 7.4. *Surface membrane IgM and IgD receptors of identical specificity appear on the same cell through differential splicing of the composite primary RNA transcript. For simplicity the leader sequence has been omitted.* ∿∿∿ = *introns.*

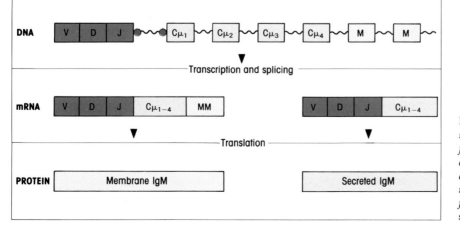

Figure 7.5. *Splicing mechanism for the switch from the membrane to the secreted form of IgM. The hydrophobic sequence encoded by the exons M—M which anchors the receptor IgM to the membrane is spliced out in the secreted form (leader sequences again omitted for simplicity).*

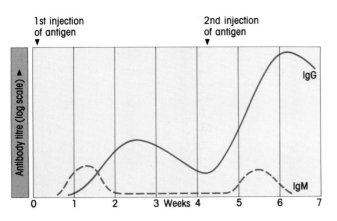

Figure 7.6. *Synthesis of IgM and IgG antibody classes in the primary and secondary responses to antigen.*

concentrations that inhibit the effects of IL-4. IL-5 promotes maturation without affecting Ig class. The notion that IL-4 was a switch factor for IgA stemmed largely from results with a given lymphoma but with no confirmatory data using normal B-cells. Rather more convincing was the 5−10-fold increase

in IgA production when transforming growth factor-β (TGFβ) was introduced into the LPS system and the demonstration of a switch from surface IgA negative to positive in Peyer's patch cells so treated. Significantly, TGFβ induced the formation of sterile transcripts consisting of a 5′ exon derived from germline sequences upstream of the α-switch region (cf. figure 7.7) spliced to the IgA class Cα gene. The 5′ exons contain stop codons in the open reading frame of the Cα gene and so cannot encode large proteins. This is now seen to be one instance of a more general phenomenon in which sterile transcripts of a C_H gene are associated with a switch to that class (figure 7.7). Perhaps the transcripts facilitate the action of the recombinase in some way or maybe they reflect an increased accessibility of that particular switch region to the enzyme. Under the influence of the recombinase, a given *VDJ* gene segment is transferred from μδ to an alternative constant region gene by utilizing the specialized switch region sequences (figure 7.7), so yielding antibodies of the same specificity but of different class.

133

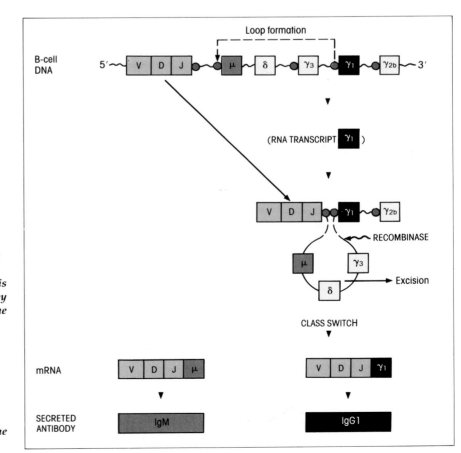

Figure 7.7. *Class-switching to produce antibodies of identical specificity but different immunoglobulin isotype (in this example from IgM to IgG₁) is achieved by a recombinase process which utilizes the specialized switch sequences (●) and leads to a loss of the intervening DNA loop (μ, δ and γ3). The role of the C_H transcript which always accompanies the phenomenon is not yet established. Rare examples of mutant clones expressing an isotypic gene 5′ of the parent heavy chain gene suggest that switching to constant region genes on the sister chromatid may sometimes occur.*

Is the specificity of antibody secreted by the progeny the same as that of the surface immunoglobulin of the clonal parent?

The answer is, often yes, often partially and sometimes no. You may think this a trifle cryptic so let's recapitulate. The clonal selection hypothesis predicts an affirmative answer to our question because it postulates that each lymphocyte is programmed to make only one antibody, that it puts the antibody as a receptor on its surface so that antigen will bind to it, and that as a result the cell is selectively triggered for antibody formation; as it only knows how to make one antibody, the specificity should be identical with the original surface receptor.

The one-cell one-antibody idea does seem O.K.

With immunofluorescent techniques, individual immunoglobulin cells can be stained for either κ or λ chains but not both, and in the heterozygous rabbit, for the maternal allotypic marker or the paternal but never both together (*allelic exclusion*). Furthermore, plasma cell tumours only produce one, and not more than one, myeloma protein. Similar restrictions apply to the staining of surface Ig on B-lymphocytes.

That these surface immunoglobulins can behave as antibodies is suggested by the ability of a small percentage of lymphocytes to bind specific antigens such as sheep cells (forming 'rosettes') or radioactive salmonella flagellin. This binding can be blocked by anti-immunoglobulin sera. Humphrey has further shown that the percentage of cells binding antigen is increased in primed and decreased in tolerant animals.

When a soluble antigen like polymerized flagellin binds to a specific cell it causes patching and capping of the surface Ig in just the same way as an anti-Ig serum (cf. p. 21). If the antigen-capped cells are now stained with fluorescent anti-Ig, all the Ig is found in the cap, there being none on the remainder of the lymphocyte surface, i.e. when antigen reacts with a cell, all the Ig molecules on the cell surface combine with the antigen showing that they have similar specificity. Exactly the same result is seen if an anti-idiotype is used for capping, i.e. all the surface Ig molecules on a given cell have the same idiotype. So far so good.

The surface antibody does appear to be related to the specificity of the secreted immunoglobulin

If the production of a given antibody depends upon its representation as a surface Ig in the pool of antigen-sensitive B-cells, then positive or negative selection for cells of that specificity prior to antigen challenge should have profound effects on subsequent reactivity. Indeed that is just what happens. Depletion of antigen-specific cells by reaction with their surface receptors abrogates the further ability of that population to respond to antigen (figure 7.8). Likewise, a high percentage of cells isolated by virtue of their specific binding to a hapten like DNP, secrete anti-DNP when stimulated under kindly conditions *in vitro*. If more is wanted, then it can be shown rather cleverly that surface and cytoplasmic Ig in secreting cells share a common idiotype. First stain the surface Ig of the living cells at 4°C with fluorescein-labelled anti-idiotype and then fix with glutaraldehyde and stain the cytoplasm of

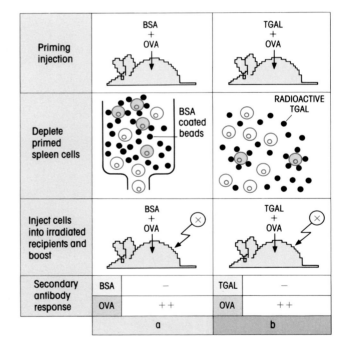

Figure 7.8. *Depletion of cells with surface receptors for antigen removes subsequent ability to respond to that antigen. (a) Primed cells (green) depleted by reaction between surface Ig on the lymphocytes and insolubilized antigen packing the column. Further control, ovalbumin-coated beads. (b) Primed cells (green) destroyed by radiation 'suicide' through binding highly radioactive antigen to surface Ig. Further control, unlabelled antigen (TGAL). BSA = bovine serum albumin; Ova = ovalbumin; TGAL = poly-lysine with poly-alanine side-chains randomly tipped with tyrosine and glutamine.*

the cytocentrifuged cells with anti-idiotype conjugated with rhodamine. Double staining proves the point. Well now, why could the initial question not be answered unequivocally in the affirmative? The answer lies in somatic mutation.

Class-switched B-cells are subject to high mutation rates after the initial response

The reader will no doubt recollect that this idea was raised in Chapter 3 when discussing the generation of diversity. The normal V region mutation rate is of the order of 10^{-5}/base pair/cell division but this rises to 10^{-3}/base pair/generation in B-cells as a result of antigenic stimulation. This process is illustrated well in figure 7.9 which charts the accumulation of somatic mutations in the immunodominant V_H/V_K antibody structure during the immune response to phenyloxazolone. With time and successive boosting the mutation rate is seen to rise dramatically, and in the context of the present discussion it is clear that mutations occurring within or adjacent to the complementarity determining hypervariable loops can give rise to cells which secrete antibodies having a different combining affinity to that of the original parent cell. Randomly, some mutated daughter cells will have higher affinity for antigen, some the same or lower and others perhaps none at all. Similarly, mutations in the framework regions may be 'silent' or, if they perturb the ability of the molecule to fold properly, give rise to non-functional molecules. Pertinently, the proportions of germinal centre B-cells with 'silent' mutations is high early in the immune response but falls dramatically with time suggesting that early diversification is followed by preferential expansion of clones expressing mutations which improve their chances of reacting with and being stimulated by antigen.

Antibody affinity

The effect of antigen dose

Other things being equal, the binding strength of an antigen for the surface antibody receptor of a B-cell will be determined by the usual affinity constant of the reaction:

$$Ag + (surface)Ab \rightleftharpoons AgAb$$

and the reactants will behave according to the Law of Mass Action (cf. p. 71).

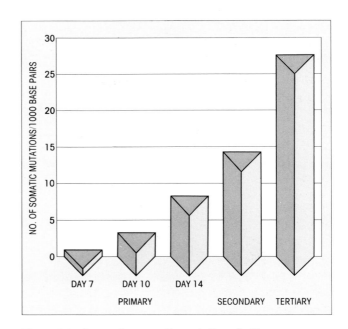

Figure 7.9. *Increasing somatic mutations in the immunodominant germ line antibody observed in hybridomas isolated following repeated immunization with phenyloxazolone. (Data from Berek C. & Apel M. (1989)* **Progress in Immunol.,** *vii, 99. Melchers F. et al. (eds). Springer Verlag, Berlin.)*

It may be supposed that when an appropriate number of antigen molecules are bound to the antibody receptors on the cell surface, the lymphocyte will be stimulated to develop into an antibody-producing clone. When only small amounts of antigen are present, only those lymphocytes with high-affinity antibody receptors will be able to bind sufficient antigen for stimulation to occur and their daughter cells will, of course, also produce high-affinity antibody. Consideration of the antigen–antibody equilibrium equation will show that, as the concentration of antigen is increased, even antibodies with relatively low affinity will bind more antigen; therefore at high doses of antigen the lymphocytes with lower-affinity antibody receptors will also be stimulated and, as may be seen from figure 7.10, these are more abundant than those with receptors of high affinity. Furthermore, there is a strong possibility that cells with the highest affinity will bind so much antigen, as to become tolerized (cf. p. 187). Thus, in summary, low amounts of antigen produce high-affinity antibodies, whereas high antigen concentrations give rise to an anti-serum with low to moderate affinity.

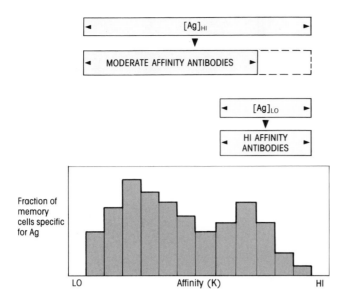

Figure 7.10. *Relationship of antigen concentration to affinity of antibodies produced. Low concentrations of antigen ([Ag]$_{LO}$) bind to and stimulate a range of high affinity memory cells and the resulting antibodies are of high affinity. High doses of antigen ([Ag]$_{HI}$) are able to bind sufficiently to the low affinity cells and to stimulate them, whilst the highest affinity cells may bind an excess of antigen and be tolerized; the resulting antiserum will have a population of low to moderate affinity antibodies.*

Maturation of affinity

In addition to being brisker and fatter, secondary responses tend to be of higher affinity, which from our point of view is a particularly felicitous state of affairs. There are probably two main reasons for this maturation of affinity after primary stimulation. First, once the primary response gets under way and the antigen concentration declines to low levels, only successively higher affinity cells will bind sufficient antigen to maintain proliferation. Second, at this stage the cells are mutating madly in the germinal centres and any mutants with an adventitiously higher affinity will bind well to antigen on follicular dendritic cells and be positively selected for by its persistent clonal expansion. The increase in somatic mutation which occurs *pari passu* with the maturation of affinity accords well with this analysis and argues against the view that high-

affinity clones arise without mutation from very small numbers of precursors in the preimmune population. Modification of antibody specificity by point mutations allows gradual diversification on which positive selection for affinity can act during clonal expansion; on the other hand, other mechanisms such as gene conversion which produce gross changes are more likely to destroy the antigen binding structure.

It is worth noting that responses to thymus-independent antigens which have poorly developed memory with very rare mutations do not show this phenomenon of affinity maturation. Overall, the ability of T-cell helpers to facilitate responses to non-polymeric, non-polyclonally activating antigens, to induce expansive clonal proliferation, to effect class switching and, lastly, to fine-tune responses to higher affinity has provided us with bigger, better and more flexible immune responses.

The monoclonal antibody revolution

First in rodents

A fantastic technological breakthrough was achieved by Milstein and Köhler who devised a technique for the production of 'immortal' clones of cells making single antibody specificities by fusing normal antibody-forming cells with an appropriate B-cell tumour line. These so-called 'hybridomas' are selected out in a tissue culture medium which fails to support growth of the parental cell types, and by successive dilutions or by plating out, single clones can be established (figure 7.11). These clones can be propagated in spinner culture or grown up in the ascitic form in mice when quite prodigious titres of monoclonal antibody can be attained. Remember that even in a good antiserum, over 90% of the Ig molecules have little or no avidity for the antigen, and the 'specific antibodies' themselves represent a whole spectrum of molecules with different avidities directed against different determinants on the antigen. What a contrast is provided by the monoclonal antibodies where all the molecules produced by a given hybridoma are identical: they have the same

Figure 7.11 continued
secreting heterohybridoma obtained by fusing a mouse myeloma with human B-cells can be used as a productive fusion partner for antibody-producing human B-cells. Other groups have turned to the well-characterized murine fusion partners and the heterohybridomas so formed grow well,

clone easily and are productive. There is some instability from chromosome loss and it appears that antibody production is maintained by translocation of human Ig genes to mouse chromosomes. Fusion frequency is even better if EBV-transformed lines are used instead of B-cells.

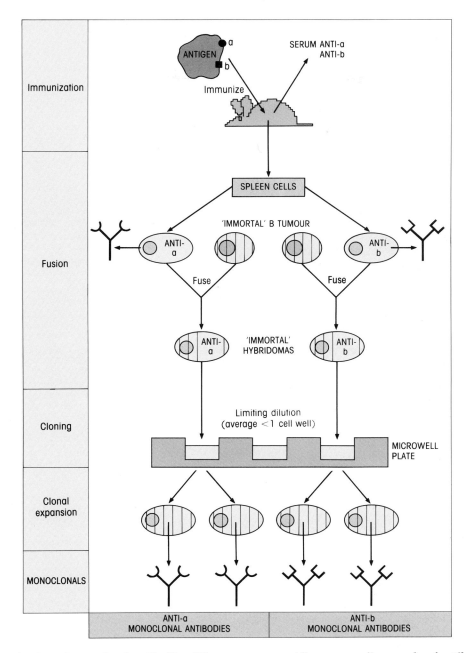

Immunization

Fusion

Cloning

Clonal expansion

MONOCLONALS

ANTIGEN
a
b

SERUM ANTI-a ANTI-b

Immunize

SPLEEN CELLS

'IMMORTAL' B TUMOUR

ANTI-a

ANTI-b

Fuse

Fuse

'IMMORTAL' HYBRIDOMAS

ANTI-a

ANTI-b

Limiting dilution
(average <1 cell well)

MICROWELL PLATE

ANTI-a
MONOCLONAL ANTIBODIES

ANTI-b
MONOCLONAL ANTIBODIES

137

Figure 7.11. *Production of monoclonal antibodies. Mice immunized with an antigen bearing (shall we say) two epitopes, **a** and **b**, develop spleen cells making anti-**a** and anti-**b** which appear as antibodies in the serum. The spleen is removed and the individual cells fused in polyethylene glycol with constantly dividing (i.e. 'immortal') B-tumour cells selected for a purine enzyme deficiency and often for their inability to secrete Ig. The resulting cells are distributed into micro-well plates in HAT (hypoxanthine, aminopterin, thymidine) medium which kills off the perfusion partners, at such a high cell dilution that **on average** each well will contain less than one hybridoma cell. Each hybridoma being the fusion product of a single antibody-forming cell and a tumour cell will have the ability of the former to secrete a single species of antibody and the immortality of the latter enabling it to proliferate continuously, clonal progeny providing an unending supply of antibody with a single specificity—the monoclonal antibody. In this example, we considered the production of hybridomas with specificity for just two epitopes, but the same technique enables monoclonal antibodies to be raised against complex mixtures of multiepitopic antigens. Fusions using rat cells instead of mouse may have certain advantages in giving a higher proportion of stable hybridomas, and monoclonals which are better at fixing human complement, a useful attribute in the context of therapeutic applications to humans involving cell depletion.*

Naturally for use in the human, the ideal solution is the production of purely human monoclonals. Human myeloma fusion partners have not found wide acceptance since they tend to have low fusion efficiencies, poor growth and secretion of Ig which dilutes the desired monoclonal. A non-

Ig class and allotype, the same variable region, structure, idiotype, affinity and specificity for a given epitope.

Whereas the large amount of non-specific, relative to antigen-specific, Ig in an antiserum means that background binding to antigen in any given immunological test may be uncomfortably high, the problem is greatly reduced with a monoclonal antibody preparation since all the Ig is antibody, thus giving a much superior 'signal:noise' ratio. By being directed towards single epitopes on the antigen, monoclonal antibodies frequently show high specificity in terms of their low cross-reactivity with other antigens. Occasionally, however, one sees quite unexpected binding to molecules which react poorly, if at all, with a specific antiserum directed to the original antigen. The reason for this has already been discussed (p. 74). Suffice it to say here that the problem can be circumvented by using a group of overlapping monoclonals reacting with the same determinant or a combination of monoclonals to more than one determinant on the same antigen.

An outstanding advantage of the monoclonal antibody as a reagent is that it provides a single standard material for all laboratories throughout the world to use in an unending supply if the immortality and purity of the cell line is nurtured; antisera raised in different animals, on the other hand, may be as different from each other as chalk and cheese. The monoclonal approach again shows a clean pair of heels relative to conventional strategies in the production of antibodies specific for individual components in a complex mixture of antigens, which, for example, one may wish to do in trying to identify which of a set of antigens on a given parasite can generate antibodies which are protective for the host. Whereas in the prehybridoma era we would have tried to purify individual antigens from the complex mixture and then raised antibodies to each component, now we would make a large number of hybridomas from the spleen of an animal immunized with the complete antigen mixture and separate the individual hybridomas by simple cloning. It must be clear that we now have in our hands a really powerful technique whose applications are truly legion. Some of these are touched upon in table 7.1 to give the reader an inkling of what is possible but the potential defies the imagination; the separation of individual cell types with specific surface markers (lymphocyte subpopulations, neural cells, etc.), diagnosis of lymphoid and myeloid malignancies, tissue typing, radioimmunoassay, serotyping of micro-organisms,

Table 7.1. *Some applications of monoclonal antibodies.*

ENUMERATION OF HUMAN LYMPHOCYTE SUBPOPULATIONS	Anti-CD3 identifies all mature T-cells Anti-CD4 identifies subset containing T-helpers Anti-CD8 identifies cytotoxic-suppressor T-cells
CELL DEPLETION	Cocktail of anti-CD3 monoclonals + complement kills T-cells in human bone marrow to prevent graft vs host reaction (p. 279)
CELL ISOLATION	Separation of murine Lyt1 + ve T-cells by monoclonal anti-Lyt1 in the FACS (p. 99)
IMMUNOSUPPRESSION	Anti-CD3 depresses T-cell function Anti-CD4 induces tolerance
PASSIVE IMMUNIZATION	High titre anti-microbial human monoclonals can give passive protection
PROBING FUNCTION OF CELL SURFACE MOLECULES	Anti-CD8 inhibits killing by cytotoxic T-cells Anti-Ia monoclonal inhibits T-cell response to macrophage-processed Ag
BLOOD GROUPING	Anti-A monoclonal provides more reliable standard reagent than conventional antisera
DIAGNOSIS IN CANCER	Monoclonal anti-T-ALL allows differentiation from non-T-ALL (cf. p. 191) Follicle centre cell lymphoma identified by peroxidase-labelled anti-common ALL in tissue sections
IMAGING	Radioactive anti-carcinoembryonic antigen (p. 297) used to localize colonic tumours or secondaries by scanning
IMMUNOASSAY	Good discrimination for assay of antigen by monoclonals to more than one site
ANALYSIS OF COMPLEX ANTIGEN MIXTURES	Identification of the 'protective' antigen in parasite suitable for vaccine production Identification of antigenic 'patch' on acetyl choline receptor involved in experimental myasthenia gravis (p. 329)
PURIFICATION OF ANTIGEN	Isolate from mixtures by monoclonal on affinity column
ANALYSIS OF EMBRYOLOGICAL RELATIONSHIPS	Separate monoclonals to neurons of neural tube and neural crest origin help to define embryological derivation of cells in nervous system
MONOCLONAL MUTANTS	Mutants lacking Fc structures used for in vivo neutralization of toxic drugs e.g. digoxin overdose, or for defining biological roles of Fc domains
GENETICALLY ENGINEERED ANTIBODIES	Transfer mouse CDRs to human Ig framework Change Fc isotype to improve particular function
FUSED HYBRIDOMAS	Producing antibodies with dual specificity
ANALYSIS OF IMMUNE RESPONSE	Hybridomas made during an immune response give data on repertoire and on mutation events (the original reason for developing the hybridoma technology)
ARTIFICIAL ENZYMES ('ABZYMES')	Monoclonal antibodies which recognize the transitional state of the reactants in a reversible reaction can simulate an enzyme — early days but big potential

elucidation of the fine structure of the antibody combining site and the basis for variability, immunological intervention with passive antibody, anti-idiotype inhibition or 'magic bullet' therapy with cytotoxic agents coupled to antitumour-specific antibody—these and many other areas are being transformed by hybridoma technology.

Abzymes

An especially interesting development with tremendous potential is the recognition that a monoclonal antibody to a stable analogue of the transition state of a given reaction can act as an enzyme ('abzyme') in catalysing that reaction. The possibility of generating enzymes to order promises a very attractive future, and some exceedingly adroit chemical manoeuvres have already extended the range of reactions which can be catalysed in this way. A recent demonstration of sequence-specific peptide cleavage with an antibody which incorporates a metal complex cofactor has raised the pulse rate of the *cognoscenti* since this is an energetically difficult reaction which has an enormous range of applications.

Curiously, an 'autoabzyme' (*sic*) which catalyses the cleavage of vasoactive intestinal peptide (the neural mediator of non-adrenergic, non-cholinergic relaxation of airway smooth muscle—no less) has been found in the serum IgG of around 16% of adult asthma patients and strenuously exercising healthy subjects. The autoantibody in non-asthmatics is bound to a small inhibitor and has a far lower affinity, but even so it does leave one wondering what else might be lurking in the murky depths of one's blood circulation.

Human monoclonals can be made

Mouse monoclonals injected into human subjects for therapeutic purposes are frightfully immunogenic and the human anti-mouse antibodies (HAMA in the trade) so formed are a wretched nuisance, accelerating clearance of the monoclonal from the blood and possibly causing hypersensitivity reactions, preventing the mouse antibody from reaching its target and, in some cases, blocking its binding to antigen. In some circumstances it is conceivable that a mouse monoclonal taken up by a tumour cell could be processed and become the MHC-linked target of cytotoxic T-cells or help to boost the response to a weakly immunogenic antigen on the tumour cell surface. In general, however, logic points to removal of the xenogeneic (foreign) portions of the monoclonal antibody and their replacement by human Ig structures using recombinant DNA technology. Chimaeric constructs, in which the V_H and V_L mouse domains are spliced onto human C_H and C_L genes (figure 7.12a), are far less immunogenic in humans although they have a tendency to provoke anti-idiotype responses;

these have to be circumvented by using chimaeric antibodies bearing different idiotypes for subsequent injections. The choicest construct so far is one in which the six CDRs of the Campath-1 rat anti-human leucocyte monoclonal were grafted to a completely human Ig framework without loss of specific reactivity (figure 7.12b).

This is not a trivial exercise, however, and the objective of fusing human B-cells to make hybridomas is still appealing, taking into account not only the gross reduction in immunogenicity, but also the fact that within a species, antibodies can be made to subtle differences such as MHC polymorphic molecules and tumour-associated antigens on other individuals, whereas xenogeneic responses are more directed to immunodominant structures common to most subjects. Notwithstanding the difficulties in finding good fusion partners, large numbers of human monoclonals have been established. A further restriction arises because the peripheral blood B-cells, which are the only B-cells readily available in the human, are not normally regarded as a good source of antibody-forming cells. If, as we are told, good primary responses with peripheral blood lymphocytes can be obtained *in vitro* by addition to the culture of the methyl O-ester of leucine which eliminates monocytes, NK cells and cytotoxic T-cells, then we have cause to hope that this approach will provide B-cells of wide specificities for human hybridomas.

Many human monoclonals are awaiting the go-ahead for clinical use; one can cite IgG anti-RhD for the prevention of rhesus disease of the newborn (p. 262), and highly potent monoclonals for protection against varicella zoster, cytomegalovirus, group B streptococci and lipopolysaccharide endotoxins of Gram-negative bacteria.

Genetically engineered antibody variants

The wiles of modern molecular biology provide us with the ability to fabricate a rich variety of modified forms of monoclonal antibodies. Reference has already been made to the 'humanizing' of rodent antibodies and a series of other possible strategies are illustrated in figure 7.12. Comment on the single heavy-chain variable-domain miniantibodies is warranted (figure 7.12d). The affinity of these domain antibodies (DABs) after antigen selection proved to be unexpectedly high—of the order of 20 nanomolar; this can be improved by site-specific mutagenesis or by transfection together with a library of V_L genes and selection of strong binders

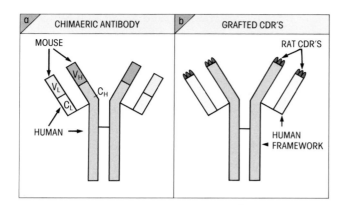

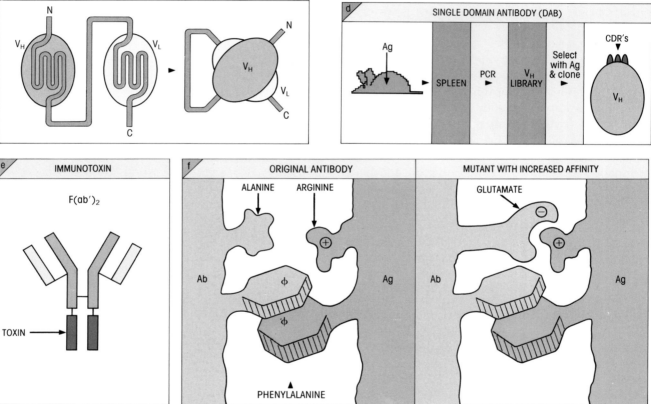

Figure 7.12. *Genetically engineered antibody variants. (a) Chimaeric antibody with mouse variable regions fused to human Ig constant region. (b) 'Humanized' rat monoclonal in which gene segments coding for all 6 CDRs are grafted on to a human Ig framework. (c) A single gene encoding V_H and V_L joined by a sequence of suitable length gives rise to an Fv antigen-binding fragment. (d) A V_H library derived from the spleen of an immunized mouse can yield single V_H domains with acceptably high affinity for the immunizing antigen. (e) Potential 'magic bullets' can be constructed by fusing the gene for a toxin (e.g. ricin) to the Fab. (f) By site-specific mutagenesis of residues in or adjacent to the complementarity determining region (CDR), it is possible to increase the affinity of the antibody at will.*

140

by antigen. The small size of the minigenes could be exploited for tissue penetration and, as the authors aggressively state, for patent busting.

CELL-MEDIATED IMMUNITY HAS TWO ARMS

In combating intracellular infections by acquired immune responses, T-cells exploit two main strategies: the first, secretion of soluble factors called *lymphokines* which activate the cells they combine with to enhance their contribution to microbicidal defence mechanisms and, second, the production of *cytolytic T-cells* which kill the infected target. Although the distinction between these strategies is not quite as clear cut as it sounds, it suits us to use them as a convenient basis for discussion.

Lymphokines are part of a complex cytokine network

Cytokines act as intercellular messengers

The triggering event in the response to an infectious agent involves the direct reaction of the foreign molecules with macrophage receptors, the complement system, antigen-specific lymphocyte receptors, and so on. Orchestration of the subsequent immune/inflammatory responses, however, largely depends upon communication between the participating and interacting cells by soluble molecules, given the generic term, *cytokines*. Lymphokines represent the contribution made through the acquired immune response to this process but because the system as a whole involves a network of all cytokines, not just those derived from lymphocytes, it only makes sense to discuss the cytokine interactions as an integrated totality. This will include relationships between cells in the immune system with cells conventionally outside the system, and also with cells controlling haematopoiesis.

Cytokine action is transient and usually short-range

The cytokines, which include the group previously called lymphokines, monokines, interleukins and interferons (see table 7.2), are low molecular weight secreted proteins, usually of the order of 15—25 kDa, which regulate the amplitude and duration of the immune-inflammatory responses. They must therefore be produced in a transient manner tightly regulated by the presence of foreign material, and it is relevant that the AU-rich sequences in the 3'-untranslated regions of the mRNA of many cytokines are correlated directly with rapid degradation and therefore short half-life. Unlike endocrine hormones, the majority of cytokines normally act locally in a paracrine or even autocrine fashion and the reader may recollect experiments showing a concentration of cytokine at the pole of the secreting cell receiving the maximum stimulus (cf. p. 124). Thus lymphokines rarely persist in the circulation but non-lymphoid cells can be triggered by bacterial products to release cytokines which may be detected in the bloodstream often to the detriment of the host. There is a growing suspicion that certain cytokines, perhaps IL-1 and TNF, may exist in membrane forms which could exert their stimulatory effects without becoming soluble.

Cytokines are highly potent, often acting at femtomolar (10^{-15} M) concentrations, combining with small numbers of high-affinity cell surface receptors to produce changes in the pattern of RNA and protein synthesis. In general, they are pleiotropic, i.e. with multiple effects on growth and differentiation of a variety of cell types (figure 7.2), and there is considerable overlapping and redundancy between them, partially accounted for by the induction of synthesis of common proteins.

Network interactions

The complex and integrated relationships between the different cytokines are mediated through cellular events. The genes for IL-3, 4, 5 and GM-CSF are all tightly linked on chromosome 5 in a region containing genes for M-CSF and its receptor and several other growth factors and receptors. Interaction may occur through a cascade in which one cytokine induces the production of another, through transmodulation of the receptor for another cytokine and through synergism or antagonism of two cytokines acting on the same cell (see figure 7.13). Despite the widespread success in cloning and sequencing individual cytokines and their receptors, the means by which target cells integrate and interpret the complex patterns of stimuli induced by these multiple soluble factors is still an unresolved puzzle.

Assessment of individual cytokines

Originally, cytokines were usually estimated by the functional effect in various biological assays of a T-cell 'soup' secreted during the proliferative response of sensitized T-cells to specific antigens or to polyclonal activators. One of the favourites used to be the measurement of migration inhibition factor (MIF; probably IL-4) which suppressed the movement of macrophages. The system, which the more historically minded can read about in greater detail in earlier editions, involved packing a mixture of lymphocytes and macrophages into capillary tubes which were then incubated overnight with antigen in dishes; the cells would migrate out of the capillaries to form a fan of cells on the floor of the dish and any reduction in the area of migration was attributable to MIF. Where possible, one used a cellular assay system thought to be entirely dependent upon the activity of a single cytokine, as for example the proliferative response of thymocytes to IL-1 and of IL-2-dependent T-cell lines for interleukin-2.

CYTOKINE	SOURCE	STIMULATORY FUNCTION‡
INTERLEUKINS		
IL-1	Mφ, fibroblasts	Proliferation activated B- & T-cells Induction PGE$_2$ & cytokines by Mφ Induction neutrophil & T-adhesion molecules on endothelial cells Induction IL-6, IFN-β1 & GM-CSF Induction fever, acute phase proteins, bone resorption by osteoclasts
IL-2	T	Growth activated T- and B-cells; activation NK cells
IL-3	T, MC	Growth & differentiation haematopoetic precursors Mast cell growth
IL-4	CD4 T, MC, BM stroma	Proliferation activated B-, T-, mast & haemopoietic precursor Induction MHC class II and FcεR on B-cells, p75 IL-2R on T-cells Isotype switch to IgG1 & IgE Mφ APC & cytotoxic function, Mφ fusion (migration inhibition)
IL-5	CD4 T, MC	Proliferation activated B-cells; production IgM & IgA Proliferation eosinophils; expression p55 IL-2R
IL-6	CD4 T, Mφ, MC, fibroblasts	Growth & differentiation B- and T-cell effectors, & haemopoietic precursors Acute phase proteins
IL-7	BM stromal cells	Proliferation pre-B, CD4- CD8- T-cells & activated mature T-cells
IL-8	Monocytes	Chemotaxis & activation neutrophils Chemotaxis T-cells
COLONY STIMULATING FACTORS		
GM-CSF	T, Mφ, fibroblasts, MC, endothelium	Growth granulocyte & Mφ colonies Activates Mφ, neutrophils, eosinophils
G-CSF	Fibroblasts, endothelium	Growth mature granulocytes
M-CSF	Fibroblasts, endothelium epithelium	Growth macrophage colonies
TUMOUR NECROSIS FACTORS		
TNF-α TBF-β	Mφ, T CD4 T	Tumour cytotoxicity; cachexia; Induction acute phase proteins Anti-viral & anti-parasitic activity Activation phagocytic cells Induction IFNγ, TNFα, IL-1, GM-CSF & IL-6 Endotoxic shock
INTERFERONS		
IFNα IFNβ	Leucocytes Fibroblasts	Anti-viral; expression MHC I
IFNγ	T (Mφ?)	Anti-viral; Mφ activation Expression MHC class I & II on Mφ & other cells Differentiation of cytotoxic T Synthesis IgG2a by activated B Antagonism several IL/4 actions
OTHER		
TGF-β	T, B	Inhibition IL-2R upregulation and IL-2 dependent T- and B-cell proliferation, Inhibition (by TGF-β1) of IL-3 + CSF induced haematopoiesis Isotype switch to IgA Wound repair (fibroblast chemotaxin) and angiogenesis Neoplastic transformation certain normal cells
CSIF	CD4 T	Inhibits IFNγ secretion
LIF	T	Proliferation embryonic stem cells without affecting differentiation chemoattraction & activation of eosinophils

Table 7.2. *Cytokines: their origin and function. Mø, macrophage; MC, mast cell; BM, bone marrow.*

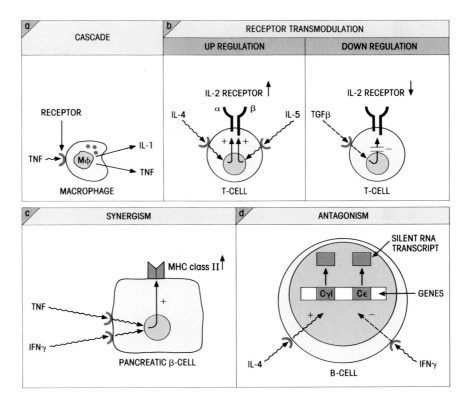

Figure 7.13. *Network interactions of cytokines. (a) Cascade: in this example TNF induces secretion of IL-1 and of itself (autocrine) in the macrophage (note all diagrams in this figure are simplified in that the effects on the nucleus are due to messengers resulting from combination of cytokine with its surface receptor); (b) receptor transmodulation showing upregulation of each chain forming the high affinity IL-2 receptor in an activated T-cell by individual lymphokines and downregulation by TGFβ; and (c) synergy of TNF and IFNγ in upregulation of surface MHC class II molecules on cultured pancreatic insulin-secreting cells and antagonism of IL-4 and IENγ on transcription of silent mRNA relating to isotype switch (cf. figure 7.7).*

The growing awareness of the pleiotropic and network effects of cytokines has alerted us to the possible pitfalls in many of these biological systems and the availability of recombinant cytokines and monoclonal antibodies has seen a burgeoning of immunoassay tests. As ever, caution must be exercised in extrapolating effects observed *in vitro* to the behaviour of a cytokine *in vivo* since on occasions this can be misleading and it is more reassuring to analyse the role in physiological and pathological responses by injection of a specific neutralizing antibody if available.

Do different T-cell subsets make different lymphokines?

There is not a broad consensus on the answer but in the mouse, long-term T-helper clones can be divided into two types with distinct cytokine secretion phenotypes (table 7.3). This makes biological sense in that T_{h1} cells producing lymphokines like IFNγ would be especially effective against intracellular infections with viruses and organisms which grow in macrophages, whereas T_{h2} cells are very good helpers for B-cells and would seem to be adapted for defence against parasites which are vulnerable to IL-4-switched IgE, IL-5-induced eosinophilia and IL-3/4-stimulated mast cell proliferation. Studies on

the infection of mice with the pathogenic protozoan *Leishmania major* do not conflict with this hypothesis. Intravenous or intraperitoneal injection of killed promastigotes leads to protection against challenge with live parasites associated with high expression of IFNγ mRNA and low levels of IL-4

Table 7.3. *Cytokine patterns of mouse T-cell clones.*

CYTOKINE PATTERNS OF MOUSE T-CELL CLONES			
	T_{H1}	T_{H2}	T_c
IFNγ			
IL-2			
TNFβ			
TNFα			
GM-CSF			
IL-3			
Met. enkephalin			
IL-4			
IL-5			
IL-6			
CSIF			

██ ++   ☐ +   ☐ Negative

$T_{h1/2}$ = T-helper-1/2; T_c = cytotoxic T-cell (from Mormann et al. (1989) Progress in Immunol., 7, 611. Melchers F. et al. (eds) Springer-Verlag, Berlin).

143

PRODUCTION OF EFFECTORS

mRNA; the reciprocal finding of low IFNγ and high IL-4 expression was made after subcutaneous immunization which failed to provide protection. Furthermore, non-vaccinated mice infected with live organisms could be saved by injection of IFNγ and anti-IL-4. These results are consistent with preferential expansion of a population of protective IFNγ-secreting T_{h1} cells by i.p. or i.v. immunization, and of non-protective T_{h2} cells producing IL-4 in the subcutaneously injected animals.

And yet, having said all that, no such clear cut patterns of secreted lymphokines have been demonstrable in human or rat T-cell clones, or even in murine cells early after immunization. We should recall that the original Mosmann/Coffman classification into T_{h1} and T_{h2} subsets was predicted on data obtained with clones which had been maintained in culture for long periods and might have been artefacts of conditions *in vitro*. It could be that, in the mouse at least, early T_h cells secrete T_{h1} and T_{h2} lymphokines and later differentiate into either T_{h1} or T_{h2} cells depending upon the nature of the antigen stimulus (figure 7.14). The ability of IFNγ, the characteristic T_{h1} lymphokine, to inhibit proliferation of T_{h2} clones, and of T_{h2}-derived CSIF to block both proliferation and cytokine release by T_{h1} cells suggest that the ideas cannot be ignored.

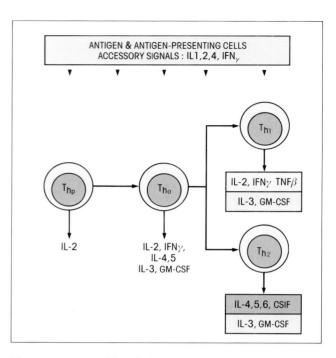

Figure 7.14. *Possible T-helper phenotypes and their interrelationships. There may be one or more intermediates on the differentiation pathways represented by the arrows. (T_{hp} = T- helper precursor; T_{ho} = early undifferentiated helper cell; other abbreviations as in tables 7.2 and 7.3.)*

Cytokines control haemopoiesis

The differentiation of stem cells to become the formed elements of blood within the environment of the bone marrow is carefully nurtured through production of cytokines by the stromal cells. These include GM-CSF, G-CSF, M-CSF, IL-6, IL-7 and LIF (see table 7.2) and many of them are also derived from T-cells and macrophages. It is not surprising, therefore, that during a period of chronic inflammation, the cytokines produced recruit new precursors into the haematopoietic differentiation pathway—a useful exercise in the circumstances. One of the lymphokines, IL-3, should be highlighted for its exceptional ability to support the early cells in this pathway, particularly in synergy with IL-6 and G-CSF.

Cytokine function in the adaptive immune response

The roles of various cytokines in the activation, proliferation and differentiation of B-cells have al-

ready been considered, but a few words on the nature of IL-6 may not be out of place. This cytokine plays an important role in the maturation of activated B-cells into plasma cells and has made previous appearances as BSF-2, BCDF and IFNβ2. It is pleiotropic with a vengeance, having major effects on haematopoiesis, thrombopoiesis, T-cell growth and differentiation, acute phase protein production, and proliferation of glomerular mesangial cells.

In so far as T-cells are concerned, amplification following activation is critically dependent upon IL-2. This lymphokine is a single peptide of molecular weight 15.5 kDa which acts only on cells which express high-affinity IL-2 receptors. These receptors are not present on resting cells, but 9 hours after polyclonal activation the genes for IL-2 receptor begin to be transcribed, and only after a further 15 hours are the IL-2 genes themselves expressed (figure 7.15).

The IL-2 receptor is composed of an α-chain (reacting with the CD25 Tac monoclonal) of low affinity, and a β-chain of intermediate affinity (figure 7.16). IL-2 binds to and dissociates from the α-chain very rapidly but the same processes involving the β-chain occur 2−3 orders of magnitude

144

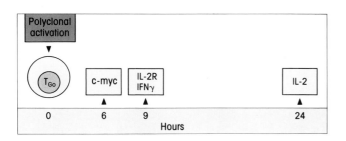

Figure 7.15. *Sequential transcription of genes for the c-myc proto-oncogene, IL-2 receptor (IL-2R), γ-interferon (IFNγ) and IL-2 following polyclonal activation of resting human T-cells. The transcriptions are unaffected by the presence of cycloheximide showing that they are independent of protein synthesis and therefore that the c-myc protein itself, for example, is not involved.*

more slowly. When the α- and β-chains form a single receptor, the α-chain binds the IL-2 rapidly and facilitates its binding at a separate site to the β-chain from which it can only dissociate slowly. Since the final affinity (K_d) is based on the ratio of dissociation to association rate constants, then $K_d = 10^{-4}$ s^{-1}/10^7 M^{-1} s^{-1} = 10^{-11} M which is a very high affinity. This could represent a general model for cytokine 2-chain receptors of which there appear to be an increasing number, although in the case of the IL-6 receptor, the second chain is not thought to bind the cytokine.

Separation of an activated T-cell population into those with high- and low-affinity IL-2 receptors showed clearly that an adequate number of high-affinity receptors were mandatory for the mitogenic action of IL-2. It is the skewed cellular distribution of these high-affinity receptors which is responsible for the asynchronous division of activated T-cells on addition of IL-2. The numbers of these receptors on the cell increase under the action of antigen and of IL-2, and as antigen is cleared, so the receptor numbers decline and, with that, the responsiveness to IL-2. It should be appreciated that although IL-2 is an immunologically non-specific T-cell growth factor, it only functions appropriately in specific responses because unstimulated T-cells do not express IL-2 receptors.

The proliferative effect of IL-2 is reinforced by the action of IL-4 and to some extent IL-6 which react with corresponding receptors on the dividing T-cells. We must not lose sight of the importance of control mechanisms, and obvious candidates to subsume this role are TGFβ, which blocks IL-2-induced proliferation (figure 7.13b) and production of TNFα and β, and the two cytokines IFNγ and CSIF which mediate the mutual antagonism of T_{h1} and T_{h2} subsets.

145

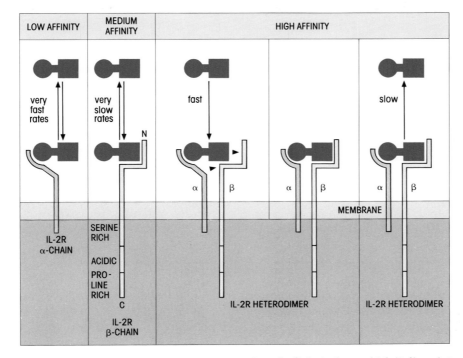

Figure 7.16. *Formation of 2-chain high affinity IL-2 receptor. IL-2 associates rapidly with the α-chain, which passes the IL-*
2 to the β-chain from which it dissociates slowly. The fast on and slow off rates give the high affinity of ligand binding.

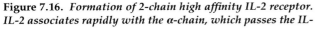

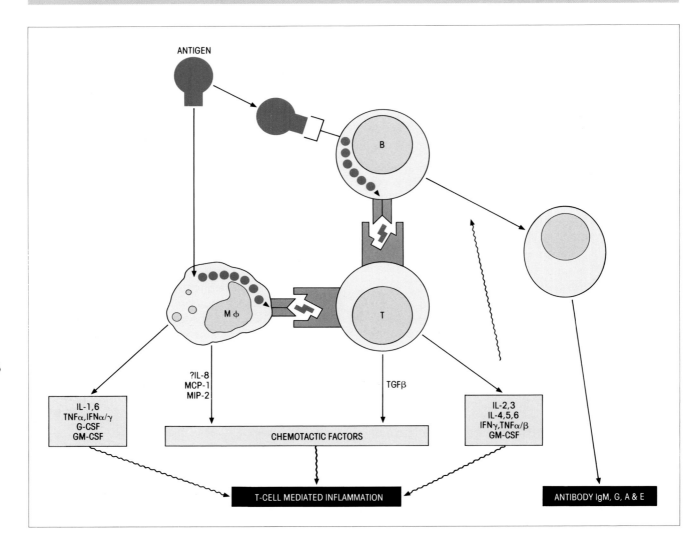

Figure 7.17. *Cytokines controlling the antibody and T-cell mediated inflammatory responses (abbreviations as in table 7.2; MCP-1 = macrophage chemotactic protein; MIP-2 =* *macrophage inflammatory protein having substantial sequence homology with IL-8). (After Nakayama N. et al. (1989)* **Current Opinion in Immunol., 2, 68.)**

Cytokines mediate chronic inflammatory responses

In addition to their role in the adaptive response, the T-cell lymphokines are responsible for generating antigen-specific chronic inflammatory reactions which deal with intracellular parasites (figure 7.17) although there is a different emphasis on the pattern of factors involved (cf. p. 218).

The initiating event is the encounter between an antigen-specific T-cell trafficking through the tissue and processed antigenic peptide, derived from the intracellular infective organism, on the surface of an antigen-presenting cell. Secreted lymphokines such as TNF induce the synthesis of adhesion molecules on adjacent vascular endothelial cells, including a homing receptor for T-cells which is characteristically related to an inflammatory site; in this way the chances of further memory T-cells in the circulation meeting the antigen provoking inflammation will be greatly enhanced. Macrophages with intracellular organisms are activated by agents such as IFNγ, GM-CSF, IL-2 and TNF and should become endowed with microbicidal powers. During this process, some macrophages may die (helped along by cytotoxic T-cells?) and release living parasites, but these will be dealt with by fresh macrophages brought to the site by chemotaxis and newly activated by local cytokines so that they have passed the stage of differentiation at which the intracellular parasites can subvert their killing mechanisms (cf. p. 212).

Virally-infected cells require a different strategy and one strand of that strategy exploits the innate interferon mechanism to deny the virus access to the cell's replicative machinery. IFNγ of course does this but note that TNFα and β both induce 2'-5'(A) synthetase, a protein also switched on by IFN and which is involved in viral protection. TNF has another string to its bow in its ability to kill certain cells, since death of an infected cell before viral replication has occurred is obviously beneficial to the host. Its cytotoxic potential was first recognized using tumour cells as targets (hence the name) and recent work with cloned products reveals a synergism between IFNγ and lymphotoxin (figure 7.18) in which IFNγ sets up the cell for destruction by inducing the formation of TNF receptors (see also figure 7.13c). It is interesting to note also that IFNγ can affect the growth of intracellular parasites in cells other than macrophages; for example, it inhibits the growth of *Rickettsia prowazekii* in mouse fibroblast cultures.

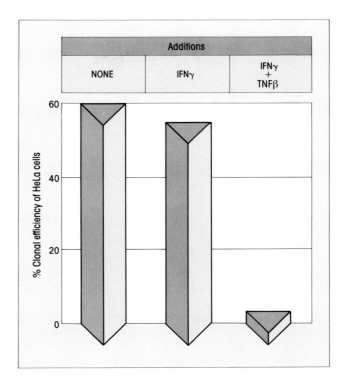

Figure 7.18. *Synergism of γ-interferon (IFNγ) and TNFβ in the growth inhibition of the HeLa tumour cell line (data from Stone-Wolff D.S. et al. (1984) J. Exp. Med. 159, 828).*

Killer T-cells

Cytolytic T-cells represent the other major arm of the cell-mediated immune response and are generally thought to be of strategic importance in the killing of virally infected cells and possibly in contributing to the postulated surveillance mechanisms against cancer cells.

The cytotoxic cell precursor cells recognize antigen on the surface of cells in association with class I MHC, and like B-cells they require help from T-cells. The mechanism by which help is proffered may, however, be quite different. As explained earlier (p.122), effective T−B collaboration is usually 'cognate' in that the collaborating cells recognize two epitopes which are physically linked (usually on the same molecule). If I may remind the reader without causing offence, the reason for this is that the surface Ig receptors on the B-cell capture native antigen, process it internally and present it to the T-helper as a peptide in association with MHC class II. Although it has been shown that linked epitopes on the antigen are also necessary for cooperation between T-helper and cytotoxic T-cell precursor (T_{cp}), the nature of T-cell recognition prevents native antigen being focused onto the T_{cp} by its receptor for subsequent processing, even if that cell were to express MHC II, which in its resting state it does not. It seems most likely that T_h and T_{cp} bind to the same antigen-presenting cell which has processed

viral antigen and displays processed viral peptides in association with both class II (for the T_h cell) and class I (for the T_{cp}) on its surface; one cannot exclude the possibility that the antigen-presenting cell could be the virally-infected cell itself. Lymphokines from the triggered T_h will be released in close proximity to the T_{cp} which is engaging the antigen-MHC signal and will be stimulated to proliferate and differentiate into a cytotoxic T-cell under the influence of IL-2 and IL-6. The possibility of a T-helper independent mechanism by which the virally infected cell triggers the antigen-specific T_{cp} through the CD2 molecule has also been mooted, but this requires greater clarification.

The frequency of the precursor cells can be measured by *limiting dilution techniques* and one such study is shown in detail in figure 7.19 because this approach is widely used to determine precursor frequency in different systems. In essence, the method depends upon the fact that if one takes several replicate aliquots of a given cell suspension which would be expected to contain *on average* one precursor per aliquot, then Poisson distribution analysis shows that 37% of the aliquots will contain *no* precursor cells (through the randomness of the

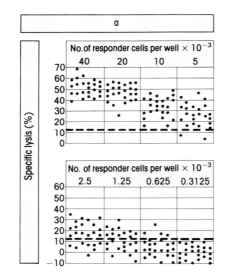

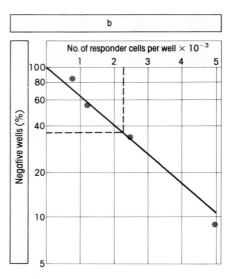

Figure 7.19. *Limiting dilution analysis of cytotoxic T-cell precursor frequency in spleen cells from a BALB/c mouse stimulated with irradiated C57BL/6 spleen cells as antigen. BALB/c splenic responder cells were set up in 24 replicates at each concentration tested together with antigen and excess of T-helper factors. The generation of cytotoxicity in each well is looked for by adding ^{51}Cr-labelled tumour cells (EL-4) of the C57BL/6 haplotype; cytotoxicity is then revealed by measuring the release of soluble ^{51}Cr-labelled intracellular material into the medium. (From Simpson E. & Chandler P. In* **Handbook of Experimental Immunology, Weir D.M. (ed.)** *(1986), figure 68.2. Blackwell Scientific Publications, Oxford, with permission.)*

(a) The points show the percentage of specific lysis of individual wells. The dotted line indicates 3 standard deviations above the medium release control, and each point above that line is counted as positive for cytotoxicity.

(b) The data replotted in terms of the percentage of negative wells at each concentration of responder cells over the range in which the data titrated (5×10^3/well to 0.625×10^3/well). The dotted line is drawn at 37% negative wells and this intersects the regression line to give a precursor (T_{cp}) frequency of 1 in 2327 responder cells. The regression line has an r^2 value of 1.00 in this experiment.

sampling). Thus, if aliquots are made from a series of dilutions of a cell suspension and incubated under conditions which allow the precursors to mature and be recognized through some amplification scheme, the dilution at which 37% of the aliquots give negative responses will be known to contain an average of one precursor cell per aliquot and one can therefore calculate the precursor frequency in the original cell suspension.

The lethal process

Cytolytic T-cells are generally of the CD8 or Ly2 subset and their binding to the target cell through T-receptor recognition of antigen plus class I MHC, is assisted by association between CD8 and class I and by other accessory molecules such as LFA-1 and CD2 (figure 6.13). MHC recognition is important for this binding but it does not seem to be involved in the signals leading to cell death, since B-cell hybridomas making anti-T3 or antibodies to the T-receptor idiotype are killed by cytolytic T-cells independently of their MHC haplotype; what does

appear to be vital is an intimate signalling to the T-receptor or the CD3 transducer.

Following activation of the killer cell, most of the cytoplasmic granules rapidly become localized between the nucleus and the target cell, together with the intracellular skeletal protein tailin which accumulates under the membrane of the cytotoxic cell, possibly protecting it from damage during the killing event. As we have argued earlier (cf. p. 15), there is evidence for exocytosis of the granule contents including perforins which cause lesions in the target cell membrane and death by colloid osmotic lysis, and TNF which kills by inducing apoptosis. The story is unfinished as yet.

Memory cells

Antibodies encoded by unmutated germ-line genes represent a form of evolutionary memory in the sense that they tend to include specificities for commonly encountered pathogens which appear in the so-called 'natural antibody' fraction of serum. Memory acquired during the adaptive immune response requires contact with antigen and ex-

148

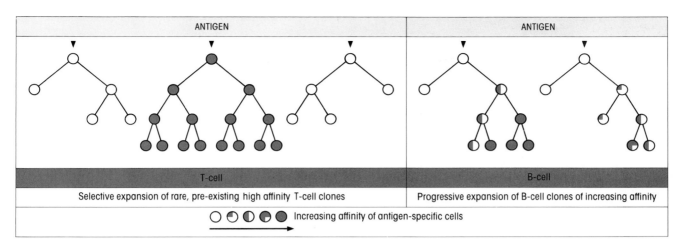

ANTIGEN	ANTIGEN
T-cell	B-cell
Selective expansion of rare, pre-existing high affinity T-cell clones	Progressive expansion of B-cell clones of increasing affinity

○ ◔ ◑ ◕ ● Increasing affinity of antigen-specific cells

Figure 7.20. *Antigen selects high affinity memory T- and B- cells by different mechanisms.*

pansion of antigen-specific memory cells as seen, for example, in the 20-fold increase in cytotoxic T-cell precursors after immunization of females with the male H-Y antigen.

Memory of early infections such as measles is long-lived and the question arises as to whether the memory cells are long-lived or are subject to repeated antigen stimulation from persisting antigen or subclinical reinfection. Panum in 1847 described a measles epidemic on the Faroe Islands in the previous year in which almost the entire population suffered from infection except for a few old people who had been infected 65 years earlier. While this evidence favours the long half-life hypothesis, recent studies show that the memory function of B-cells transferred to an irradiated syngeneic recipient is lost within a month unless antigen is given. The physiological relevance of these results has been challenged on the basis of the artificiality of the transfer environment and, in contrast, blockade of T-helper function in mice by doses of anti-CD4, which completely inhibit the generation of memory as well as primary and secondary responses, leaves established B-cell memory intact for at least 6 weeks. On the other hand, foci of antigen in the form of complexes adhering to follicular dendritic cells in germinal centres do persist for some months and this is the anatomical site considered to be entrusted with the production of memory B-cells.

The memory population is not simply an expansion of corresponding naive cells

In general, memory cells are more readily stimu-

lated by a given dose of antigen because they have a higher affinity. In the case of B-cells we have been satisfied by the evidence linking mutation and antigen selection to the creation of high affinity memory cells within the germinal centre of secondary lymph node follicles. The receptors for antigen on memory T-cells also have higher affinity but since they do not undergo somatic mutation during the priming response, it would seem that pre-existing receptors of relatively higher affinity in the population of naive cells proliferate selectively through preferential binding to the antigen (figure 7.20).

Intuitively one would not expect to improve on affinity to the same extent that somatic mutation can achieve for the B-cells, but none the less memory T-cells augment their binding avidity for the antigen-presenting cell through increased expression of accessory adhesion molecules, CD2, LFA-1, LFA-3 and ICAM-1 (table 7.4). Since several of these molecules also function to enhance signal transduction, the memory T-cell is more readily triggered than its naive cell counterpart.

An important phenotypic change in the isoform of the leucocyte common antigen CD45R, derived by differential splicing, allows a useful distinction to be made between naive and memory cells. Monoclonal antibodies to CD45RA molecules which express exon A, define naive T-cells and monoclonals which only react with the lower molecular weight form CD45RO, identify the memory cells capable of responding to recall antigens (table 7.4). Virgin B-cells lose their surface IgM and IgD and switch receptor isotype on becoming memory cells

149

Table 7.4. *Phenotype and function of naïve and memory human T-cells.*

Phenotype	Naïve	Memory	Activated
CD45RA	++	+	+
CD45RO	+	++	++
CD29 (VLA-β)	+	++	++
LFA-1	+	++	++
CD2	+	++	++
LFA-3	+	++	+++
ICAM-1	+	++	+++
IL-2Rα	+	+	+++
MHC class II	+	+	+++
Function			
Response to recall antigens	±/−	++	
Response to alloantigens	+	++	
Response to mitogens	++	++	
Helper activity	+	++	
Secretion of IL-2	++	+	
Secretion of IL-4	±/−	++	
Secretion of IFN-γ	±/−	++	

███ +++	▒▒ ++	☐ +	☐ ±/−

and the differential expression of these surface markers has greatly facilitated the separation of B- and T-cells into naïve and memory populations for the purposes of further study.

SUMMARY

Antibody-forming cells can be detected by immunofluorescent and plaque techniques. Ig peptide chains are synthesized as a single unit starting at the N-terminal end. The switch from membrane-bound to secreted IgM involves loss by RNA-splicing of the hydrophobic membrane 'anchor'.

IgM antibody responses reach an early peak and decline; IgG levels are quantitatively much higher and more persistent and dominate the secondary response. Generally speaking, T-dependent antigens through the action of T-helper cells and their soluble factors, give bigger antibody responses than T-independent antigens, and furthermore, involve isotype class-switching and the generation of memory. Individual lymphokines are related to specific class switches. Sterile transcripts of a C_H gene are associated with a switch to that class.

The evidence that one cell is programmed to make one antibody and that this provides the receptor for selection by antigen, is sound. However, the final specificity of the progeny may differ somewhat from that of the parent due to the fact that class-switched B-cells undergo surprisingly high mutation rates as they mature into memory cells. Selection of high-affinity cells arising by mutation leads to higher affinity antibody responses. Low doses of antigen provoke higher affinity antibody responses than high doses.

Immortal hybridoma cell lines making monoclonal antibodies provide powerful new immunological reagents and insights into the immune response. Applications include enumeration of lymphocyte subpopulations, cell depletion, immunoassay, cancer diagnosis and imaging, purification of antigen from complex mixtures, and recently the use of monoclonals as artificial enzymes (abzymes). Human monoclonals are valuable for passive antimicrobial protection and for immunosuppressive treatment. Intriguing genetically engineered variants can be made including single heavy chain domain antibodies (DABs).

The T-cell-mediated immune response has two arms: T-helpers which make a range of soluble effector molecules (lymphokines) and cytotoxic T-cells which are themselves responsible for direct killing, usually of virally-infected cells.

T-helpers belong to the CD4 subset in the human, L3T4 in the mouse, and their activation may be followed by proliferation or selected lymphokine release.

Lymphokines act as intercellular messengers as part of a complex cytokine network. Cytokine action is transient and usually short range. They are highly potent and act through receptors on the target cell. They have multiple effects on different cells and overlap in their activities. The network interactions result from a cascade through one cytokine inducing production of another, transmodulation of the receptor for another cytokine and through synergism or antagonism of two cytokines. Cytokines contribute to the control of haemopoiesis, macrophage activation and chronic inflammation, and growth and differentiation during the adaptive immune response.

IL-4 supports growth of B- and T-cells, the switch to IgE synthesis and the immobilization of macrophages. IL-5 is also a B-cell growth factor and induces eosinophilia, IL-6 has many effects including late-stage B-cell growth activity and induction of acute phase proteins in the liver. IL-7 is a growth factor for early T-cells while IL-8 is a chemoattractant for neutrophils. TGFβ down-regulates expression of IL-2 receptors and promotes wound healing. GM-CSF promotes growth of myeloid colonies from bone marrow stem cells in agar, but IL-3 is a panspecific haemopoietin which acts on all haemopoietic precursors and even on mature cells. γ-Interferon has a multiplicity of effects; it induces the differentiation of myeloid cells and promotes expression of class II MHC molecules on endothelial cells, a variety of epithelial cells and many tumour cell lines so facilitating interactions between T-lymphocytes and non-lymphoid cells. γ-Interferon also plays a role as a major macrophage activating factor stimulating a full range of microbicidal mechanisms which enable the phagocytes to kill intracellular organisms.

γ-Interferon also acts synergistically with the cellular poison, lymphotoxin (TNFβ) by inducing the expression of lymphotoxin receptors in the target cell.

Cytotoxic lymphocytes develop from precursors which are activated by antigen plus MHC class I and are expanded and mature by the action of IL-2 and ill-defined maturation factors produced by helper T-cells. The precursor frequency can be estimated by the method of limiting dilution analysis.

Cytolytic T-cells which belong to the CD8 (or Ly2) subsets, bind to their targets through recognition of antigen + class I by the T-cell receptor; interaction with class I is facilitated by CD8. A rapid rearrangement of cytoplasmic granules with cytotoxic potential occurs and exocytosis releases the contents onto the membrane of the target cell. Lesions are produced and the twilight and demise of the cell ensues.

Further reading

Goding J.W. (1986) *Monoclonal Antibodies: Principles and Practice*. Academic Press, London.
Lennox E.S. (ed.) (1984) Clinical applications of monoclonal antibodies. *Brit. Med. Bull.* Churchill Livingstone, UK.
Mayforth R.D. & Quintans J. (1990) Designer and catalytic antibodies. *New Engl. J. Med.* **323**, 173.
Mitchison N.A. & O'Malley C. (1987) Three-cell-type clusters of T-cells with antigen-presenting cells best explain the epitope linkage and non-cognate requirements of the *in vivo* cytolytic response. *Eur. J. Immunol.*, **17**, 1579.
Pick E. (ed.) Series *Lymphokines*. Academic Press, New York.

CHAPTER 8

THE ACQUIRED IMMUNE RESPONSE
III – Control

Antigen is a major factor in control

The acquired immune response evolved so that it would come into play when contact with an infectious agent was first made. The appropriate antigen-specific cells expand, the effectors eliminate the antigen and then the response quietens down and leaves room for reaction to other infections. Feedback mechanisms must operate to limit antibody production; otherwise, after antigenic stimulation, we would become overwhelmed by the responding clones of anti-body-forming cells and their products, a clearly unwelcome state of affairs as may be clearly seen in multiple myeloma where control over lymphocyte proliferation is lost. It makes sense for antigen to be a major regulatory factor and for antibody production to be driven by the presence of antigen, falling off in intensity as the antigen concentration drops. There is abundant evidence to support this view. Antigens can stimulate lymphocytes through their surface receptors directly as witnessed by proliferation of T-cell clones presented with antigen *in vitro* and formation of a clone of antibody-forming cells from a single B-cell precursor cultured with antigen and T-cell soluble factors under limiting-dilution conditions. Furthermore, clearance of antigen by injection of excess antibody during the course of an immune response leads to a dramatic drop in antibody synthesis and the number of antibody-secreting cells.

Antibody exerts feedback control

A useful control mechanism is to arrange for the product of a reaction to be an inhibitor and this type of negative feedback is seen with antibody. Thus we see examples of antibody diverting antigen to immunogenically inoffensive sites in the body to prevent primary sensitization in the protection against rhesus immunization afforded by administration of anti-D to mothers at risk (p. 262) and the inhibitory effect of maternal antibody on the peak titres obtained on vaccinating infants. Removal of circulating antibody by plasmapheresis during an on-going response leads to an increase in synthesis, whereas injection of preformed IgG antibody markedly hastens the fall in the number of antibody-forming cells (figure 8.1) consistent with feedback control on overall synthesis. It is unlikely that this is achieved by simple neutralization of antigen since whole IgG is so much more effective that its F(ab')$_2$ fragment in switching off the reaction even allowing for the longer half-life of the complete immunoglobulin. A clue to the underlying mechanism comes from the finding that cross-linking of IgM on the resting B-cell surface by an IgG anti-μ has no discernable effect whereas the F(ab')$_2$ fragment of this anti-μ induces proliferation (figure 8.2). The current view is that a complex of antigen with IgG antibody could block the productive phase of the T-dependent B-cell response by cross-linking

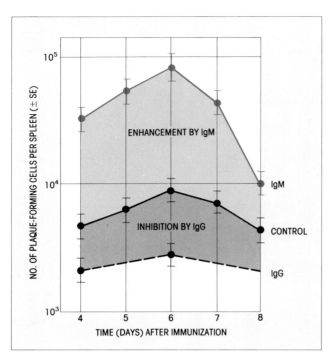

Figure 8.1. *Time course of enhancement of antibody response to sheep red cells (SRBC) due to injection of preformed IgM, and of suppression by preformed IgG antibodies. Mice received medium containing monoclonal IgM anti-SRBC, IgG anti-SRBC or medium alone i.v. 2 hours prior to immunization with 10^5 SRBC. (Data provided by J. Reiter, P. Hutchings, P. Lydyard and A. Cooke.)*

the antigen and Fcγ surface receptors (figure 8.2c).

In complete contrast, injection of IgM antibodies enhances the response (figure 8.1), but since antibodies of this isotype appear at an early stage after antigen challenge, they would be useful in boosting the initial response.

T-cell regulation

T-helper cells

We have deliberated at length on the role of T-helper cells in the facilitation of cytotoxic T-cell and B-cell responses, and in the production of class-switching and memory responses. We should perhaps note that the T-helpers do not expand B-cell and Tc-cell clone sizes indefinitely since the maturation factors inhibit the action of the proliferative lymphokines.

Different T-cells have surface receptors for the Fc regions of the various Ig classes and a role for these in isotype-specific help has been sought. Thus T-cell lines from Peyer's patches produced many more IgA-producing B-cells from Peyer's patch precursors than did splenic T-cell lines. However, the bias was for help to IgA-precommitted B-cells rather than inducing a class-switch to IgA since Peyer's patch T-cells did not markedly enhance IgA production by splenic B-cells. Evidence for the production of IgE-binding factors from Fcε-receptor bearing T-cells which enhance B-cell secretion of IgE has been obtained; intriguingly, lipocortin produced by CD8 T-cells under the influence of steroids, or following immunization with mycobacteria is said to block glycosylation of the IgE-binding factor so that it now becomes a *suppressor* of IgE synthesis.

T-suppressor cells

We have now raised the question of suppression as distinct from help and perhaps it is inevitable that Nature, having evolved a functional set of T-cells

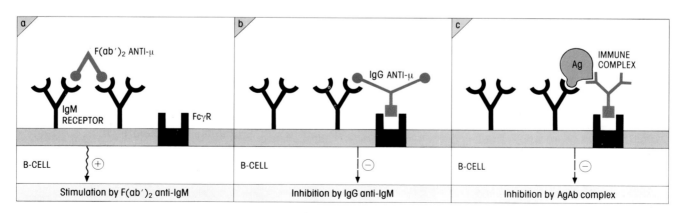

Figure 8.2. *Cross-linking of surface IgM antigen receptor and IgG Fc receptor leads to inhibition of B-cell function. This can* *be observed at the level of* **c-myc** *induction (cf. p. 188). IL-4 blocks this effect.*

which promote immune responses, should also develop an opposite set whose job would be to prevent the helpers from getting out of hand. Suppressor T-cells were first brought to the serious attention of the immunological fraternity by a phenomenon colourfully named by its discoverer, 'infectious tolerance'. Quite surprisingly it was shown that if mice are made unresponsive by injection of a high dose of sheep red cells, their T-cells will suppress specific antibody formation in normal recipients to which they have been transferred (figure 8.3). It may not be apparent to the reader why this result was at all surprising, but at that time antigen-induced tolerance was regarded essentially as a negative phenomenon involving the depletion or silencing of clones rather than a state of *active* suppression. Over the years, T-suppressors have been shown to modulate a variety of humoral and cellular responses, the latter including delayed-type hypersensitivity, cytolytic T-cells and antigen-specific T-cell proliferation. However, suppressor systems are not exactly straightforward.

Initiation is by suppressor-inducer cells

There is a general agreement that the suppressor circuits are initiated by cells of helper phenotype, i.e. CD4, called suppressor-inducer cells. Taking a broad view, the helper cells may be looked upon as general inducers of all the effector cells for cell-mediated and humoral immunity and it would be consistent with such a scheme that the T-suppressors should be generated by and react against cells occupying this pivotal position (figure 8.4). The $CD4^+$ population displays heterogeneity when analysed for cell surface markers by monoclonal antibodies; proliferative responses to recall antigens and help for human B-cell stimulation by the polyclonal activator pokeweed mitogen (PWM) resides

in the UCHL1 positive set (CD45 Ro-memory, cells) while the ability to induce suppression in PWM responses is a property of the UCHL1$^-$, Leu8$^+$ T-cells (the labels refer to the monoclonal antibodies used).

Class II MHC restriction of induction

Murine suppressor-inducers are characterized by surface expression of the notorious class II-related I-J determinants. Now the I-J story is very confused but we will try to make some sense out of it because the polymorphism it defines is linked in a clear way with the function of the suppressor circuits. Originally I-J was identified by antisera obtained by reciprocal hyperimmunization of the B10.A(3R) and (5R) strains with unfractionated spleen cells. After appropriate absorptions, the antisera so obtained recognized a subset of the total T-cell population which proved to be associated with suppressor activity. Since the 3R and 5R strains only differed as a result of a recombination event mapping close to I-E, I-J was thought to be encoded by genes in this region. Unfortunately, DNA sequencing showed that this region was already fully occupied with genes for I-E and C4 and there was no room for a further gene product. Some considerable light was shed on this conundrum by experiments which showed that bone marrow cells of H-2^b haplotype developing in the thymus of H-2$^{b\times k}$ hosts developed I-J molecules of *host* (i.e. H-2^b *and* H-2^k) phenotype and vice versa. Thus the I-J specificity is imposed by the I-E region haplotype rather than being encoded by it. Since the thymus selects for T-cells with receptors which recognize host MHC, it is possible that the I-J antisera are directed to the determinants (idiotype) on the T-cell receptors restricted to I-E molecules, and maybe also to the T-cell receptors which are anti-idiotypic to them.

155

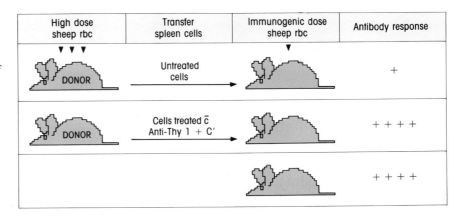

Figure 8.3. *Demonstration of T-suppressor cells. Spleen cells from a donor injected with a high dose of antigen, depress the antibody response of a syngeneic animal to which they have been transferred. The effect is lost if the spleen cells are first treated with anti-Thy 1 serum plus complement showing that the suppressors are T-cells (after Gershon R.K. & Kondo K. (1971) Immunology 21, 903: in these studies recipient mice were first thymectomized, irradiated and reconstituted with bone marrow and thymocytes).*

High dose sheep rbc	Transfer spleen cells	Immunogenic dose sheep rbc	Antibody response
DONOR	Untreated cells		+
DONOR	Cells treated c̄ Anti-Thy 1 + C'		+ + + +
			+ + + +

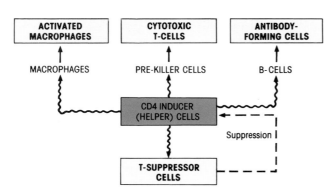

Figure 8.4. *Immunoregulatory feedback circuit showing the central position of CD4 cells in the induction (~~~→) of T-dependent responses and in the generation of T-suppressors. The inducer population is heterogeneous.*

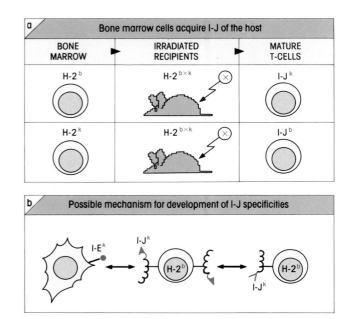

Figure 8.5. *The nature of I-J on suppressor T-cells. Stem cells acquire the I-J haplotype of the environment within which they mature (note they also acquire the I-J specificity of their own haplotype). One explanation is that I-J collectively describes idiotypes on the suppressor cells (and the complementary anti-idiotypic cells) selected by the host class II molecules during ontogeny.*

On this view, anti I-J is an anti-idiotypic serum reacting with the series of idiotypically related receptors associated with I-E recognition (figure 8.5 may help!). However, caution rather than over-confidence is advised since the mysteries of I-J have not yet been convincingly solved.

None the less there are many examples of immune responses, e.g. leishmania, polyglutamyl, alanyl, tyrosyl peptide and lactate dehydrogenase β, where T-suppression has been linked to the I-E haplotype and this, together with the fact that most, but by no means all, T-helper clones are I-A rather than I-E restricted, has led to Klein's suggestion that in the majority of cases (but not necessarily in all), T-helpers use I-A and suppressors I-E. Strands of evidence which accord with this hypothesis derive from the enhancement of antigen-specific proliferation of putatively suppressed T-cells resulting from addition of anti-I-E, as with the mouse liver F-protein and lactate dehydrogenase responses (figure 8.6). The human disease, lepromatous leprosy, is very informative in this respect. These patients carry large numbers of bacteria in their tissues, make buckets of useless antibodies and manifest a selective T-cell unresponsiveness to *Mycobacterium leprae* but not to *M.tuberculosis*. In 10% of lepromatous patients, addition of anti-HLA-DQ (a human class II molecule) to the culture medium resulted in a greatly improved proliferative response to *M.leprae* suggesting the release of cells from the grip of DQ-mediated suppression. The fact that DQ is structurally homologous with I-A rather than I-E is a slight hiccup for the hypothesis unless there was a flip over from DR to DQ for suppressor purposes during evolution, but the main point is

that the overall class II restriction of the phenomenon remains a dominant feature.

Detailed analysis of murine responses to antigens such as hen egg-white lysozyme tells us that certain determinants can evoke very strong suppressor rather than helper responses depending on the mouse strain, and also, that T-suppressors directed to one determinant can switch off helper and antibody responses to other determinants on the same molecule. Thus mice of $H-2^b$ haplotype respond poorly to lysozyme because they develop dominant suppression; however, if the three N-terminal amino acids are removed from the antigen, $H-2^b$ mice now make a splendid response showing that the T-suppression directed against the determinant associated with the N-terminal region had switched off the response to the remaining determinants on the antigen. This must imply that the antigen itself must act as a form of bridge to allow communication between T-suppressor and cells reacting to the other determinants, as might occur through these cells binding to an antigen-presenting cell expressing several different processed determinants of the same antigen on its surface (figure 8.8).

156

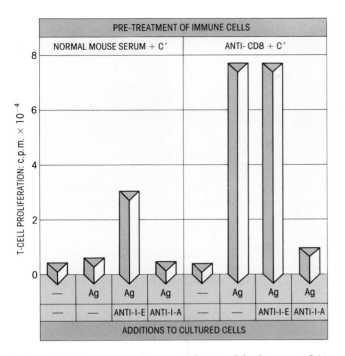

PRE-TREATMENT OF IMMUNE CELLS

Figure 8.6. *Low responsiveness to lactate dehydrogenase β in B10.A. (2R) mice is due to active suppression by I-E restricted, CD8⁺ T-suppressors. Left: lymph node cells from immunized animals showed increased proliferation to antigen when cultured in the presence of anti-I-E. Right: removal of CD8 cells prior to culture revealed a high proliferative response to antigen which was restricted to I-A. Data from Baxevanis C.V., Nagy Z.A. & Klein J. (1981)* **Proc. Nat. Acad. Sci., 78, 3809.**

The effectors of suppression

There is little doubt that T-suppression as an operational act is real enough but there has been a sharp conflict of view within the immunological fraternity about the nature of the cells which mediate suppression: do they belong to a dedicated subpopulation or does suppression represent the functional behaviour of normally helpful lymphocytes conditioned by a particular set of signals received from neighbouring cells? The issue is still open but we can usefully examine some of the features of the effector cells. Thus, cells which mediate suppression are far more vulnerable than helpers to adult thymectomy, X-irradiation and cyclophosphamide. For example, adult thymectomy in the mouse has little effect on the T-helper population but does lead to a fall in the T-suppressors, thereby increasing the response to T-independent antigens and preventing the fall-off in IgE antibody to haptens coupled with Ascaris extracts which occurs in intact animals.

They are classically of the CD8⁺, I-J⁺ phenotype in the mouse and belong to the CD8⁺ subset in the human. To look at some examples, the B10.A (2R) mouse strain has a low immune response to lactate dehydrogenase β (LDHβ) associated with the possession of the I-Eβ gene of *k* rather than *b* haplotype. Lymphoid cells taken from these animals after immunization with LDHβ proliferate poorly *in vitro* in the presence of antigen but if CD8⁺ cells are depleted, the remaining CD4⁺ cells give a much higher response (figure 8.6). Adding back the CD8⁺ cells reimposed the active suppression. In a study of human populations in Japan who were either spontaneously or deliberately exposed to a variety of antigens, there was a tendency for responders to a given antigen to fall into low or high categories (figure 8.7). Analysis of responses to streptococcal cell wall, *M.leprae*, cedar pollen and hepatitis B surface antigens showed that low responsiveness was inherited dominantly and was linked to HLA class II indicative of active suppression; supportive evidence was obtained from the demonstration that depletion of CD8 cells increased the T-cell response to antigen of peripheral blood cells *in vitro*.

Reports of successful cloning of T-cells with suppressor activity are now appearing; they have the CD8 phenotype and rearranged T-cell receptor genes. They are said to bind antigen but this may be restricted to cases involving organic moieties such as NP (4-hydroxy-3-nitrophenylacetate) coupled to carrier where the hapten itself will not be modified by processing. Both the CD4⁺ suppressor inducer (Ts₁) and the CD8⁺ effector of suppression (Ts₃) are antigen-specific and are thought to be linked by an idiotype-specific transducing Ts₂-cell (figure 8.8). Conceivably, Ts₂ suppressors could be linked to the major regulatory immunoglobulin idiotypes to be discussed shortly since neonatal suppression of the B-cell idiotype by treatment with anti-μ serum or anti-idiotype prevents the development of the anti-idiotype Ts₂ cells normally seen in the suppression of delayed type hypersensitivity induced by azobenzene arsonate.

The suppressor circuit is probably completed by release of a soluble suppressor factor which is taken up by antigen-presenting cells. This still mysterious factor is thought to be a heterodimer with one chain binding antigen and the other said to express I-J and lipomodulin determinants (lipomodulin is a phospholipase inhibitor whose phosphorylated form, lipocortin, mediates production of IgE-suppressor factor). Whatever its constitution finally proves to be, uptake by antigen-presenting cells

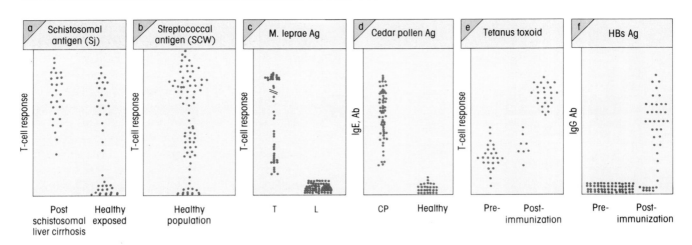

| a | Schistosomal antigen (Sj) | b | Streptococcal antigen (SCW) | c | M. leprae Ag | d | Cedar pollen Ag | e | Tetanus toxoid | f | HBs Ag |

Figure 8.7. *Polymorphism of immune responsiveness to natural antigens or vaccines in humans. Proliferative response of peripheral T-cells specific to* **Schistosoma japonicum** *antigen (a), streptococcal cell wall antigen (b),* **Mycobacterium leprae** *antigen in patients with tuberculoid leprosy (T) or lepromatous leprosy (L) (c) or tetanus toxoid in*

healthy individuals pre and post immunization (e). IgE levels specific to cedar pollen antigen among patients with cedar pollinosis (CP), or healthy controls (d). IgG levels specific to hepatitis B virus surface antigen in healthy vaccines, pre- and post-immunization (f).

158

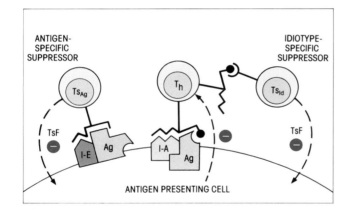

Figure 8.8. *Possible mechanism for interaction of antigen and idiotype-specific suppressors operating through an antigen-presenting cell (tongue in cheek). For those likely to read the literature on this topic, one suppressor loop is thought to involve a cascade starting with the inducer (Ts₁; antigen-specific) which through a soluble factor TsF₁, triggers the transducer (Ts₂; idiotype-specific) which itself produces TsF₂ leading to recruitment of the effector (Ts₃). This scheme is not identical to that in the diagram and time will tell how many different suppressor systems operate* **in vivo** *and how complex they will prove to be.*

could lead to loss of ability to present antigen if, for example, they blocked production of costimulatory signals such as IL-1. It seems to me that interaction of suppressors with antigen on the surface of antigen-presenting cells would account for the regulation of helper cells binding to other determinants on the same antigen as discussed earlier

and also explain how suppressors recognizing antigen plus I-E could influence helpers binding to antigen plus I-A (assuming it needs explaining) (figure 8.8). Such a reaction could also be responsible for *antigenic competition*, the situation in which one T-dependent antigen can block the response to another.

Other modes of suppression readily suggest themselves, such as mutual antagonism of Th1 and Th2 cells by IFNγ and cytokine synthesis inhibitory factor (p. 144) and downregulation of IL-2 receptors by TGFβ. Suppression of T-helpers will of course indirectly affect antibody production but we should not ignore reports of MHC class II-restricted cytotoxic cells which could liquidate antigen-specific B-cells which express high levels of processed antigen and are class II positive.

It is important not to lose track of the so-called 'natural suppressor cells' such as those provoked by total lymph node irradiation (cf. p. 286) and I would like to draw attention to a report that NK cells can inhibit the one-way mixed lymphocyte reaction (p. 279) or the primary IgM response to sheep cells *in vitro*, by suppressing dendritic cells which have already reacted with the antigen; this offers a further opportunity for feedback control since IFNγ and IL-2 produced by T-helpers can activate NK cells.

Further complexity is introduced by the controversial concept of the *'contrasuppressor' cell* which competes with and antagonizes the action of suppressors for T-helpers. The mouse effector is an

Ly1$^+$ I-J$^+$ T-cell with binding sites for the lectin *Vicia villosa* and there is evidence for a CD8$^+$ (T8$^+$) cell with the same lectin-binding ability subserving a similar function in the human. Make no mistake, suppression is still a murky area, and is not for the unwary.

Effector T-cells are guided to the appropriate target by MHC surface molecules

One may well ask why the complicated process of MHC recognition by T-cells evolved; why can't the T-cell just see the antigen alone without all this MHC fuss? The reason is that a T-cell works by recognizing antigen on the surface of a cell with which it is going to communicate and it is pointless for it to perceive either free antigen or antigen idly sitting on some basement membrane. The role of the MHC molecules is to make sure that the T-cell makes contact with antigen on the surface of the *appropriate* target cell.

Let us explore this point by looking at the role of cytotoxic T-cells in viral infection. When a cell is first infected with virus, there is an eclipse phase during which the machinery of the cell is being switched for viral replication and the only marker of the complete microbe is the processed viral antigen peptide on the cell surface. At this stage, killing of the cell by a cytotoxic T-cell will prevent viral replication.

How does the killer T-cell know when it has reached its target? It has to recognize two features before striking: one is the presence of viral peptide and the other is its location on the surface of a body cell; it does not want to dissipate its efforts on extracellular free virus. This dual recognition function is carried out by the T-cell receptor which identifies both the surface viral antigen and the class I MHC molecules which are present on nearly every cell in the body and can therefore be used as markers for cells as such. Thus the killer cell operates on the basis that:

surface **viral** antigen + *class I MHC* = **virally** infected *cell*

In other words, processed viral antigen is the code for 'viral infection' and class I molecules are the code for 'cell', and that is why T-cell receptors have to see both antigens.

The situation is quite different with intracellular bacteria and protozoa which do not go through an eclipse phase after phagocytosis by macrophages but are held as infectious entities; lysis by cytotoxic T-cells will merely release the organisms, not kill them. A separate strategy utilizing the delayed-type hypersensitivity T-cell population is required and, in this case, the effector T-lymphocyte recognizes the infected macrophage by the presence of microbial antigen on the surface in association with a class II molecule which is now a code for 'macrophage'. This interaction triggers the release of lymphokines which enable the macrophage to kill the intracellular parasites (p. 121). Similarly, in T$-$B cooperation, the B-cell is recognized through its class II molecule associated with the foreign antigen while T-cells mediating suppression utilize I-J and possibly I-E in the mouse and equivalent molecules in the human. In summary, each antigen-specific T-lymphocyte subset has to communicate with a particular cell type in order to make the *appropriate* immune response and it does so by recognizing not only processed foreign antigen but also the particular MHC molecule used as a marker of that cell (table 8.1).

159

Table 8.1. *Guidance of T subpopulations to appropriate target cell by MHC molecules.*

Function	Cell interaction	MHC marker on target cell
T-help	T-B	II
T-proliferation	T-macrophage	II
T-delayed sensitivity	T-macrophage	II
T-suppression	T-T	I-J(II?)
T-cytotoxic	T-infected cell	I

Idiotype networks

Jerne's network hypothesis

The hypervariable loops on the immunoglobulin molecule which go to form the antigen combining site have individual characteristic shapes which can be recognized by the appropriate antibodies as idiotypic determinants (cf. p. 39). There are hundreds of thousands, if not more, of different idiotypes in one individual.

Jerne reasoned brilliantly that the great diversity of idiotypes would to a considerable extent mirror the diversity of antigenic shapes in the external world. Thus, he said, if lymphocytes can recognize a whole range of foreign antigenic determinants, they should be able to recognize the idiotypes on other lymphocytes. They would therefore form a large network or series of networks depending upon idiotype—anti-idiotype recognition between lymphocytes of the various T- and B-subsets (figure 8.9) and the response to an external antigen perturbing this network would be conditioned by the state of the idiotypic interactions.

Evidence for idiotypic networks

Anti-idiotype can be induced by autologous idiotypes

There is no doubt that the elements which can form an idiotypic network are present in the body. Individuals can be immunized against idiotypes on their own antibodies, and such autoanti-idiotypes have been identified during the course of responses induced by antigens. For example, when certain strains of mice are injected with pneumococcal vaccines, they make an antibody response to the phosphoryl choline groups in which the germ-line-encoded idiotype T15 dominates. If the individual antibody-forming cells are examined by plaque assays at different times after immunization, waves of T15$^+$ and of anti-T15 (i.e. autoanti-idiotype) cells are demonstrable. Similarly, immunization with the acetylcholine agonist BISQ followed by fusion of the spleen cells to produce hybridomas, yielded a series of anti-BISQ monoclonals (idiotypes) and a smaller number of anti-idiotypic monoclonals of which a surprising proportion behaved as internal images of BISQ in their ability to stimulate acetylcholine receptors (figure 8.10).

A network is evident in early life

If the spleens of fetal mice which are just beginning to secrete immunoglobulin are fused with myeloma cells to produce hybridomas, an unusually high proportion are inter-related as idiotype—anti-idiotype pairs. This high level of idiotype connectivity is not seen in later life and suggests that these early cells, mostly a B-cell subset bearing the T-cell marker CD5, are programmed to synthesize germ-

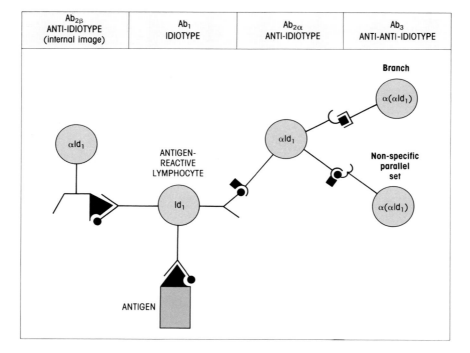

Figure 8.9. *Elements in an idiotypic network in which the antigen receptors on one lymphocyte reciprocally recognize an idiotype on the receptors of another. T-helper, T-suppressor and B-lymphocytes interact through idiotype—anti-idiotype reactions; either stimulation or suppression may result. One of the anti-idiotype sets, Ab$_{2\beta}$, may bear an idiotype of similar shape to (i.e. provides an **internal image** of) the antigen. The same idiotype (●) may be shared by two receptors of different specificity (since the several hypervariable regions provide a number of potential idiotypic determinants and a given idiotype does not always form part of the epitope binding site, i.e. the paratope), so that the anti-(anti-Id$_1$) does not necessarily bind the original antigen. (The following abbreviations are often employed: α as a prefix = anti; Id = idiotype; Ab$_1$ = Id; Ab$_{2\alpha}$ = αId not involving the paratope; Ab$_{2\beta}$ = internal image αId involving the paratope; Ab$_3$ = α(αId).)*

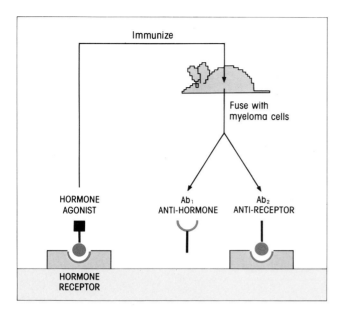

Immunize

HORMONE
AGONIST

Fuse with
myeloma cells

Ab₁
ANTI-HORMONE

Ab₂
ANTI-RECEPTOR

HORMONE
RECEPTOR

Figure 8.10. *The spontaneous production of autoanti-idiotype during immunization with a hormone agonist. Hybridomas obtained from the immunized mouse secrete anti-hormone and anti-idiotype which reacts with the hormone receptor; this indicates a close relationship between hormone, receptor, anti-hormone and anti-idiotype implying some connection between autoantibodies within the idiotype network and hormone systems.*

line gene specificities which have network relationships and that the network may be concerned with the stability of the Ig gene pool and possibly the amplification of the antibody repertoire by anti-idiotype-driven mutation in the non-CD5 B-cell population. The specificities of these 'early' hybridomas are very similar to those of the 'natural' antibodies which appear spontaneously in germ-free animals not exposed to exogenous antigens, and it is noteworthy that several are IgM with low affinity for self-components such as DNA, IgG and cytoskeletal proteins, hinting perhaps at the use of these body components as points of reference to maintain the V genes encoding individual members of the idiotype network. Of course, by no means are all the CD5 B specificities anti-self; many are directed to polysaccharide antigens of common pathogens, e.g. phosphoryl choline.

T-cells can also do it

It seems likely that similar interactions will be established for early T-cells possibly linking with the B-cell network. Certainly, anti-idiotypic reactivity can be demonstrated in T-cell populations. For example, let us divide a sample of T-cells from the peripheral blood of individual X into two; one half is cultured with irradiated lymphocytes from individual Y of the same species and gives rise to proliferating T-cell blasts directed against the allogeneic MHC class II of Y. If these blasts are now added back to the remaining (resting) half of X's cells, they induce a T-cell proliferation, i.e. the resting cells contain a population of T-cells which spontaneously recognize the idiotype of the expanded autologous T-blasts. Take another interesting experiment: a T-cell population which has been polyclonally activated (e.g. by concanavalin A which stimulates T-cells independently of their antigen specificity) can be analysed by limiting dilution (cf. p. 149) for the frequency of cells reacting to specified antigens. In wells with relatively small numbers of T-cells, a surprising degree of degeneracy in the recognition of antigen was uncovered in that for every antigen tested, the frequency of specific clones approached 1%. This is startling and has interesting implications, but the relevant point comes next. As the number of cells in each well was increased, antigen reactivity was largely lost. The interpretation is that the population of T-cells contains naturally-occurring anti-idiotype suppressors which are likely to be present together with the antigen-reactive cell in wells with high T-cell numbers, whereas at low cell numbers it is likely that wells containing single antigen-specific lymphocytes will be unaccompanied by suppressors. The physiological significance of this is not completely obvious but it does suggest that when T-cells with complementary idiotype/anti-idiotype receptors come together, suppression results. We hinted previously that idiotypic interactions may come into play in immune suppression. As an illustration, when active suppression to the p-azobenzene arsonate group is induced by intravenous injection of hapten-conjugated lymphocytes, antigen-specific Ts_1 suppressors bearing the major cross-reactive idiotype CRI_A (p. 40) appear first, but these give rise to second-order Ts_2 anti-idiotype suppressor cells.

Regulation by idiotype interactions

There has been a series of investigations based on the following protocol. Antigen is injected into animal₁ and the antibody produced, Ab_1 (idiotype), is purified and injected into animal₂. Ab_2 (anti-idiotype) so formed is purified and used to immunize animal₃ and so on (figure 8.11). Consistently, it is found that Ab_2 (anti-Id_1) recognizes an idiotype

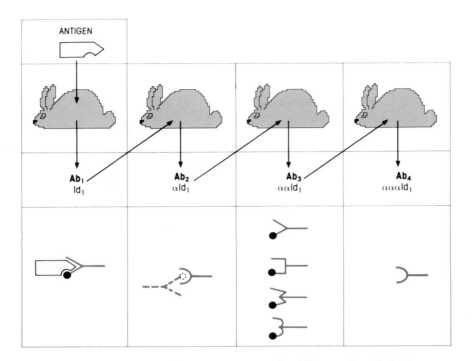

Figure 8.11. Ab_1 *produced by the antigen is injected into a second animal to produce* Ab_2; *this in turn is purified and injected into animal$_3$ and so on.* Ab_2 *and* Ab_4 *both react with an idiotype (●) on* Ab_1 *and* Ab_3 *but only a fraction of* Ab_3 *reacts with the original antigen. Bona & Paul* (**Immunol. Today** *1982, 3, 230) interpret the results in terms of a common regulatory idiotype* Id_1 *shared by many antibodies other than those reacting with the original antigen but recruited by the injection of anti-Id_1* (Ab_2) *which stimulates the range of lymphocytes whose receptors bear this common or cross-* *reacting idiotype. On this basis, one can understand the paradoxical finding of Oudin & Cazenave that not all the Ig molecules bearing a given Id in response to an antigen can function as specific antibody since they belong to the non-specific parallel set. The presence of large amounts of* Id_1 *in* Ab_3 *also suggests that the linear relationship through the cross-reacting* Id_1 *is dominant, with relatively insignificant branching through the variety of 'private' idiotypes on* Ab_2 *molecules (cf. figure 8.9) because of the low frequency of such idiotypes and their anti-idiotypes.*

(Id_1) on Ab_1 which is also strongly present in Ab_3. Ab_4 behaves like Ab_2 in seeing the common idiotype on Ab_1 and Ab_3. None the less, although Ab_1 and Ab_3 share idiotypes, only a small fraction of Ab_3 reacts with the original antigen. This is the result one would expect if the idiotype was a cross-reacting Id (public Id) present on a variety of antibodies (and by implication B-cell receptors) of different specificities. As may be seen in figure 8.11, the anti-Id_1 (Ab_2), when injected into animal$_3$, would react with all B-cells bearing Id_1 and presumably trigger them to produce Id_1 antibodies, only a fraction of which have specificity for the original antiserum.

Such frequently occurring and usually germ-line-encoded idiotypes seem to be provoked fairly readily with anti-Id and are therefore candidates for regulatory Id which can be under some degree of control by a limited idiotypic network. Germane to this idea are the observations that, late in immunization, antibodies with utterly distinct specificities, directed against totally different epitopes on the same antigen, often bear a common or cross-reacting idiotype. Presumably, the first clone of B-cells to be expanded which bears a dominant cross-reacting Id can generate a population of regulatory T-helper cells which recognize this Id as well as antigen. Processing of internalized Ig receptor plus antigen leads to expression of peptides derived from the idiotype and antigen in association with MHC class II; these B-cells can then access the full repertoire of antigen-specific and idiotype-specific T-helpers. The latter may be of two types, one recognizing the native receptor idiotype (non-MHC-restricted) and the other, processed idiotype (MHC-restricted) (figure 8.12). From the complex mixture of B-lymphocytes activated by the other epitopes on the antigen, these T-helpers will selectively recruit those with Id positive receptors. We can now see how the antigen and idiotype specific T-helpers synergize in the antibody response, the latter expanding Id positive clones induced by the former.

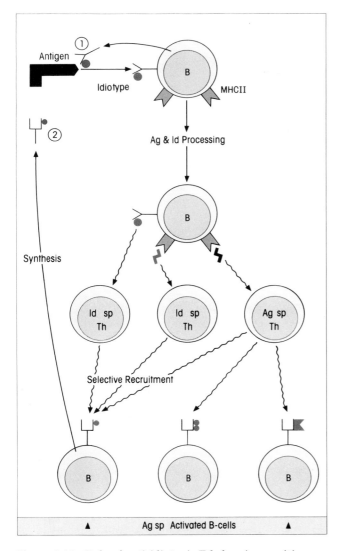

Figure 8.12. *Role of anti-idiotypic T-helper in recruiting antibodies with specificities for the different epitopes on an antigen but bearing the same public or cross-reacting idiotype. The first expanded B-cell clone bearing a cross-reacting Id induces αId T-helpers which are assumed to selectively recruit Id⁺ B-cells already activated by antigen; if resting Id⁺ cells were recruited the amount of non-specific Ig synthesized might be wastefully high. It is also possible that recruitment might operate via anti-idiotypic antibodies which could act on Id⁺ B-cells to increase their surface class II and improve their 'cooperability' with T-helpers. It is worth considering whether memory αId T-helpers could be responsible for the phenomenon of 'original antigenic sin' in which a second infection with influenza virus involving an antigenically related but not identical strain generates antibodies with a higher titre for the strain which produced the first infection.*

While there would be a large measure of agreement with the view that relatively closed Id—anti-Id circuits involving major germ-line idiotypes con-

tribute to a regulatory system, there is probably much less support for a full 'Jernerian' network extending functionally to the myriad private idiotypes. Given that regulation can occur through interaction with public or cross-reactive idiotypes, what is its importance relative to antigen-mediated control? Although the answer will vary with different antigens, it may turn out that in general the antigen-directed systems will dominate, with idiotypic networks providing accessory amplification and suppressive loops since (i) it seems most likely that antigen recognition and elimination were the driving forces behind the evolutionary selection for an adaptive immune response and therefore one wants the system to be sensitive to the presence and concentration of antigen, and (ii) there would seem to be little point in Id and anti-Id squabbling about control of the response after antigen had been eliminated. The Id network could allow the response to 'tick over' for extended periods and maintain the memory-cell population, while the presence of primed T-helpers directed against a common Id on the various memory B-cells specific for a given antigen would increase their rate of mobilization during a secondary response.

The germ-line idiotypic network may have a fundamental role to play in the maintenance of the *V* gene repertoire and in determining the initial state of the immune system before the encounter with antigen as we shall discuss in the next chapter.

Manipulation of the immune response through idiotypes

Quite low doses of anti-idiotype, of the order of nanograms, can greatly enhance the expression of the idiotype in the response to a given antigen, whereas doses in the microgram range lead to a suppression (figure 8.13). Thus the idiotypic network provides interesting opportunities to manipulate the immune response, particularly in hypersensitivity states such as autoimmune disease, allergy and graft rejection. However, normally the B-cell response is so diverse that suppression by anti-Id is likely to prove difficult; even when the response is dominated by a public Id and that Id is suppressed, compensatory expansion of Id negative clones ensures that the fall in the total antibody titre is relatively undramatic (cf. figure 8.13). Perhaps ways can be developed to restrict this Id negative compensation, particularly if the total number of idiotypes is small as might perhaps be the case with IgE antibody synthesis in patients with atopic al-

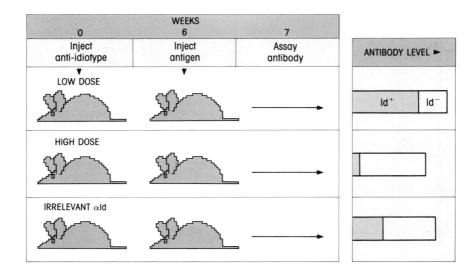

WEEKS		
0	6	7
Inject anti-idiotype	Inject antigen	Assay antibody

Figure 8.13. *Modulation of a major idiotype in the antibody response to antigen by anti-idiotype. In the example chosen, the idiotype is present in a substantial proportion of the antibodies produced in controls injected with irrelevant anti-Id plus antigen (i.e. this is a public or cross-reacting Id; p. 40). Pretreatment with 10 µg of a monoclonal anti-Id greatly expands the Id$^+$ antibody population whereas prior injection of 10 µg of anti-Id completely (or almost completely) suppresses expression of the idiotype without having any substantial effect on total antibody production due to a compensatory increase in Id$^-$ antibody clones.*

lergy. Conceivably, T-helper cells may express a narrow spectrum of idiotypes thereby being more susceptible to suppression by Id autoimmunization which in any case may produce far more widespread effects within the internal network than treatment with anti-Ids from other species which may see only a small part of the system. In this respect, reports that 'vaccination' with irradiated lines of helper T-cells specific for brain or thyroid antigens prevents the induction of experimental autoimmunity against the relevant organ, are encouraging. Sporadic success has been obtained with the strategy of autoimmunizing rats of strain A with antibodies (AαB) raised in A against the transplantation antigens of strain B so that the T-cell-mediated rejection of a subsequent strain B graft is suppressed, presumably because the anti-idiotypic response (anti-[AαB]) inactivates lymphocytes capable of recognizing the graft by virtue of the AαB receptors on their surface. Presumably success is only sporadic because the assumption that T-cell receptors and antibody recognizing the graft antigen share idiotypes, is unlikely to be true very often, bearing in mind that one receptor recognizes processed antigen and the other, native antigen. A totally different approach would be to use monoclonal anti-Id of the 'antigen internal image' set (figure 8.9) to stimulate antigen-specific T-suppressors capable of turning off B-cells directed to other epitopes on the antigen through bridging by the antigen itself (cf. figure 8.8).

Since we know that under suitable conditions anti-Id can also stimulate antibody production, it might be possible to use 'internal image' monoclonal anti-Ids as 'surrogate' antigens for immunization in cases where the antigen is difficult to obtain in bulk—for example, antigens from parasites such as filaria or the weak embryonic antigens associated with some cancers. Another example is where protein antigens obtained by chemical synthesis or gene cloning fail to fold into the configuration of the native molecule; this is not a problem with the anti-Id which by definition has been selected to have the shape of the antigenic epitope.

At this stage, if the reader is feeling a little groggy, try a glance at figure 8.14 which attempts a summary of the main factors currently thought to modulate the immune response.

The influence of genetic factors

Some genes affect general responsiveness

Mice can be selectively bred for high or low antibody responses through several generations to yield two lines, one of which consistently produces high-titre antibodies to a variety of antigens and the other,

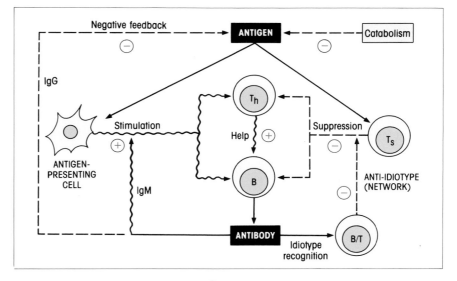

Figure 8.14. *Regulation of the immune response. T_h = T-helper cell; T_s = T-suppressor cell. T-help for cell-mediated immunity will be subject to similar regulation. Some of these mechanisms may be interdependent; for example, one could envisage anti-idiotypic antibody acting in concert with a suppressor T-cell by binding to its Fc receptor, or suppressor T-cells with specificity for the idiotype on T_h or B-cells. To avoid too many confusing arrows, I have omitted the recruitment of B-cells by anti-idiotypic T-helpers and direct activation of anti-idiotype T-suppressors by idiotype-positive T-helpers.*

antibodies of relatively low titre (figure 8.15; Biozzi & colleagues). Out of the ten or so different genetic loci involved, one or more affect macrophage behaviour. The two lines are comparable in their ability to clear carbon particles or sheep erythrocytes from the blood by phagocytosis, but macrophages from the high responders retain a far higher proportion of added antigen on their surface (cf. p. 113). On the other hand, the low responders survive infection by *Salmonella typhimurium* better and their macrophages support much slower replication of listeria (cf. p. 210) showing a dichotomy in the ability of macrophages to subserve humoral as compared with cell-mediated immunity.

Immune response linked to immunoglobulin genes

A large proportion of the antibodies made by the A/J strain of mice in response to the hapten p-azophenylarsonate, bear a major cross-reacting idiotype (CRI_A) somewhat coarsely referred to often as the ARS idiotype. Breeding experiments have shown that the capacity to produce this idiotype is inherited and is linked to the genetic markers for the immunoglobulin constant region, i.e. as might be expected, the gene encoding the idiotype occurs on the chromosome carrying the genes for the constant region. Thus, since we inherit genes which enable us to make particular antibodies one might suppose that the capacity to produce an antibody response would be limited by the repertoire of specificities encoded by the genes on this chromosome. However, since the mechanisms for generating antibody diversity from the available genes

are so powerful, immunodeficiency is unlikely to occur as a consequence of a poor Ig variable region gene repertoire. Just occasionally we see holes in the repertoire due to absence of a gene; failure to respond to the sugar polymer α1-6, dextran is a feature of animals without the V_{dex} gene and mice lacking the $V_{\alpha2}$ T-cell receptor gene cannot mount a cytotoxic T-cell response to the male (H-Y) antigen.

The immune response can be influenced by the major histocompatibility complex

There was much excitement when it was first discovered that the antibody responses to a number of thymus-dependent antigenically simple substances are determined by genes mapping to the MHC. For example, mice of the H-2^b haplotype respond well to the synthetic branched polypeptide (T,G)-A--L (cf. figure 7.8b), whereas H-2^k mice respond poorly.

It was said that mice of the H-2^b haplotype (i.e. a particular set of H-2 genes) are high responders to (T,G)-A--L because they possess the appropriate immune response (Ir) gene. With another synthetic antigen, (H,G)-A--L, having histidine in place of tyrosine, the position is reversed, the 'poor (T,G)-A--L responders' now giving a good antibody response and the 'good (T,G)-A--L responders' a weak one, showing that the capacity of a particular strain to give a high or low response varies with the individual antigen (table 8.2). These relationships are only apparent when antigens of highly restricted structure are studied because the response to each single determinant is controlled by an Ir gene and it is highly unlikely that the different determinants on

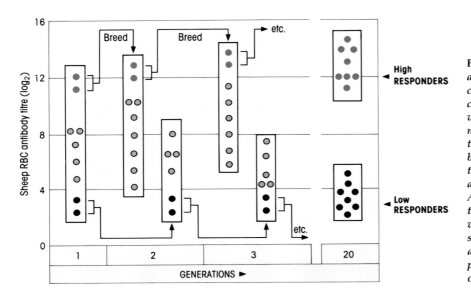

Figure 8.15. *Breeding of high and low antibody responders (after Biozzi and colleagues). A group of wild mice (with crazy mixed-up genes) are immunized with sheep red blood cells (RBC), a multideterminant antigen. The antibody titre of each individual mouse is shown by a circle. The male and female giving the highest titre antibodies (●) were bred and their litter challenged with antigen. Again, the best responders were bred together and so on for 20 generations when all mice were high responders to sheep RBC and a variety of other antigens. The same was done for the poorest responders (●) yielding a strain of low responder animals.*

Table 8.2. *H-2 haplotype linked to high, low and intermediate immune responses to synthetic peptides.*

ANTIGEN	H-2 HAPLOTYPE				
	b	k	d	a	s
(TG)-A--L	Hi	Lo	Int	Lo	Lo
(HG)-A--L	Lo	Hi	Int	Hi	Lo

Table 8.3. *Mapping of the Ir gene for (H,G)-A--L responses by analysis of different recombinant strains.*

Strain	H-2 region					(H,G)-A--L Response
	K	I-A	I-E	S	D	
A	k	k	k	b	b	Hi
A.TL	s	k	k	k	b	Hi
B.IO.A(4R)	k	k	b	b	b	Hi
B.IO	b	b	b	b	b	Lo
A.SW	s	s	s	s	s	Lo

a complex antigen will all be associated with consistently high or consistently low responder Ir genes; rather one would expect an average of randomly high and low responder genes since the various determinants on most thymus-dependent complex antigens are structurally unrelated. Thus H-2 linked immune responses have been observed not only with relatively simple polypeptides, but also with transplantation antigens from another strain and auto-antigens where merely one or two determinants are recognized as foreign by the host. With complex antigens in the majority of cases, H-2 linkage is usually only seen when the dose administered is so low that just one immunodominant determinant is recognized by the immune system. In this way, reactions controlled by Ir genes are distinct from the overall responsiveness to a variety of complex antigens which is a feature of the Biozzi mice (above).

The Ir genes map to the I region and control T—B cooperation

Table 8.3 gives some idea of the type of analysis used to map the Ir genes. The three high responder strains have individual *H-2* genes derived from prototypic pure strains which have been interbred to produce recombinations within the H-2 region. The only genes they have in common are *I-A^k* and *H-2D^b*; since the B.10 strain bearing the *H-2D^b* gene is a low responder, high reponse must be linked in this case to possession of *I-A^k*. The I-region molecules must almost certainly represent the Ir gene product since a point mutation in the I-A subregion in one strain led to a change in the class II molecule at a site affecting its polymorphic specificity and changed the mice from high to low responder status with respect to their thymus-dependent antibody response to antigen *in vivo*. The mutation also greatly reduced the proliferation of T-cells from immunized animals when challenged *in vitro* with antigen plus appropriate presenting cells, and there is a good correlation between antigen-specific T-cell proliferation and the responder status of the host. The implication that responder status may be linked to the generation of T-helpers is amply borne out by adoptive transfer studies showing that irradiated

$(H\text{-}2^b \times H\text{-}2^k)$ F1 mice make good antibody responses to (T,G)-A--L when reconstituted with antigen-primed B-cells from another F1 plus T-cells from a primed $H\text{-}2^b$ (high responder); T-cells from the low responder $H\text{-}2^k$ mice only supported poor antibody responses. This also explains why these H-2 gene effects are seen with thymus-dependent but not T-independent antigens.

Three mechanisms have been proposed to account for class-II-linked high and low responsiveness:

1 *Defective presentation*. In a high responder, processing of antigen and its recognition by a corresponding T-cell leads to lymphocyte triggering and clonal expansion (figure 8.16a). Although there is (and has to be) considerable degeneracy in the specificity of the class II groove for peptide binding, variation in certain key residues can alter the strength of binding to a particular peptide and convert a high to a low responder because the MHC fails to present antigen to the reactive T-cell (figure 8.16b). Sometimes the natural processing of an antigen in a given individual does not produce a peptide which fits well into their MHC molecules. A recent study showed that a cytotoxic T-cell clone restricted to HLA-A2, which recognized residues 58−68 of influenza A virus matrix protein, could cross-react with cells from an Aw69 subject pulsed with the same peptide; none the less, the clone failed to recognize Aw69 cells infected with influenza A virus. Interestingly, individuals with the HLA-Aw69 class I MHC develop immunity to a different epitope on the same protein.

2 *Defective T-cell repertoire*. It is now accepted that T-cells capable of recognizing self-MHC molecules and their complexes with processed self-antigens, will be rendered unresponsive (cf. tolerance induction, p. 181) so creating a 'hole' in the T-cell repertoire. If there is a cross-reaction, i.e. similarity in shape at the T-cell recognition level between a foreign antigen and a self-molecule which has already induced unresponsiveness, the host must lack T-cells specific for the foreign antigen and will therefore be a low responder (figure 8.16c). To take a concrete example, mice of DBA/2 strain respond well to the synthetic peptide polyglutamyl, polytyrosine (GT), whereas BALB/c do not, although both have identical class II genes. BALB/c B-cell blasts express a structure which mimics GT and the presumption would be that self-tolerance makes these mice unresponsive to GT. This was confirmed by showing that DBA/2 mice made tolerant by a

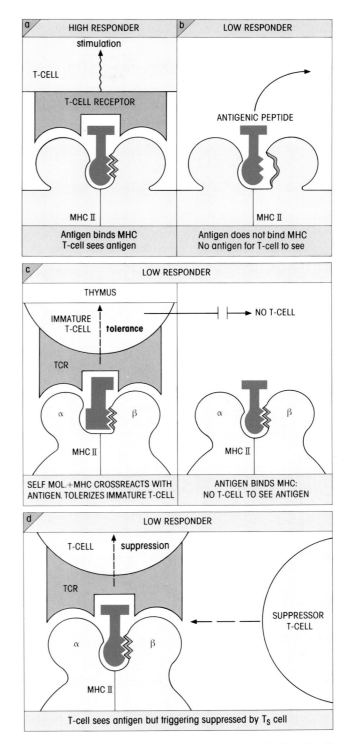

Figure 8.16. *Different mechanisms can account for low T-cell response to antigen in association with MHC class II.*

small number of BALB/c haemopoietic cells were changed from high to low responder status. To round off the story in a very satisfying way, DBA/2 mice injected with BALB/c B-blasts, induced by the polyclonal activator lipopolysaccharide, were found to be primed for GT.

3 *T-suppression*. I would like to refer again to the MHC class II-restricted low responsiveness to relatively complex antigens occurring within families (p. 157), since it illustrates the notion that low responder status can arise as an expression of CD8 T-suppressor activity (figure 8.16d). Low response was dominant in class II heterozygotes, indicating that suppression can act against T-helpers restricted to any other class II molecule. In this it differs from models **1** and **2** above where high response is dominant in a heterozygote because the factors associated with the low responder gene cannot influence the activity of the high responder. Overall, it seems likely that each of the three models may provide the basis for class II-linked Ir gene phenomena in different circumstances.

Factors influencing the genetic control of the immune response are summarized in figure 8.17.

168

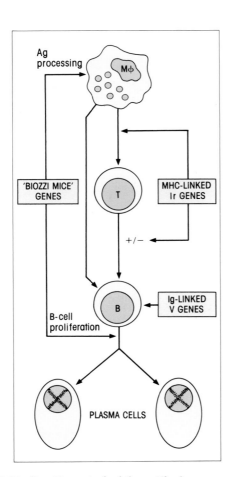

Figure 8.17. *Genetic control of the antibody response.*

Are there regulatory immuno-neuroendocrine networks?

There is a danger, as one focuses more and more on the antics of the immune system, of looking at the body as a collection of myeloid and lymphoid cells roaming around in a big sack and of having no regard to the integrated physiology of the organism (Are there really people who are so myopic? I can hear you say). Within the wider physiological context, attention has been drawn increasingly to interactions between immunological and neuro-endocrine systems.

Immune processes can be influenced by neuroendocrine factors

Immunological cells have the receptors which enable them to receive signals from a whole range of hormones: corticosteroids, insulin, growth hormone, oestradiol, testosterone, β-adrenergic agents, acetylcholine, endorphins and enkephalins. There is an extensive literature concerning their influence on immune function, but by and large, glucocorticoids, androgens, oestrogens and progesterone depress immune responses whereas growth hormone, thyroxine and insulin do the opposite. To give one example, 10–15-fold variations in blood glucocorticoid levels induced by adrenalectomy and stress were mirrored reciprocally by changes in the number of antibody-secreting cells. Sex differences are especially notable in autoimmune diseases.

Immunological organs are innervated by autonomic and primary sensorial neurons, and neonatal (but not adult) sympathectomy with 6-hydroxydopamine and surgical denervation of the spleen enhance immune responses. Mast cells and nerves often have an intimate anatomical relationship and nerve growth factor causes mast cell degranulation. The gastrointestinal tract also has extensive innervation and a high number of immune effector cells. In this context, the ability of substance P to stimulate, and of somatostatin and vasoactive intestinal peptide (VIP) to inhibit, proliferation of Peyer's patch lymphocytes may prove to have more than a trivial significance. The pituitary hormone prolactin has been brought to our attention from two convergent experimental observations: first, inhibition of prolactin secretion by bromocryptine suppresses T-helper activity, and second, cyclosporin A which is a selective inhibitor of T-helper cells is said to displace prolactin from its receptors in lymphocytes.

It is not easy at this stage to see just how these diverse neuroendocrine effects fit into the regulation of immune responses but at a more physiological level, stress and circadian rhythms modify the functioning of the immune system and there is a very popular observation concerning modulation of the delayed-type hypersensitivity Mantoux reaction in the skin by hypnosis. Elegant demonstration of nervous system control is provided by studies showing suppression of conventional immune responses and enhancement of NK cell activity by classical Pavlovian conditioning. There is every possibility that the numerous investigations alleging an adverse effect of psychological factors such as bereavement upon immune function are leading us with tiny faltering steps to a new age of 'psychoimmunology'.

Immunological influences on neuroendocrine mechanisms

Glucocorticoid levels in the blood are reported to increase to immunosuppressive levels at the time of the peak response to antigen challenge. Interleukin-1 (figure 8.18) and a not fully characterized lymphokine are capable of stimulating glucocorticoid synthesis and do so through the pituitary—adrenal axis. There seems to be an interaction between inflammation and nerve growth in regions of wound healing and repair. Mast cells are often abundant, IL-6 induces neurite growth and IL-1 enhances production of nerve growth factor in sciatic nerve explants.

IL-1 increases slow-wave sleep when introduced into the lateral ventricle of the brain and both IL-1

and interferon produce pyrogenic effects through their action on the temperature-controlling centre. The significance of IgFc binding to pituitary ACTH-producing cells has still not been revealed.

Circuits

Two network interactions between the immune and neuroendocrine systems have been reasonably well established. The first would involve the increased synthesis of glucocorticoids under the influence of IL-1, a lymphokine and possibly a thymus hormone, generated during the immunological response. In turn, the glucocorticoids would exert feedback suppression by influencing several processes including production of IL-1 and IL-2 (figure 8.19a).

A second circuit involves the seemingly intimate relationships between hormone receptor, hormone, anti-hormone and anti-idiotype (figure 8.19b). This point has come to our attention already in discussing the production of anti-receptor antibodies during immunization with an acetylcholine agonist (figure 8.10) and is of relevance to the pathogenesis of autoimmune disorders directed against hormone receptors (see p. 319).

169

(see p. 319)

Effects of diet, exercise, trauma and age on immunity

Malnutrition diminishes the effectiveness of the immune response

The greatly increased susceptibility of under-

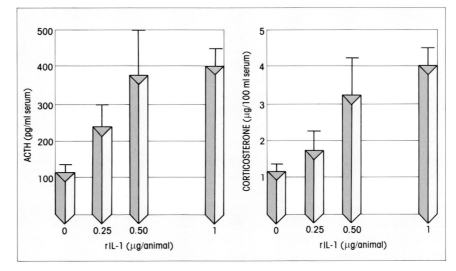

Figure 8.18. *Enhancement of ACTH and corticosterone blood levels in C3H/HeJ mice 2 hours after injection of recombinant IL-1 (values are means ± S.E.M. for groups of 7—8 mice). The significance of the mouse strain used is that they lack receptors for bacterial lipopolysaccharide (LPS) so the effects cannot be attributed to LPS contamination of the IL-1 preparation. (Reprinted from Besedovsky H., del Rey A., Sorkin E. & Dinarello C.A. (1986) Science, 233, 652, with permission. Copyright 1986 by the AAAS.)*

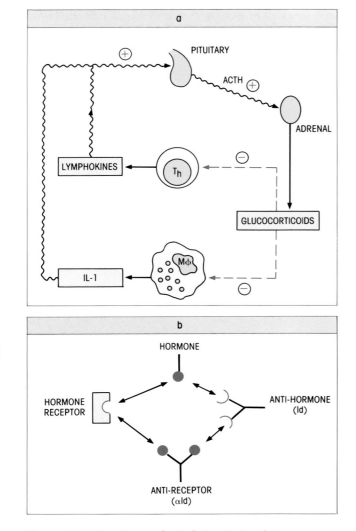

Figure 8.19. *Two immunological circuits involving neurological and endocrinological systems. (a) Glucocorticoid feedback through IL-1 and lymphokine production (after Besedovsky and colleagues). (b) Autoantibodies to hormones and their receptors (cf. figure 8.10).*

activity of thymus hormones and has a major effect on cell-mediated immunity, perhaps as a result.

Moderate restriction of total calorie intake and/or marked reduction in fat intake, ameliorates age-related diseases such as autoimmunity. Oils with an n-3 double bond such as fish oils are also protective, but it is too complex to be confident about the mechanisms at this stage.

Other factors

Exercise, particularly severe exercise, induces stress and raises plasma levels of cortisol, catecholamines, IFNα, IL-1, β-endorphin and metenkephalin. It can lead to reduced IgA levels, immune deficiency and increased susceptibility to infection. Maniacal joggers and other such like masochists—you have been warned!

Multiple traumatic injury, surgery and major burns are also immunosuppressive and so contribute to the increased risk of sepsis. Corticosteroids produced by stressful conditions, the immuno-suppressive prostaglandin E_2 released from damaged tissues and bacterial endotoxin derived from disturbance of gut flora, are all factors which influence the outcome after trauma. A novel suppressive peptide, SAP, appears in serum within hours of a burn and awaits characterization.

Accepting that the problem of understanding the mechanisms of ageing is a tough nut to crack, it is a trifle disappointing that the easier task of establishing the influence of age on immunological phenomena is still not satisfactorily accomplished. Perhaps the elderly population is skewed towards individuals with effective immune systems which give a survival advantage. Be that as it may, there is a general belief that T-cell-mediated functions, such as delayed type hypersensitivity reactions to common skin test antigens and polyclonal responses to mitogens *in vitro*, decline with age and so, it is thought, does T-suppression although this is a notoriously elusive function to measure.

Most B-cell responses to exogenous antigens are not dramatically changed with the passage of time but one of the few well-founded observations concerns the relative increase in agalactosyl oligosaccharides on the Cγ2 domains of IgG (cf. p. 331) from the age of 40 years onwards. Does this give us a clue to the increased prevalence of autoantibodies in our senior citizens?

nourished individuals to infection can be attributed to many factors: poor sanitation and personal hygiene, overcrowding and inadequate health education. But in addition there are gross effects of protein–calorie malnutrition on immuno-competence. The widespread atrophy of lymphoid tissues and the 50% reduction in circulating CD4 T-cells underlies serious impairment of cell-mediated immunity. Antibody responses may be intact but they are of lower affinity; phagocytosis of bacteria is relatively normal but the subsequent intra-cellular destruction is defective. Zinc deficiency is rather interesting; this greatly affects the biological

SUMMARY

Regulation of the antibody response is strongly influenced by antigen concentration; since the response is largely antigen driven, as effective antigen levels fall through catabolism and antibody elimination, the synthesis of antibody wanes. IgG acts as a feedback inhibitor of antibody synthesis, whereas IgM antibodies, which appear early, enhance the response.

T-cells regulate B-lymphocyte responses not only through cooperative help but also by T-cell suppressor networks which are initiated by inducer cells of T-helper phenotype. There is class II restriction governing these interactions and some evidence that I-E (DQ in the human) restriction tends to dominate for suppression. Effector T-cells are guided to their targets by MHC surface molecules, cytotoxic T-cells by class I, T-helpers and T-suppressors by class II.

Lymphocytes can interact with the idiotypes on the receptors of other lymphocytes to form a network (Jerne). Idiotypes which occur frequently and are shared by a multiplicity of antibodies (public or cross-reacting Id) are targets for regulation by anti-idiotypes in the network thus providing a further mechanism for control of the immune response. An idiotype network involving CD5 B-cells is evident in early life. T-cell idiotypic interactions can also be demonstrated. The network offers the potential for therapeutic intervention to manipulate immunity.

A number of varied genetic factors influence the immune response. Approximately ten genes control the overall antibody response to complex antigens: some affect macrophage antigen handling and some the rate of proliferation of differentiating B-cells. Genes coding for antibodies of given specificities may be inherited together with (i.e. linked to) genetic markers for the heavy chain. Immune response genes linked to the major histocompatibility locus define the class II products on the T- and B-cells and antigen-presenting cells which control the interactions required for T—B collaboration. Class II-linked high and low responsiveness may be due to defective presentation by MHC, a defective T-cell repertoire caused by tolerance to MHC + self peptides and T-suppression.

Immunological, neurological and endocrinological systems can all interact and regulatory interdependent circuits are being described.

Malnutrition, exercise, trauma and age can all act to impair immune mechanisms.

Further reading

Blalock J.E. & Bost K.L. (eds) (1988) Neuroimmunoendocrinology. *Progr. Allergy*, **43**, Karger, Basel.

Dorff M. & Benacerraf B. (1984) Suppressor cells and immunoregulation. *Ann. Rev. Immunol.*, **2**, 127.

Male D.K., Champion B. & Cooke A. (1987) *Advanced Immunology*. Gower Medical Publishing, London.

Moller G. (ed.) (1984) Idiotype networks. *Immunol. Rev.*, **79**.

Schwartz R. (1986) Immune response genes of the murine MHC. *Adv. Immunol.*, **38**, 31.

THE ACQUIRED IMMUNE RESPONSE

IV – Development

T-CELL DEVELOPMENT

The multipotential haemopoietic stem cell gives rise to the formed elements of the blood

Haemopoiesis originates in the early yolk sac but as embryogenesis proceeds, this function is taken over by the fetal liver and finally by the bone marrow where it continues throughout life. The haemo-poietic stem cell which gives rise to the formed elements of the blood (figure 9.1) can be shown to be multipotent, to seed other organs and to renew itself through the creation of further stem cells. Thus an animal can be completely protected against the lethal effects of high doses of irradiation by injection of bone marrow cells which will repopulate its lymphoid and myeloid systems. The stem cells differentiate within the micro-environment of sess-ile stromal cells which produce various growth fac-tors such as IL-3, IL-4, IL-6, IL-7, GM-CSF and so on. The importance of this interaction between un-differentiated stem cells and the micro-environment which guides their differentiation is clearly shown by studies on mice homozygous for mutations at the W or the Sl loci which, amongst other defects, have severe macrocytic anaemia. W/W lack myeloid progenitors and can be restored by injection of normal bone marrow stem cells, whereas Sl/Sl, which have normal stem cells but a defective stromal

micro-environment, can be corrected by trans-plantation of a normal spleen fragment (figure 9.2).

We have come a long way towards the goal of isolating highly purified populations of haemato-poietic stem cells. In the mouse, the most likely candidate is the cell with the following surface phenotype: high expression of MHC, low positivity for Thy1, clearly positive for Sca-1 (recognized by a monoclonal antibody reacting with stem cells) and for the adhesion molecule PGP-1, and negative for B220, Mac-1, Gr-1 and CD8 (markers for B-cells, macrophages, granulocytes and cytotoxic T-cells re-spectively. Low-level expression of CD4 may have implications for the aetiology of AIDS. Impressively, less than 100 of such cells can prevent death in a lethally irradiated animal.

The thymus provides the environment for T-cell differentiation

The gland is organized into a series of lobules based upon meshworks of epithelial cells derived embryo-logically from an outpushing of the gut endoderm of the third pharyngeal pouch and which form well-defined cortical and medullary zones (figure 9.3). Monoclonal antibodies raised against thymic epi-thelial cells reveal six staining patterns by im-munofluorescence, which show marked species consistency. There is shared antigen expression between subcapsular, perivascular and medullary epithelium and distinct antigens in the cortical epi-

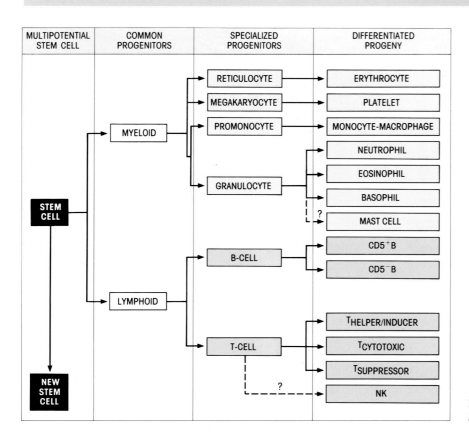

Figure 9.1. *The multipotential haemopoietic stem cell and its progeny.*

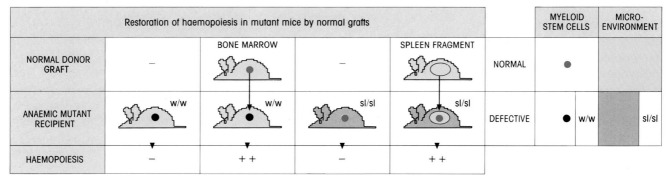

Figure 9.2. *Haemopoiesis requires normal bone marrow stem cells differentiating in a normal micro-environment. (The W locus codes for the c-kit oncogene, a tyrosine kinase membrane receptor on stem cells; Sl locus might encode the ligand for this receptor.)*

thelial cells, one of which is the IL-4 receptor. This framework of cells provides the micro-environment for T-cell differentiation and produces a series of peptide hormones of which four have been well characterized and sequenced: thymulin, α_1 and β_4-thymosin, and thymopoietin (and its active pentapeptide TP-5). They mostly seem capable of promoting the appearance of T-cell differentiation markers and a variety of T-cell functions on culture with bone marrow cells *in vitro*, but while it seems clear that they will be concerned with the many

differentiation steps within the thymus, the details of how they operate and integrate *in vivo* are still lacking.

The specialized large epithelial cells in the outer cortex are known as 'nurse' cells because they can each be associated with large numbers of lymphocytes which do appear to be lying within their cytoplasm. The epithelial cells of the deep cortex have branched dendritic processes rich in class II MHC. They connect through desmosomes to form a network through which cortical lymphocytes must

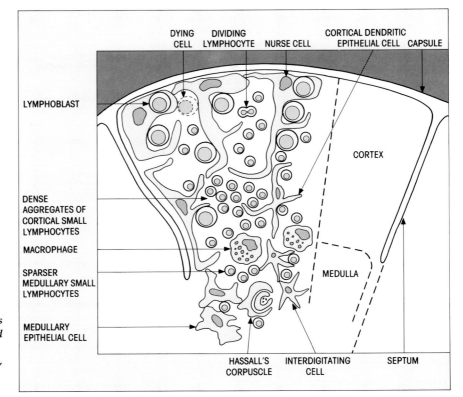

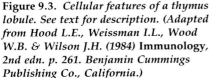

*Figure 9.3. Cellular features of a thymus lobule. See text for description. (Adapted from Hood L.E., Weissman I.L., Wood W.B. & Wilson J.H. (1984) **Immunology**, 2nd edn. p. 261. Benjamin Cummings Publishing Co., California.)*

175

pass on their way to the medulla (figure 9.3). The cortical lymphocytes are densely packed compared with those in the medulla, many are in division and a surprising number are in the throes of dying as evidenced by their pyknotic nuclei. On their way to the medulla, the lymphocytes pass a cordon of 'sentinel' macrophages at the cortico-medullary junction. A number of bone-marrow-derived inter-digitating dendritic cells are present in the medulla and the epithelial cells have broader processes than their cortical counterparts and express high levels of both class I and class II MHC. Whorled, possibly degenerate aggregates of epithelial cells form the highly characteristic Hassall's corpuscles beloved of histopathology examiners.

A fairly complex relationship with the nervous system awaits discovery; the thymus is richly innervated with both adrenergic and cholinergic fibres, while the neurotransmitter oxytocin, vasoppressin and neurophysin are synthesized endogenously by subcapsular, perivascular and medullary epithelial cells and nurse cells. Acute stress leads to an indecently rapid loss of cortical thymocytes and an increase in epithelial cells expressing both cortical and medullary markers — surely intrathymic epithelial stem cells? The destruction of cortical thymocytes is at least partly due to the cytolytic action of steroids, the relative invulnerability of the medullary lymphocytes being attributable to their possession of a 20α-hydroxyl steroid dehydrogenase. The distinctive nature of the two main compartments in the gland is emphasized by the selective atrophy induced by a number of agents; thus the primary target of organotin is the immature cortical thymocyte, dioxin interacts with a receptor on cortical epithelial cells, while the immunosuppressive drug cyclosporin A causes atrophy of all the medullary elements thereby blocking differentiation of cortical to medullary thymocyte with intriguing consequences.

There is a general view that the thymus involutes with age, but this may be less extreme than the description in many textbooks since quite large normal thymuses can be found in adults at autopsy while involution in other samples could be due to stress associated with illness before death.

Bone marrow stem cells become immunocompetent T-cells in the thymus

The evidence comes from experiments on the reconstitution of irradiated hosts. An irradiated animal is restored by bone marrow grafts through the immediate restitution of granulocyte precursors; in the longer term also through reconstitution of the T- and B-cells destroyed by irradiation. However, if the animal is thymectomized before irradiation, bone marrow cells will not reconstitute the T-lymphocyte population (figure 9.4).

By day 11−12 in the mouse embryo, lymphoblastoid stem cells from the bone marrow begin to colonize the periphery of the epithelial thymus rudiment. If the thymus is removed at this stage and incubated in organ culture, a whole variety of mature T-lymphocytes will be generated. This is not seen if 10-day thymuses are cultured and shows that the lymphoblastoid colonizers give rise to the immunocompetent small lymphocyte progeny.

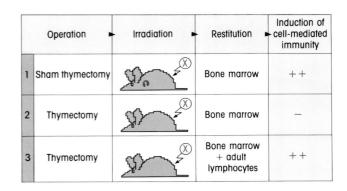

	Operation	Irradiation	Restitution	Induction of cell-mediated immunity
1	Sham thymectomy	Ⓧ	Bone marrow	+ +
2	Thymectomy	Ⓧ	Bone marrow	−
3	Thymectomy	Ⓧ	Bone marrow + adult lymphocytes	+ +

Figure 9.4. *Maturation of bone marrow stem cells under the influence of the thymus to become immunocompetent lymphocytes capable of cell-mediated immune reactions. X-irradiation (X) destroys the ability of host lymphocytes to mount a cellular immune response but the stem cells in injected bone marrow can become immunocompetent and restore the response (1) unless the thymus is removed (2), in which case only already immunocompetent lymphocytes are effective (3). Incidentally, the bone marrow stem cells also restore the levels of other formed elements of the blood (red cells, platelets, neutrophils, monocytes) which otherwise fall dramatically after X-irradiation and such therapy is crucial in cases where accidental or therapeutic exposure to X-rays or other anti-mitotic agents seriously damages the haemopoietic cells.*

Differentiation is accompanied by changes in surface markers

The incoming prothymocyte attracted to the thymus by thymotaxin, a chemotactic factor, stains positively for the enzyme TdT (figure 9.5) which is thought to be involved in the insertion of nucleotide sequences at the N-terminal region of *D* and *J* variable region segments to increase diversity of the T-cell receptors (cf. p. 59). The cortical thymocytes soon express the surface markers CD2 and CD7 and, under the influence of IL-1 and perhaps through engagement of CD2 with LFA-3 on stromal cells, the gene encoding IL-2 is activated. This in turn induces expression of the full IL-2 receptor and a massive autocrine expansion of the cortical thymocytes is set in train. CD1 and CD5 together with CD3, the invariant signal transducing complex of the T-cell receptor, next appear and then the cells begin to express T-cell receptor variable chains. At this stage the cells do not stain for surface CD4 or CD8, the markers of the helper/inducer and cytotoxic/suppressor subsets respectively, but subsequently, the cells which have rearranged their α- and β-T-cell receptor genes now become double positive CD4$^+$8$^+$. Finally the cells traverse the corticomedullary junction to the medulla where the CD4 and CD8 markers segregate in parallel with differentiation into separate immunocompetent populations of T-helpers and cytotoxic T-cell precursors (figure 9.5).

The precise lineage of NK cells is still in doubt. They express the markers CD2, 3 and 8 which are normally restricted to T-cells, they have IL-2 receptors and are driven to proliferate by IL-2 and they

can produce IFNγ. Their T-receptor *V* genes are not rearranged but they must be related to T-cells in some way.

Receptor rearrangement

The rearrangement of *V, D, J* and *C* region genes required to generate the T-cell receptor (p. 58) has not yet taken place at the prothymocyte stage. The Lyf-1 gene for TdT and the recombinase activator gene are transcribed at the pre-T stage and, by day 15, cells with the γδ TCR1 can be detected in the mouse thymus followed on day 19 by the appearance of TCR2 αβ-cells (figure 9.6). Mice expressing rearranged γ and δ transgenes do not rearrange any further γ or δ gene segments, indicating that once a cell expresses a given V, D, J combination, it suppresses rearrangement of the γδ genes on the sister chromatid (remember each cell contains two chromosomes for each γ and δ cluster, one from each parent). Thus each cell expresses only a single γδ receptor and the process by which the homologous genes on the sister chromatid are suppressed is called *allelic exclusion* (cf. p. 185). Shorter γ and δ transgene constructs which lack a *cis*-acting 'silencer' region greatly inhibited the generation of

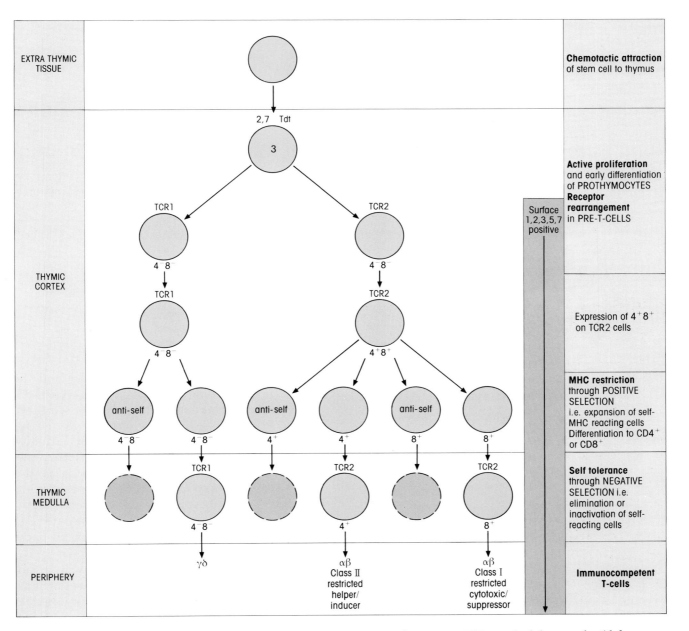

Figure 9.5. *Differentiation of T-cells within the thymus gland. Numbers refer to CD designation. TCR1, γδ receptors.* *TCR2, αβ receptors. TdT, terminal deoxynucleotidyl transferase.*

177

αβ T-cell clones while enhancing the number of γδ-cells.

γδ-T-cells in the mouse, unlike the human, predominate in association with epithelial cells. A curious feature of the cells leaving the fetal thymus is the restriction in V-gene utilization. Thus virtually all of the first wave of fetal γδ cells express the same V-genes and colonize the skin; the second wave use the same δ-gene combination but a different γ V-J pair and they seed the female reproductive organs

(figure 9.7). In adult life, there is far more receptor diversity due to a high degree of junctional variation (cf. p. 59) although the intraepithelial cells in the intestine and those in encapsulated lymphoid tissue form two distinct groups with respect to single V gene usage. By contrast, αβ T-cells are much more heterogeneous in V-gene expression.

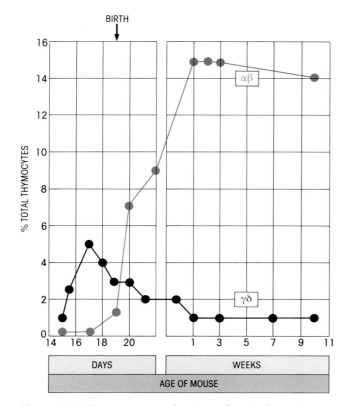

Figure 9.6. *The appearance of mature αβ and γδ receptor positive T-cells in the thymus with time. (Data reproduced from Tonegawa et al. (1989) Progress in Immunology 7, 243. Melchers F. et al. (eds). Springer-Verlag, Berlin.)*

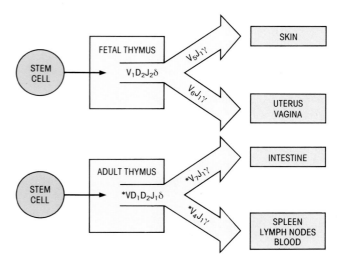

Figure 9.7. *Predominant development of mouse γδ T-cell subsets in fetal and adult thymus. Adult receptors show a high degree of junctional diversity*. (Reference as in figure 9.6.)*

Cells are positively selected for self-MHC restriction in the thymus

The ability of T-cells to recognize antigenic peptides in association with self-MHC is developed in the thymus gland. If an (H-2^k × H-2^b) F1 animal is sensitized to an antigen, the primed T-cells can recognize that antigen on presenting cells of either H-2^k or H-2^b haplotype, i.e. they can use either parental haplotype as a recognition restriction element. However, if bone marrow cells from the (H-$2^{k×b}$) F1 are used to reconstitute an irradiated F1 which had earlier been thymectomized and given an H-2^k thymus, the subsequently primed T-cells can only recognize antigens in the context of H-2^k, not of H-2^b (figure 9.8). Thus it is the phenotype of the thymus that imprints H-2 restriction on the differentiating T-cells.

It will also be seen in figure 9.8 that incubation of the thymus graft with deoxyguanosine, which destroys the cells of macrophage and dendritic cell lineage, has no effect on imprinting suggesting that

this function is carried out by epithelial cells. These cells are rich in surface MHC molecules and the current view is that double positive (CD4$^+$8$^+$) T-cells bearing receptors which recognize self-MHC on the epithelial cells are positively selected for differentiation to CD4$^+$8$^-$ or CD4$^-$8$^+$ single positive cells. The evidence for this comes largely from transgenic mice in which the appropriate genes are introduced artificially into fertilized eggs. Since this is a very active area, I would like to cite some experimental examples; non-professionals may need to hang on to their haplotypes, put on their ice-packs and concentrate.

One highly sophisticated study starts with a cytotoxic T-cell clone raised in H-2^b females against male cells of the same strain. The clone recognizes the male antigen, H-Y, and this is seen in association with the H-2D^b self-MHC molecules, i.e. it reacts with the H-2^b/Y complex. The α- and β-clones forming the T-cell receptor of this clone are now introduced as transgenes into mice with severe combined immunodeficiency (SCID) which lack the ability to rearrange their own germ-line variable region receptor genes; thus the only T-cell receptor which could possibly be expressed is that of the transgene, provided of course, we are looking at females rather than males in whom the clone would be eliminated by self-reactivity. If the transgenic SCID females bear the original H-2^b haplotype (e.g. F1 hybrids between b × d haplotypes) then the anti-H^b/Y receptor is amply expressed on CD8$^+$ cytotoxic precursor cells (table 9.1a), whereas H-2$^{d/d}$ trans-

Figure 9.8. *Imprinting of H-2 T-helper restriction by the thymus. Host mice were F1 crosses between strains of haplotype H-2^b and H-2^k. They were thymectomized and grafted with 14 day fetal thymuses, irradiated and reconstituted with F1 bone marrow. After priming with the antigen, keyhole limpet haemocyanin (KLH), the proliferative response of lymph node T-cells to KLH on antigen-presenting cells of each parental haplotype was assessed. In some experiments the thymus lobes were cultured in deoxyguanosine (dGuo) which destroys intrathymic cells of macrophage/ dendritic cell lineage. (From Lo D. & Sprent J. (1986)* **Nature 319,** *672.)*

Thymectomize b × k mice	Graft with thymus of haplotype	Irradiate and reconstitute with b × k bone marrow	Prime with KLH	Proliferative response of primed T-cells to KLH on antigen-presenting cells of haplotype	
				H-2^b	H-2^k
	b × k	⟶		+ +	+ +
	b	⟶		+ +	−
	dGuo-treated b	⟶		+ +	−
	k	⟶		−	+ +
	dGuo-treated k	⟶		−	+ +

genics lacking H-2^b produce only double CD4$^+$8$^+$ thymocytes with no single CD4$^+$8$^-$ or CD4$^-$8$^+$ cells. Thus as CD4$^+$8$^+$ cells express their TCR transgene, they only differentiate into CD8$^+$ immunocompetent cells if they come into contact with thymic epithelial cells of the MHC haplotype recognized by their receptor. We say that such self-recognizing thymocytes are being *positively selected*.

In another example, genes coding for an αβ-receptor from a T-helper clone (2B4) which responds to moth cytochrome c in association with the class II molecule I-Eα^k,β^b (remember I-E has an α and β chain), are transfected into H-2^k and H-2^b mice. H-2^k express the I-E molecule on the surface of their antigen-presenting cells, but H-2^b do not. In the event, the frequency of circulating CD4$^+$ T-cells

bearing the 2B4 receptor was 10 times greater in the H-2^k relative to H-2^b strains, again speaking for positive selection of double positive thymocytes which recognize their own thymic MHC. In a further twist to the story, positive selection only occurred in mice manipulated to express I-E on their cortical rather than their medullary epithelial cells, showing that this differentiation step is affected before the developing thymocytes reach the medulla.

The induction of immunological tolerance is necessary to avoid self-reactivity

In essence, lymphocytes recognize foreign antigens through complementariness in shape mediated by the intermolecular forces we have described previously (p. 68). To a large extent the building blocks used to form microbial and host molecules are the same, so it is the assembled shapes of *self* and *non-self* molecules which must be discriminated by the immune system if potentially disastrous auto-reactivity is to be avoided. The restriction of each lymphocyte to a single specificity makes the job of establishing self-tolerance that much easier simply because it just requires a mechanism which functionally deletes self-reacting cells and leaves the remainder of the repertoire unscathed. The most radical difference between self and non-self molecules lies in the fact that, in early life, the developing lymphocytes are surrounded by self and normally only meet non-self antigens at a later stage. With its customary efficiency, the blind force

Table 9.1. *Positive and negative selection in severe combined immunodeficiency (SCID) transgenic mice bearing the αβ receptors of an H-2D^b T-cell clone cytotoxic for the male antigen H-Y.*

Phenotype	a Positive selection Transgenic females		b Negative selection Transgenic H-2b	
	H-2$^{b/d}$	H-2$^{d/d}$	Males	Females
CD4$^-$8$^-$ TCR$^-$	+	+ +	+ + +	+
CD4$^+$8$^+$ TCR$^\pm$	+ +	+ +	−	+ + +
CD4$^-$8$^+$ TCR^{++}	+	−	−	+
CD4$^+$8$^-$ TCR^{++}	−	−	−	−

The pluses represent a crude measure of the relative numbers of T-cells in the thymus having the phenotype indicated. (Based on data from von Boehmer H. et al. (1989) **In Progress in Immunology 7,** *297. Melchers F. et al. (eds), Springer Verlag, Berlin.)*

of evolution has exploited this temporal difference to establish the mechanisms of immunological tolerance to host constituents as we shall now see.

The discovery of neonatal tolerance

Over 40 years ago Owen made the intriguing observation that non-identical (dizygotic) twin cattle, which shared the same placental circulation and whose circulations were thereby linked, grew up with appreciable numbers of red cells from the other twin in their blood; if they had not shared the same circulation at birth, red cells from the twin injected in adult life would be rapidly eliminated by an immunological response. From this finding Burnet and Fenner conceived the notion that potential antigens which reach the lymphoid cells during their developing immunologically immature phase can in some way specifically suppress any future response to that antigen when the animal reaches immunological maturity. This, they considered, would provide a means whereby unresponsiveness to the body's own constituents could be established and thereby enable the lymphoid cells to make the important distinction between 'self' and 'non-self'. On this basis, any foreign cells introduced into the body around the perinatal period should trick the animal into treating them as 'self' components in later life and the studies of Medawar and his colleagues have shown that *immunological tolerance* or unresponsiveness can be artificially induced in this way. Thus neonatal injection of CBA mouse cells into newborn A strain animals suppresses their ability to immunologically reject a CBA graft in adult life (figures 9.9 and 9.10). Tolerance can

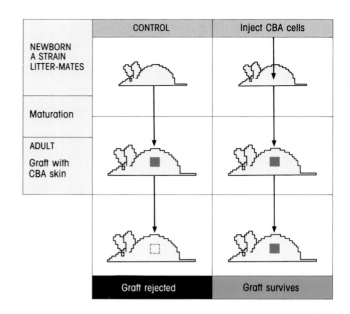

Figure 9.9. *Induction of tolerance to foreign CBA skin graft in A strain mice by neonatal injection of antigen (after Billingham R., Brent L. & Medawar P.B. (1953)* **Nature 172,** *603). The effect is antigen specific since the tolerant mice can reject third-party grafts normally.*

also be induced with soluble antigens; for example, rabbits injected with bovine serum albumin at birth fail to make antibodies on later challenge with this protein.

Persistence of antigen is required to maintain tolerance. In Medawar's experiments the tolerant state was long lived because the injected CBA cells survived and the animals continued to be chimaeric (i.e. they possessed both A and CBA cells). With non-living antigens such as BSA, tolerance is gradu-

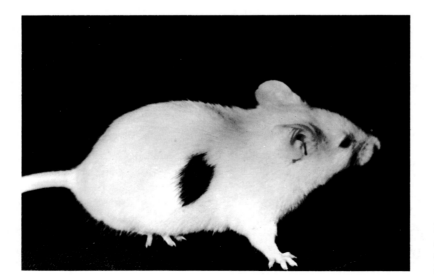

Figure 9.10. *CBA skin graft on fully tolerant A strain mouse showing healthy hair growth eight weeks after grafting (courtesy of Prof. L. Brent).*

CHAPTER 9

ally lost, the most likely explanation being that, in the absence of antigen, newly recruited immunocompetent cells which are being generated throughout life are not being rendered tolerant. Since recruitment of newly competent T-lymphocytes is drastically curtailed by removal of the thymus, it is of interest to note that the tolerant state persists for much longer in thymectomized animals.

Induction of self-tolerance in the thymus

If stem cells in bone marrow of H-2^k haplotype are cultured with fetal thymus of H-2^d origin, the maturing cells become tolerant to H-2^d as shown by their inability to give a mixed lymphocyte proliferative response when cultured with stimulators of H-2^d phenotype; third-party responsiveness is not affected. Further experiments with deoxyguanosine-treated thymuses showed that the cells responsible for tolerance induction were deoxyguanosine-sensitive, bone-marrow derived macrophages or dendritic cells which are abundant at the corticomedullary junction (table 9.2).

Intra-thymic clonal deletion leads to self-tolerance

There seems little doubt that self-reactive T-cells can be physically deleted within the thymus gland. If we look back at the experiment in table 9.1b we can see that SCID males bearing the transgenes coding for the αβ receptor reacting with the male H-Y antigen do not possess any thymic cells expressing this receptor whereas the females which lack H-Y do. In other words, self-reactive cells undergo a *negative selection* process in the thymus. A similar phenomenon is seen when the thymic cells bear certain self-components which react with a whole family of V_β receptors, probably by recognizing non-variable structures on a V_β segment. An example of such a 'superantigen' (cf. p. 117) is the 1-E molecule which reacts with receptors belonging to the V_β17a family; strains which cannot express 1-E because of a defect in the E_α gene, possess mature T-cells utilizing V_β17a, whereas strains which express 1-E normally delete their V_β17a positive T-cells. Likewise mice of the Mls[a] genotype delete V_β6-bearing cells, the Mls being a locus encoding a B-cell product which induces strong proliferation in T-cells from a strain bearing a different Mls allele. Even exogenous superantigens such as staphylococcal enterotoxin B which activates the V_β3 and V_β8 T-cell families in the adult, will eliminate these cells when incubated with early immature thymocytes. Even more enlightening is the fact that under these circumstances, the V_β3 and V_β8 thymocytes can actually be seen to undergo programmed cell death (apoptosis, cf. p. 15). The phenomenon seems to be linked to intracellular calcium mobilization since calcium ionophores do the same thing. An interesting clue comes from the observation that when double positive CD4[+]8[+] thymocytes have their receptors engaged by a TCR antibody, only half mobilize Ca[++] and only half are eliminated, whereas an anti-CD3 mobilizes Ca[++] in all and each one dies (cf. figure 9.11); this implies that signalling between the TCR (αβ and probably γδ) and the CD3 complex during differentiation is crucially related to the negative selection tolerance process.

If we pause for breath and try to bring things together in a coherent way, we seem to be saying that early engagement of the T-cell receptor of differentiating double-positive CD4[+]8[+] thymocytes with self-MHC on cortical epithelial cells leads to expansion and positive selection for clones which recognize self-MHC, perhaps with a whole range of affinities, but that engagement of the TCR of more mature cells with high affinity for self MHC (+ self peptide) on bone-marrow-derived medullary cells will lead to elimination and hence negative selection. To put it bluntly, it looks as though thymic epithelial cells are concerned (as one of their jobs) with establishing the specificity of MHC restriction whereas the macrophage/dendritic cells (and B-cells) may be concerned with tolerance induction to self. This view finds support rather neatly in the

181

Table 9.2. *Induction of tolerance in bone marrow stem cells by incubation with deoxyguanosine-sensitive macrophages or dendritic cells in the thymus. These inducing cells can be replaced by progenitors in the bone marrow inoculum (Jenkinson E.J., Jhittay P., Kingston R. & Owen J.J. (1985) Transplantation 39, 331) or by adult dendritic cells from spleen showing that it is the stage of differentiation of the immature T-cell rather than any special nature of the thymic antigen presenting cell which leads to tolerance (Matzinger P. & Guerder S. (1989) Nature 338, 74).*

Bone marrow cells	Incubate with H-2^d thymus	Tolerance induction to H-2 haplotype		
		k	d	b
k	Untreated	+	+	−
k	d Guo-treated	+	−	−
k + d	d Guo-treated	+	+	−

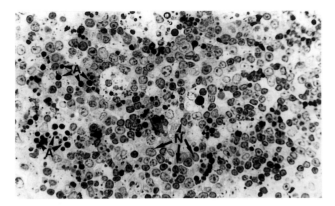

a

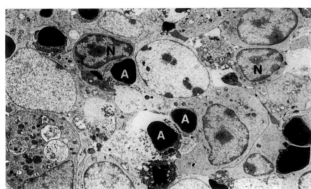

b

Figure 9.11. *Histological appearance of cells induced to undergo apoptosis in intact fetal thymus lobes after short-term exposure to anti-CD3. (a) Toluidine blue-stained 1μm sections. (b) Electron micrograph taken from the same anti-CD3 treated culture as in (a). A and N indicate representative apoptotic and normal lymphocytes respectively. Note the highly condensed state of the nuclei of the apoptotic lymphocytes. (Photographs kindly donated by Prof. J.J.T. Owen, from Smith et al. (1989) Nature, 337, 181. Reproduced by permission from Macmillan Journals Ltd., London.)*

following: a hybrid antibody which links the TCR to MHC by reacting with both $V_\beta 8$ and class I or II MHC, when added to cultures of early thymocytes, leads to an increase in the number of $V_\beta 8$ positive T-cells, whereas in cultures of more mature thymocytes there is a reduction in these cells.

T-cell tolerance can be due to clonal anergy

A $CD4^+$ T-helper clone responds to stimulation by its corresponding antigenic peptide present on an appropriate cell by proliferation and cytokine synthesis. If the peptide is first added to a fixed antigen-presenting cell, the helper-clone becomes unresponsive; recognition of peptide/MHC does

impart a signal which leads to Ca^{++} mobilization but the IL-2 gene is not activated. We have already entertained the idea that engagement of the T-cell receptor plus a costimulatory signal from an antigen-presenting cell are both required for T-cell stimulation, but now we are going further and saying that when the costimulatory signal is lacking, the T-cell becomes tolerized or anergic, or if you prefer, paralysed.

This happens *in vivo*. When a transgene construct of $I-E^b$ attached to an insulin promoter is introduced into a mouse which normally fails to express I-E, the $I-E^b$ transgene product appears on the β-cells of the pancreas and induces tolerance to itself. Whereas the expression of I-E on bone-marrow-derived cells in the thymic medulla deletes T-cells bearing $V_\beta 17a$ receptors, the cells are not lost in the tolerant transgenic mouse expressing pancreatic I-E, i.e. there is a state of clonal anergy, not deletion. The altered immunological status of these cells is revealed by their inability to proliferate when their receptors are cross-linked by an antibody to $V_\beta 17a$.

Lack of communication can cause unresponsiveness

It takes two to tango: if the self-molecule cannot engage the T-cell receptor there can be no response. The anatomical isolation of molecules like the lens protein of the eye and myelin basic protein in the brain virtually precludes them from contact with lymphocytes except perhaps for minute amounts of breakdown metabolic products which leak out and may be taken up by antigen-presenting cells, but at concentrations way below that required to trigger the corresponding naive T-cell.

Molecules that are specifically restricted to particular organs which do come into contact with circulating lymphocytes represent another special case. Common cellular components expressed in the MHC class II positive tolerance-inducing cells of the thymic medulla will presumably delete their self-reacting lymphocyte counterparts. Organ-specific molecules, such as thyroid peroxidase, are by definition not present in these thymic cells and since the cells they are associated with do not normally express MHC class II, there is no opportunity for clonal deletion or paralysis of the thyroid specific helper T-cells. We are left with a situation in which the body has self-reactive T-cells, which can be demonstrated, and the corresponding organ-specific potential antigen, but they do not communicate because of the lack of class II molecules.

There is another subtle form of silent or uncommunicative unresponsiveness in which an animal rendered tolerant by a high dose of protein can fail to have tolerized all antigen-specific cells if natural processing by antigen-presenting cells does not produce a high enough concentration of a given peptide to tolerize or activate them. However, if the animal is now immunized with the peptide itself, these naive cells will be stimulated and their progeny, having an increased affinity (cf. p. 71) and thereby being capable of recognizing lower concentrations of peptide, can now be stimulated by the original antigen. This may sound a trifle tortuous but the principle could have important implications for the induction of autoimmunity by cross-reacting T-cell epitopes (cf. figure 14.10).

Immunological silence would also result if an individual has no genes coding for lymphocyte receptors directed against particular self-determinants; analysis of the experimentally induced autoantibody response to cytochrome *c* suggests that only those parts of the molecule which show species variation are autoantigenic whereas the highly conserved regions where the genes have not altered for a much longer time appear to be silent, supposedly because the autoreactive specificities have had time to disappear.

Do T-suppressors contribute to self-tolerance?

Frankly, we do not know, but it seems likely that if autoimmunity is induced in a normal animal either actively by injection of an antigen cross-reacting with self, or passively by injection of autoreactive T-cells (cf. p. 321, 343), the self-reacting clones are usually squashed by T-suppression. In a nutshell, suppressors probably do not prevent autoimmunity but they may reverse it.

B-CELL DEVELOPMENT

B-cells differentiate in the fetal liver and then in bone marrow

The B-lymphocyte precursors, pro-B-cells, are present among the islands of haemopoietic cells in fetal liver by 8—9 weeks of gestation in man and 14 days in the mouse. Production of B-cells wanes and is taken over by the bone marrow for the remainder of life. Using the modified culture conditions recently introduced by Whitlock and Witte, it is now possible to grow bone marrow cells *in vitro* and achieve the growth of pre-B and B-cells. Although pre-B cells comprise only a minor subpopulation of the cells in those cultures, it is possible to analyse the different stages in their development by rescue with the Abelson murine leukaemia virus (A-MuLV), a replication-defective retrovirus capable of transforming pre-B cells at various points in their development into clones.

Phenotypic changes in differentiating B-cells

After the rearrangement of Ig genes which occurs during the pre-B-cell stage, the early rapidly dividing pre-B cells display cytoplasmic μ chains but no light chains (figure 9.12). Two genes, *pre-B1* and *λ5*, with homology for the V_L and C_L segments of λ-light chains respectively, are temporarily transcribed to form a 'pseudo-light chain' whose function is obscure. Subsequently, the true light chains are expressed and, in the immature B-cell, the receptor for which the cell is finally programmed is inserted into the plasma membrane as a specific IgM molecule.

At the next stage of differentiation, the cell develops a commitment to producing a particular antibody class and either bears surface IgM alone or in combination with IgA or IgG. The further addition of surface IgD now marks the readiness of the virgin B-cell for priming by antigen. Some cells, therefore, bear surface Ig of three different classes; M, G and D or M, A and D, but all Ig molecules on a single cell have the same idiotype and therefore are derived from the same V_H and V_L genes presumably by splicing of a long RNA transcript. IgD is lost on antigenic stimulation so that memory cells lack this Ig. At the terminal stages in the life of a fully mature plasma cell, virtually all surface Ig is shed. Injection of anti-μ (anti-IgM heavy chain) into chick embryos prevents the subsequent maturation of IgM and IgG antibody-producing cells, whereas anti-γ inhibits only IgG development. Although we have seen earlier that T-helpers can induce class-switching, it is also the case that some isotype switching probably occurs independently of antigen as a result of microenvironmental factors. In the embryonic chicken bursa, a regular switch from IgM to IgG is observed and it seems possible that local influences in the gut will prove to be responsible for the predominant development of IgA bearing cells. These cells are

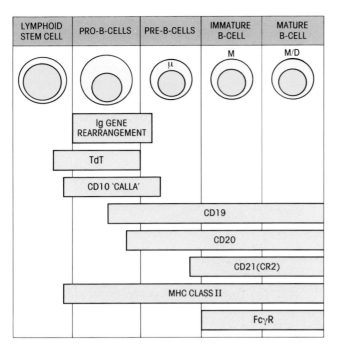

| LYMPHOID STEM CELL | PRO-B-CELLS | PRE-B-CELLS | IMMATURE B-CELL | MATURE B-CELL |

Figure 9.12. *Differentiation markers of developing B-cells. The boxes show the time of appearance of the surface markers, many of them defined by monoclonal antibodies (see table 6.1 for list of CD members).*

184

generated in Peyer's patches, pass into the blood via the thoracic duct and return to populate the diffuse lymphoid tissue in the lamina propria of the gut.

There are marked differences between CD5 positive and negative B-cells

We have previously drawn attention to the sub-population of B-cells which, in addition to surface Ig, express the T-cell marker CD5 in the human and its homologue, Ly1 in the mouse. The progenitors of this subset move from the bone marrow to the peritoneal cavity fairly early in life, at which stage they are the most abundant B-cell type and pre-dominate in their contribution to the idiotype network and to the production of low-affinity multi-specific IgM autoantibodies and the so-called 'natural' antibodies to bacterial carbohydrates which seemingly arise slightly later in the neonatal period without obvious exposure to conventional antigens. It has been suggested that the CD5 popu-lation form an inward-looking world in which the component B-cells recognize and stimulate each other ceaselessly through their idiotypic receptor interactions with relatively limited responses to

external antigens, characterized by T-independence and lack of affinity maturation. The protective IgM polysaccharide antibodies produced by CD5 cells are generally highly restricted in their usage of V_H and V_L genes and therefore tend to express particular dominant idiotypes. Very early injection of BALB/c mice with IgM antibodies to the major anti-phosphoryl choline (T15) and anti-dextran (J558) idiotypes greatly augmented the subsequent re-sponse to immunization with these two antigens. By contrast, injection of IgG anti-idiotype, or of the idiotype itself, resulted in impairment of these re-sponses and it seems clear that these early-appearing cells do much to shape the adult repertoire of the CD5 population.

The low-affinity self-reactivity of many $CD5^+$ B-cells is enigmatic. Is recognition of self more important than non-self? There is little evidence for this in the case of CD5 negative B-cells and even the $CD5^+$ cells develop specificities against extrinsic antigens. As discussed earlier, this comfy internal self-contemplation may be linked to maintenance of the V-gene pool and to subsequent development of adult specificities. The autoantibodies normally produced by these cells do not cause tissue damage; they could play a role in self-tolerance induction. Although IgM autoantibodies in mice with spon-taneous autoimmune disease are made by $CD5^+$ B-cells, we are uncertain whether it is these cells which undergo a switch to produce the high affinity IgG autoantibodies associated with pathogenesis. The striking differences between $CD5^+$ and con-ventional B-cells come into sharp focus when they are tabulated (table 9.3).

The sequence of immunoglobulin gene rearrangements

By analysis of Abelson-MuLV-transformed clones of pre-B cells, it has proved possible to unravel the orderly cascade of Ig gene rearrangements which occur during differentiation.

1 Initially, the *D-J* segments on *both* heavy chain coding regions (one from each parent) rearrange (figure 9.13).

2 A *V-DJ* recombinational event now occurs on one chain. If this proves to be a *non-productive* rearrangement (i.e. adjacent segments are joined in an incorrect reading frame or in such a way as to generate a termination codon downstream from the splice point), then a second *V-DJ* rearrangement

Table 9.3. *Comparison of two mouse B-cell subsets.*

	CD5 (Ly-1) B	CONVENTIONAL B
ONTOGENY	Arise first	Arise later
MAIN LOCATION	Peritoneal (PerC) & Pleural Cavities	Lymphoid Organs
ADULT POPULATION	Self-replenishing (no new entrants)	Constantly renewed
ADULT SOURCE FOR ADOPTIVE TRANSFER	Mature Ly-1 B (PerC)	Ig- progenitors (BM, spleen)
DEVELOPMENTAL REGULATION	Feedback inhibition by mature Ly-1 B	?
DEVELOPMENT IMPAIRED	Xid (CBA/N)[1]	me^v (motheaten)[2]
PHENOTYPE:		
IgM	+++	+
IgD	+	+++
B220/6B2	+	+++
CD5 (Ly-1)	+	−
CD11a (MAC-1)	+ (only in PerC)	−
CD23 (Fcε R)	−	+
Size	large	small
ANTIBODY PRODUCTION:		
Serum IgM, IgG3	+++	+
IgG1	+	+++
IgG2a, IgG2b	+ − ++	++ − +++
IgM autoantibody	+++	?
IgM anti-bacterial ab	+++	+ − +++
Anti-hapten, anti-protein	?	+++
T-dependence	−	++
Affinity maturation	−	++

1 *CBA/N mice have X-linked immunodeficiency gene (Xid) associated with defective CD5 B-cell maturation and poor response to type II T-independent antigens.*
2 *Motheaten mice have widespread autoimmunity and most of their B-cells are CD5+ (from Herzenberg L.A. & Stall A. (1989) Progress in Immunology 7, 409. Melchers F. et al. (eds). Springer Verlag, Berlin).*

will occur on the sister heavy chain region. If a productive rearrangement is achieved, the pre-B cell expresses cytoplasmic μ chains.

3 The next set of Ig gene rearrangements occur on the κ light chain gene loci and these involve *V-J* recombinations on first one and then the other κ allele until a productive $V_κ$-*J* rearrangement is accomplished. Were that to fail, an attempt would be made to achieve productive rearrangement of the λ alleles.

4 The IgM molecule now prohibits any further gene shuffling.

Allelic exclusion

Since each cell has chromosome complements derived from each parent, the differentiating B-cell has four light and two heavy chain gene clusters to choose from. Once the *V.D.J.* DNA rearrangement has occurred within one light and one heavy chain cluster, the V genes on the other four chromosomes are held by some mechanism in the embryonic state so that the cell is able to express *only one light and one heavy chain*. This so-called *allelic exclusion* is essential for clonal selection to work since the cell is then only programmed to make the one antibody it uses as a cell surface receptor to recognize antigen. Furthermore, this gene exclusion mechanism prevents the formation of molecules containing two different light or two different heavy chains which would have non-identical combining sites and therefore be functionally monovalent with respect to the majority of antigens; such antibodies would be non-agglutinating and would tend to have low avidity because the bonus effect of multivalency could not operate.

Two mechanisms have been postulated to account for allelic exclusion. The stochastic (random) model proposed that because of a high probability of un-productive rearrangement, only one functional allele was likely to be created. The feedback model proposed that the creation of a functional Ig some-how inhibited subsequent rearrangement at allelic loci. Studies with transgenic mice in which a pre-rearranged μ-gene was successfully injected into fertilized mouse embryos, have provided support for the feedback model. Thus the presence of a functional transmembrane μ-gene represses heavy chain gene rearrangements in pre-B cells (figure 9.13). Furthermore, the formation of associated heavy and light chains inhibits any subsequent light chain gene rearrangement.

Different specific responses can appear sequentially

The responses to given antigens in the neonatal period appear sequentially as though each species were programmed to rearrange its V genes in a definite order (figure 9.14). Early in ontogeny there is a bias favouring the rearrangement of the V_H genes most proximal to the DJ segment.

The induction of tolerance in B-lymphocytes

Tolerance can be caused by clonal deletion and clonal anergy

Just as for T-cells, so both mechanisms can operate on B-cells to prevent the reaction to self. Excellent

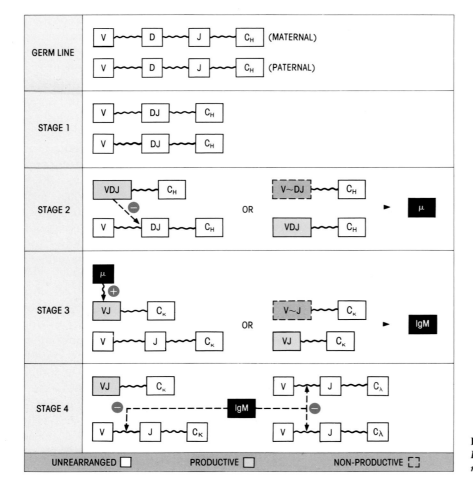

Figure 9.13. *Postulated sequence of B-cell gene rearrangements and mechanism of allelic exclusion (see text).*

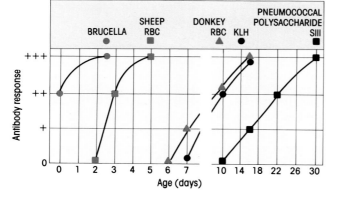

Figure 9.14. *Sequential appearance of responsiveness to different antigens in the neonatal rat. (RBC = red blood cell; KLH = keyhole limpet haemocyanin.)*

evidence for deletion comes from mice bearing transgenes coding for IgM which binds to H-2K molecules of all H-2 haplotypes except *d* and *f*. Mice of H-2^d haplotype express the transgenic IgM abundantly in the serum while 25–50% of total B-

cells bear the transgenic idiotype. H2^d × H2^k F1 crosses completely failed to express the transgene either in the serum or on B-cells, i.e. B-cells programmed for anti-H-2K^k were expressed in H-2^d mice but deleted in mice positive for H-2K^k which in these circumstances acts as an autoantigen.

Tolerance through B-cell anergy was clearly demonstrated in another study in which double transgenic mice were made to express both lysozyme and a high-affinity antibody to lysozyme. The animals were completely tolerant and could not be immunized to make anti-lysozyme; nor did the transgenic antibody appear in the serum although it was abundantly present on the surface of B-cells. These anergic cells could bind antigen to their surface receptors but could not be activated. Like the aged roué wistfully drinking in the visual attractions of some young belle, these tolerized lymphocytes can 'see' the antigen but lack the ability to do anything about it.

Whether deletion or anergy is the outcome of the encounter with self may depend upon concentration and ability to cross-link Ig receptors. In the first of the two B-cell tolerance models above, the H-2K^k autoantigen would be richly expressed on cells in contact with the developing B-lymphocytes and could effectively cause cross-linking. In the second case, the lysozyme, masquerading as a 'self' molecule, is essentially univalent with respect to the receptors on an anti-lysozyme B-cell and would not readily bring about cross-linking.

Tolerance may result from helpless B-cells

With soluble proteins at least, T-cells are more readily tolerized than B-cells (figure 9.15) and, depending upon the circulating protein concentration, a number of self-reacting B-cells may be present in the body which cannot be triggered by T-dependent self-components since the T-cells required to provide the necessary T–B help are already tolerant—you might describe the B-cells as helpless. If we think of the determinant on a self-component which combines with the receptors on a self-reacting B-cell as a hapten and another determinant which has to be recognized by a T-cell as a carrier (cf. figure 6.15), then tolerance in the T-cell to the carrier will prevent the provision of T-cell help and the B-cell will be unresponsive. Take C5 as an example; this is normally circulating at concentrations which tolerize T- but not B-cells. Some strains of mice are congenitally deficient in C5 and their T-cells can help C5 positive strains to make antibodies to C5, i.e. the C5 positive strains still have inducible B-cells but they are helpless and need non-tolerized T-cells from the C5 negative strain (figure 9.16).

It is likely that self-tolerance in both B- and T-cells involves all the mechanisms we have discussed to varying degrees and these are summarized in figure 9.17. Remember that throughout the life of an animal, new stem cells are continually differentiating into immunocompetent lymphocytes and what is early in ontogeny for them can be late for the host; this means that self-tolerance mechanisms are still acting on early lymphocytes even in the adult.

The overall response in the neonate

Lymph node and spleen remain relatively underdeveloped in the human even at birth except where there has been intra-uterine exposure to antigens as in congenital infections with rubella or other organ-

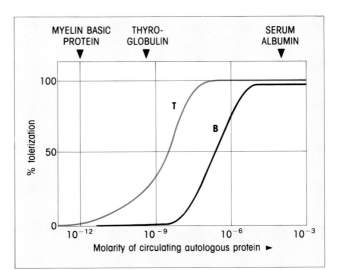

Figure 9.15. *Relative susceptibility of T- and B-cells to tolerance by circulating autologous molecules. Those circulating at low concentration induce no tolerance; at intermediate concentration, e.g. thyroglobulin, T-cells are moderately tolerized; molecules such as albumin which circulate at high concentrations tolerize both B- and T-cells.*

DONORS	TRANSFER T-HELPERS	C5 POSITIVE NORMAL RECIPIENTS	IMMUNIZE WITH C5	ANTI-C5
C5 DEFICIENT			►	++
NORMAL			►	–

○ Tolerized   ◑ Non-tolerant

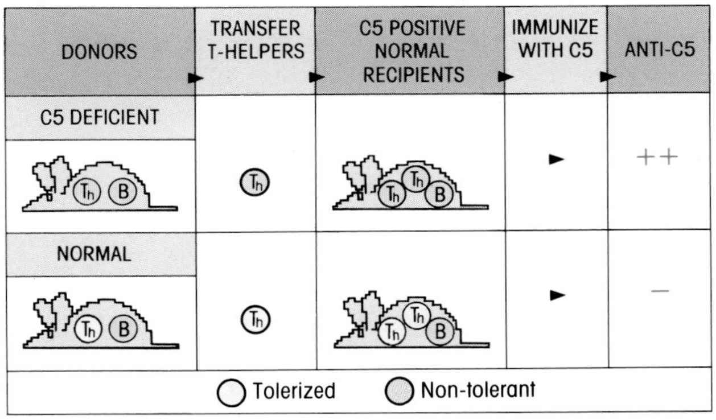

Figure 9.16. *Circulating C5 tolerizes T- but not B-cells leaving them helpless. Animals with congenital C5 deficiency do not tolerize their T-helpers and can be used to break tolerance in normal mice.*

isms. The ability to reject grafts and to mount an antibody response is reasonably well developed by birth but the immunoglobulin levels with one exception are low particularly in the absence of intra-uterine infection. The exception is IgG which is acquired by placental transfer from the mother, a process dependent upon Fc structures specific to this Ig class. This material is catabolized with a half-life of approximately 30 days and there is a fall in IgG concentration over the first three months accentuated by the increase in blood volume of the growing infant. Thereafter the rate of synthesis

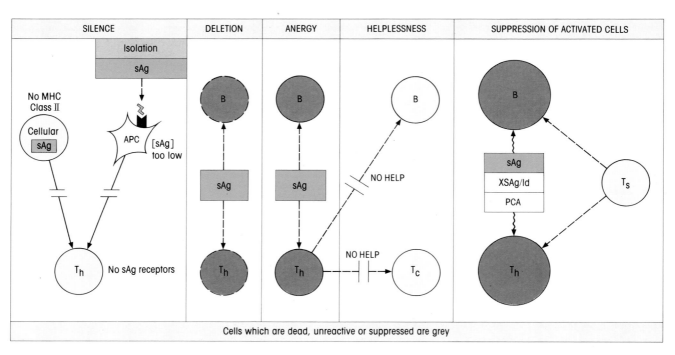

SILENCE	DELETION	ANERGY	HELPLESSNESS	SUPPRESSION OF ACTIVATED CELLS

Cells which are dead, unreactive or suppressed are grey

188   *Figure 9.17. Mechanisms of self-tolerance (see text). sAg, self antigen; XS Ag/Id, cross-reacting antigen or idiotype; PCA,*   *polyclonal activator; APC, antigen-presenting cell; T_h, T-helper; T_s, T-suppressor; T_c, cytotoxic T-cell precursor.*

overtakes the rate of breakdown of maternal IgG and the overall concentration increases steadily. The other immunoglobulins do not cross the placenta and the low but significant levels of IgM in cord blood are synthesized by the baby (figure 9.18). IgM reaches adult levels by nine months of age. Only trace levels of IgA, IgD and IgE are present in the circulation of the newborn.

UNREGULATED DEVELOPMENT GIVES RISE TO LYMPHOPROLIFERATIVE DISORDERS

The cells involved in immune responses may undergo malignant transformation, giving rise to leukaemia, lymphoma or myeloma characterized by uncontrolled proliferation.

Deregulation of the c-*myc* proto-oncogene is a characteristic feature of many B-cell tumours

The realization that viral oncogenes are almost cer-

tainly derived from normal host genes concerned in the regulation of cellular proliferation, has led to the identification of many of these so-called proto-oncogenes. One of them, c-*myc* appears to be of crucial importance for entry of the lymphocyte, and probably many other cells, from the resting G_0 stage to the cell cycle. As we have earlier noted, increased expression of c-*myc* is an early event associated with lymphocyte activation and it has been established that there is a strong relationship between the level of c-*myc* mRNA and the proliferative capacity of a cell population. It is also generally believed that shutdown of c-*myc* expression is linked to exit from the cycle and return to G_0.

Thus deregulation of c-*myc* expression will prevent cells from leaving the cycle and consign them to a fate of continuous proliferation. This is just what is seen in the neoplastic B-lymphoproliferative disorders where the malignant cells express high levels of c-*myc* protein usually associated with a reciprocal chromosomal translocation involving the c-*myc* locus. For example, Burkitt's lymphoma is a B-cell neoplasia with a relatively high incidence among African children in whom there is an association with the Epstein-Barr virus (EBV); in most cases studied, the c-*myc* gene located on chromosome 8 band q24 is joined by a reciprocal

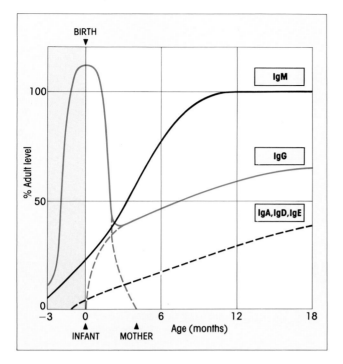

Figure 9.18. *Development of serum immunoglobulin levels in the human (after Hobbs J.R. (1969) In* Immunology and Development, *Adinolfi M. (ed.), p. 118. Heinemann, London).*

translocation event to the μ-heavy chain gene on chromosome 14 band q32 (figure 9.19). The two genes are connected in a transcriptionally opposing fashion so that c-*myc* is transcribed from the normal c-*myc* promoters, not those belonging to the μ chain. It is suggested that the normal mechanisms which down-regulate c-*myc* can no longer work on the translocated gene and so the cell is held in the cycling mode. Less frequently, c-*myc* translocates to the site of the kappa (chromosome 2) or lambda (chromosome 22) loci.

Chromosome translocations are common in lymphoproliferative disorders

Most lymphomas and leukaemias have visible chromosome abnormalities bound up with translocations to B-cell immunoglobulin or T-cell receptor gene loci but not necessarily involving c-*myc*. A reciprocal translocation between the μ-chain gene on chromosome 14 and the *bcl*-2 oncogene on chromosome 18 has been identified in a follicular B-cell lymphoma, and another between the T-cell α-gene on chromosome 14 (q11) and another presumed oncogene on chromosome 11 in a T-acute lymphoblastic leukaemia (T-ALL). In a further case of T-cell leukaemia, an inversion on chromosome 14 brought the μ-chain locus at band q32 to the T-receptor α-gene at q11 with the possibility of producing a chimaeric receptor consisting of $V_HC_\alpha/V_\beta C_\beta$ chains.

The lack of proliferative control engendered by deregulation of c-*myc* and other similar events induced by chromosomal translocations is permissive for the vulnerability to induction of neoplasia but is not in itself sufficient to bring about malignant transformation. Thus, transgenic mice harbouring a c-*myc* gene driven by the μ-heavy chain enhancer (E_μ-*myc* mice) have hyperplastic expansions of the pre-B cell population in the bone marrow and spleen during the pre-neoplastic period and yet do not develop tumours until 6–8 weeks of age and then they are monoclonal not polyclonal, suggesting that a random second event is required before autonomy is achieved. Indeed, if the E_μ-*myc* transgenic mice are now infected with viruses carrying the v-*raf* oncogene, they rapidly develop lymphomas. It is generally thought that whereas factors like c-*myc* can make a cell competent for mitosis, it is only

189

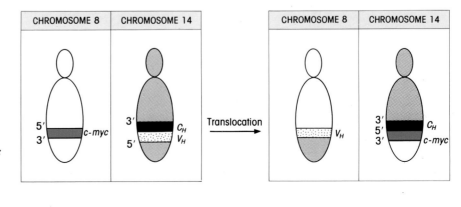

Figure 9.19. *Translocation of the c-myc gene to the μ-chain locus in Burkitt's lymphoma.*

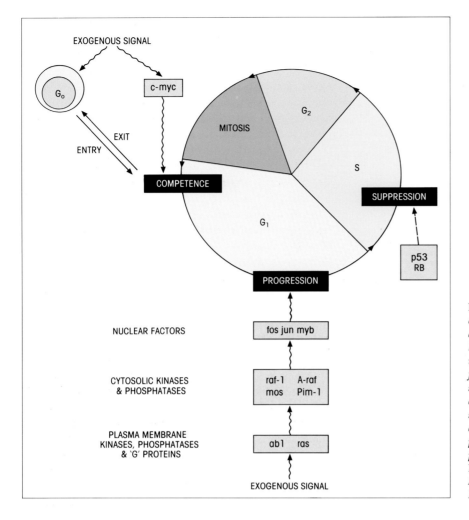

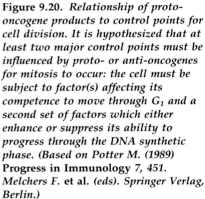

Figure 9.20. *Relationship of proto-oncogene products to control points for cell division. It is hypothesized that at least two major control points must be influenced by proto- or anti-oncogenes for mitosis to occur: the cell must be subject to factor(s) affecting its competence to move through G_1 and a second set of factors which either enhance or suppress its ability to progress through the DNA synthetic phase. (Based on Potter M. (1989)* **Progress in Immunology 7, 451.** *Melchers F. et al. (eds). Springer Verlag, Berlin.)*

through the additional upregulation of progression genes like *fos*, *jun* and *myb* or the loss of suppressor gene products like p53 which allow cell division to occur. The way in which two such events may synergize in the process of malignant transformation and the associated unfettered cell proliferation is indicated in figure 9.20.

Different lymphoid malignancies show maturation arrest at characteristic stages in differentiation

Lymphoid cells at almost any stage in their differentiation or maturation may become malignant and proliferate to form a clone of cells which are virtually 'frozen' at a particular developmental stage because of defects in maturation. The malignant cells bear the markers one would expect of normal lymphocytes reaching the stage at which maturation had been arrested. Thus, chronic lymphocytic leukaemia cells resemble mature B-cells in expressing surface class II and Ig, albeit of a single idiotype in a given patient. Using monoclonal antibodies directed against the terminal deoxynucleotidyl transferase (figure 9.22a), class II MHC, Ig and specific antigens on cortical thymocytes, mature T-cells and non-T, non-B acute lymphoblastic leukaemia cells, it has been possible to classify the lymphoid malignancies in terms of the phenotype of the equivalent normal cell (figure 9.21).

Susceptibility to malignant transformation is high in lymphocytes at an early stage in ontogeny. If we look at Burkitt's lymphoma, the EBV-induced translocation of the c-*myc* to bring it under control of the *IgH* gene complex is most likely to occur at the pro-B-cell stage since the chromatin structure of the

190

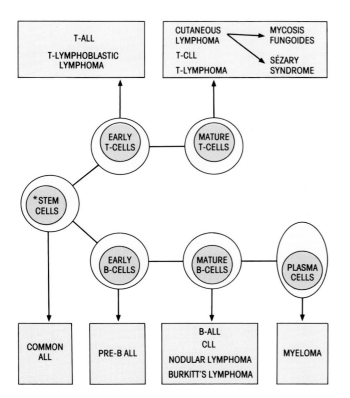

Figure 9.21. *Cellular phenotype of human lymphoid malignancies. ALL, acute lymphoblastic leukaemia; CLL, chronic lymphocytic leukaemia. (After Greaves M.F. & Janossy G.)*

Ig locus opens up for transcription as signalled by the appearance of sterile C_μ transcripts. Furthermore, the cell is likely to escape immunological recognition because in its undifferentiated resting form it has downregulated its EBV-encoded antigens and MHC class I polymorphic specificities, and the adhesion molecules LFA-1, LFA-3 and ICAM-1.

At one time it was thought that maturation arrest occurred at the stage when the cell first became malignant, but we now know that the tumour cells can be forced into differentiation by agents such as phorbol myristate acetate and the current view is that cells may undergo a few differentiation steps after malignant transformation before coming to a halt. The demonstration of a myeloma protein idiotype on the cytoplasmic μ chains of pre-B cells in the same patient certainly favours the idea that the malignant event had occurred in a pre-B cell whose progeny formed the plasma cell tumour. However, an alternative explanation could be transfection of normal pre-B cells by an oncogene complex from the myeloma cells possibly through a viral vector. With the exciting discovery of a C-type retrovirus associated with certain human T-cell leukaemias (HTLV), this is an interesting possibility. The virus is likely to have the same relationship to the T-cell as EB virus does to the B-cell, although what that is exactly is still unknown.

Immunohistological diagnosis of lymphoid neoplasias

With the availability of a range of monoclonal antibodies and improvements in immuno-enzymatic technology, great strides have been made in exploiting, for diagnostic purposes, the fact that malignant lymphoid cells display the markers of the normal lymphocytes which are their counterpart.

Leukaemias

This point can be made rather well if one looks at the markers used to distinguish between the various types of leukaemia (table 9.4). Whereas T-ALL and B-ALL cases have a poor prognosis, the patients positive for the common acute lymphoblastic leukaemia antigen (CALLA; figure 9.22b) who include most childhood leukaemias, belong to a prognostically favourable group, many of whom are curable with standard therapeutic combinations of vincristine, prednisone and L-asparaginase. Bone marrow transplantation may help in the management of patients with recurrent ALL provided a remission can first be achieved.

Table 9.4. *Classification of lymphocytic leukaemia by immuno-enzymatic staining.*

Lymphocyte marker	Common ALL	Pre-B ALL	B-cell ALL	T-cell ALL	Chronic lymphocytic leukaemia
*CALLA	+	+	−	−	−
Cytoplasmic μ	−	+	−	−	−
Surface μ	−	−	+	−	+
Surface $\kappa + \lambda$	−	−	−	−	−
Pan-B	−	+	+	−	+
TdT	+	+	−	+	−
CD5	−	−	+	+	+
CD2	−	−	−	+	−
HLA-DR	+	+	+	−	+

* Antigen-specific for lymphoid precursor cells and pre-B cells.

192

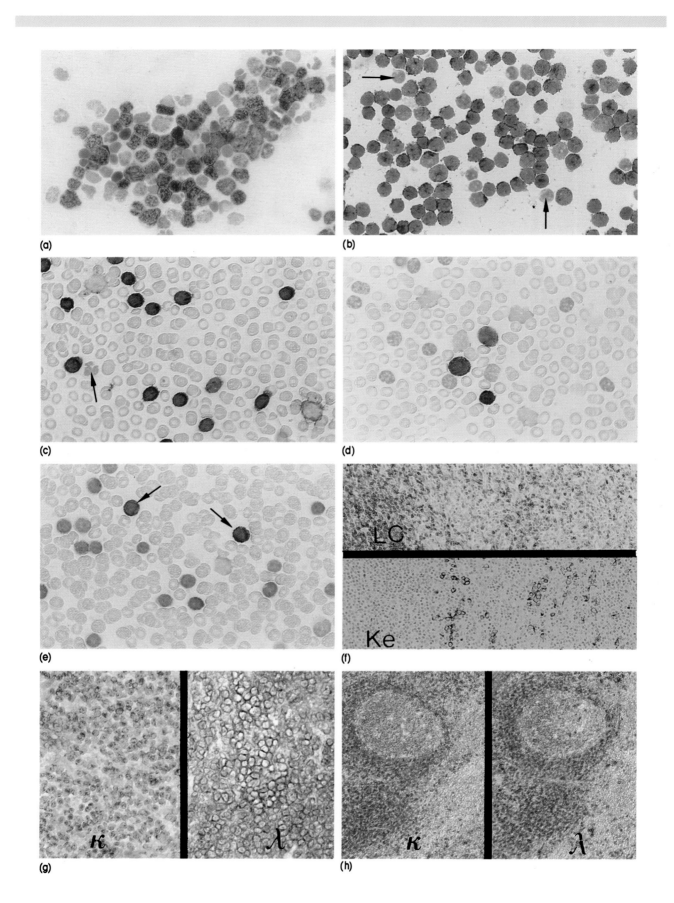

(a)

(b)

(c)

(d)

(e)

(f)

LC

Ke

(g)

κ   λ

(h)

κ   λ

CHAPTER 9

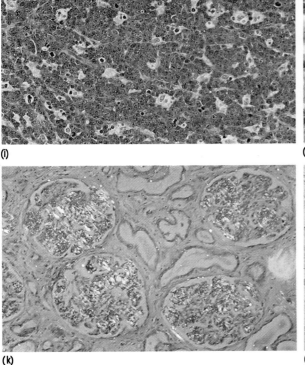
(i)

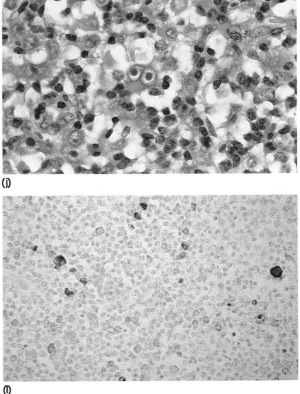
(j)

(k)

(l)

Figure 9.22 facing page and above. *Immunodiagnosis of lymphoproliferative disorders. (a) Cytocentrifuged blast cells from a case of acute lymphoblastic leukaemia stained by anti-terminal deoxynucleotidyl transferase (TdT) using an immuno-alkaline phosphatase method (cells treated first with mouse monoclonal anti-TdT, then anti-mouse Ig and finally with an immune complex of mouse anti-alkaline phosphatase + alkaline phosphatase before developing the enzymic reddish-purple colour reaction). Many strongly stained blast cells are seen together with unlabelled normal marrow cells. (b) Immuno-alkaline phosphatase staining of bone marrow cells from a case of acute lymphoblastic leukaemia, using monoclonal antibody specific for the common-acute lymphoblastic leukaemia antigen (anti-CALLA; antibody J5). The majority of cells are strongly labelled. Two non-reactive cells are indicated by arrows. (c, d, e) Immuno-alkaline phosphatase labelling of blood smears from a case of chronic lymphocytic leukaemia with three monoclonal antibodies (anti-HLA-DR, anti-CD3 antigen, and anti-CD1 antigen): (c) HLA-DR antigen is present on all the leukaemic cells seen, but absent from a polymorph (arrowed); (d) three normal*

T-cells are labelled for the CD3 antigen, but the leukaemic cells are negative; (e) CD1 antigen is strongly expressed on two normal lymphocytes (arrowed), but also weakly expressed on the CLL cells. This pattern is typical of chronic lymphocytic leukaemia. (f) A case of gastric carcinoma (stained at the bottom using anti-cytokeratin, Ke) with a heavy lymphocytic infiltrate (top, stained with anti-leucocyte common antigen, LC). (g) Diffuse follicle centre type B-cell lymphoma showing λ light chain restriction; compare with (h) a reactive lymph node staining for both κ and λ light chains. (i) Burkitt's lymphoma showing 'starry sky' appearance. (j) Hodgkin's disease showing mixed cellularity and characteristic binucleate Reed—Sternberg cell with massive prominent nucleoli in the centre of the figure. (k) Amyloid deposits in kidney glomeruli visualized by Congo Red staining under polarized light. (l) A case of malignant lymphoma associated with macroglobulinaemia, showing lymphoplasmacytoid cells stained by the brown immunoperoxidase reaction for cytoplasmic IgM.

((a)—(e) very kindly provided by Dr D. Mason, and (f)—(l) by Prof. P. Isaacson.)

Chronic lymphocytic leukaemia is uncommon in people under 50 and is usually relatively benign, although the 10—20% of patients with a circulating monoclonal Ig have a bad prognosis. Excessive numbers of CLL small lymphocytes are found in the blood (figure 9.22c, d and e) and, being derived from a single clone, they can be stained only with anti-κ or anti-λ. Their weak expression of CD5 strongly suggests that they may be derived from the equivalent of the Ly1 B-cell population in the mouse, especially since they can be encouraged to make the IgM polyspecific autoantibodies typical of this subset, if pushed by phorbol ester stimulation.

Lymphomas

The extensive use of markers has greatly helped in the diagnosis of non-Hodgkin lymphomas. In the first place, the sometimes difficult distinction between a lymphoproliferative condition and carcinoma can be made with ease by using monoclonal antibodies to the leucocyte common antigen which will react with all lymphoid cells whether in paraffin or cryostat sections, and antibodies to cytokeratin which recognize most carcinomas (figure 9.22f). Second, the cell of origin of the lymphoma can be ascertained by panels of monoclonals which differentiate the cellular elements which form normal lymphoid tissue (table 9.5).

The majority of non-Hodgkin lymphomas are of B-cell origin and the feature which gives the game away to the diagnostic immunohistologist is the synthesis of monotypic Ig, i.e. of one light chain only (figure 9.22g); in contrast, the population of cells at a site of reactive B-cell hyperplasia will stain for both κ and λ chains (figure 9.22h).

Follicle centre cell lymphomas (figure 9.22g) imitating the reactive germinal centre account for over 50% of the B-lymphomas. They exhibit monotypic surface Ig and the larger centrocytes and centroblasts which make up two-thirds of the cases contain cytoplasmic Ig. They stain for MHC class II and weakly for CALLA (cf. table 9.4). Morphologically similar cells make up tumours variously labelled 'mantle zone lymphoma' or 'small cleaved cell lymphoma' but differ from follicle centre cells in positive surface staining for IgM *and* IgD, and CD5 and negativity for CALLA. Burkitt lymphoma lympho-blastoid cells (figure 9.22i) exhibit the common ALL antigen and surface IgM.

The overall prognosis for patients with non-Hodgkin lymphoma is poor even though improved by combined chemotherapy. Transplanted patients are 35 times more likely to develop lymphoma than normals, and there are indications that this cannot necessarily be attributed to the long-term immunosuppression.

Hodgkin's disease attacks the gross architecture of lymphoid tissue and is characterized by the binucleate giant cells known as Reed–Sternberg cells (figure 9.22j) whose lineage is still disputed. Therapy depends upon the stage of the disease: patients with disease localized to lymphoid tissue above the diaphragm respond well to radiotherapy, while those with more widespread disease are treated more aggressively.

Plasma cell dyscrasias

Multiple myeloma

This is defined as a malignant proliferation of a clone of plasma cells in the bone marrow secreting a monoclonal Ig. The myeloma or 'M' component in serum is recognized as a tight band on paper electrophoresis (all molecules in the clone are of course identical and have the same mobility) and as an abnormal arc on immunoelectrophoresis with a 'bump' caused by the monoclonal protein (figure 9.23a and b). Since Ig-secreting cells produce an excess of light chains, it is to be expected that free

Marker	Follicle centre cells	Mantle zone cells	Plasma cells	T-cells	Macrophages	Interdigitating cells (T-cell area)	Follicular dendritic cells
Cytoplasmic Ig	±	−	+	−	−	−	−
J chain	±	−	±	−	−	−	−
Leucocyte common Ag (LCA)	+	+	+	+	+	+	?
HLA-DR	+	+	−	−	±	+	?
CALLA	+	−	−	−	−	−	−
Lysozyme	−	−	−	−	+	−	−
α1-Antitrypsin	−	−	−	−	+	−	−
S-100	−	−	−	−	−	+	−
Surface Ig	+	+	−	−	−	−	−
T-cell	−	−	−	+	−	±	−
Pan B-cell	+	+	±	−	−	−	−
C3b receptor	−	±	−	−	−	−	+

Table 9.5. *Immunohistochemical markers of normal lymphoid tissue (from Isaacson P.G. & Wright D.H. (1986). In* Immunochemistry: Modern Methods and Applications, *2nd edn. Polak J.M. & Noorden S. van (eds) Wright, Bristol, UK, with permission).*

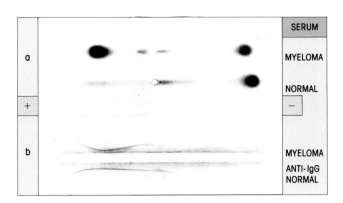

Figure 9.23. *Myeloma serum with an 'M' component. (a) Agar gel electrophoresis showing strong band in γ-globulin region. (b) Immunoelectrophoresis against anti-IgG serum revealing the 'bump' or 'bow' in the precipitin arc. (Courtesy of Prof. F.C. Hay.)*

light chains are present in the plasma of multiple myeloma patients, and indeed they can be recognized in the urine and give rise to amyloid deposits (see below). The characteristic 'punched out' osteolytic lesions in bones are thought to be due to release of osteoclastic factors by the abnormal plasma cells in the marrow. If untreated, the disease is rapidly progressive. With chemotherapy, the mean survival time from diagnosis is now about 5 years.

'M' bands have been found in the sera of a number of individuals who have no clinical signs of myeloma; the comparative rarity with which invasive multiple myeloma develops in these people and the constant level of the monoclonal protein over a period of years suggests the presence of benign tumours of the lymphocyte-plasma cell series.

Amyloid

Between 10 and 20% of patients with myeloma develop widespread amyloid deposits which contain the variable region of the myeloma light chain. Being identical, the variable region fragments polymerize and form the characteristic amyloid fibrils which are recognizable by their birefringence on staining with Congo Red (figure 9.22k). Other components in amyloid have not yet been characterized. The fibrils are relatively resistant to digestion and accumulate in the ground substance of connective tissue where they can lead to pathological changes in the kidneys, heart and brain. Amyloid can also be formed secondarily to chronic inflammatory

conditions such as rheumatoid arthritis and familial Mediterranean fever but in this case involves the polymerization of a unique substance, Amyloid A (AA) protein derived from the N-terminal part of a serum precursor (SAA) of molecular weight 90 000. SAA behaves as an acute phase protein in that its concentration increases rapidly in response to tissue injury or inflammation. Levels rise with age and the minority of individuals with high values are those most likely to develop amyloid.

Waldenström's macroglobulinaemia

This disorder is produced by the unregulated proliferation of cells of an intermediate appearance called lymphoplasmacytoid cells which secrete a monoclonal IgM, the Waldenström macroglobulin (figure 9.22l). Remarkably, many of the monoclonal proteins have autoantibody activity, anti-DNA, anti-IgG (rheumatoid factor) and so on. It has been suggested that they are of the same lineage as CLL cells. Since the IgM is secreted in large amounts and is confined to the intravascular compartment, there is a marked rise in serum viscosity, the consequences of which can be temporarily mitigated by vigorous plasmapheresis. The disease runs a fairly benign course and the prognosis is quite good, although the appearance of lymphoplasmacytoid tumour cells in the blood is an ominous sign.

Heavy chain disease

Heavy chain disease is a rare condition in which quantities of abnormal heavy chains are excreted in the urine — γ chains in association with malignant lymphoma and α chains in cases of abdominal lymphoma with diffuse lymphoplasmacytic infiltration of the small intestine. The amino acid sequences of the N-terminal regions of these heavy chains are normal but they have a deletion extending from part of the variable domain through most of the C_H1 region so that they lack the structure required to form cross-links to the light chains. One idea is that the defect arises through faulty coupling of V and C region genes (cf. p. 58).

Immunodeficiency secondary to lymphoproliferative disorders

Immunodeficiency is a common feature in patients with lymphoid malignancies. The reasons for this

195

are still obscure but it seems as though the malignant cells interfere with the development of the corresponding normal cells, almost as though they were producing some cell-specific chalone or transfecting suppressor factor.

Thus in multiple myeloma the levels of normal B-cells and of non-myeloma Ig may be grossly depressed and the patients susceptible to infection with pyogenic bacteria. Although the lineage of the Reed−Sternberg cell is still contentious, the main candidates are either T-cell or macrophage, and feedback suppressive influences on the normal counterpart would accord with the defects in cell-mediated immunity which are so striking even in early stage I or stage II patients. In fact, half the deaths in this malignant lymphoma are accounted for by infections with intracellular organisms such as *Pneumocystis* or cytomegalovirus.

THE EVOLUTION OF THE IMMUNE RESPONSE

Recognition of self is fundamental for multicellular organisms

The multiplicity of life forms which inhabit our planet have arisen from selective forces operating on 'selfish genes' driven by the chance establishment of mechanisms which optimized their replication and survival. As an example of the stringency of such mechanisms we have only to look at bacteria which use restriction endonucleases to cleave the DNA of invading viruses; they protect their own DNA by methylating the specific nucleotide sequences recognized by the enzyme. Primitive discriminatory processes must come into play when amoebocytes, which are so widespread through invertebrate phylogeny, feed by recognizing non-self material for phagocytosis and digestion. Where survival of cellular DNA is increased by organized aggregation of identical cells into a multicellular organism it is essential that each such colony maintains its individuality. It is not surprising, therefore, that mechanisms for the recognition and subsequent rejection of non-self can be identified as far down the evolutionary scale as the sponges commonly regarded as the most primitive of present-day animals (figure 9.24a). A like phenomenon has been studied in more detail in the colonial tunicate *Botryllus schosseri* which occur as subtidal individual cells or colonies which on meeting fuse or reject, the fusion resulting in establishment of a parabiotic multi-individual colony. Genetically identical members fuse and establish a common blood supply, but when different individuals fuse, although an initial vascular anastomosis is formed, this is rapidly plugged by inflammatory blood cells, both within the blood vessel and in the perivascular tunic. Cytotoxic cells, macrophages and other blood cells stream in and pinch off the blood vessel—truly transplantation in the wild! Rejection is controlled by a single gene locus with many alleles and if a homozygous colony (say of genotype *AA*) fuses with a heterozygote (*AB*), it is the homozygote which is preferentially absorbed. This contributes to an impressive polymorphism and contrasts with the rules of graft rejection in vertebrates, for whom transplantation has a somewhat different significance. The evolution and range of the molecular mechanisms exploited for self/non-self discrimination from the lowliest organisms, through creatures such as the earthworm (figure 9.24b) to the human, have yet to be clarified but there are indications that the structural motif of the cellular adhesion molecule, N-CAM, which as we shall see is a member of the supergene family including MHC and lymphocyte antigen receptors, can be traced back a long way into the invertebrates.

Invertebrates have humoral defence mechanisms

In many phyla, phagocytosis is augmented by coating with agglutinins and bactericidins in the body fluids of non-immunized animals. Furthermore, it now appears that antisomes (as they are called) with some specificity can be *induced* by antigen administration; figure 9.25 provides an example of the response to a synthetic aromatic hapten on a carrier in the earthworm.

B- and T-cell responses are well defined in the vertebrates

Both B- and T-cell responses can be elicited even in the lowliest vertebrate studied; the California hagfish. This unpleasant cyclostome (which preys upon moribund fish by entering their mouths and eating the flesh from the inside) was originally considered 'the negative hero of the phylogeny of immunity'

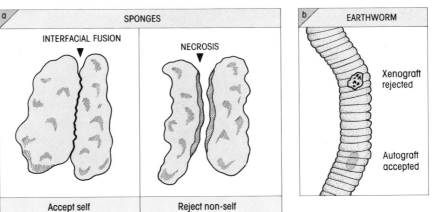

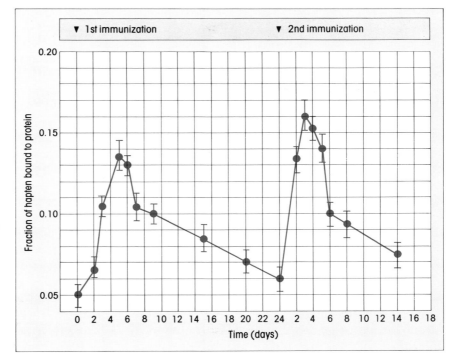

Figure 9.24. *Recognition and rejection of non-self. (a) Parabiosed fingers of sponge from the same colony are permanently united but members of different colonies reject each other by 7–9 days. (b) A xenograft of body wall tissue from the earthworm* **Eisenia** *onto the earthworm* **Lumbricus** *is completely destroyed by 50 days.*

Figure 9.25. *Induction of protein specifically binding the hapten intensain after injection of earthworms with a hapten-KLH conjugate (10.5 μg for the first immunization and 6 μg for the second immunization). Each point represents the mean ± SD based upon results from at least six immunized earthworms. (Reprinted from Châteaureynaud-Duprat P. et al. (1985)* **Immunology** *56, 751, with permission.)*

since, unlike the lamprey, a more advanced cyclostome, it appeared incapable of reacting immunologically. It now transpires that hagfish can make antibodies to haemocyanin and reject allografts, provided they are maintained at temperatures approaching 20°C (in general, poikilotherms make antibodies better at higher temperatures). The antibodies were present in a 28S macroglobulin fraction, but further up the evolutionary scale in the cartilaginous fishes, well-defined 18S and 7S immunoglobulins with heavy and light chains have now been defined.

The toad, *Xenopus*, is a pliable, if unlovely, species for study since it is possible to make transgenics and cloned tadpoles fairly readily and it has a less complex lymphoid system than mammals, characterized by a small number of lymphocytes and a restricted antibody repertoire not subject to somatic mutation. Furthermore, positive and negative thymic selection have been demonstrated in frogs and I must say that if I belonged to an immunological laboratory which was strapped for funds, I would give serious consideration to the possibility of working with amphibian systems.

ACQUIRED RESPONSE — DEVELOPMENT

Mechanisms for the generation of antibody diversity receive quite different emphasis as one goes from one species to another. We are already familiar with the mammalian system where multiple V genes are greatly amplified by a variety of recombinational events involving multiple D and J segments. The horned shark also has many V genes but the opportunities for combinatorial joining are tightly constrained by close linkage between individual, V, D, J and C segments and this may be a factor in the restricted antibody response of this species. In sharp contrast, there seems to be only one operational V gene at the λ light chain locus in the chicken but this undergoes extensive somatic diversification possibly utilizing non-functional adjoining V pseudogenes in a somatic gene-conversion-like process.

The evolution of distinct B- and T-cell lineages was accompanied by the development of separate sites for differentiation

The differential effects of neonatal thymectomy and bursectomy in the chicken on subsequent humoral and cellular responses paved the way for the eventual recognition of the separate lymphocyte lineages which subserve these functions. Like the thymus, the bursa of Fabricius develops as an embryonic outpushing of the gut endoderm, this time from hind- as distinct from fore-gut, and provides the micro-environment to cradle incoming stem cells and direct their differentiation to immunocompetent B-lymphocytes. As may be seen from table 9.6, bursectomy had a profound effect on humoral antibody synthesis, but did not unduly influence the cell-mediated reactions responsible for tuberculin skin reactivity and graft rejection. On the other hand, thymectomy grossly impaired cell-mediated reactions and had some effect on antibody production.

The distinctive anatomical location of the B-cell differentiation site in a separate lymphoid organ in the chicken was immensely valuable to progress in this field because it allowed such experiments to be carried out. However, many years went by in a fruitless search for an equivalent bursa in mammals before it was realized that the primary site for B-cell generation was in fact the bone marrow itself (a nameless immunologist regularly slays his students by recalling that 'the bursa is strictly for the birds').

Cellular recognition molecules exploit gene superfamilies

The immunoglobulin superfamily

When nature fortuitously chances upon a protein structure ('motif' is the buzz word) which successfully mediates some useful function, the selective forces of evolution make sure that it is widely exploited. Thus, all the molecules involved in antigen recognition which we have described at such (painful!) length in Chapter 3 are members of a gene superfamily related by sequence and presumably a common ancestry. All polypeptide members of this family which includes heavy and light Ig chains, T-cell receptor α and β chains, class I and class II peptides and β_2-microglobulin, are composed of one or more immunoglobulin homology units. Each unit is roughly 110 amino acids in length and is characterized by certain conserved residues around the two cysteines found in every domain and the alternating hydrophobic and hydrophilic amino acids which give rise to the familiar anti-parallel β-pleated strands with interspersed short variable lengths having a marked propensity to form reversed turns — the 'immunoglobulin fold' in short (cf. p. 42).

Attention has been drawn to a very important feature of the Ig domain structure, namely the mutual complementarity which allows strong interdomain non-covalent interactions such as those between V_H and V_L and the two C_H3 regions which form the IgG pFc' fragment. Gene duplication and

All X-irradiated after birth	Peripheral blood lymphocyte count	Ig conc.	Antibody	Delayed skin reaction to tuberculin	Graft rejection
Intact	14 800	+ +	+ + +	+ +	+ +
Thymectomized	9 000	+ +	+	−	+
Bursectomized	13 200	−	−	+	+

Table 9.6. *Effect of neonatal bursectomy and thymectomy on the development of immunological competence in the chicken. (From Cooper M.D., Peterson R.D.A., South M.A. & Good R.A. (1966) J. Exp. Med. 123, 75, with permission of the editors.)*

diversification can create mutual families of inter-acting molecules such as T-cell receptors with MHC, and IgA with the poly-Ig receptor (figure 9.26). On this basis, it is not surprising that the domain homology units are turning up in other surface molecules concerned in cell—cell interactions such as CD8 and Ly2 which associate with class I MHC, and CD4 and L3T4 which help focus the helper cell onto target class II MHC. Likewise the intercellular adhesion molecules ICAM-1 and N-CAM (figure 9.26) are richly endowed with these domains and the long evolutionary history of N-CAM, hinted at above, strongly suggests that these structures made a relatively early appearance in phylogeny as mediators of intercellular recognition. A recent trawl of the protein sequence database revealed, in addition to the 279 known members of the Ig super-family, a further six new ones of which two were EB virus proteins. Some family!

The integrin superfamily

Leucocyte adherence to vascular endothelial cells, which precedes emigration into extravascular sites of inflammation, depends upon interaction between the leucocyte receptors LFA-1, Mac-1 and p150,95, and endothelial cell ligands. It transpires that these receptors belong to another structural superfamily called the *integrins* which also include a number of haematopoietic cell-surface molecules concerned with adhesion to extracellular matrix proteins, their function being to direct these cells to particular tissue sites.

Integrins tend to be heterodimers with unique but related α-chains which can be grouped into subsets (table 9.7), each of which has a common β-chain. A feature of this family is that many, if not all, members are receptors for ligands containing the sequence Arg.Gly.Asp. or something closely related.

The VLA subfamily took its name from VLA-1 and -2 which appeared as very late antigens (VLA) on T-cells, 2—4 weeks after *in vitro* activation. However, VLA-3, -4, and -5 belong to the same family but are not 'very late' and are found to different extents on lymphocytes, monocytes, platelets and probably haematopoietic progenitors. To give an example of the possible function of these molecules, it is reasonable to expect that fibronectin receptors would anchor differentiating cells to the stroma during haemopoiesis until they were ready to emi-grate. Although weakly expressed or absent from most normal tissue and blood cells, VLA-3 is

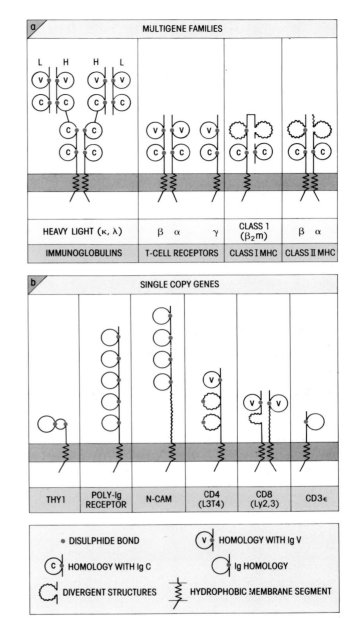

199

Figure 9.26. *The immunoglobulin gene superfamily, a series of surface molecules involved in cell—cell recognition which all share a common structure, the **immunoglobulin homology unit**, suggesting evolution from a single primordial ancestral gene. (a) Multigene families involved in antigen recognition (the single copy β₂-microglobulin is included because of its association with class I). (b) Single copy genes. Thy 1 is present on T-cells and neurones. Poly-Ig transports IgA across mucosal membranes. N-CAM is an adhesion molecule binding neuronal cells together. Other molecules now included in this superfamily are α1B glycoprotein, a human plasma protein; neurocytoplasmic protein 3 (NP3), a brain-specific molecule; OX-2, of unknown function present on lymphocytes and neurones; and the CD3 δ chain. (Reprinted by permission from* **Nature** *323, 15, copyright © 1986, MacMillan Magazines Limited.)*

Subfamily	Receptor	Ligand
1	VLA-1 VLA-2 VLA-3 VLA-4 VLA-5	? Collagen Laminin, collagen, fibronectin ? Fibronectin
2	Vitronectin receptor GP IIb/IIIa	Vitronectin Fibronectin, vitronectin fibrinogen, von Willebrand factor
3	LFA-1 Mac-1 (CR3) p 150, 95	ICAM-1 iC3b iC3b

abundantly expressed on many haematopoietic cell malignancies and may facilitate the invasive attachment of metastasizing cells.

This may be a good point to pause for breath and summarize the main types of leucocyte receptors which fall into four groups: (i) leucocyte adherence to endothelial cells (integrin family); (ii) interaction of lymphocytes with antigens (Ig superfamily); (iii) lymphocyte homing through high endothelial venules (another family ?); (iv) leucocyte adherence to extracellular matrix (integrins again). Two points to note are that the Ig and integrin families meet dramatically in the ICAM-1/LFA-1 interaction (cf. figure 6.13) and Ig family members on non-leucocytic cells such as N-CAM may have a powerful role in intercellular recognition.

SUMMARY

Ontogeny

Multipotential stem cells from the bone marrow give rise to all the formed elements of the blood. The differentiation of T-cells occurs within the micro-environment of the thymus. Differentiation to immunocompetent T-cell subsets is accompanied by changes in the surface phenotype which can be recognized with monoclonal antibodies. T-cell receptor (TCR) genes rearrange in the thymus cortex, TCR1 γδ before TCR2 αβ. The thymus epithelial cells positively select T-cells with affinity for their MHC haplotype on the developing T-cells so they are restricted to the recognition of antigen in the context of that haplotype. High affinity T-cells which react with self-antigens presented by cortico-medullary macrophages and interdigitating dendritic cells are eliminated by negative selection.

Self-tolerance can also be achieved by paralysis (anergy) and by failure to present a self-antigen to lymphocytes either because of compartmentalization or lack of class-II on the antigen-presenting cell. T-suppression is probably more concerned in reversing autoimmunity rather than preventing it.

B-cells differentiate in the fetal liver and then in the bone marrow to become immunocompetent B-cells after passing through pre-B and immature B-cell stages. Some class-switching can occur before contact with antigen as a result of micro-environmental factors. A minor population expressing the T-cell marker CD5, or in the mouse Ly1 predominate in early life, show a high level of idiotype-anti-idiotype connectivity, produce low affinity, IgM polyreactive antibodies, many of them autoantibodies, and are responsible for the 'natural' IgM antibacterial antibodies which appear spontaneously. The sequence of Ig variable gene rearrangements is DJ, VDJ then V-J_κ and, if unproductive, V-J_λ. If the rearrangement at any stage is unproductive, i.e. does not lead to an acceptable gene reading frame, the allele on the sister chromosome is rearranged. The mechanisms of allelic exclusion ensure that each lymphocyte is programmed for only one antibody. Responses to different antigens appear sequentially with age. B-cell tolerance is induced by clonal deletion, clonal anergy, and 'helplessness' due to preferential tolerization of T-cells' needs to cooperate in B-cell stimulation. Maternal IgG crosses the placenta and provides a high level of passive immunity at birth. The antigen-independent differentiation within primary lymphoid organs and antigen-driven maturation in secondary lymphoid organs are summarized in figure 9.27.

Lymphoproliferative disorders

Deregulation of the c-*myc* proto-oncogene is a characteristic feature of many B-cell tumours and keeps them in the cell cycle. This is associated with translocation of the c-*myc* gene to Ig heavy or light chain loci. Other B- and T-cell tumours show different translocations but always to a locus relating to an antigen receptor. A second signal is required for malignancy since mice transfected with μ-chain enhancer linked to c-*myc* have hyperplastic B-cells but do not readily produce tumours unless transfected with a further oncogene which allows progression from the G1 to the S phase of the mitotic cycle. Different lymphoid malignancies show maturation arrest at characteristic stages in differentiation. Be-

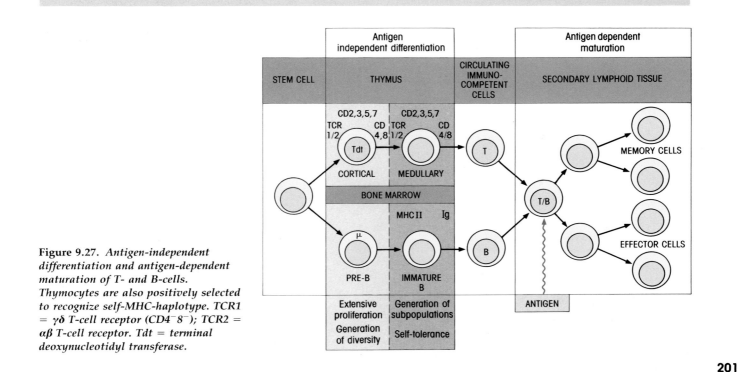

Figure 9.27. *Antigen-independent differentiation and antigen-dependent maturation of T- and B-cells. Thymocytes are also positively selected to recognize self-MHC-haplotype. TCR1 = γδ T-cell receptor (CD4⁻8⁻); TCR2 = αβ T-cell receptor. Tdt = terminal deoxynucleotidyl transferase.*

cause the B-cell tumours express the phenotypic markers of their normal counterparts, it is now possible to make a diagnosis of lymphoid malignancy based on the origin of the tumour cell using the batteries of available monoclonal antibodies and modern immuno-enzymatic cytochemical tests. The features of the various B- and T-cell tumours are discussed. Immunodeficiency often occurs because the tumour cells inhibit the development of their normal cellular counterpart.

Phylogeny

Recognition of self is of fundamental importance for multicellular organisms, even lowly forms like sponges and earthworms. Invertebrates have humoral defence mechanisms and there is some evidence of inducible 'anti-some' production. B- and T-cell responses are well defined in the vertebrates and the evolution of these distinct lineages was accompanied by the development of separate sites for differentiation. The success of the immunoglobulin domain structure, possibly through its ability to give non-covalent mutual binding, has been exploited by evolution to produce the very large Ig gene superfamily of recognition molecules including Ig, T-cell receptors, MHC class I and II, β_2-microglobulin, CD4, CD8, the poly-Ig receptor and Thy 1. Another superfamily, the integrins, which include LFA-1 and the VLA molecules, are concerned with leucocyte binding to endothelial cells and extracellular matrix proteins.

Further reading

Ferrick A. *et al.* (1989) Thymic ontogeny and selection of αβ and γδ cells. *Immunol. Today*, **10**, 403 (very good summary of coverage of this central theme at the 7th Int. Congress of Immunology).

Forbes I.J. & Leong A.S-Y (1987) *Essential Oncology of the Lymphocyte.* Springer-Verlag, Berlin.

Hemler E. (1988) Adhesive protein receptors on haemopoietic cells. *Immunol. Today*, **9**, 109.

Horton J. & Lackie A. (1989) Evolution of immunity. In *Immunology*, I.M. Roitt, J. Brostoff & D.K. Male (eds), p. 91, 2nd edn. Gower Medical Publishing, London.

Stein H. & Mason D.Y. (1985) Immunological analysis of tissue sections in diagnosis of lymphoma. In *Recent Advances in Haematology*, A.V. Hoffbrand (ed.), 4, 127. Churchill Livingstone, Edinburgh.

IMMUNITY TO INFECTION
I – Adversarial Strategies

We are engaged in constant warfare with the microbes which surround us and the processes of mutation and evolution have tried to select micro-organisms which have evolved means of evading our defence mechanisms. In this chapter, we look at the varied, often ingenious, adversarial strategies which we and our enemies have developed over very long periods of time.

EXTRACELLULAR BACTERIA SUSCEPTIBLE TO KILLING BY PHAGOCYTOSIS AND COMPLEMENT

Bacterial strategies to avoid death

The variety and ingenuity of these escape mechanisms are most intriguing and, as with virtually all infectious agents, if you can think of a possible avoidance strategy, some microbe will already have used it.

Poor innate adherence. The cell walls of bacteria are multifarious (figure 10.1) and in some cases are inherently resistant to a number of microbicidal agents, but a common mechanism by which virulent forms escape phagocytosis is by synthesis of an outer capsule which does not adhere readily to phagocytic cells (figure 10.2i). For example, as few

as 10 encapsulated pneumococci can kill a mouse, but if the capsule is removed by treatment with hyaluronidase, 10 000 bacteria are required for the job.

Poor activation of complement. In the absence of antibody, complement is activated through surface stabilization of the C3bBb convertase. Most bacterial capsules tend to be poor activators of the alternative complement pathway and selective pressures have obviously favoured the synthesis of capsules whose surface components do not favour stable binding of the convertase complex (figure 10.2ii).

Resistance to insertion of terminal complement components. Gram-positive organisms (cf. figure 10.1) have evolved thick peptidoglycan layers which prevent the insertion of the lytic C5b-9 membrane attack complex into the bacterial cell membrane. Many capsules do the same (figure 10.2iii).

Complement deviation. Some species manage to avoid lysis by deviating the complement activation site either to a secreted decoy protein or to a position on the bacterial surface distant from the cell membrane (figure 10.2iv).

Acceleration of complement breakdown. Certain bacterial surface molecules, notably those rich in sialic acid, are grossly unsporting in their ability to bind factor H which acts as a focus for the degra-

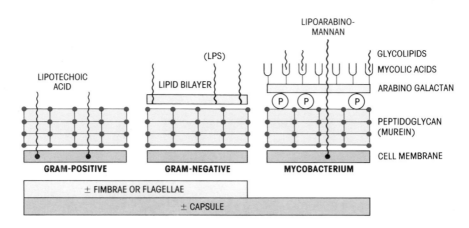

LIPOARABINO-MANNAN

GLYCOLIPIDS
MYCOLIC ACIDS
ARABINO GALACTAN

(LPS)

LIPOTECHOIC ACID

LIPID BILAYER

PEPTIDOGLYCAN (MUREIN)

CELL MEMBRANE

GRAM-POSITIVE   GRAM-NEGATIVE   MYCOBACTERIUM

± FIMBRAE OR FLAGELLAE

± CAPSULE

Figure 10.1. *The structure of bacterial cell walls. All types have an inner cell membrane and a peptidoglycan wall which can be cleaved by lysozyme and lysosomal enzymes. The outer lipid bilayer of Gram-negative bacteria which is susceptible to the action of complement or cationic proteins, sometimes contains lipopolysaccharide (LPS; also known as endotoxin; composed of O-specific oligosaccharide side-chains attached to a basal core polysaccharide, itself linked to the mitogenic moiety, lipid A; 148 O antigen variants of* **Escherichia coli** *are known). The mycobacterial cell wall is highly resistant to breakdown. When present, capsules may protect the bacteria from phagocytosis.*

204 dation of C3b by factor I (cf. p. 8). Other bacteria may secrete enzymes which degrade peptides such as C5a, which play an essential role in the acute inflammatory response (figure 10.2v).

Bacterial toxins. Bacteria may secrete exotoxins which interfere with phagocytosis, often by poisoning the leucocytes (figure 10.2vi).

External colonization. Presumably some organisms try to avoid undue provocation of phagocytic cells by adhering to and *colonizing the external mucosal surfaces* of the body.

The host counter-attack

The defence mechanisms exploit the specificity and variability of the antibody molecule. Antibodies can defeat these devious attempts to avoid engulfment by neutralizing the anti-phagocytic molecules and by binding to the surface of the organisms to focus the site for fixation of complement, so 'opsonizing' them for ingestion by polymorphs and macrophages or preparing them for the terminal membrane attack complex.

Toxin neutralization

Circulating antibodies act to neutralize the soluble anti-phagocytic molecules and other exotoxins (e.g. phospholipase C of *Clostridium welchii*) released by bacteria. Combination near the biologically active site of the toxin would stereochemically block reaction with the substrate, particularly if it were macromolecular; combination distant from the active site may also cause inhibition through allosteric conformational changes. In its complex with antibody, the toxin may be unable to diffuse away rapidly and will be susceptible to phagocytosis, especially if the complex can be increased in size by the action of naturally occurring autoantibodies to complexed IgG (anti-globulin factors) and C3b (immunoconglutinin, not to be confused with bovine *conglutinin* which is a non-antibody molecule which combines with the carbohydrate portion of C3b).

Opsonization of bacteria

Encapsulated bacteria which resist phagocytosis become extremely attractive to polymorphs and macrophages when coated with antibody and their rate of clearance from the bloodstream is strikingly enhanced (figure 10.3). The less effective removal of coated bacteria in complement-depleted animals emphasizes the synergism between antibody and complement for opsonization which is mediated through specific high affinity receptors for IgG and C3b on the phagocyte surface (figure 10.4). It is clearly advantageous that the subclasses which bind strongly to these Fc receptors (e.g. IgG_1 and IgG_3 in the human) also fix complement well, it being appreciated that the heterodimer of C3b bound to IgG

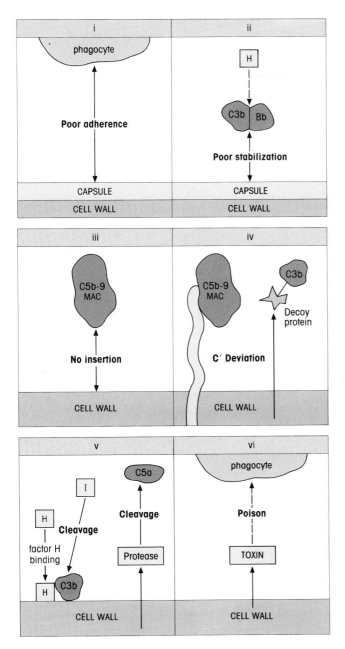

Figure 10.2. *Avoidance strategies by extracellular bacteria (see text).*

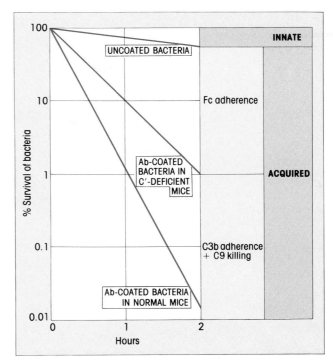

Figure 10.3. *Effect of opsonizing antibody and complement on rate of clearance of virulent bacteria from the blood. The uncoated bacteria are phagocytosed rather slowly (innate immunity) but on coating with antibody, adherence to phagocytes is increased many-fold (acquired immunity). The adherence is less effective in animals temporarily depleted of complement. This is a hypothetical but realistic situation; the natural proliferation of the bacteria has been ignored.*

Fd is a very efficient opsonin because it engages two receptors simultaneously. Complexes containing C3b may show immune adherence to the CR1 complement receptors on primate red cells and rabbit platelets to provide aggregates which are transported to the liver for phagocytosis.

Some elaboration on complement receptors may be pertinent at this stage. The CR1 receptors for C3b are also present on neutrophils, macrophages, B-cells and follicular dendritic cells in lymph nodes.

Together with the CR3 receptor, they have the main responsibility for clearance of complexes containing C3. The CR1 gene is linked in a cluster with C4b-binding protein and factor H, all of which subserve a regulatory function by binding to C3b or C4b to disassemble the C3/C5 convertases and act as co-factors for the proteolytic inactivation of C3b and C4b by factor I.

CR2 receptors for C3d, C3dg and iC3b are present on B-cells and follicular dendritic cells and may well transduce accessory signals for B-cell activation especially in the germinal centres (cf. p. 126). Their affinity for EB virus provides the means for entry of the virus into the B-cell.

CR3 receptors on polymorphs, macrophages and NK cells all bind the inactivated form C3bi. They are related to LFA-1 and CR4 (whose function is uncertain) in being members of an integrin sub-family of two-chain proteins of which the β chain is always 95 kDa molecular weight.

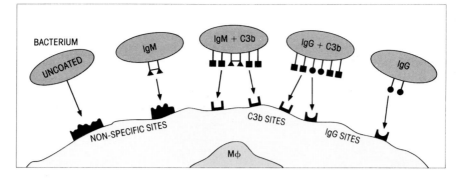

Figure 10.4. *Immunoglobulin and complement coats greatly increase the adherence of bacteria (and other antigens) to macrophages and polymorphs. Uncoated or IgM (▲—▲) coated bacteria adhere to non-specific sites including the pectin-like mannose-binding receptor, but there are high affinity receptors for IgG (Fc) (●) and iC3b (■, CR1 and CR3 types) on the macrophage surface which considerably enhance* *the strength of binding. The augmenting effect of complement is due to the fact that two adjacent IgG molecules can fix many C3b molecules thereby increasing the number of links to the macrophage (cf. 'bonus' effect of multivalency; p. 72). Although IgM does not bind specifically to the macrophage, it promotes adherence through complement fixation.*

Some further effects of complement

Some strains of Gram-negative bacteria which have a lipoprotein outer wall resembling mammalian surface membranes in structure are susceptible to the bactericidal action of fresh serum containing antibody. The antibody initiates the development of a complement-mediated lesion which is said to allow access of serum lysozyme to the inner peptidoglycan wall of the bacterium to cause eventual cell death. Activation of complement through union of antibody and bacterium will also generate the C3a and C5a anaphylatoxins leading to extensive transudation of serum components including more antibody, and to the chemotactic attraction of polymorphs to aid in phagocytosis as described earlier (cf. figure 2.18).

The secretory immune system protects the external mucosal surfaces

Adherence to the epithelial cells of the mucous membranes is essential for viral infection and bacterial colonization. IgA antibodies afford protection in the external body fluids, tears, saliva, nasal secretions and those bathing the surfaces of the intestine (so-called 'coproantibodies') and lung, by coating bacteria and viruses and preventing such adherence to mucosal surfaces. It might be anticipated that in order to fulfil this function, secretory IgA molecules would themselves have very little innate adhesiveness for cells, and certainly no high

affinity Fc receptors for this Ig class have yet been described.

If an infectious agent succeeds in penetrating the IgA barrier, it comes up against the next line of defence of the secretory system (p. 110) which is manned by IgE. It is worth noting that most serum IgE arises from plasma cells in mucosal tissues and in the lymph nodes that drain them. Although present in low concentration, IgE is bound very firmly to the Fc receptors of the mast cell (p. 49) and contact with antigen leads to the release of mediators which effectively recruit agents of the immune response and generate a local acute inflammatory reaction. Thus histamine, by increasing vascular permeability, causes the transudation of IgG and complement into the area while chemotactic factors for neutrophils and eosinophils attract the effector cells needed to dispose of the infectious organism coated with specific IgG and C3b (figure 10.5). Engagement of the Fcγ and C3b receptors on local macrophages by these complexes will lead to secretion of peptides which will further reinforce these vascular permeability and chemotactic events.

Where the opsonized organism is too large for phagocytosis, these cells can kill by an extracellular mechanism after attachment by their Fcγ receptors. This phenomenon, termed antibody-dependent cell-mediated cytotoxicity (ADCC) has been discussed earlier (p. 28) and there is evidence for its involvement in parasitic infections (p. 216). There are obvious parallels between the ways in which complement-derived anaphylatoxins and IgE utilize

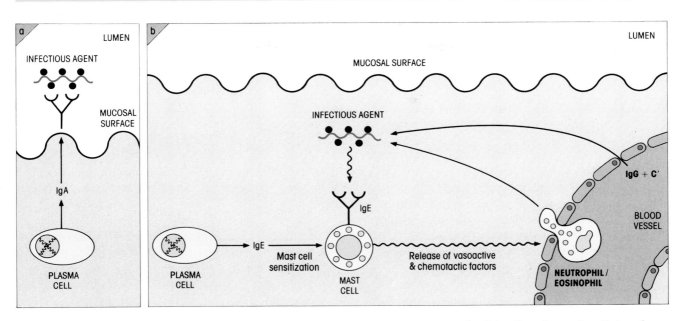

Figure 10.5. *Defence of the mucosal surfaces. IgA prevents adherence of organisms to the mucosa. IgE recruits agents of the immune response by firing the release of mediators from mast cells.*

the mast cell to cause-local amplification of the immune defences.

Some specific examples

First let us see how these considerations apply to the defence against infection by common organisms such as streptococci and staphylococci. β-Haemolytic streptococci were classified by Lancefield according to their carbohydrate antigen and the most important from the standpoint of human disease are those belonging to group A. However, the most important virulence factor is the surface M-protein (variants of which form the basis of the Griffith typing). This protein is an acceptor for factor H which facilitates C3b breakdown and binds fibrinogen and its fragments which cover sites that may act as complement activators. It thereby inhibits opsonization and the protection afforded by antibodies to the M-component is attributable to the striking increase in phagocytosis which they induce. High-titred antibodies to the streptolysin O exotoxin (ASO) are indicators of recent streptococcal infection. The erythrogenic toxin elaborated by strains which give rise to scarlet fever is neutralized by antibody and the erythematous intradermal reaction to the injected toxin is only seen in individuals lacking antibody (Dick reaction). Antibody also neutralizes bacterial enzymes like hyaluronidase which act to spread the infection.

A growing body of evidence is tending to incriminate *Streptococcus mutans* as an important cause of dental caries. The organism has a constitutive enzyme, glucosyltransferase, able to convert sucrose to dextran which is utilized for adhesion to the tooth surface. Passive transfer of IgG, but not IgA or IgM, antibodies to *S. mutans* in monkeys conferred protection against caries. It is thought that IgG antibody and complement in the gingival crevicular fluid bathing the tooth opsonize the bacteria to facilitate phagocytosis and killing by polymorphonuclear leucocytes. Curiously, a single treatment with a monoclonal anti- *S. mutans* kept teeth free of the micro-organism for 1 year, perhaps due to a shift in bacterial ecology with the place vacated by *S. mutans* being filled by another organism from the oral flora.

Virulent forms of staphylococci, of which *S. aureus* is perhaps the most common, resist phagocytosis. This may be due partly to capsule formation *in vivo* and partly to the elaboration of factors such as a coagulase enzyme which could protect the bacterium by a barrier of fibrin. It has been suggested that the ability of a cell wall component, protein A, to combine with the Fc portion of IgG (other than subclass IgG3) is responsible for inhibition of phagocytosis by virulent strains, but IgG—protein A complexes fix complement and one study reports that protein A actually increases complement-mediated phagocytosis. We must return an open verdict on that issue. It seems to be accepted that *S. aureus* is readily phagocytosed in the presence of *adequate* amounts of antibody but a small proportion of the ingested bacteria survives and they are difficult organisms to eliminate completely. Where the infection is inadequately controlled, severe lesions may occur in the immunized host as a consequence of type IV delayed hypersensitivity reactions. Thus, staphylococci were found to be avirulent when injected into mice passively immunized with antibody but caused extensive tissue damage in animals previously given sensitized T-cells (Glynn).

Other examples where antibodies are required to overcome the inherently anti-phagocytic properties of bacterial capsules are seen in immunity to infection by pneumococci, meningococci and *Haemophilus influenzae*. *Bacillus anthrax* possesses an anti-phagocytic capsule composed of a gamma polypeptide of D-glutamic acid but although anticapsular antibodies effectively promote uptake by polymorphs, the exotoxin is so potent that vaccines are inadequate unless they also stimulate anti-toxin immunity. In addition to releasing such lethal exotoxins, *Pseudomonas aeruginosa* also produces an elastase that inactivates C3a and C5a; as a result only minimal inflammatory responses are made in the absence of neutralizing antibodies.

The ploy of diverting complement activation to insensitive sites is seen rather well with different strains of Gram-negative organisms which vary in the number of O-specific oligosaccharide side-chains attached to the lipid-A-linked core polysaccharide of the endotoxin (cf. figure 10.1). Variants with long side-chains are relatively insensitive to killing by serum through the alternative complement pathway (p. 19); as the side-chains become shorter and shorter, the serum sensitivity increases. Although all variants activate the alternative pathway, only those with short or no side-chains allow the cytotoxic membrane attack complex to be inserted near to the outer lipid bilayer (figure 10.2iv). On the other hand, antibodies focus the complex to a more vulnerable site.

The destruction of gonococci by serum containing antibody is dependent upon the formation of the membrane attack complex and rare individuals lacking C8 or C9 are susceptible to *Neisseria* infection. *N. gonorrhoeae* specifically binds complement proteins and prevents their insertion in the outer membranes, but antibody, like a ubiquitous 'Mr Fixit', corrects this situation, at least so far as the host is concerned. With respect to the infective process itself, IgA produced in the genital tract in response to these organisms inhibits the attachment of the bacteria, through their pili, to mucosal cells, but seems unable to afford adequate protection against reinfection. This could be due to the existence of multiple cross-reacting serotypes but might also be a reflection of the ability of gonococcal protease to split IgA_1 dimers. Meningococci which frequently infect the nasopharynx, *Haemophilus influenzae* and *Strep. pneumoniae* have similar unfair proteases.

Cholera is caused by the colonization of the small intestine by *Vibrio cholerae* and the subsequent action of its enterotoxin. The B subunits of the toxin bind to specific GM1 monosialoganglioside receptors and translocate the A subunit across the membrane where it activates adenyl cyclase. The increased cAMP then causes fluid loss by inhibiting uptake of sodium chloride and stimulating active Cl^- secretion by intestinal epithelial cells. Locally synthesized IgA antibodies against *V. cholerae* lipopolysaccharide and the toxin provide independent protection against cholera, the first by inhibiting bacterial adherence to the intestinal wall, the second by blocking attachment of the toxin to its receptor. In accord with this analysis is the epidemiological data showing that children who drink milk with high titres of IgA antibodies specific for either of these antigens are less likely to develop clinical cholera.

I thought it might be helpful to summarize the ways in which antibody can parry the different facets of bacterial invasion (figure 10.6).

BACTERIA WHICH GROW IN AN INTRACELLULAR HABITAT

Bacterial gambits

Some strains of bacteria such as the tubercle and leprosy bacilli, and listeria and brucella organisms, escape the wrath of the immune system by cheekily fashioning an intracellular life within one of its strongholds, the macrophage no less. Mononuclear phagocytes are a good target for such organisms in the sense that they are very mobile and allow wide dissemination throughout the body. Entry of opsonized bacteria is facilitated by phagocytic uptake after attachment to Fcγ and C3b receptors but once inside they defy the mighty macrophage by

208

Antibody to fimbrae lipoteichoic acids and some capsules
Attachment
Trigger complement through Gram – ve outer lipid bilayers
Proliferation of organisms
Block metabolic transport mechanisms, e.g. receptor for iron-chelating compounds
Antibody to M proteins and capsules. Opsonization via Fc and C3 receptors
Avoidance of phagocytosis
Neutralize immunorepellents
Damage to host
Antibody to toxins Neutralization
Toxic
Invasive
Neutralize spreading factors, e.g. hyaluronidase

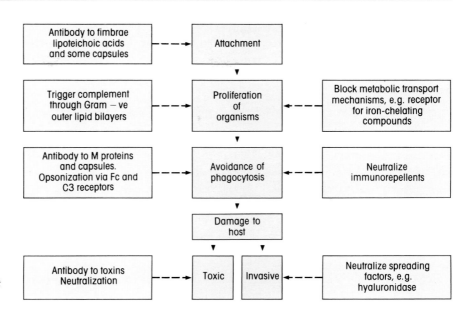

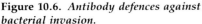

Figure 10.6. *Antibody defences against bacterial invasion.*

subverting the killing mechanisms in a variety of ways. Organisms such as *Mycobacterium tuberculosis* inhibit fusion of the lysosomes with the phagocytic vacuole containing the ingested bacterium (figure 10.7). Mycobacterial lipids such as lipoarabinomannan obstruct priming and activation of the macrophage and also protect the bacteria from attack by scavenging reactive oxygen intermediates such as superoxide anion, hydroxyl radicals and hydrogen peroxide (cf. p. 7). Organisms such as *Listeria monocytogenes* use a special lysin to escape from their phagosomal prison to lie happily free within the cytoplasm; some rickettsias and the protozoon *Trypanosoma cruzi* can do the same. *Legionella* are said to inhibit the respiratory burst further confirming the view that if there is a mechanism available to inhibit, some micro-organisms will eventually find a way to do it.

Defence is by cell-mediated immunity (CMI)

In an elegant series of experiments, Mackaness has demonstrated the importance of CMI reactions for the killing of these intracellular parasites and the establishment of an immune state. Animals infected with moderate doses of *M. tuberculosis* overcome the infection and are immune to subsequent challenge with the bacillus. Surprisingly, if they are given an unrelated organism such as *Listeria monocytogenes at the same time* as the second infection with tubercle bacillus, they are resistant and can kill the listeria which have been engulfed by macrophages. Without the prior immunity to *M. tuberculosis* or the second challenge with this organism, the animal would have succumbed to listeria infection.

Mϕ
LYSOSOME
PHAGOSOME
Intracellular bacterium
1 Inhibit lysosome fusion
2 Resist oxidative & lysosomal attack
3 Escape from phagosome

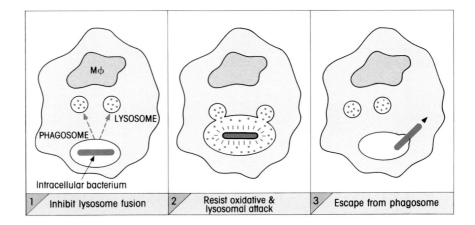

Figure 10.7. *Evasion of phagocytic death by intracellular bacteria.*

Thus the triggering of a specific secondary immune response to one organism may endow the animal with a simultaneous but transient non-specific resistance to unrelated microbes of similar growth habits.

This immunity—both specific and non-specific—can be transferred to a normal recipient with T-lymphocytes but not macrophages or serum from an immune animal (Figure 10.8). In support of this view that the specific immunity is mediated by T-cells is the greater susceptibility to infection with tubercle and leprosy bacilli of mice in which the T-lymphocytes have been depressed by thymectomy plus anti-lymphocyte serum. In human leprosy, the disease presents as a spectrum ranging from the *tuberculoid* form with few viable organisms, to the *lepromatous* form characterized by an abundance of *M. leprae* within the macrophages. As Turk has emphasized, the tuberculoid state is associated with an active T-lymphocyte system giving good antigen-specific transformation of lymphocytes and cell-mediated dermal hypersensitivity responses, although still not good enough to completely eradicate the bacilli. In the lepromatous form, there is poor T-cell reactivity and the paracortical areas in the lymph nodes are depleted of lymphocytes although there are numerous plasma cells which contribute to a high level of circulating antibody. Clearly CMI rather than humoral immunity is important for the control of the leprosy bacillus.

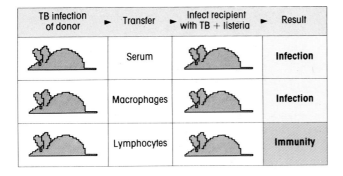

Figure 10.8. *Transfer of specific and non-specific immunity by lymphocytes from an immune animal. The syngeneic recipient of the lymphocytes resisted simultaneous challenge with tubercle and listeria organisms. The recipients were not immune to listeria given without the tubercle. The immunity was mediated by T-cells since lymphocytes lost their power to confer passive immunity on the recipients if treated with a cytotoxic anti-T cell serum plus complement prior to injection. Serum or macrophages were ineffective in transferring immunity (after Mackaness).*

Activated macrophages kill intracellular parasites

When monocytes first settle down in the tissue to become 'resident' macrophages they are essentially down-regulated with respect to expression of surface receptors and function. They can be activated in several stages (figure 10.9). Macrophages (Mφ) taken from sites of inflammation induced by complement or non-immunological stimuli such as thioglycollate, are considerably increased in size, acid hydrolase content, secretion of neutral proteinases and phagocytic function. If I may give one example, the C3b receptors on resident Mφ are not freely mobile in the membrane so cannot permit the 'zippering' process required for phagocytosis (p. 4); consequently, they bind but do not ingest C3b-coated red cells. Inflammatory Mφ, on the other hand, have C3 receptors which display considerable lateral mobility and the C3 opsonized erythrocytes are readily phagocytosed.

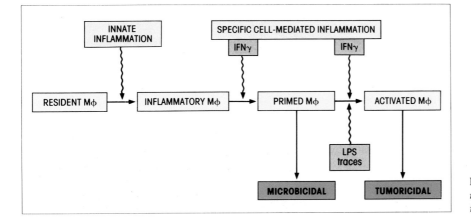

Figure 10.9. *Stages in the activation of macrophages (Mφ) for microbicidal and tumoricidal function.*

However, the ability to kill obligate intracellular microbes only comes when the cells are stimulated to a further stage of activation usually mediated by macrophage activating factor(s) such as IFNγ released from stimulated lymphokine-producing T-cells.

Striking changes on surface components accompany activation. In mouse macrophages there is an increase in class II MHC (dramatic), Fc receptors for IgG2b and binding sites for tumour cells; the mannose receptor, the F4/80 marker and IgG2a receptors all decline while the Mac-I component associated with the CR3 iC3b receptor remains unchanged. The activated macrophage is undeniably a remarkable and formidable cell, capable of secreting the 60-odd substances which are concerned in chronic inflammatory reactions (figure 10.10) — not the sort to meet in an alley on a dark night!

The mechanism of the Mackaness phenomenon now becomes clear. The specificity of the CMI lies at the level of the initial reaction of the primed T-cell with the challenge antigen presented in processed form on the surface of the infected macrophage; the subsequent release of lymphokines activates the macrophage and endows it with the ability to kill almost any organism it has phagocytosed (figure 10.11).

Recreation of the phenomenon *in vitro* using T-cell cytokines and infected macrophages has supported the general thrust of this argument but has also revealed complexities. When bone-marrow-derived macrophages were cultured for 9 days in serum-free medium and then activated with various lymphokines before infection with mycobacteria, only IFNγ was tuberculostatic. If macrophages were infected *before* lymphokine treatment, only IL-4 and IL-6 were anti-mycobacterial activators whereas IFNγ now antagonized these effects. It would seem that IFNγ preferentially targets freshly immigrant monocytes whereas IL-4 can help macrophages which are already infected. If, despite this assistance, a macrophage still fails to destroy its unwanted guests, the host can deploy cytotoxic CD8, and to a lesser extent CD4, cells to kill the macrophage and release the live mycobacteria; these should now be taken up by new phagocytic cells freshly activated by IFNγ and summarily disposed of (figure 10.11).

In the face of these potential CMI defences, why do some individuals fail to eradicate their infections with mycobacteria and other intracellular facultative bacteria and so suffer from TB and leprosy and so on? One important clue is provided by the demonstration that inbred strains of mice differ dramatically in their susceptibility to infection by various mycobacteria, *Leishmania donovani* and *Salmonella*

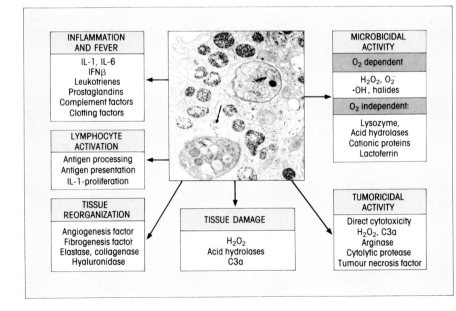

Figure 10.10. *The role of the activated macrophage in the initiation and mediation of chronic inflammation with concomitant tissue repair, and in the killing of microbes and tumour cells. It is possible that macrophages differentiate along distinct pathways to subserve these different functions.*

The electron micrograph shows a highly activated macrophage with many lysosomal structures which have been highlighted by the uptake of thorotrast; one (arrowed) is seen fusing with a phagosome containing the protozoon **Toxoplasma gondii** *(courtesy of Prof. C. Jones).*

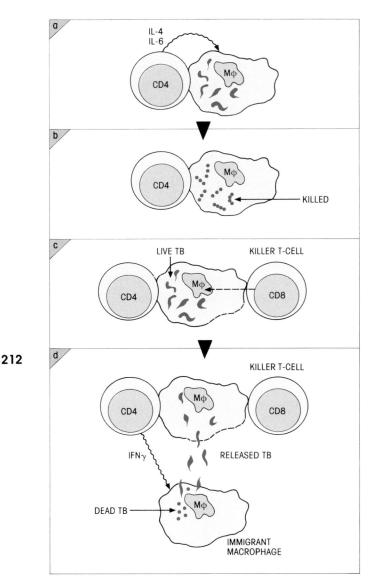

Figure 10.11. *The 'lymphokine connection': non-specific macrophage killing of intracellular bacteria triggered by a specific T-cell mediated immunity reaction accounts for the Mackaness phenomenon.*

typhimurium. Control of the resistance/susceptibility phenotype is by two alleles of a single autosomal dominant gene, *Bcg*, and resistance is linked to a T-cell-independent enhanced state of macrophage priming for bactericidal activity. Moreover, macrophages from resistant strains had increased MHC class II expression and induced better stimulation of T-cells, whereas macrophages from susceptible strains tended to have suppressor effects on T-cell proliferation to mycobacterial antigens. Naturally, the human counterpart to the *Bcg* gene is being actively sought.

Yet to be identified is the role played by the TCR1 T-cells bearing γδ-receptors which have an eerie, almost compelling, relationship to mycobacterial antigens. Limiting dilution analysis indicates that almost every γδ-T-cell in the peripheral blood of normal individuals is stimulated by mycobacterial lysates. These cells accumulate at the site of reversal reactions and in the skin test lesions of leprosy patients, and can lyse target cells presenting mycobacterial antigens. In the mouse, a high percentage of γδ-cells react to the 65 kDa heat shock protein and we have earlier drawn attention to the exaggerated involvement of these cells in the course of immune responses to mycobacteria.

Where the host has difficulty in effectively eliminating such organisms, the chronic CMI response to local antigen leads to the accumulation of densely packed macrophages which release angiogenic and fibrogenic factors and stimulate the formation of granulation tissue and ultimately fibrosis. The activated macrophages, perhaps under the stimulus of IL-4, transform to epithelioid cells and fuse to become giant cells. The resulting structure, termed a granuloma, represents an attempt by the body to isolate a site of persistent infection. Let us leave this particular subject on a cryptic note by remarking that the frequency of γδ-T-cells in the granulomatous lesions of leprosy is increased 5–8 fold. Lines from these lesions proliferate *in vitro* to mycobacterial antigens and the supernatants induce adhesion and aggregation of bone marrow monocytes in the presence of GM-CSF, suggesting a possible role in stimulating granuloma formation.

IMMUNITY TO VIRAL INFECTION

Genetically controlled constitutional factors which render a host or certain of his cells non-permissive (i.e. resistant to takeover of their replicative machinery by virus) play a dominant role in influencing the vulnerability of a given individual to infection. Macrophages may readily take up viruses non-specifically and kill them. However, in some instances the macrophages allow replication and if the virus is capable of producing cytopathic effects in various organs, the infection may be lethal; with non-cytopathic agents such as lymphocytic choriomeningitis, Aleutian mink disease and equine infectious anaemia viruses, a persistent infection will result.

212

CHAPTER 10

Antigenic drift and shift

In the course of their constant duel with the immune system, viruses are continually changing the structure of their surface antigens. They do so by processes termed 'antigenic drift' and 'antigenic shift', the nature of which may be made more apparent by consideration of different influenza strains. The surface of the influenza virus contains a haemagglutinin by which it adheres to cells prior to infection, and a neuraminidase which releases newly formed virus from the surface sialic acid of the infected cell; of these the haemagglutinin is the more important for the establishment of protective immunity. Minor changes in antigenicity of the haemagglutinin occur through point mutations in the viral genome (drift) but major changes arise through wholesale swapping of genetic material with reservoirs of different viruses in other animal hosts (shift). When alterations in the haemagglutinin are sufficient to render previous immunity ineffective, new influenza epidemics break out (figure 10.12).

Over the last 50 years epidemics have been associated with the emergence by antigenic shift of the A/PR8 strain in 1933 with the structure H_0N_1 (the official nomenclature assigns numbers to each haemagglutinin and neuraminidase major variant), A/FM1 in 1947 (H_1N_1), A/Singapore in 1957 (H_2N_2) and A/Hong Kong in 1968 (H_3N_2); note that each new epidemic was associated with a fundamental change in the haemagglutinin.

Mutant forms can be favoured by selection pressure from antibody. In fact one current strategy for generating mutants in a given epitope is to grow the virus in tissue culture in the presence of a monoclonal antibody which reacts with that epitope; only mutants which do not bind the monoclonal will escape and grow out. This principle underlies the antigenic variation characteristic of the common cold rhinoviruses. The site for attachment and penetration of mucosal cells bearing ICAM-1 is a hydrophobic pocket lying on the floor of a canyon which antibodies are too large to penetrate. Antibodies react with the rim of the canyon and mutations in the rim enable the virus to escape from the host immune response without affecting the conserved site for binding to the target cell. Two points occur to me. Anyone thinking of becoming a virus in their next reincarnation would be well advised to design a canyon for their attachment site even if it has to be large enough to allow penetration

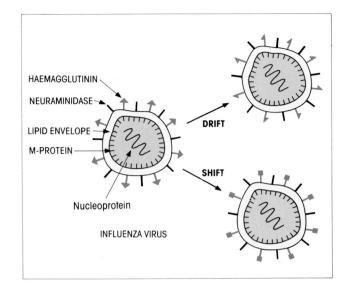

Figure 10.12. *Antigenic drift and shift in influenza virus. The changes in haemagglutinin structure caused by drift may be small enough to allow protection by immunity to earlier strains. This may not happen with radical changes in the antigen associated with antigenic shift and so new virus epidemics break out.*

by an antibody, since concave surfaces on antigens are notoriously lacking in immunogenicity. The other point, just gossip really, is that hydrophobic drugs have been synthesized which fit the rhinovirus canyon and cause a change in conformation which prevents binding to cells. Furthermore, since host proteins have very different folds to those of the viral capsid molecule, the drugs have limited cytotoxicity.

Playing games with the complement system

Blocking of complement-mediated induction of the inflammatory response and viral killing is achieved by an abundant vaccinia virus product structurally related to C4b binding protein. For its part, *Herpes simplex* type I subverts the complement cascade by producing a C3-binding molecule which augments decay of the alternative pathway C3bBb convertase.

Several viruses utilize complement receptors to gain entry into cells especially since engagement of the complement receptor alone on a macrophage is a feeble activator of the respiratory burst. Flavivirus coated with iC3b enters through the CR3 receptors. As noted previously, EB virus infects B-cells by binding to the CR2 surface receptors. Ominously,

HIV coated with antibody and complement is more virulent than unopsonized virus.

Protection by serum antibody

The antibody molecule can neutralize viruses by a variety of means. It may stereochemically inhibit combination with the receptor site on cells, thereby preventing penetration and subsequent intracellular multiplication, the protective effect of antibodies to influenza viral haemagglutinin providing a good example. Similarly, antibodies to the measles haemagglutinin prevent entry into the cell but spread of virus from cell to cell is stopped by antibodies to the fusion antigen. Antibody may destroy a free virus particle directly through activation of the classical complement pathway or produce aggregation, enhanced phagocytosis and intracellular death by mechanisms already discussed.

Relatively low concentrations of circulating antibody can be effective and one is familiar with the protection afforded by poliomyelitis antibodies, and by human γ-globulin given prophylactically to individuals exposed to measles. The most clear-cut protection is seen in diseases with long incubation times where the virus has to travel through the bloodstream before it reaches the tissue which it finally infects. For example, in poliomyelitis the virus gains access to the body via the gastrointestinal tract and eventually passes through the circulation to reach the brain cells which become infected. Within the blood, the virus is neutralized by quite low levels of specific antibody while the prolonged period before the virus infects the brain allows time for a secondary immune response in a primed host.

Local factors

With other viral diseases, such as influenza and the common cold, there is a short incubation time related to the fact that the final target organ for the virus is the same as the portal of entry and no intermediate stage involving passage through the body occurs. There is little time for a primary antibody response to be mounted and in all likelihood the rapid production of interferon is the most significant mechanism used to counter the viral infection. Experimental studies certainly indicate that after an early peak of interferon production, there is a rapid fall in the titre of live virus in the lungs of

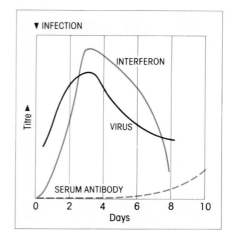

Figure 10.13. *Appearance of interferon and serum antibody in relation to recovery from influenza virus infection of the lungs of mice (from Isaacs A. (1961)* **New Scientist 11, 81).**

mice infected with influenza (figure 10.13). Antibody, as assessed by the *serum* titre, seems to arrive on the scene much too late to be of value in aiding recovery. However, recent investigations have shown that antibody levels may be elevated in the *local* fluids bathing the infected surfaces, e.g. nasal mucosa and lung, despite low serum titres and it is the production of anti-viral antibody (most prominently IgA) by locally deployed immunologically primed cells which is of major importance for the *prevention* of subsequent infection. Unfortunately, in so far as the common cold is concerned, a subsequent infection is likely to involve an antigenically unrelated virus so that general immunity to colds is difficult to achieve.

Cell-mediated immunity gets to the intracellular virus

We emphasized the general point in Chapter 2 that to a first approximation, antibody dealt with extracellular infective agents and cell-mediated immunity with intracellular ones. The same holds true for viruses which try to shelter from antibody in an intracellular habitat. Local or systemic antibodies can block the spread of cytolytic viruses which are released from the host cell they have just killed, but alone they are usually inadequate to control those viruses which modify the antigens of the cell membrane and bud off from the surface as infectious particles because they are also capable of spreading to adjacent cells without becoming exposed to antibody (figure 10.14). Included in this group are:

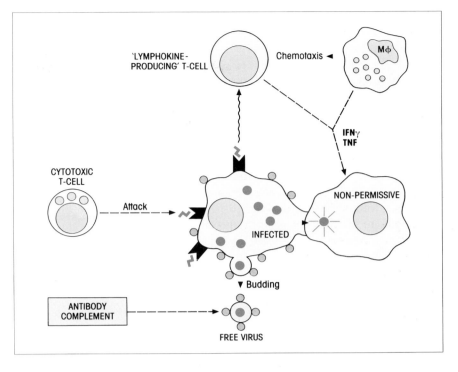

Figure 10.14. *Control of infection by 'budding' viruses. Cytotoxic T-cells kill virally infected targets directly after recognition of new surface antigen. Interaction with a (separate?) subpopulation of T-cells releases lymphokines which attract macrophages and prime contiguous cells with interferon and TNF to make them resistant to viral infection. Free virus released by budding from the cell surface is neutralized by antibody (which is usually thymus dependent pointing to yet another contribution by the T-cell to viral immunity).*

215

oncorna (= oncogenic RNA virus, e.g. murine leukaemogenic), orthomyxo (influenza), paramyxo (mumps, measles), toga (dengue), rhabdo (rabies), arena (lymphocytic choriomeningitis), adeno, herpes (simplex, varicella zoster, cytomegalo, Epstein—Barr, Marek's disease), pox (vaccinia), papova (SV40, polyoma) and rubella viruses. The importance of cell-mediated immunity for recovery from infection with these agents is underlined by the inability of children with primary T-cell immunodeficiency to cope with such viruses, whereas patients with Ig deficiency but intact cell-mediated immunity are not troubled in this way.

T-lymphocytes from a sensitized host are directly cytotoxic to cells infected with viruses from this group, the new surface antigens on the target cells being recognized by specific receptors on the aggressor lymphocytes. Cytotoxic T-cells are less strain-specific, i.e. show broader cross-reaction, than antibody and, strikingly, of course are haplotype specific, i.e. they do not attack cells infected with the same virus but carrying different class I major histocompatibility antigens (cf. figure 4.13). They can usually be detected in the peripheral blood lymphocytes of individuals who have recovered from infection with influenza, cytomegalovirus or Epstein—Barr virus by re-exposure *in vitro* to appropriately infected cells. In the case of cytomegalovirus, for example, the targets are cells with the

'early antigen' on their surface expressed within 6 hours of infection. In fact, provided the surface antigens are expressed before the virus has replicated, as is usually the case, it is clearly advantageous for the cytotoxic cell to strike as soon as the viral antigen appears. That cytolytic T-cells may be important in viral infection in the human is suggested by studies on volunteers showing that high levels of cytotoxic activity before challenge with live influenza correlated with low or absent shedding of virus.

After a natural infection, both antibody and cytotoxic T-cells are generated and subsequent protection is long lived. By contrast, injection of killed influenza produces antibodies but no cytotoxic T-cells and protection is only short term. There have also been some studies showing that influenza-specific cytotoxic T-cell clones can reduce lung virus titres in infected mice. Remember, peptide fragments of the viral proteins make cells into good targets for the cytotoxic T-cells which develop spontaneously during influenza infection (cf. figure 4.15).

A number of studies on transfer of protection to lymphocytic choriomeningitis, vaccinia, ectromelia and cytomegalovirus infections focus on CD8 rather than CD4 T-cells as the major defensive force. The knee-jerk response would be to implicate cytotoxic cells but it is becoming increasingly clear that CD8 cells also produce some cytokines. This may well be crucial when viruses escape the cytotoxic mechanism and manage to sidle laterally into an adjacent cell. CMI can now play some new cards: if T-cells (CD8?) stimulated by viral antigen release lymphokines such as IFNγ and macrophage or monocyte chemotaxin, the mononuclear phagocytes attracted to the site will be activated to secrete TNF which will synergize with the IFNγ to render the contiguous cells non-permissive for the replication of any virus acquired by intercellular transfer (figure 10.14). IFNγ may also increase the non-specific cytotoxicity of NK cells (p. 14) for infected cells. This generation of 'immune interferon' (IFNγ) and TNF in response to non-nucleic acid viral components provides a valuable back-up mechanism when dealing with viruses which are intrinsically poor stimulators of interferon synthesis.

The neutralization of free virus particles by antibody is relatively straightforward but the interaction with infected cells is rather more complex. Access to the surface antigens by T-cells cannot be blocked by coating with antibody since T-cells recognize processed, and antibody, native antigen molecules. None the less, these antibodies should be able to initiate antibody-dependent cell-mediated cytotoxicity (ADCC; p. 260) and this has been reported with herpes, vaccinia and mumps-infected target cells while Oldstone has described the complement-mediated killing of measles-infected cells by F(ab')$_2$ antibody fragments via the alternative pathway. Antibody can play a different tune, however, since in the case of measles-infected cells, although 10^6 antibody molecules per cell permit complement-mediated cytotoxicity, 10^5 molecules do not kill but cause capping and shedding of surface antigen (cf. p. 216).

IMMUNITY TO PARASITIC INFECTIONS

The diverse organisms responsible for the major parasitic diseases are listed in figure 10.15. The numbers affected are truly horrifying and the sum of misery they engender is too large to comprehend. To be successful, a parasite must avoid wholesale killing of the human host and yet at the same time escape destruction by the immune system. In practice, each type of parasite is virtually a world unto itself in the complexity of the mechanisms by which this is achieved.

The host responses

A wide variety of defensive mechanisms are deployed by the host but the rough generalization may be made that a humoral response develops when the organisms invade the bloodstream (malaria, trypanosomiasis) whereas parasites which grow within the tissues (e.g. cutaneous leishmaniasis) usually elicit cell-mediated immunity (table 10.1).

Humoral immunity

Antibodies of the right specificity present in adequate concentrations and affinity are effective in providing protection against blood-borne parasites such as *Trypanosoma brucei* and the sporozoite and merozoite stages of malaria. Thus individuals receiving IgG from solidly immune adults in malaria endemic areas are themselves protected against infection, the effector mechanisms being opsonization and phagocytosis, and complement-dependent lysis.

A marked feature of the immune reaction to helminthic infections such as *Trichinella spiralis* in man and *Nippostrongylus brasiliensis* in the rat is the eosinophilia and the high level of IgE antibody produced. In man, serum levels of IgE can rise from normal values of around 100 ng/ml to as high as 10 000 ng/ml. These changes have all the hallmarks of response to Th2-type lymphokines (cf. p. 143) and it is notable that in animals infected with helminths, injection of anti-IL-4 greatly reduces IgE production and anti-IL-5 suppresses the eosinophilia. This exceptional increase in IgE has encouraged the view that it represents an important line of defence. One can see that antigen-specific triggering of IgE-coated mast cells would lead to exudation of serum proteins containing high concentrations of protective antibodies in all the major Ig classes and the release of eosinophil chemotactic factor. It is relevant to note that schistosomules, the early immature form of the schistosome, have been killed in cultures containing both specific IgG and eosinophils, which induce a form of antibody-dependent cell-mediated cytotoxicity by binding through their FcγRII receptors to the IgG-coated organism (figure 10.16); after 12 hours or so, the major basic protein forming the electron-dense core of the eosinophilic granules is released on to the parasite and brings about its destruction. A contribution to this process from CMI is emerging since eosinophils can express class

216

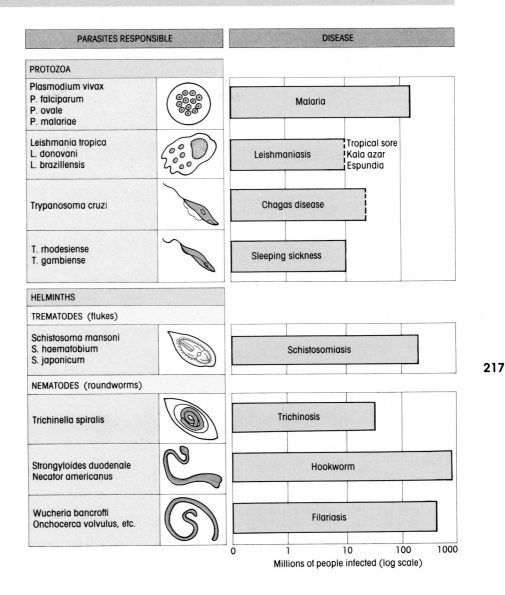

PARASITES RESPONSIBLE	DISEASE

PROTOZOA

Plasmodium vivax P. falciparum P. ovale P. malariae	Malaria
Leishmania tropica L. donovani L. brazillensis	Leishmaniasis — Tropical sore Kala azar Espundia
Trypanosoma cruzi	Chagas disease
T. rhodesiense T. gambiense	Sleeping sickness

HELMINTHS

TREMATODES (flukes)

| Schistosoma mansoni
S. haematobium
S. japonicum | Schistosomiasis |

NEMATODES (roundworms)

Trichinella spiralis	Trichinosis
Strongyloides duodenale Necator americanus	Hookworm
Wucheria bancrofti Onchocerca volvulus, etc.	Filariasis

0   1   10   100   1000
Millions of people infected (log scale)

Figure 10.15. *The major parasites in man and the sheer enormity of the numbers of people infected.*

217

II MHC and their IgG-mediated ADCC is strongly enhanced by GM-CSF and TNF. Further evidence for an involvement of this cell comes from the experiment in which the protection afforded by passive transfer of antiserum *in vivo* was blocked by pretreatment of the recipient with an anti-eosinophil serum. It has recently been found that eosinophils can also kill IgE-coated schistosomules but the mechanism is different because activation of the IgE (FcεRII) receptors now triggers release of platelet activating factors and the eosinophil peroxidase. This dichotomy in Fcγ and Fcε receptor pathways is also evident from reports that IgE but not IgG can mediate schistosome killing by macrophages or platelets. Further complication: engagement of the eosinophil receptor for secretory IgA releases the peroxidase plus a neurotoxic protein

derived from the granules. There is no telling what will happen next.

Two further points are in order. The IgE-mediated reactions may be vital for recovery from infection, whereas the resistance in vaccinated hosts may be more dependent upon preformed IgG and IgA antibodies. Furthermore, the ability to deal with certain helminths may be skewed more towards production of Th1-type lymphokines, such as IFNγ, than the Th2 which favour IgE production.

Cell-mediated immunity

Aside from infections of cattle with the protozoon *Theilaria parva* which modifies the antigenic composition of the cells it parasitizes, no prominent defensive role for cytotoxic T-cells has been

PARASITE	TRYPANOSOMA BRUCEI	PLASMODIUM	TRYPANOSOMA CRUZI	LEISHMANIA
HABITAT	Free in blood	Inside red cell	Inside macrophage	Inside macrophage
ANTIBODY				
Importance	+ + + +	+ + +	+ +	+
Mechanism	Lysis with complement. Opsonizes for phagocytosis	Blocks invasion. Opsonizes for phagocytosis	Limits spread in acute infection	Limits spread
Means of evasion	Antigenic variation	Intracellular habitat	Intracellular habitat	Intracellular habitat
CELL MEDIATED				
Importance	−	+ (?)	+ + + (Chronic phase)	+ + + +
Mechanism	−	Direct and lymphokine mediated macrophage activation	Macrophage activation by lymphokines and killing by metabolites of O_2	

Table 10.1. *The relative importance of antibody and cell-mediated responses in protozoal infections.*

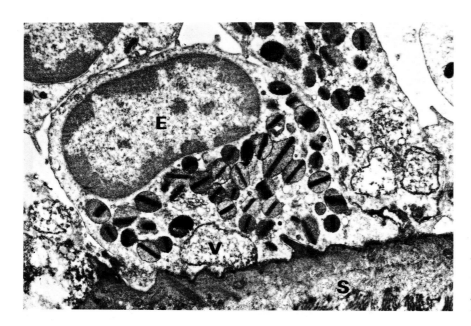

Figure 10.16. *Electron micrograph showing an eosinophil (E) attached to the surface of a schistosomulum (S) in the presence of specific antibody. The cell develops large vacuoles (V) which appear to release their contents on to the parasite (× 16 500). (Courtesy of Drs D.J. McLaren & C.D. Mackenzie.)*

apparent. Lymphokine-producing T-cells, on the other hand, are of special importance for the activation of macrophages to kill intracellular organisms such as *Toxoplasma gondii*, *Trypanosoma cruzi* and *Leishmania* spp. which normally subvert the macrophage microbicidal mechanisms (see below). The whole effect can be witnessed *in vitro* when γ-interferon is added to cultures of macrophages support-

ing the intracellular growth of *Leishmania donovani* and *T. cruzi*.

In vivo, the balance of lymphokines produced may be of the utmost importance. Infection of mice with *Leishmania major* is instructive in this respect; the organism produces fatal disease in susceptible mice but other strains are resistant. As discussed earlier in Chapter 7, in susceptible mice there is

CHAPTER 10

excessive stimulation of Th2-like cells producing IL-4 which do not help to eliminate the infection, whereas resistant strains are characterized by the expansion of Th1-type cells which secrete IFNγ in response to antigen presented by macrophages harbouring *living* protozoa. CD4 clones which recognize only lysates of the organism do not confer protection even though they produce IFNγ, a point to be borne in mind in designing vaccines. As for CD8 cells, little ripples here and there betoken an important contribution yet to be revealed.

Eliminating worm infestations of the gut is a more tricky operation and the combined forces of cellular and humoral immunity are required to expel the unwanted guest. One of the models studied is the response to *Nippostrongylus brasiliensis*; transfer studies in rats (Ogilvie) have shown that, although antibody produces some damage to the worms, T-cells from *immune* donors are also required for vigorous expulsion which is probably achieved through a combination of mast cell-mediated stimulation of intestinal motility and lymphokine activation of the innumerable intestinal goblet cells. These secrete a complex mixture of densely glycosylated high molecular weight molecules which form a visco-elastic gel around the worm so protecting the colonic and intestinal surfaces from invasion (figure 10.17). Another model, this time of *Trichinella spiralis* infection in mice, again hints at a duality of T-subset lymphokine responses. One strain, which expels adult worms rapidly, makes large amounts of IFNγ and IgG2a antibody, while in contrast, more susceptible mice made miserly amounts of IFNγ and favoured IgG1, IgA and IgE antibody classes. Clearly the protective strategy varies with the infection.

Organisms such as malarial plasmodia, and incidentally rickettsiae and chlamydiae, which live in cells which are not professional phagocytes may be eliminated through activation of intracellular defence mechanisms by IFNγ released from CD8 positive T-cells.

Evasive strategies by the parasite

Resistance to effector mechanisms

Two tricks to pre-empt the complement defences are of interest. *T. cruzi* has elegantly created a DAF-

219

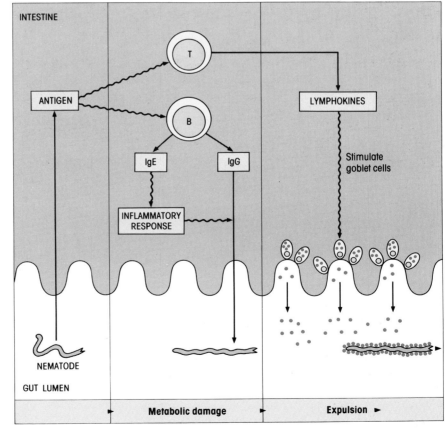

Figure 10.17. *The expulsion of nematode worms from the gut. The parasite is first damaged by IgG antibody passing into the gut lumen possibly as a consequence of IgE-mediated inflammation and possibly aided by accessory ADCC cells. Lymphokines released by antigen-specific triggering of T-cells stimulate proliferation of goblet cells and secretion of mucous materials which coat the damaged worm and facilitate its expulsion from the body by increased gut motility induced by mast cell mediators.*

INTESTINE

T

ANTIGEN

B

IgE

IgG

INFLAMMATORY RESPONSE

LYMPHOKINES

Stimulate goblet cells

NEMATODE

GUT LUMEN

Metabolic damage

Expulsion ▶

like molecule (cf. p. 240) which accelerates the decay of C3b. The cercarii of *Schistosoma mansoni* activate complement directly but eject the bound C3 by shedding their glycocalyx. In a similar fashion, malarial sporozoites shed their circumsporozoite antigen when it binds antibody and *Trypanasoma brucei* releases its surface antigens into solution to act as decoy proteins (p. 203). In each case, these shedding and decoy systems are well suited to parasites or stages in the parasite life cycle which are only briefly in contact with the immune system.

We have already mentioned the way in which different protozoal parasites hide away from the effects of antibody by using the interior of a macrophage as a sanctuary. To do this they must block the normal microbicidal mechanisms and they use similar methods to those deployed by intracellular obligate and facultative bacteria (cf. p. 208). *Toxoplasma gondii* inhibits phagosome—lysosome fusion by lining up host cell mitochondria along the phagosome membrane. *Trypanosoma cruzi* escapes from the confines of the phagosome into the cytoplasm while *Leishmania* parasites are surrounded by a lipophosphoglycan which protects them from the oxidative burst by scavenging oxygen radicals, but which can nevertheless still kill them if the macrophages are appropriately activated.

Avoiding antigen recognition by the host

Some parasites *disguise* themselves to look like the host. This can be achieved by molecular mimicry as instanced by cross-reactivity between *Ascaris* antigens and human collagen. Another way is to cover the surface with host protein. Schistosomes are very good at that; the adult worm takes up host red-cell glycoproteins, MHC molecules and IgG and lives happily in the mesenteric vessels of the host, despite the fact that the blood which bathes it contains antibodies which can prevent reinfection.

Another very crafty ruse, rather akin to moving the goal posts in football, is *antigenic variation* in which the parasites escape from the cytocidal action of humoral antibody on their cycling blood forms by the ingenious trick of altering their antigenic constitution. Figure 10.18 illustrates how the trypanosome continues to infect the host, even after fully protective antibodies appear, by switching to the expression of a new antigenic variant which these antibodies cannot inactivate; as antibodies to the new antigens are synthesized, the parasite escapes again by changing to yet a further variant and so on. The same phenomenon has been observed with *Plasmodium* spp. and this may explain why, in hyperendemic areas, children are subjected to repeated attacks of malaria for their first few years and are then solidly immune to further infection. Immunity must presumably be developed against all the antigenic variants before full protection can be attained, and indeed it is known that IgG from individuals with solid immunity can effectively terminate malaria infections in young children.

Of course, antigenic variation poses a big problem for vaccine development and a number of investi-

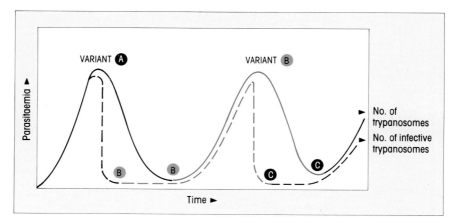

Figure 10.18. *Antigenic variation during chronic trypanosome infection. As antibody to the initial variant A is formed, the blood trypanosomes become complexed prior to phagocytosis and are no longer infective, leaving a small number of viable parasites which have acquired a new antigenic constitution. This new variant (B) now multiplies until it, too, is neutralized by the primary antibody response* *and is succeeded by variant C (after A.R. Gray, see further reading list). At any time, only one of the variant surface glycoproteins (VSG) is expressed and covers the surface of the protozoon to the exclusion of all other antigens. Nearly 9% of the genome (approx. 1000 genes) is devoted to generation of VSGs. Switching occurs by insertion of a duplicate gene into a new genomic location in proximity to the promoter.*

gators in the malaria field have turned their attention to the invariant antigens of the sporozoite which is the form with which the host is first infected; this rapidly goes to the liver to emerge later as a merozoite which infects the red cells. The sporozoite has a characteristic antigen with multiple tetrapeptide repeats. *Plasmodium falciparum*, for example, has 37 repeats of the tetrapeptide asparagyl-alanylasparagylproline (NANP). Field trials of vaccines with polymers of NANP and similar tetrapeptides from other species have not so far been spectacularly successful. Because the sporozoite only takes 30 minutes to reach the liver, and, notwithstanding the shedding phenomenon alluded to above, the antibody has to act fast so that inactivation is limited by diffusion events and hence dependent on the concentration of antibody molecules. The destruction of blood stage malaria by reactive oxygen intermediates has maintained interest in forms of therapy such as BCG and *Corynebacterium parvum* injection which non-specifically stimulate their production.

Deviation of the host immune response

Immunosuppression has been found in most of the parasite infections studied. During infection by *T. brucei*, for example, antibody and cell-mediated immunity is only 5—10% of the normal value while T-suppressor activity is prominent presumably related to an excessive load of antigen.

The ability of certain helminths to activate IgE producing B-cells polyclonally is good for the parasite and correspondingly not so good for the host, since a high concentration of irrelevant IgE binding to a mast cell will crowd out the parasite-specific IgE molecules and diminish the possibility of triggering the mast cell by specific antigen to initiate a protective defensive reaction.

Immunopathology

Where parasites persist chronically in the face of an immune response, the interaction with foreign antigen frequently produces tissue damaging reactions. One example is the immune-complex-induced nephrotic syndrome of Nigerian children associated with quartan malaria. Increased levels of TNF are responsible for pulmonary changes in acute malaria, cerebral malaria in mice and severe wasting of cattle with trypanosomiasis. Another example is the liver damage resulting from T-cell-

mediated granuloma formation around schistosome eggs (cf. figure 12.7o). It has even been argued that the delayed-type hypersensitivity reaction helps the eggs to escape from the intestinal blood capillaries into the gut lumen to continue the cycle outside the body, although others hold that it leads to eventual destruction of the eggs with resolution of the chronic inflammation.

Cross-reaction between parasite and self may give rise to autoimmunity and this has been proposed as the basis for the cardiomyopathy in Chagas' disease. It is also pertinent that the non-specific immunosuppression which is so widespread in parasitic diseases, tends to increase susceptibility to bacterial and viral infections and, in this context, the association between Burkitt's lymphoma and malaria has been ascribed to an inadequate host response to the Epstein—Barr virus.

SUMMARY

Immunity to infection involves a constant battle between the host defences and the mutant microbes trying to evolve evasive strategies. *Bacteria* try to avoid phagocytosis by surrounding themselves with capsules, secreting exotoxins which kill phagocytes or impede inflammatory reactions, deviating complement to inoffensive sites or by colonizing relatively inaccessible locations. Antibody combats these tricks by neutralizing the toxins, making complement deposition more even on the bacterial surface, and overcoming the anti-phagocytic nature of the capsules by opsonizing them with Ig and C3b.

The secretory immune system protects the external mucosal surfaces. IgA inhibits adherence of bacteria. IgE bound to mast cells can initiate the influx of protective IgG, complement and polymorphs to the site by a miniature acute inflammatory response.

Intracellular bacteria such as tubercle and leprosy bacilli grow within macrophages. They defy killing mechanisms by blocking macrophage activation, scavenging oxygen radicals, inhibiting lysosome fusion, having strong outer coats and by escaping from the phagosome into the cytoplasm. They are killed by cell-mediated immunity: specifically sensitized T-helpers release lymphokines on contact with infected macrophages which powerfully activate the formation of reactive oxygen intermediates (ROI) and other microbicidal mechanisms.

Viruses try to avoid the immune system by

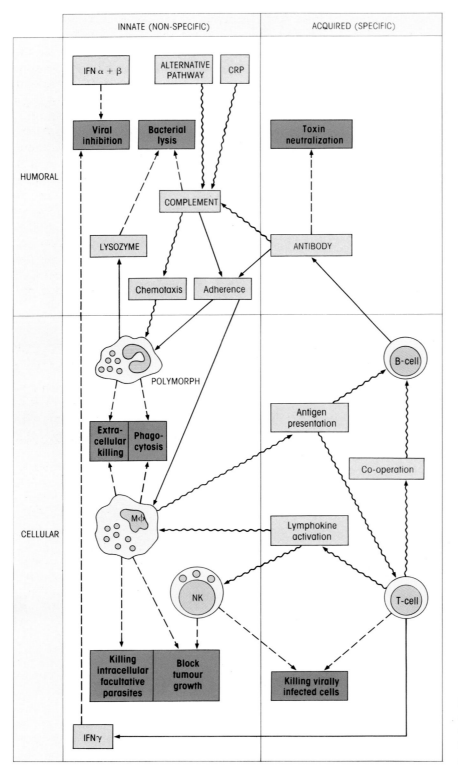

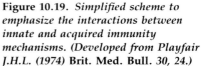

Figure 10.19. *Simplified scheme to emphasize the interactions between innate and acquired immunity mechanisms. (Developed from Playfair J.H.L. (1974) Brit. Med. Bull. 30, 24.)*

changes in the antigenicity of their surface antigens. Point mutations bring about minor changes (antigenic drift) but radical changes leading to endemics can result from wholesale swapping of genetic ma-

terial with different viruses in other animal hosts (antigenic shift). Some viruses subvert the function of the complement system to their own advantage. Antibody neutralizes free virus and is particularly effective when the virus has to travel through the bloodstream before reaching its final target. Where the target is the same as the portal of entry, e.g. the lungs, interferon is dominant in recovery from infection. Antibody is important in preventing re-infection. 'Budding' viruses which can invade lateral cells without becoming exposed to antibody are combatted by cell-mediated immunity. Infected cells express a processed viral antigen peptide on their surface in association with MHC class I a short time after entry of the virus and rapid killing of the cell by cytotoxic T-cells prevents viral multiplication which depends upon the replicative machinery of the intact host cell. T-cells and macrophages producing γ-interferon and TNF bathe the contiguous cells and prevent them from becoming infected by lateral spread of virus.

Diseases involving *protozoal parasites* and *helminths* affect hundreds of millions of people. Antibodies are usually effective against the blood-borne forms. IgE production is notoriously increased in worm infestations and can lead to mast-cell-mediated influx of Ig and eosinophils; schistosomes coated with IgG or IgE are killed by adherent eosinophils through extracellular mechanisms involving release of cationic proteins and peroxidase. Organisms such as *Leishmania* spp., *Trypanosoma cruzi* and *Toxoplasma gondii* hide from antibodies inside macrophages and use the same strategies as intracellular parasitic bacteria to survive, and like them are killed when the macrophages are activated by lymphokines produced during cell-mediated immune responses. Expulsion of intestinal worms requires the coordinated action of antibody and the release of mucin by lymphokine-stimulated goblet cells.

Some parasites avoid recognition by disguising themselves as the host either through molecular mimicry or by absorbing host proteins to their surface. Other organisms such as *Trypanosoma brucei* and various malarial species have the extraordinary ability to cover their surface with a dominant antigen which is changed by genetic switch mechanisms to a different molecule as antibody is formed to the first variant. Most parasites also tend to produce non-specific suppression of host responses.

Chronic persistence of parasite antigen in the face of an immune response often produces tissue-damaging immunopathological reactions such as immune complex nephrotic syndrome, liver granulomata and autoimmune lesions of the heart. Generalized immunosuppression increases susceptibility to bacterial and viral infections.

As the features of the response to infection are analysed, we see more clearly how the specific acquired response operates to amplify and enhance innate immune mechanisms; the interactions are summarized in figure 10.19.

Further reading

Alt F., Marrack P. & Roitt I.M. (eds) (1991) Immunity to infection. *Current Opinion in Immunol.*, **3**, Issues 1 & 3. Current Science, London. (Brief surveys of major developments.)

Baron S. (ed.) (1986) *Medical Microbiology*, 2nd edn. Addison-Wesley Publishers, Menlo Park, California, USA.

Frank M.M. (1989) Evasion strategies of microorganisms. In *Progress in Immunology*, 7, 194 (and many other contributions). Melchers F. *et al.* (eds). Springer Verlag, Berlin.

Gray A.R. (1969) Antigenic variation in trypanosomes. *Bull. World Health Organisation*, **41**, 805.

Mims C.A. & White D.O. (1984) *Viral Pathogenesis and Immunology*. Blackwell Scientific Publications, Oxford. (One of the best accounts of the interaction between virus and host.)

Underdown B.J. & Schiff J.M. (1986) IgA: strategic defense initiative at the mucosal surface. *Ann. Rev. Immunol.*, **4**, 389.

CHAPTER 11

IMMUNITY TO INFECTION

II – Prophylaxis and Immunodeficiency

The control of infection is approached from several directions. One method of breaking the chain of infection has been achieved in the UK with rabies and psittacosis by controlling the importation of dogs and parrots respectively. Improvements in public health—water supply, sewage systems, education in personal hygiene—prevent the spread of cholera and many other diseases. And of course when other measures fail we can fall back on the induction of immunity.

PASSIVELY ACQUIRED IMMUNITY

Temporary protection against infection can be established by giving preformed antibody from another individual of the same or a different species. As the acquired antibodies are utilized by combination with antigen or catabolized in the normal way, this protection is gradually lost.

Horse globulins containing anti-tetanus and anti-diphtheria toxins have been extensively employed prophylactically, but at the present time the practice is more restricted because of the complication of serum sickness developing in response to the foreign protein. This is more likely to occur in subjects already sensitized by previous contact with horse globulin; thus individuals who have been given horse anti-tetanus (e.g. for immediate protection after receiving a wound out in the open) are later advised to undergo a course of active immu-

nization to obviate the need for further injections of horse protein in any subsequent emergency.

Maternally acquired antibody

In the first few months of life while the baby's own lymphoid system is slowly getting under way, protection is afforded by maternally derived antibodies acquired by placental transfer and by intestinal absorption of colostral immunoglobulins. The major immunoglobulin in milk is secretory IgA and this is not absorbed by the baby but remains in the intestine to protect the mucosal surfaces. In this respect it is quite striking that the sIgA antibodies are directed against bacterial and viral antigens often present in the intestine, and it is presumed that IgA-producing cells, responding to gut antigens, migrate and colonize breast tissue (as part of the MALT immune system; p. 110) where the antibodies they produce appear in the milk.

Pooled human γ-globulin

Preparations of pooled human adult γ-globulin are of value to modify the effects of chicken pox or measles, particularly in individuals with defective immune responses such as premature infants, children with primary immunodeficiency or protein malnutrition or patients on steroid treatment. Contacts with cases of infectious hepatitis and smallpox may also be afforded protection by γ-globulin, especially when in the latter case the material is derived from the serum of individuals vaccinated some weeks previously. Human anti-tetanus immunoglobulin is preferable to horse anti-toxin which can cause serum reactions.

Isolated γ-globulin preparations tend to form small aggregates spontaneously and these can lead to severe anaphylactic reactions when administered intravenously on account of their ability to aggregate platelets and to activate complement and generate C3a and C5a anaphylatoxins. For this reason the material is always injected intramuscularly. Preparations free of aggregates are available and separate pools with raised antibody titres to selected organisms such as vaccinia, *Herpes zoster*, tetanus and perhaps rubella would be welcome. This need may ultimately be satisfied as it becomes possible to produce human monoclonal antibodies on demand.

Cultured antibodies made to order

The techniques for producing human monoclonal antibodies to predetermined specificities still leave something to be desired but they are improving steadily. Restlessly we look to recombinant DNA technology to engineer antibodies of very high affinity. We described different approaches to the production of antibodies which circumvent the need for intervention by a host immune system such as the single chain Fv (V_H-V_L) construct and the single V_H domain antibodies. The latter being so small may well be capable of reaching cell receptors on viruses which are tucked away at the bottom of protein canyons where they might be inaccessible to the Fv of an intact antibody. It should be possible to generate high affinities from these single domain antibodies and, in one experiment, random mutation of four central residues in the CDR3 of anti-lysozyme yielded one mutant, out of a very large number, with higher affinity than the parent.

VACCINATION

Herd immunity

In the case of tetanus, active immunization is of benefit to the individual but not to the community since it will not eliminate the organism which is formed in the faeces of domestic animals and per-

sists in the soil as highly resistant spores. Where a disease depends on human transmission, immunity in just a proportion of the population can help the whole community if it leads to a fall in the reproduction rate (i.e. the number of further cases produced by each infected individual) to less than one; under these circumstances the disease will die out, witness for example the disappearance of diphtheria from communities in which around 75% of the children have been immunized (figure 11.1). In contrast, focal outbreaks of poliomyelitis have occurred in communities which object to immunization on religious grounds.

Strategic considerations

The objective of vaccination is to provide effective immunity by establishing adequate levels of antibody and a primed population of cells which can rapidly expand on renewed contact with antigen and so provide protection against infection. Sometimes, as with polio infection, a high blood titre of antibody is required; in mycobacterial diseases such as TB, a macrophage-activating cell-mediated immunity is most effective, whereas with influenza

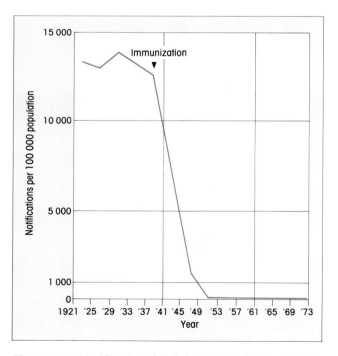

Figure 11.1. *Notification of diphtheria in England and Wales per 100 000 population showing dramatic fall after immunization. (Reproduced from* **Immunisation** *by G. Dick, 1978, Update Books; with kind permission of author and publishers.)*

virus infection, cytotoxic T-cells probably play a significant role. The site of the immune response evoked by vaccination may also be most important. For example in cholera, antibodies need to be in the gut lumen to inhibit adherence to and colonization of the intestinal wall.

Eradication of the infectious agent is not always the most practical goal. To take the example of malaria, the blood-borne form releases molecules which trigger TNF and other cytokines from monocytes and the secretion of these mediators is responsible for the unpleasant effects of the disease. Accordingly, an antibody response targeted to these released antigens with structurally conserved epitopes may be a more realistic strategy than running after the more elusive antigen-swapping parasite itself. Under these circumstances life with the parasite might be acceptable.

In addition to an ability to engender effective immunity, a number of mundane but none the less crucial conditions must be satisfied for a vaccine to be considered successful. The antigens must be readily available, the preparation should be stable under extreme climatic conditions, preferably not requiring refrigeration, it should be cheap and, certainly, safe. Clearly the first contact with antigen during vaccination should not be injurious and the manoeuvre is to avoid the pathogenic effects of infection while maintaining protective immunogens.

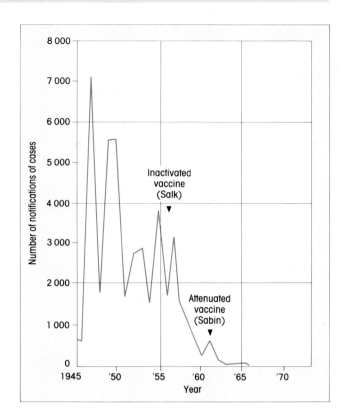

Figure 11.2. *Notifications of paralytic poliomyelitis in England and Wales showing the beneficial effects of community immunization with killed and live vaccines. (Reproduced from* **Immunisation** *by G. Dick, 1978, Update Books; with kind permission of author and publishers.)*

Killed organisms as vaccines

The simplest way to destroy the ability of microbes to cause disease yet maintain their antigenic constitution is to prevent their replication by killing in an appropriate manner. Parasitic worms and, to a lesser extent, protozoa are extremely difficult to grow up in bulk to manufacture killed vaccines. This problem does not arise for many bacteria and viruses and, in these cases, the inactivated micro-organisms have generally provided safe antigens for immunization. Examples are typhoid (in combination with the relatively ineffective paratyphoid A and B), cholera and killed poliomyelitis (Salk) vaccines. The success of the Salk vaccine was slightly marred by a small rise in the incidence of deaths from poliomyelitis in 1960–61 (figure 11.2) but this has now been attributed to poor antigenicity of one of the three different strains of virus used and present-day vaccines are far more potent. Care has to be taken to ensure that important protective antigens are not

destroyed in the inactivation process. During the production of an early killed measles vaccine, the fusion antigen which permits cellular spread of virus was inactivated; as a result, incomplete immunity was produced and this left the individual susceptible to the development of immunopathological complications on subsequent natural infection. The dangers of incomplete immunity are especially worrying in areas where measles is endemic and the immune response is relatively enfeebled due to protein malnutrition. Since the widespread correction of this dietary deficiency is unlikely in the near future, it is worth considering whether non-specific stimulation by immunopotentiating drugs or thymus hormones at the time of vaccination might provide a feasible solution.

This idea of supplementing a deficient adaptive immune response with some synergistic treatment has surfaced in other contexts. Thus, the antibiotic polymyxin B is too toxic for normal use; however, if certain end groups are removed, the molecule loses its toxicity but still retains its ability to disturb the outer wall of Gram-negative bacteria thereby allowing potentially lytic antibodies and complement to reach previously inaccessible bacterial inner membranes. Another curious phenomenon which might be exploited is the finding that the amoeba *Entamoeba histolytica*, which is resistant to lysis by antibody and complement, shows greatly increased susceptibility if treated with an otherwise non-toxic protein inhibitor.

Live attenuated organisms have many advantages as vaccines

The objective of attenuation is to produce a modified organism which mimics the natural behaviour of the original microbe without causing significant disease. In many instances the immunity conferred by killed vaccines, even when given with adjuvant (see below), is often inferior to that resulting from infection with live organisms. This must be partly because the replication of the living microbes confronts the host with a larger and more sustained dose of antigen and that, with budding viruses, infected cells are required for the establishment of good cytotoxic T-cell memory. Another significant advantage of using live organisms is that the immune response takes place largely at the site of the natural infection. This is well illustrated by the nasopharyngeal IgA response to immunization with polio vaccine. In contrast with the ineffectiveness of parenteral injection of killed vaccine, intranasal administration evoked a good local antibody response; but whereas this declined over a period of 2 months or so, per oral immunization with *live attenuated* virus established a persistently high IgA antibody level (figure 11.3).

Classical methods of attenuation

The objective of attenuation, that of producing an organism which causes only a very mild form of the natural disease, can be equally well attained by using strains which are virulent for another species, but avirulent in man. The best example of this was Jenner's remarkable demonstration that cowpox would protect against smallpox. Since then, a global effort by the World Health Organization combining extensive vaccination and selective epidemiological control methods, has eradicated the human disease.

Attenuation itself can be achieved by modifying the conditions under which an organism grows.

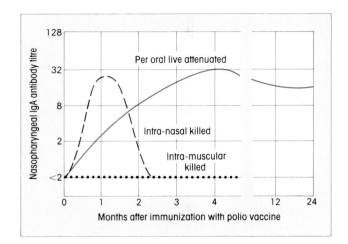

Figure 11.3. *Local IgA response to polio vaccine. Local secretory antibody synthesis is confined to the specific anatomical sites which have been directly stimulated by contact with antigen. (Data from Ogra P.L. et al. (1975) In* **Viral Immunology and Immunopathology**, *p. 67. Notkins A.L. (ed.). Academic Press, New York.)*

Pasteur first achieved the production of live but non-virulent forms of chicken cholera bacillus and anthrax by such artifices as culture at higher temperatures and under anaerobic conditions, and was able to confer immunity by infection with the attenuated organisms. A virulent strain of *Mycobacterium tuberculosis* became attenuated by chance in 1908 when Calmette and Guérin at the Institut Pasteur, Lille, added bile to the culture medium in an attempt to achieve dispersed growth. After 13 years of culture in bile-containing medium, the strain remained attenuated and was used successfully to vaccinate children against tuberculosis. The same organism, BCG (Bacille, Calmette, Guérin), is widely used today for immunization of tuberculin-negative individuals; it will also bestow a reasonable degree of protection against *Mycobacterium leprae* provided the response to the group i cross-reacting antigens have not been subverted by exposure to suppressive species of mycobacteria in the local environment. Attenuation by cold adaptation of influenza and other respiratory viruses seems hopeful; the organism can grow at the lower temperatures (32–34°C) of the upper respiratory tract, but fails to produce clinical disease because of its inability to replicate in the lower respiratory tract (37°C).

Attenuation by recombinant DNA technology

Genetic recombination is being used to develop

228

various attenuated strains of viruses such as influenza with lower virulence for man and some with an increased multiplication rate in eggs (enabling newly endemic strains of influenza to be adapted for rapid vaccine production). The potential is clearly quite enormous.

The tropism of attenuated organisms for the site at which natural infection occurs is likely to be exploited dramatically in the near future to establish gut immunity to typhoid and cholera using attenuated forms of *Salmonella* strains and *Vibrio cholerae* in which the virulence genes have been identified and modified by genetic engineering.

Microbial vectors for other genes

An ingenious trick is to use a virus as a 'piggy-back' for genes from another virus particularly one that cannot be grown successfully, or which is inherently dangerous. Large DNA viruses such as vaccinia can act as carriers for one or many foreign genes while retaining infectivity for animals and cultured cells. The proteins encoded by these genes are appropriately expressed with respect to glycosylation and secretion, and are processed for MHC presentation by the infected cells thus effectively giving rise to both humoral and cell-mediated immunity. An example of a construct in which vaccinia is a vector for an inserted foreign gene is described in figure 11.4.

A wide variety of genes has been expressed by vaccinia virus vectors and it has been demonstrated that the products of genes coding for viral envelope proteins such as influenza virus haemagglutinin, vesicular stomatis virus glycoprotein, HIV-I gp120 and herpes simplex virus glycoprotein D, could be correctly processed and inserted into the plasma membrane of infected cells. Hepatitis surface antigen (HBsAg) was secreted from recombinant vaccinia virus infected cells as the characteristic 22 nm particles. It is an impressive approach and chimpanzees have been protected against the clinical effects of hepatitis B virus, while mice inoculated with the influenza haemagglutinin recombinant generated cytotoxic T-cells and were protected against influenza infection. Spectacular neutralizing antibody titres were produced by a recombinant with the gene encoding rabies virus glycoprotein and protected animals against a severe intracerebral challenge. It is even possible to make a vector with two inserts.

No system is trouble-free and some recombinants grow poorly *in vivo*. Furthermore, immunodeficient individuals have difficulty in clearing the virus, although the resistance of nude mice lacking T-cells to 10^8 plaque-forming units of recombinant vaccinia expressing the IL-2 gene suggests a way round this problem. There is also the objection that a viral vaccine which produces occasional but serious side-effects should not be used in a world free of smallpox. Perhaps less virulent strains can be developed, but in any case the real issue, as ever, is whether the recombinant vaccine causes more problems than the disease for which a vaccine is sought. For veterinary use, of course, there is no problem and excellent results have been obtained with rinderpest in cattle, for example. Although based on the same principles as those used for vaccinia virus, there may be a more favourable climate regarding the acceptance of hybrid polio viruses as potential vaccines, and HIV, hepatitis A and foot and mouth disease virus genes have all been inserted into the polio genome and shown to produce neutralizing antibodies.

Attention has turned to BCG as a vehicle for antigens required to evoke CD4-mediated T-cell immunity. The organism is avirulent, has a low frequency of serious complications, can be administered any time after birth, has strong adjuvant properties, gives long-lasting CMI after a single injection and is a bargain at around US$ 0.05 a shot. The development of shuttle vectors which can replicate in *E. coli* as plasmids and in mycobacteria as phages has allowed foreign DNA to be introduced into *M. smegmatis* and BCG vaccine strains. We can expect many advances on this front: thus incorporation of a gene for kanamycin resistance into the plasmid provides a selectable marker for transformed bacteria, while inclusion of a signal sequence permits secretion of the recombinant protein.

There is an attractive possibility that the oral route of vaccination may be applicable not only for the establishment of gut mucosal immunity but also for providing systemic protection. For example, *Salmonella typhimurium* not only invades the mucosal lining of the gut, but also infects cells of the mononuclear phagocyte system throughout the body thereby stimulating the production of humoral and secretory antibodies as well as cell-mediated immunity. Attenuated *Salmonella* can be made to express proteins from *Shigella*, cholera, malaria, sporozoites and so on, and it is entirely feasible to consider these as potential oral vaccines. Thus, the circumsporozoite antigen construct given orally to mice inhibits the development of the parasite liver

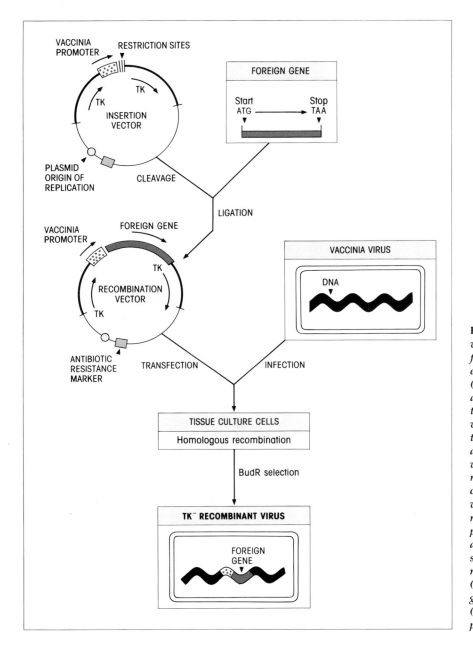

Figure 11.4. *Construction of vaccinia virus recombinants that express a foreign gene. The gene in question, say encoding hepatitis surface antigen (HBsAg), is first inserted into an appropriate vector so that it is adjacent to a vaccinia promoter and flanking vaccinia DNA sequences (in this case thymidine kinase—TK) which determines the site of recombination with the virus. The plasmid is replicated and then used to transfect cells that are simultaneously infected with vaccinia. Homologous recombination inserts the promoter plus foreign gene into the viral genome and the resulting TK⁻ recombinant is selected by picking viral plaques resistant to 5-bromodeoxyuridine (BUdR). TK is not essential for viral growth. (Reproduced from B. Moss (1985)* Immunology **Today** *6, 243, with permission.)*

stages; that this occurred in the absence of antibody supports the view that CMI can be effective.

Constraints on the use of attenuated vaccines

Attenuated vaccines for poliomyelitis (Sabin), measles and rubella have gained general acceptance. None the less, with certain vaccines there is a very small, but still real, risk of developing complications such as the encephalitis which can occur following measles immunization; note, however, that the natural infection carries a far greater risk of encephalitis (*c.* 1:2000)! With live viral vaccines there is a possibility that the nucleic acid might be incorporated into the host's genome or that there may be reversion to a virulent form, although this will be unlikely if the attenuated strains contain several mutations. Another disadvantage of attenuated strains is the difficulty and expense of maintaining appropriate cold storage facilities especially in out-of-the-way places. In diseases such as viral hepatitis and cancer, the dangers associated with live vaccines would make their use unthinkable. It cannot be emphasized too often, that the risk of complication must be balanced against the expected chance of contracting the disease with its own complications. Where this is minimal some may prefer to avoid general vaccination and to rely upon a crash course backed up if necessary by passive immunization in the localities around isolated outbreaks of infectious disease.

It is important to recognize those children with immunodeficiency before injection of live organisms; a child with impaired T-cell reactivity can become overwhelmed by BCG and die. Perhaps this is only a sick story, but it is said that in one particular country there are no adults with T-cell deficiency. The reason? All children had been immunized with live BCG as part of a community health programme(!). The extent to which children with partial deficiencies are at risk has yet to be assessed. It is also inadvisable to give live vaccines to patients being treated, with steroids, immunosuppressive drugs or radiotherapy or who have malignant conditions such as lymphoma and leukaemia; pregnant mothers must also be included here because of the vulnerability of the fetus.

The deviating influence of maternally derived IgG antibody has been discussed in an earlier chapter. Injection of preformed (monoclonal) IgM antibody at the time of immunization with a malaria vaccine seemed to overcome this problem in young mice, but it remains to be seen whether this can be developed into a practical strategy. Preliminary results suggest that infants of 4−6 months can be seroconverted by inhaled aerosol measles vaccine which presumably evades the maternal antibody; this will have singular relevance in endemic measles areas where almost split-second timing is required with conventional immunization as passively acquired antibody wanes.

Vaccines containing individual protective antigens

A whole parasite or bacterium usually contains many antigens which are not concerned in the protective response of the host but may give rise to problems by suppressing the response to protective antigens or by provoking hypersensitivity as we saw in the last chapter. Vaccination with the isolated protective antigens may avoid these complications and identification of these antigens then opens up the possibility of producing them synthetically in circumstances where bulk growth of the organism is impractical or isolation of the individual components too expensive.

Identification of protective antigens is greatly facilitated if one has an experimental model. If protection is antibody-mediated, one can try out different monoclonal antibodies and use the successful ones to pull out the antigen. Where antigenic variation is a major factor, desperate attempts are being made to identify some element of constancy which could provide a basis for vaccination, again using monoclonal antibodies with their ability to recognize a single specificity in a highly complex mixture. If protection is based primarily on T-cell activity, the approach would then be through the identification of individual T-cell clones capable of passively transferring protection.

The use of purified components

Bacterial exotoxins such as those produced by diphtheria and tetanus bacilli have long been used as immunogens. First, they must of course be detoxified and this is achieved by formaldehyde treatment which fortunately does not destroy the major immunogenic determinants (figure 11.5). Immunization with the *toxoid* will therefore provoke the formation of protective antibodies which neutralize the toxin by stereochemically blocking the active site and encourage removal by phagocytic cells. The toxoid is generally given after adsorption to aluminium hydroxide which acts as an adjuvant and produces higher antibody titres. In the case of cholera, a vaccine which combines the B subunit of cholera toxin with killed vibrios is reported to stimulate gut mucosal antibody formation when given orally, the response being said to equal that seen after clinical cholera. Generally speaking it must be said that the emphasis now is to move towards gene cloning of individual proteins once they have been identified immunologically and biochemically. Purified pneumococcal and meningococcal polysaccharide vaccines are in a differ-

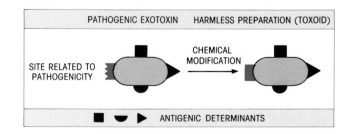

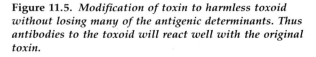

Figure 11.5. *Modification of toxin to harmless toxoid without losing many of the antigenic determinants. Thus antibodies to the toxoid will react well with the original toxin.*

231

INFECTION — PROPHYLAXIS AND IMMUNODEFICIENCY

ent category but they will normally require coupling to some immunogenic carrier protein since they fail to stimulate T-helpers or induce adequate memory.

Antigens can be synthesized through gene cloning

Recombinant DNA technology enables us to make genes encoding part or the whole of a protein peptide chain almost at will, and express them in an appropriate vector. We have already ruminated upon vaccinia virus and other recombinant vectors but very often we wish to utilize the gene product on its own to be incorporated into an adjuvant. Baculovirus vectors in moth cell lines produce large amounts of glycosylated recombinant protein. The product secreted by yeast cells expressing the HbsAg gene is immunogenic and is available as a commercial vaccine. A promising vaccine cocktail against *Schistosoma mansoni* is the combination of the p28-I antigen, a glutathione-S-transferase, together with the parasite paramyosin, both produced as recombinant proteins.

The potential of gene cloning is clearly vast and in principle economical, but there are sometimes difficulties in identifying a good expression vector, in obtaining correct folding of the peptide chain to produce an active protein, and in separating the required product from the culture melange in an undenatured state. It could be instructive to follow one particular study on production of a vaccine against ovine cysticercosis. This disease in sheep is caused by larval tapeworms (*Taenia ovis*) and an extract of the early larval oncosphere stage will immunize completely against reinfection. Immune sera reacted strongly on Western immunoblots with oncosphere antigens of molecular weight 47–52 kDa (figure 11.6) and when cut out of the gel, this fraction gave good protection. Antibodies affinity-purified from the 47–52 kDa immunoblots were used to screen a cDNA expression library to identify two clones producing antigen linked to β-galactoside. Although one of the fusion proteins generated antibodies, it could not protect against infection suggesting that the antigen may have been denatured. When glutathione-S-transferase from *S. japonicum* was used as the fusion partner, the antigen could be isolated under non-denaturing conditions and now gave almost complete protection when administered to sheep in the adjuvant saponin. A valuable vaccine is on its way.

One restriction to gene cloning is that carbohydrate antigens cannot be synthesized directly by recombinant DNA technology although preliminary attempts to clone the cohort of genes which encode the cascade of synthetic enzymes needed to produce complex carbohydrates are under way.

Antigens can be mimicked by synthetic peptides

B-cell epitopes

Small peptide sequences corresponding with important epitopes on a microbial antigen can be synthesized readily and economically; long ones are rather expensive to manufacture. One might predict that although the synthetic peptide has the correct linear *sequence* of amino acids, its random structure would make it a poor model for the *conformation* of the parent antigen and hence a poor vaccine for evoking humoral immunity. Curiously this does not always seem to be a serious drawback. The 20 amino acid peptide derived from the foot and mouth virus-specific protein (VP1) evokes a good neutralizing response. The explanation has been forthcoming from X-ray structural analysis which shows the peptide sequence to be in a 'loop' region with blurred electron density indicative of dramatic disorder. In this case, the epitope is linear and evidently the flexibility of the loop structure may approach that of the free peptide which can thus mimic the epitope on the native VPI molecule and stimulate a protective antibody response when used as a vaccine (figure 11.7a, b). Where the epitope is linear but is restricted in conformation by adjacent structures in the intact protein, immunization with free peptide tends to produce antibodies of disappointing affinity for the protein itself for reasons outlined in figure 11.7c.

T-cell epitopes

Although short peptides may not have the conformation to stimulate adequate B-cell responses, they can prime antigen-specific T-cells which recognize the primary sequence rather than the tertiary configuration of the protein. If the primed T-cells mediate CMI and possibly act to help B-cells make antibody, they could enable the host to mount an effective response on subsequent exposure to natural infection and this would prove to be a useful prophylactic strategy. This seems to have been the case when a peptide sequence from polio virus VPI induced poor neutralizing antibody but did prime the recipient for a good response to infection.

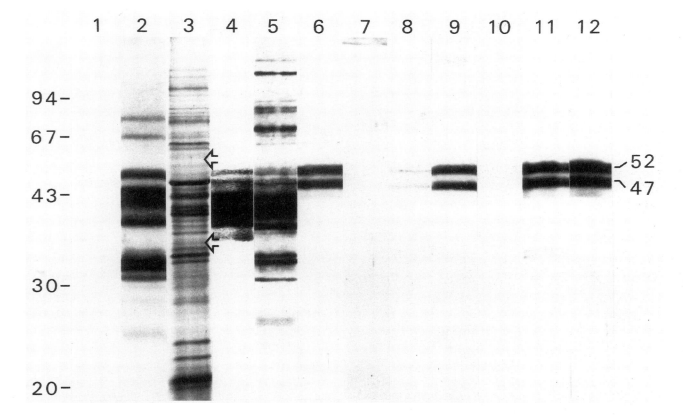

Figure 11.6. *Identification of* **T. ovis** *oncosphere antigens using immunoblotting of preparations separated by SDS-PAGE (cf. figure 5.23). Lanes were probed with: (1) preimmunization sheep sera; (2) sera from sheep immunized with oncosphere extract; (4) sheep immunized with gel cut-out fraction in lane 3; (5) rabbit hyperimmune to extract; (6) rabbit affinity-purified antibodies eluted from* blots of 47–52 kDa antigens; (7) sheep immunized with β-galactosidase; (8) sheep immunized with clone β-gal-45S; (9) same using clone β-gal-45W; (10) same using glutathione-S-transferase (GST); (11) same using clone GST-45S; (12) same using clone GST-45W. (Reproduced from Johnson K.S. et al. (1989) Nature, 338, 585, with permission).*

233

A major worry about peptides as T-cell vaccines is the variation in ability to associate with the different polymorphic forms of MHC molecules present in an outbred population, which contributes to the immune response (IR) gene effect described earlier (p. 165). This may be seen graphically in figure 11.8, it being clear that strains of mice with different H-2 haplotype may respond to quite different sequences in the core protein of hepatitis B virus. The same effects would be expected with individuals of differing HLA tissue types in human populations. One either has to use a cocktail of peptides in a general vaccine to cover HLA variation, or if that is too difficult, go back to a gene-cloned version of the whole protein antigen. Residues 378–398 of the malaria circumsporozoite protein provide an exception in being virtually a universal T-cell epitope recognizable by all individuals so far tested.

Making the peptides immunogenic

Immunogenicity of peptides for B-cells is invariably bound up with a dependence on T-cell help and failure to provide linked T-cell epitopes is thought to be responsible for poor antibody responses to the foot and mouth disease VPI loop peptide in cattle and pigs, and to NANP polymers of malarial circumsporozoite antigens in man (cf. p. 221). When the general T-cell carrier, peptide 378–398 (v.supra) was coupled to $(NANP)_3$ tetramer repeat, good antibody responses were obtained in all strains of mice tested. Furthermore, after priming with this synthetic peptide, whole sporozoites would boost antibody titres. This brings up two points: first, in order for the natural infection to boost, the T- and B-cell epitopes must both be present and, secondly, they must be linked so that the T-cell epitope is taken up for processing by the lymphocyte which

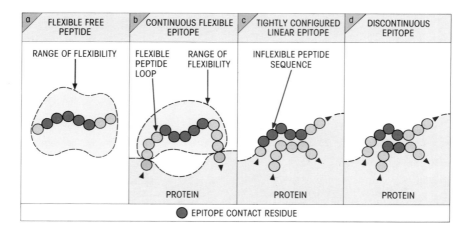

| a FLEXIBLE FREE PEPTIDE | b CONTINUOUS FLEXIBLE EPITOPE | c TIGHTLY CONFIGURED LINEAR EPITOPE | d DISCONTINUOUS EPITOPE |

RANGE OF FLEXIBILITY — FLEXIBLE PEPTIDE LOOP — RANGE OF FLEXIBILITY — INFLEXIBLE PEPTIDE SEQUENCE — PROTEIN — PROTEIN — PROTEIN

● EPITOPE CONTACT RESIDUE

Figure 11.7. *Structural basis for peptide mimicry of protein epitopes. (a) The free peptide is very flexible and can adopt a large number of structures in solution. (b) If the peptide sequence is present as a linear epitope on a part of a protein which is a flexible loop or chain, this will also exist in a variety of structures resembling the free peptide to a fair extent and will behave comparably as an antigen and as an immunogen (vaccine) so that the peptide will raise antibodies which react well with the native protein. (c) If the linear epitope on the protein is structurally constrained (i.e. inflexible), it represents only one of the many structures adopted by the free peptide; thus if this peptide is used for immunization, only a minority of the B-cells stimulated will be complementary in shape to the native protein, so the peptide would be a poor vaccine for humoral immunity to microbes containing the protein antigen. (Note, however, it would be good for Western immunoblots where the protein has been denatured after SDS treatment and the peptide structure is relatively free.) Preformed antibodies to the protein would react with the peptide albeit with lower affinity because energy must be used to constrain the peptide to the one structure which fits the antibody—just like the force used to restrain a madman in a strait-jacket. Where the sequence has a comparable degree of constraint in both peptide and protein as in the disulphide-bonded loops in diphtheria toxin and hepatitis B surface antigen, anti-peptide sera react reasonably well with the native protein. (d) Most commonly, the epitopes are discontinuous and even if, with difficulty, we can predict the contact residues, the techniques for designing a peptide with appropriate structure are not available at present.*

recognizes the B-cell epitope (figure 6.18). This does not always imply that the link in the infectious agent must be covalent since mice primed with the core antigen of hepatitis B virus gave excellent responses to the surface antigen when challenged with whole virions, i.e. an interstructural relationship may function in this regard as well as an intramolecular one. In contrast, animals immunized with an HBs B-cell peptide coupled with a streptococcal peptide T-cell carrier require boosting with the original vaccine but do not receive a boost from natural infection. In passing, it is worth noting that the presentation of a peptide such as the foot and mouth disease virus VPI loop in the form of an octamer coupled to a poly-L-lysine backbone produces responses of far greater magnitude than the monomer, a strategy which has proved successful with several other peptides. Is the poly-L-lysine a carrier, or are the multiple peptide units acting as carriers for each other?

Having said this, the evidence is mounting that the majority of protein determinants are discontinuous, i.e. involve amino acid residues far apart in the primary sequence but brought close to each other by peptide folding (cf. p. 66). In such cases, peptides which represent linear sequences of the primary structure will, at best, only mimic part of a determinant and generate low affinity responses. Defining a discontinuous determinant by X-ray crystallography and site-related mutagenesis takes a long time and by computer analysis, perhaps even longer. Even when armed with this information, synthesis of a configured peptide which will topographically mimic the contact residues which constitute such an epitope remains an awesome challenge.

Idiotypes can be exploited as epitope-specific vaccines

The attempt to produce molecules which act as substitute or 'surrogate' epitopes may be of considerable importance for parasite vaccines if one wishes to separate determinants on an individual antigen that stimulate T-helpers and protective antibodies from those which may activate T-sup-

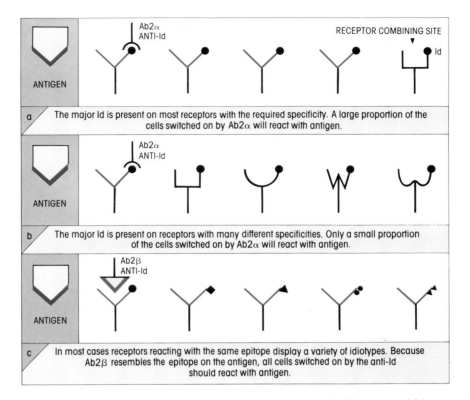

ANTIGEN	Ab2α ANTI-Id ... RECEPTOR COMBINING SITE ... Id
a	The major Id is present on most receptors with the required specificity. A large proportion of the cells switched on by Ab2α will react with antigen.
ANTIGEN	Ab2α ANTI-Id
b	The major Id is present on receptors with many different specificities. Only a small proportion of the cells switched on by Ab2α will react with antigen.
ANTIGEN	Ab2β ANTI-Id
c	In most cases receptors reacting with the same epitope display a variety of idiotypes. Because Ab2β resembles the epitope on the antigen, all cells switched on by the anti-Id should react with antigen.

235

Figure 11.8. *The theoretical reactivity of anti-idiotypes to cross-reacting regulatory idiotypes (Ab2α), or those which behave as internal images of the antigen (Ab2β), with lymphocyte receptors. The final response will reflect the range of receptors switched on by anti-Id. (a) If the major Id is present on most receptors with the required specificity, a large proportion of the cells switched on by Ab2α will react with antigen. (b) If the major Id is present on receptors with many different specificities, only a small proportion of the cells switched on by Ab2α will react with antigen. (c) In most cases receptors reacting with the same epitope display a variety of idiotypes. Because Ab2β resembles the epitope on the antigen, many cells switched on by the anti-Id should react with antigen.*

pressors or cross-react with self. As we have discussed, one problem with peptides as surrogate determinants is the difficulty in triggering lymphocyte receptors which recognize conformational epitopes characteristic for the native rather than the unfolded protein antigen. One solution is to produce antiidiotypes which act as 'internal images' of the determinant and therefore possess an acceptable conformation at the outset.

If the reader trundles back to figure 8.9, it will be seen that there are two main categories of anti-idiotype: Ab2α which recognize cross-reacting, presumably regulatory, idiotypes and Ab2β which are thought to behave as internal images of the antigenic determinant. In those instances where the major Id is mostly associated with a given specificity (e.g. murine T15 Id is largely present on antibodies to phosphoryl choline), then Ab2α anti-Ids could provide useful potential vaccines particularly for carbohydrates which are notoriously poor immunogens in the very young. In general, the Ab2β are capable of stimulating a wider range of lymphocytes (figure 11.8). Although the internal image anti-idiotypes concerned with the majority of microbial antigens are probably rather poorly represented in the B-cell repertoire, they can be pulled out by monoclonal antibody technology and grown up in substantial amounts using the approach described in figure 11.9.

Comparison of a monoclonal anti-Id internal image surrogate for HBsAg protective *a* determinant, with a peptide composed of residues 139–147 of HBsAg also meant to mimic the *a* determinant, very reassuringly showed mutual interference in competing for antibodies to HBsAg (figure 11.10). Interestingly, the anti-Id had a higher affinity for HBsAg antisera but reacted with a smaller proportion of the available antibodies than the peptide. This suggests that the anti-Id has a better fixed conformation but is restricted in the number of contact residues available for binding to the spectrum of antibodies in a polyclonal serum. This

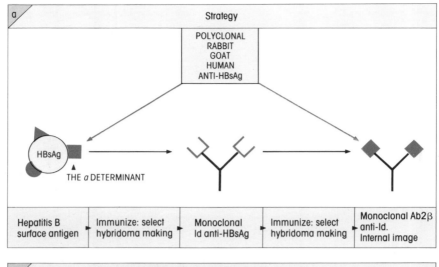

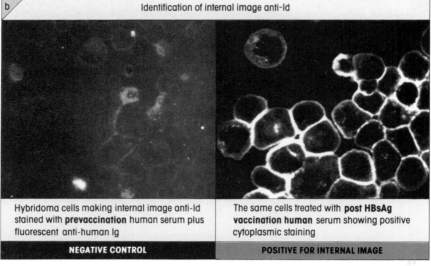

Figure 11.9. *Production of monoclonal anti-idiotype behaving as an internal image of the protective* **a** *determinant of hepatitis B surface antigen (HBsAg). A monoclonal anti-HBsAg is used to generate a range of anti-Id hybridomas; the internal image clones are selected by their ability to behave like the original antigen in reacting with a variety of polyclonal anti-HBsAg from different species. For simplicity the Ab2β is shown as identical in shape with the antigen epitope, but this need not be so; it has to be capable of* substituting for the antigen to provide a sufficient number of contact points with the antibody and theoretically does not need to look exactly like the antigen; indeed when Ab2β anti-Ids mimic carbohydrate antigens or acetylcholine and other hormone agonists, they obviously cannot be structurally identical. (See Roitt I.M. et al. (1985) **Immunology Today 6**, 265, for a more detailed analysis.) (a) Strategy. (b) Identification of internal image anti-Id (based on Thanavala Y.M. et al. (1985) **Immunology 55, 197**).

implies that a cocktail of monoclonal anti-Ids mimicking any given epitope would be needed for effective immunization. As a general point, it is also preferable to target immunization against more than one epitope because a single epitope can alter by mutation during the course of an infection; furthermore, a lone epitope is more likely to show up Ir gene deficiency (cf. p. 165) in an outbred population giving rise to inadequate immunity in these individuals, although if the surrogate epitope is presented on a carrier this would not pose a problem. It should be stressed that vaccines based on anti-Ids are still in a very experimental stage although one has been reported to protect chimpanzees against hepatitis B infection.

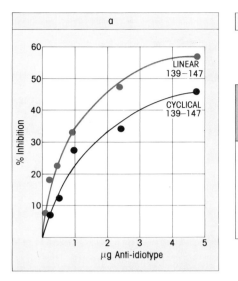

	b			
	Anti-HBs antiserum			
	Human convalescent pool		**Rabbit**	
Antigen	Antibody-combining sites (pmol per 10 μl serum)	K	Antibody-combining sites	K
Cyclical 139–147	97	7.2×10^7	110	3.3×10^7
Linear 139–147	119	8.0×10^6	106	9.0×10^6
2F10 anti-idiotype	7.7	1.4×10^8	7.2	9.0×10^8
4D4 anti-idiotype	—	—	6.7	2.0×10^8
2E7 anti-idiotype	5.4	5.8×10^8	12.1	3.5×10^8
3H1 anti-idiotype	—	—	—	—

Figure 11.10. *Comparison of reactions of anti-HBsAg with monoclonal internal image anti-idiotype and peptide surrogates for HBsAg a determinant. (a) Inhibition of binding of monoclonal anti-HBsAg to the linear and cyclic peptide representing HBsAg residues 139–147 by anti-Id. (b) Affinities and combining capacities of polyclonal anti-HBs for HBsAg peptides and monoclonal anti-Id (from Thanavala Y.M. et al. (1986) J. Exp. Med. 164, 227).*

Adjuvants

For practical and economic reasons, prophylactic immunization should involve the minimum number of injections and the least amount of antigen. We have referred to the undoubted advantages of replicating attenuated organisms in this respect but non-living organisms, and especially purified products, frequently require an adjuvant which by definition is a substance incorporated into or injected simultaneously with antigen which potentiates the immune response (Latin *adjuvare*—to help). The mode of action of adjuvants may be considered under several headings:

Depot effects

Free antigen usually disperses rapidly from the local tissues draining the injection site and an important function of the so-called repository adjuvants is to counteract this by providing a long-lived reservoir of antigen, either at an extracellular location or within macrophages. The most common adjuvants of this type used in man are aluminium compounds (phosphate and hydroxide) and Freund's incomplete adjuvant (in which the antigen is incorporated in the aqueous phase of a stabilized water in paraffin oil emulsion). Both types increase the antibody response but the emulsions tend to produce higher and far more sustained antibody levels with a broadening of the response to include more of the epitopes in the antigen preparation. Because of the life-long persistence of oil in the tissues and the occasional production of sterile abscesses, and the unpalatable fact that paraffin oil produces tumours in mice, attention has been focused on the replacement of incomplete Freund's with different types of oils such as squalene or biodegradable peanut oil. It is claimed that antibody titres are comparable to those obtained with Freund's and that no long-term adverse effects in man have yet been encountered.

Macrophage activation

Under the influence of the repository adjuvants, macrophages form granulomata which provide sites for interaction with antibody-forming cells. The maintenance by the depot of consistent antigen concentrations, particularly on the macrophage surface, ensures that as antigen-sensitive cells divide within the granuloma, their progeny are highly likely to be further stimulated by antigen. Virtually all adjuvants stimulate macrophages which are thought to act by improving immunogenicity through an increase in the amount of antigen on their surface and the efficiency of its presentation to lymphocytes, by the provision of accessory signals to direct lymphocytes towards an immune response rather than tolerance, and by the secretion of soluble stimulatory factors (e.g. interleukin-1) which influence the proliferation of lymphocytes.

Specific effects on lymphocytes

In mice, alum tends to stimulate helper cells of the Th2 family whereas complete Freund's adjuvant favours the Th1 subset. It will be recalled that complete Freund's is made from the incomplete adjuvant by addition of killed mycobacteria (cf. p. 131), the active component being the water-soluble muramyl dipeptide (MDP; N-acetylmuramyl-L-alanyl-D-isoglutamine) which acts on macrophages, B- and T-cells, inducing a variety of cytokines. Hydrophilic MDP analogues with aqueous antigen preferentially stimulate antibody responses, but if administered in a hydrophobic microenvironment such as mineral oil or incorporation into liposomes, CMI is the major outcome. Lipophilic MDP derivatives enhance CMI without the need for the water-in-oil emulsion. The immunopotentiating and other effects of the mycobacterial component in complete Freund such as the development of delayed type hypersensitivity, the production of persisting granulomas and the provocation of autoimmune disease, are so striking that their use in man is not normally countenanced; undoubtedly hope lies in the exploration of suitable MDP analogues.

Looking at other materials with adjuvant properties, BCG is a potent stimulator of T- and B-cells and macrophages. Levamisole boosts delayed hypersensitivity and isoprinosine is said to overcome the IL-2 defect in autoimmune MRL mice bearing the lymphoproliferative (lpr) gene while polyanions such as poly A:U, and the fungal polysaccharide lentinan, promote T-helper cells. Pertussis toxin, an exotoxin from *Bordetella pertussis*, potentiates cell-mediated immunity partly through its ability to alter recirculation of T-lymphocytes. By contrast, purified lipid A from bacterial lipopolysaccharide is a B-cell mitogen with a preferential effect on Bμ cells. Its conjugate with MDP should have interesting properties.

Although the role of modulatory cytokines in these interactions is unclear, it is of interest that polylysine-stabilized poly-I:C, which produces good interferon levels in primates, is said to be an effective adjuvant for immunization to influenza virus.

Anti-tumour action

This will be discussed in Chapter 13 but one may summarize by saying that the major effect is mediated through cytotoxic and cytostatic actions of activated macrophages on tumours, with the stimulation of specific T-cell immunity to the tumour antigens as a further possibility.

New approaches to the presentation of antigen

Recent interest has centred on the use of small lipid membrane vesicles (*liposomes*) as agents for the presentation of antigen to the immune system. It may be that the liposome acts as a storage vacuole within the macrophage or perhaps fuses with the macrophage membrane to provide a suitably immunogenic complex. Proteins anchored in the lipid membrane by hydrophobic means give augmented cell-mediated immunity. One envisages the possibility of selecting the type of lymphocyte activated by incorporating accessory signalling agents into the liposome membrane, e.g. MDP derivatives, polyanions or levamisole to stimulate T-cells, components of ascaris or *Bordetella pertussis* to exaggerate IgE production, T-cell soluble factors for the triggering of Bγ cells, C3b for homing to lymph node follicles and so on.

Another innovation is the ISCOM (immunostimulating complex), a hydrophobic matrix of the adjuvant saponin, with antigen, cholesterol and phosphatidyl choline. Antigens with a transmembrane hydrophobic region, such as surface molecules of lipid-containing viruses, are powerfully immunogenic in this vehicle and may engender cytotoxic T-cell responses.

It may be useful to focus on the notion floated earlier that polymeric antigens tend to be more immunogenic and to note a novel form of solid matrix of the Cowan strain of *Staphylococcus aureus* which can bind several molecules of monoclonal antibody which can in turn immobilize several molecules of antigen. Using a variety of monoclonals, one can purify onto their binding sites appropriate antigens from a mixture to give a multivalent subunit vaccine. One could also incorporate cholera toxin to give good mucosal immunity; one could do lots of things such as keeping an eye open for advances in controlled delivery of antigens using water soluble glasses.

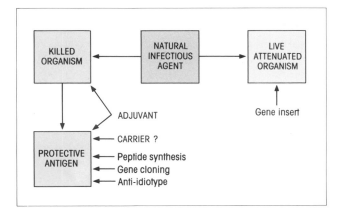

Figure 11.11. *Strategies for vaccination.*

The overall strategies for vaccination are summarized in figure 11.11.

PRIMARY IMMUNODEFICIENCY STATES IN THE HUMAN

In accord with the dictum that 'most things that can go wrong, do so', a multiplicity of immunodeficiency states in man have been recognized. These are classified in table 11.1 together with some of the most clear-cut (and correspondingly rare) examples. We have earlier stressed the manner in which the interplay of complement, antibody and phagocytic cells constitutes the basis of a tripartite defence mechanism against pyogenic (pus-forming) infections with bacteria which require prior opsonization before phagocytosis. It is not surprising then, that deficiency in any one of these factors may predispose the individual to repeated infections of this

type. Patients with T-cell deficiency of course present a markedly different pattern of infection, being susceptible to those viruses and moulds which are normally eradicated by cell-mediated immunity.

A relatively high incidence of malignancies, and of autoantibodies with or without autoimmune disease, has been documented in patients with immunodeficiency but the reason for this association is not yet clear, although failure of T-cell regulation or inability to control key viral infections are among the suggestions canvassed.

Deficiencies of innate immune mechanisms

Phagocytic cell defects

In chronic granulomatous disease the monocytes and polymorphs fail to produce reactive oxygen intermediates due to a defect in the cytochrome b_{-245} normally activated by phagocytosis. The cytochrome has 92 and 22 kDa subunits and in the X-linked form of the disease, the protein is not expressed because of a lesion in the gene encoding the larger of the subunits. The 30% of chronic granulomatous disease patients who inherit their disorder in an autosomal recessive pattern express a defective form of the cytochrome. Patients with one variant of the X-linked disease have residual amounts of cytochrome b and their condition can be improved by treatment with γ-interferon. Many bacteria help to bring about their own destruction by generating H_2O_2 through their own metabolic processes, but if they are catalase positive, the peroxide is destroyed and the bacteria will survive. Thus polymorphs from these patients readily take up catalase positive staphylococci in the presence

Table 11.1. *Classification of immunodeficiency states with examples.*

Deficiency	Example	Immune response		Infection	Treatment
		Humoral	Cellular		
Complement	C3 deficiency	Normal	Normal	Pyogenic bacteria	Antibiotics
Myeloid cell	Chronic granulomatous disease	Normal	Normal	Catalase-positive bacteria	Antibiotics
B-cell	Infantile sex-linked a-γ-globulinaemia (Bruton)	↓	Normal	Pyogenic bacteria *Pneumocystis carinii*	γ-Globulin
T-cell	Thymic hypoplasia (DiGeorge)		↓	Certain viruses *Candida*	Thymus graft
Stem cell	Severe combined deficiency (Swiss-type)	↓	↓	All the above	Bone marrow graft

of antibody and complement but fail to kill them intracellularly.

In Chediak—Higashi disease, the lysosomes are deficient in elastase and cathepsin G and the patients suffer from pyogenic infections which can be fatal. Beige mice which represent a murine model of this disease have neutrophils which lack azurophilic granules. Among other rare conditions, myeloperoxidase deficiency is associated with susceptibility to systemic candidiasis, while a defective polymorph response to chemotactic stimuli characterizes the lazy leucocyte syndrome. Lack of the CD18 β-subunit of the integrins produces a leucocyte adhesion deficiency causing impaired chemotaxis and recurrent bacterial infection. Allogeneic bone marrow grafts used to correct the disease are surprisingly well tolerated possibly because of the LFA-1 defect. Seizing on this clue, one group has increased allogeneic bone marrow survival in general to 50% by treating recipients with monoclonal anti-LFA-1. In a totally different disorder, congenital agranulocytosis, it is encouraging to report that daily infusion of recombinant G-CSF raises the granulocyte counts in the majority of patients.

Complement system deficiencies

Defects in control proteins

The importance of complement in defence against infections is emphasized by the occurrence of repeated life-threatening infection with pyogenic bacteria in a patient lacking factor I, the C3b inactivator. Because of his inability to destroy C3b there is continual activation of the alternative pathway through the feedback loop leading to very low C3 and factor B levels with normal, C1, 4 and 2.

Each red blood cell is bombarded daily with 1000 molecules of C3b generated through the formation of fluid phase alternative pathway C3 convertase from the spontaneous hydrolysis of the internal thioester of C3. There are several regulatory components on the red cell surface to deal with this. The C3 convertase complex is dissociated by decay-accelerating factor (DAF) and by CR1 complement receptors (not forgetting factor H from the fluid phase, cf. p. 8) after which the C3b is dismembered by factor I in concert with CR1, membrane cofactor protein (MCP) or factor H (figure 11.12). There are also two inhibitors of the membrane attack complex, homologous restriction factor (HRF) which is a C8b binding protein, and MAC inhibitory factor

(MACIF). DAF, HRF and MACIF bind to the membrane through glycosyl phosphatidylinositol anchors. In a condition known as paroxysmal nocturnal haemoglobinuria (PNH) there is a defect in the ability to synthesize these anchors and, in the absence of these complement regulators, serious lysis of the red cells occurs. In the less severe type II PNH, there is a defect in DAF, but in the type III form associated with deficiency of MACIF, susceptibility to spontaneous complement-mediated lysis is greatly increased (figure 11.12). The erythrocytes can be normalized by adding back the deficient factor.

An inhibitor of active C1 is grossly lacking in *hereditary angioedema* and this can lead to recurring episodes of acute circumscribed non-inflammatory oedema mediated by a vasoactive C2 fragment (figure 11.13). The patients are heterozygotes and synthesize small amounts of the inhibitor which can be raised to useful levels by administration of the synthetic anabolic steroid danazol or, in critical cases, of the purified inhibitor itself. ε-Aminocaproic acid, which blocks the plasmin-induced liberation of the C2 kinin, provides an alternative treatment.

Deficiency of components of the complement pathway

Failure to generate the classical C3-convertase through deficiencies in C1q, C1r, C4 and C2 has been reported in a small number of cases associated with an unusually high incidence of SLE-like syndromes (cf. p. 330) perhaps due to a decreased ability to mount an adequate host response to infection with a putative aetiological agent or to eliminate antigen—antibody complexes effectively (cf. p. 265). Permanent deficiencies in C5, C6, C7, C8 and C9 have all been described in man, yet in virtually every case the individuals are healthy and not particularly prone to infection apart from an increased susceptibility to disseminated *Neisseria gonorrhoeae* and *N. meningitidis*. Thus full operation of the terminal complement system does not appear to be essential for survival and adequate protection must be largely afforded by opsonizing antibodies and the immune adherence mechanism.

B-cell deficiency

In Bruton's congenital a-γ-globulinaemia the production of immunoglobulin in affected males is

240

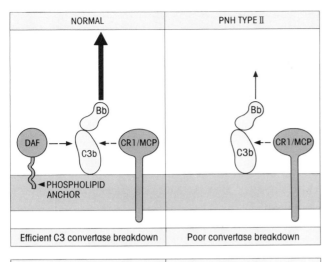

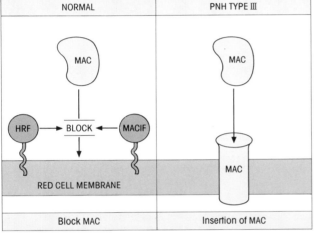

Figure 11.12. *Paroxysmal noctural haemoglobinuria (PNH). Inability to synthesize the glycosyl phosphatidylinositol anchors deprives the red cell membrane of complement control proteins and renders the cell susceptible to complement-mediated lysis. Type II is associated with a DAF defect and the more severe type III with MACIF deficiency. (DAF decay accelerating factor; CR1 complement receptor type 1; MCP membrane cofactor protein; HRF=homologous restriction factor; MAC=membrane attack complex; MACIF=MAC inhibitory factor.)*

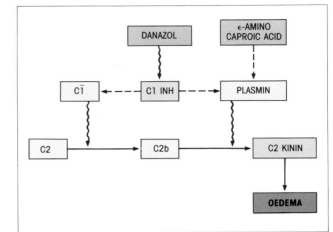

Figure 11.13. *C1 inhibitor deficiency and angioedema. C1 inhibitor stoichiometrically inhibits C$\overline{1}$, plasmin, kallikrein and activated Hageman factor and deficiency leads to formation of the vasoactive C2 kinin by the mechanism shown. The synthesis of C1 inhibitor can be boosted by methyl-testosterone or preferably the less masculinizing synthetic steroid, Danazol; alternatively, attacks can be controlled by giving ε-aminocaproic acid to inhibit the plasmin.*

241

grossly depressed and there are few lymphoid follicles or plasma cells in lymph node biopsies. In many cases there is a failure of V_H gene rearrangement with production of truncated chains of composition DJμ. The children are subject to repeated infection by pyogenic bacteria — *Staphylococcus aureus*, *Streptococcus pyogenes* and *pneumoniae*, *Neisseria meningitidis*, *Haemophilus influenzae* — and by a rare protozoon, *Pneumocystis carinii*, which produces a strange form of pneumonia. Cell-mediated immune responses are normal and viral infections such as measles and smallpox are readily brought under control. Therapy involves the repeated administration of human γ-globulin to maintain adequate concentrations of circulating immunoglobulin.

IgA deficiency due to a failure of IgA-bearing lymphocytes to differentiate into plasma cells, is encountered with relative frequency. IgA antibodies are often detectable but it is uncertain whether these antibodies prevented development of the IgA system or whether lack of tolerance resulting from an absent IgA system allowed the body to make antibodies to exogenous determinants immunologically related to IgA.

The most common form of immunodeficiency, not surprisingly known as common, variable immunodeficiency, is characterized by recurrent pyogenic infections and probably includes many entities. The marrow contains normal numbers of immature B-cells, but a third of the patients lack circulating B-cells with surface Ig and, of the remainder, half have subnormal numbers. Where present they are unable to differentiate to plasma cells in some cases or to secrete antibody in others. T-cells are, however, also affected; each lymphocyte has a low surface 5-nucleotidase, the T_M cells lack the characteristic non-specific esterase spot, around 30% have poor responses to the polyclonal T-cell activator phytohaemagglutinin (PHA) and a small proportion have T-cells of phenotype CD8$^+$, MHC class II$^+$ with marked suppressor activity for B-cells. An excess of such cells, revealed by their ability to suppress pokeweed-driven immuno-globulin synthesis by HLA-identical normal lymphocytes, is a feature of the chronic graft-vs-host disease which follows allogeneic bone marrow transplantation in man.

Transient hypogammaglobulinaemia of infancy, characterized by recurrent respiratory infections, is associated with low IgG levels which often return somewhat abruptly to normal by 4 years of age. There is a deficiency in the number of circulating lymphocytes and in their ability to generate help for Ig production by B-cells activated by pokeweed mitogen, but this becomes normal as the disease resolves spontaneously.

Immunoglobulin deficiency occurs naturally in human infants as the maternal IgG level wanes and may become a serious problem in very premature babies.

T-cell deficiency

The DiGeorge and Nezelof syndromes are characterized by a failure of the thymus to develop properly from the third and fourth pharyngeal pouches during embryogenesis (DiGeorge children also lack parathyroids and have severe cardiovascular

abnormalities). Consequently, stem cells cannot differentiate to become T-lymphocytes and the 'thymus dependent' areas in lymphoid tissue are sparsely populated; in contrast lymphoid follicles are seen but even these are poorly developed (figure 11.14). Cell-mediated immune responses are undetectable and although the infants can deal with common bacterial infections they may be overwhelmed by vaccinia (figure 11.15) or measles, or by BCG if given by mistake. Humoral antibodies can be elicited but the response is subnormal, presumably reflecting the need for the cooperative involvement of T-cells. (The similarity of this condition to neonatal thymectomy and of B-cell deficiency to neonatal bursectomy in the chicken should not go unmentioned.) Treatment by grafting neonatal thymus leads to restoration of immunocompetence but unless graft and donor are well matched, the thymus is ultimately rejected by the ungrateful host cells it has helped to maturity; in any event, some matching between the major histocompatibility antigens on the non-lymphocytic thymus cells and peripheral cells is essential for the proper functioning of the T-lymphocytes (p. 178).

Complete absence of the thymus is pretty rare and more often one is dealing with a 'partial DiGeorge' in which the T-cells may rise from 6% at birth to around 30% of the total circulating lymphocytes by the end of the first year; antibody responses are adequate. Selective T-cell depression can arise from deficiency in the enzyme, purine nucleoside

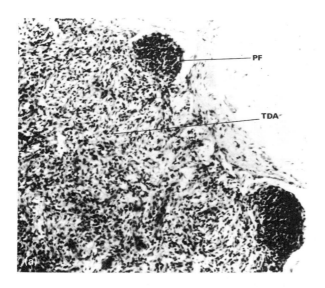
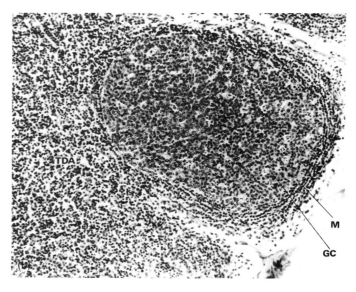

Figure 11.14. *Lymph node cortex. (a) From patient with DiGeorge syndrome showing depleted thymus-dependent area (TDA) and small primary follicles (PF); (b) from normal subject: the populated T-cell area and the well-developed* *secondary follicle with its mantle of small lymphocytes (M) and pale staining germinal centre (GC) provide a marked contrast. (DiGeorge material kindly supplied by Dr D. Webster; photograph by Mr C.J. Sym.)*

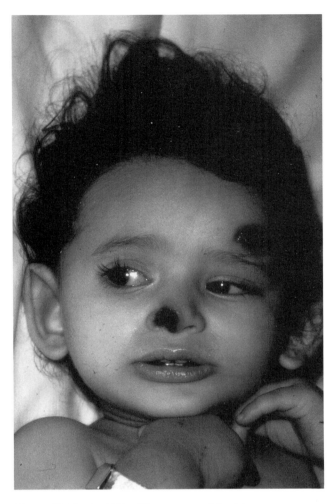

Figure 11.15. *A child with severe combined immuno-deficiency showing skin lesions due to infection with vaccinia gangrenosum resulting from smallpox immunization. Lesions were widespread over the whole body. (Reproduced by kind permission of Professor R.J. Levinsky and the Medical Illustration Department of the Hospital for Sick Children, Great Ormond Street, London.)*

phosphorylase which allows accumulation of toxic metabolites such as dGTP to which activated T-cells are particularly sensitive. The poor T-cell responses make these patients susceptible to infection with varicella and vaccinia viruses but, despite having less than 10% circulating T-cells, they have normal B-cell immunity suggesting that T−B collaboration can operate at much lower T-cell levels in the human than in the mouse.

Cell-mediated immunity is depressed in immunodeficient patients with ataxia telangiectasia or with thrombocytopenia and eczema (Wiskott−Aldrich syndrome) and it is of great interest that in both conditions about 10% of the patients so far studied have died of malignancies of the lymphoid

system or of epithelial tumours. Wiskott−Aldrich males lack a cell-surface molecule, sialophorin (CD43). Normal T-cells proliferate in response to IgG anti-CD43 in the presence of mononuclear phagocytes, independently of the CD3/TCR system. Wiskott−Aldrich is associated with a low IgM and a poor response to many polysaccharides, and they have few B-cells bearing surface idiotypes for poly-saccharide antigens. The response of these B-cells, which mature late in B-cell development, requires T-cell help elicited in a non-specific manner inde-pendent of the CD3/TCR receptor. The question arises quite naturally: is CD43 the non-specific receptor for polysaccharides capable of transducing this message for non-specific T-cell help?

Ataxia telangiectasia is a human autosomal recess-ive disorder of childhood characterized by progress-ive cerebella ataxia with degeneration of Purkinje cells, and a hypersensitivity to X-rays, which, together with the unduly high incidence of cancer, has been laid at the door of a defect in DNA repair mechanisms. This presumably accounts for the clustering of chromosome breaks around genes of the Ig supergene family, especially TCR and IgH, and the associated cellular and Ig deficiency.

The concomitant lack of IgE with IgA may be partly responsible for the greater susceptibility to upper respiratory infections in ataxia telangiectasia as compared with individuals deficient in IgA alone.

Isolated cases of T-cell deficiency have been de-scribed where the serum contains a lymphocytotoxic antibody which presumably must be selective for T- rather than B-lymphocytes. T-cells from some patients with mucocutaneous candidiasis are unable to produce the cytokine, macrophage migration inhibition factor (MIF), when stimulated *in vitro* and it is conceivable that other selective failures of lymphokine synthesis may be uncovered.

Also for the collector are the rare cases of CD3 deficiency probably arising from mutation in the ζ−chain necessary for transport of the CD3 com-plex to the cell surface. Another small subgroup with CMI deficiency have defective couplings be-tween the TCR antigen receptor and the signal-transducing G-protein machinery involving inositol triphosphate and mobilization of intracellular calcium stores.

Combined immunodeficiency

When there is a defect in the recombinase enzymes which are essential for the generation of T- and B-

243

cell receptors, T- and B-lymphocytes will fail to become immunocompetent and this will give rise to a severe combined immunodeficiency (SCID) of cellular and humoral responses. The SCID mouse with a similar recombinase defect and its utility as a host for functioning human lymphoid tissue grafts has been introduced earlier. Note that on infection with listeria, these mice develop large numbers of macrophages activated through IFNγ produced by NK cells.

Normal immune function can be established in the children by grafting with histocompatible bone marrow from a sibling. Cells from other donors too readily initiate a potentially lethal graft-vs-host reaction (cf. p. 279) even when reasonably well matched, unless steps are first taken to rid the graft of any immunocompetent T-lymphocytes. Some patients lack the enzyme adenosine deaminase which affects both B- and T-cells but predominantly the latter, by accumulation of toxic metabolites of the purine (dATP). The comparable immunodeficiency seen in acute lymphocytic leukaemia patients treated with the adenosine deaminase inhibitor deoxycoformacin attests to the validity of this analysis. Half the SCID patients do reasonably well on transfusions of normal red cells containing the enzyme whereas others with a longer-standing more severe deficiency which might have affected the thymus epithelium, also require treatment with the enzyme modified by polyethylene glycol which extends its half-life. These patients are excellent candidates for gene therapy since the disease is fatal if untreated, it can be corrected by marrow from an HLA-identical sibling and the gene has been cloned. The next step will be autotransplantation of stem cells transfected with the gene, possibly by a retroviral vector.

The rapidly fatal variant of severe combined immunodeficiency associated with lack of myeloid cell precursors is termed reticular dysgenesis. A recent exciting piece of detective work has identified an autosomal recessive MHC class II immunodeficiency involving both CMI and humoral immunity which can now be traced to a defect in the trans-acting regulatory protein, RF-X, which binds to the HLA class II promoter. Expression of class II is preserved on thymic medullary, but not cortical, cells, and this leads to the establishment of self-tolerance, a situation so closely parallel with that described in mice carrying an I-E construct with 5'-flanking region lacking the X-box (p. 179).

An attempt has been made to summarize the cellular basis of the various deficiency states in figure 11.16.

Recognition of immunodeficiencies

Defects in immunoglobulins can be assessed by quantitative estimations; levels of 2 g/l arbitrarily define the practical lower limit of normal. The humoral immune response can be examined by first screening the serum for natural antibodies (A and B isohaemagglutinins, hetero-antibody to sheep red cells, bactericidins against *E. coli*) and then attempting to induce active immunization with diphtheria, tetanus, pertussis and killed poliomyelitis—but no live vaccines.

Patients with T-cell deficiency will be hypo- or unreactive in skin tests to such antigens as tuberculin, *Candida*, tricophytin, streptokinase/streptodornase and mumps. Active skin sensitization with dinitrochlorobenzene may be undertaken. The reactivity of peripheral blood mononuclear cells to phytohaemagglutinin is a good indicator of T-lymphocyte reactivity as is also the one-way mixed lymphocyte reaction (see Chapter 13). Enumeration of T-cells is most readily achieved by counting the number of cells forming spontaneous rosettes with sheep erythrocytes (figure 2.6e) or staining with a CD3 monoclonal antibody (cf. figure 2.6c).

In vitro tests for complement and for the bactericidal and other functions of polymorphs are available while the reduction of nitroblue tetrazolium (NBT) provides a measure of the oxidative enzymes associated with active phagocytosis.

SECONDARY IMMUNODEFICIENCY

Immune responsiveness can be depressed non-specifically by many factors. Cell-mediated immunity in particular may be impaired in a state of malnutrition even of the degree which may be encountered in urban areas of the more affluent regions of the world. Iron deficiency is particularly important in this respect.

Viral infections are not infrequently immunosuppressive, and in the case of measles in man, Newcastle disease in chickens and rinderpest in cattle, this has been attributed to a direct cytotoxic effect of virus on the lymphoid cells. In lepromatous leprosy and malarial infection there is evidence for a

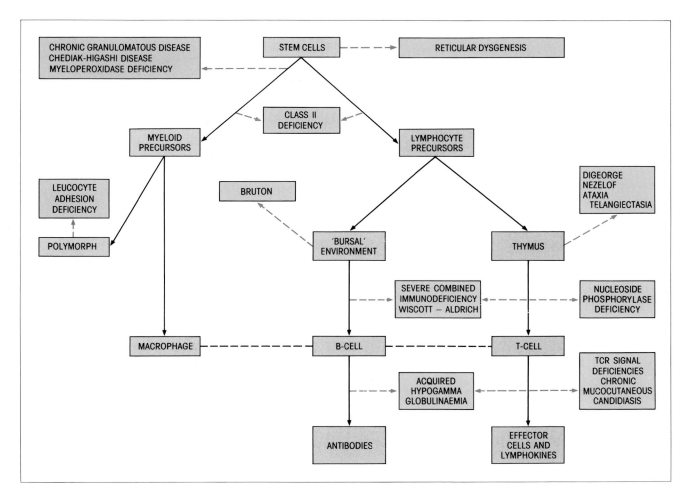

Figure 11.16. *The cellular basis of immunodeficiency states. The arrow indicates the cell type or differentiation process* which is defective. Complement deficiencies have not been included.

constraint on immune responsiveness imposed by distortion of the normal lymphoid traffic pathways and, additionally, in the latter instance, macrophage function appears to be aberrant. Plasma factors from patients with secondary syphilis which block phytohaemagglutinin transformation of lymphocytes from normal subjects could be responsible for the general reduction in CMI seen in this disease.

Many agents such as X-rays, cytotoxic drugs and corticosteroids, although often used in a non-immunological context, can none the less have dire effects on the immune system (p. 286). B-lymphoproliferative disorders like chronic lymphatic leukaemia, myeloma and Waldenström's macroglobulinaemia are associated with varying degrees of hypo-γ-globulinaemia and impaired antibody responses. Their common infections with pyogenic bacteria contrast with the situation in

Hodgkin's disease where the patients display all the hallmarks of defective cell-mediated immunity—susceptibility to tubercle bacillus, *Brucella, Cryptococcus* and herpes zoster virus.

Acquired immunodeficiency syndrome (AIDS)

AIDS is a particularly unpleasant fatal disease which is achieving endemic proportions and has thereby caused widespread alarm (and knowledge of immunology) amongst the public. In parts of Africa where the incidence is fearful, transmission is largely by heterosexual contact, but in the remainder of the world, the majority of cases so far have occurred in male homosexuals with other groups at risk including intravenous drug abusers, haemophiliacs receiving factor VIII derived from pooled plasma and infants of sexually promiscuous or drug-addicted mothers. None the less, the number of infected heterosexuals is steadily increasing. Death is usually due to pulmonary infection, but serious complications involving the nervous system are appearing in about 30% of cases. In essence, there is a sudden onset of immunodeficiency associated with opportunistic infections involving, most commonly, *Pneumocystis carinii*, but also cytomegalovirus (figure 11.17), EB and herpes simplex viruses, fungi such as *Candida*, *Aspergillus* and *Cryptococcus*, and the protozoon *Toxoplasma*; additionally, there is exceptional susceptibility for Kaposi's sarcoma. There is also an AIDS-related complex (ARC) characterized by fever, weight loss and lymphadenopathy.

AIDS results from infection by a human immunodeficiency virus (HIV)

Transmission of the disease is through infection with blood or semen containing the HIV-1 virus or the related HIV-2 which has been isolated from various body fluids of AIDS patients. HIV-1 shows considerable resemblance to the oncogenic human T-cell leukaemia virus (HTLV-1) which is closely linked to the production of a T-cell leukaemia of high prevalence in Japan. Whereas HTLV-1 induces lymphoproliferation, HIV-1 is a member of the lentivirus group which cause destruction of the cells they infect; these include a simian SIV isolated from the African green monkey and thought by some to provide a possible gene pool from which the AIDS virus might have arisen, the visna virus responsible for cns and lung lesions in sheep, and viruses which cause equine infectious anaemia and caprine arthritis. All are RNA retroviruses which utilize a reverse transcriptase to convert their genetic RNA into the corresponding DNA which is integrated into the host cell. HIV-1 is a budding virus whose genome is relatively complex (figure 11.18).

HIV infects CD4 positive cells

The envelope glycoprotein gp120 of HIV binds avidly to cell-surface CD4 molecules and initiates fusion with the cell, involving gp41, and infection. Helper T-cells with their abundant CD4 are a major target for infection but the presence of even relatively low densities of CD4 on macrophages, follicular dendritic cells and microglia makes them susceptible to infection, and in the latter case is suspected to be a major factor in the cerebral complications of the disease. There is also a worry that complexes of virus with antibody may facilitate entry into macrophages through Fc receptors.

After the viral complementary DNA is integrated into host DNA, it can remain latent for long periods. Mitogens can activate HIV from long-term latently infected T-cell cultures through the induction of cellular proteins which normally bind to the core transcriptional enhancer NFκB sequences regulating expression of IL-2 and IL-2Rα receptor genes.

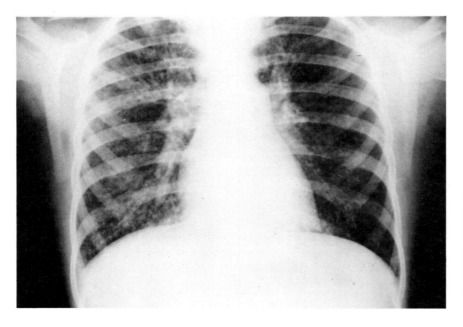

Figure 11.17. *Viral pneumonia due to cytomegalovirus; radiograph showing extensive diffuse pneumonitis in both lung fields, characteristic of viral infection. (Reproduced from Infectious Diseases Illustrated, Lambert H.P. and Farrar W.E. (eds) (1982) p.2.2. W.B. Saunders and Gower Medical Publishing, with permission.)*

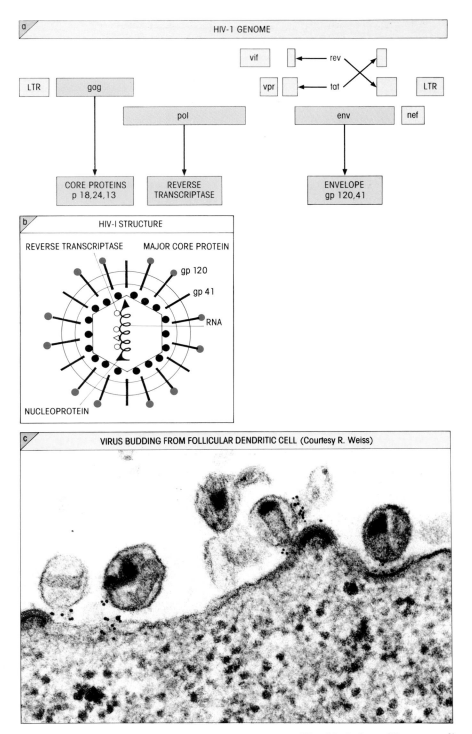

Figure 11.18. *Characteristics of the HIV-1 AIDS virus. (a) HIV-1 genome.* **tat** *= master switch, turns on all viral gene expression;* rev *= gene responsible for expression of structural proteins;* nef *= gene downregulating viral gene expression;* vif *= gene controlling infectivity by free, not cell-bound, virus;* **LTR** *= long terminal repeats concerned in regulation of viral expression, contains regions reacting with products of* **tat** *and* **nef** *genes and in addition the TATAA promoter sequence, NFκB core enhancer elements and Sp-1 binding sites. Mice bearing the* **tat** *transgene develop Kaposi sarcoma-like skin lesions. (Genes encoding structural proteins coloured, regulatory genes, grey.) (b) HIV-1 structure. (c) Electron micrograph of CBL-1 isolate of human immunodeficiency virus type I (HIV-1), isolated from patient with lymphoma. Mature and budding virus particles can be seen at the surface of CCRF-CEM human leukaemia cells that are used for HIV-1 propagation. Colloidal gold particles indicate binding of human serum antibodies from an AIDS patient. (× 121 500.) (Courtesy of D. Robertson & R.A. Weiss.)*

The labels within figure (a):

HIV-1 GENOME

vif — rev — LTR
gag — vpr — tat
LTR — pol — env — nef

CORE PROTEINS p 18,24,13 — REVERSE TRANSCRIPTASE — ENVELOPE gp 120,41

(b) HIV-I STRUCTURE

REVERSE TRANSCRIPTASE — MAJOR CORE PROTEIN
gp 120
gp 41
RNA
NUCLEOPROTEIN

(c) VIRUS BUDDING FROM FOLLICULAR DENDRITIC CELL (Courtesy R. Weiss)

247

INFECTION — PROPHYLAXIS AND IMMUNODEFICIENCY

However, there is a consensus sequence [(G/A) GGGANT (T/C)(T/C)(C/A)C] in the core κB elements of various cellular genes and the HIV enhancer region and, as a result, the mitogen induced κB binding proteins can activate replication of the latent virus. Antigens and agents which induce stress responses are also implicated in the induction of HIV re-expression and it may be pertinent that a portion of the κB binding sites in the HIV-LTR (cf. figure 11.18a) resemble the cellular heat shock core sequence. TNFα upregulates HIV replication, also apparently through κB sites, and this cytokine is present in elevated concentrations in the plasma of HIV infected individuals particularly in the advanced stage.

To digress for a moment, the HTLV-I virus is constitutively expressed in the CD4 T-cells it infects and produces a 40 kDa trans-acting regulatory protein termed Tax. Like the product of the *tat* gene in HIV, this activates its long terminal repeat (LTR) and consequently the expression of viral genes under its control through the core κB element. However, because of the close similarity to the κB sequences in the IL-2 and IL-2Rα enhancers, these two genes are also upregulated by Tax. We thus have the interesting situation in which, during a normal immune response with its feedback mechanisms operating, there is a temporary production of κB-binding factors with transient expression of IL-2 and its receptor whereas in T-cells infected by HTLV-I, there is a continuing expression of Tax and hence permanent production of IL-2 and IL-2R leading to immortalization and proliferation of leukaemic cells. On the other hand, κB-binding proteins induced by a normal immune response or by TNFα in a CD4 cell latently infected with HIV, will result in viral replication and cell death, assuming the cytopahtic effect of HIV infection on T-cells in culture is mirrored *in vivo*.

The AIDS infection depletes helper-T-cells

The drastic and often complete destruction of the helper-cell population as AIDS progresses suggests that the assumption is reasonable. There is a corresponding fall in the peripheral blood CD4 count (figure 11.19), and a drop in the CD4:CD8 ratio since CD8 cells are largely unaffected.

How this comes about is not as obvious as one would imagine especially since it happens over a time span of several years. Current estimates are that only one in a hundred or so of the surviving peripheral CD4 cells in AIDS patients are positive for

the viral genome. Activation of latent virus should make the host cell vulnerable to execution by the cytopathic effects of virus or by CD4 or CD8 cytotoxic T-cells which have been demonstrated in AIDS patients. The relatively low incidence of CD4 T-cell infection implies that under these circumstances, transmission of virus to uninfected cells is relatively inefficient; do effector cells leave so few infectious survivors after attacking a T-cell with reproductive virus, or do they create an environment by cytokine release that reduces intercellular transmission? Later in the disease, circulating gp120 by binding to surface CD4 on uninfected helper-cells could inhibit their interaction with class II on antigen-presenting cells, or make them vulnerable to gp120 specific cytotoxic T-cells or ADCC. Either way, T-helper responses would wane severely.

The consequences for cell-mediated immune responses as exemplified by the depressed delayed-type skin reactivity to common antigens (figure 11.20) and the failure to produce cytomegalovirus-specific cytotoxic T-cells, are quite devastating and leave the patient wide open to diseases caused by normally non-pathogenic (i.e. opportunistic) agents such as *Pneumocystis carinii* and cytomegalovirus.

AIDS patients also have hypergammaglobulin-aemia and large numbers of B-cells which spontaneously secrete Ig in culture suggesting that they are polyclonally stimulated; this would make them refractory to immunization with new antigens or to triggering stimuli from anti-IgM. The polyclonal activation might be a result of the ability of AIDS virus to infect follicular dendritic cells, or of the production of some T-cell factor, or stimulation by viruses such as EBV and cytomegalovirus which cannot be controlled by the ailing T-cells.

Diagnosis of AIDS

An individual with opportunistic infections, lymphopenia, low CD4 but relatively normal CD8 in the peripheral blood, raised IgG and IgA levels and poor skin tests to common recall antigens may well have AIDS particularly if they come from a group at risk. IFNγ and neopterin, a degradation product of GTP induced in macrophages by IFNγ, are good indicators of CMI and are significantly increased in AIDS infection preceding subsequent loss of CD4 cells. Confirmation of the diagnosis comes from lymph node biopsy, showing profound abnormalities and drastic changes in germinal centres, and the demonstration of viral antibodies by enzyme-linked immunosorbent assay (ELISA) or by

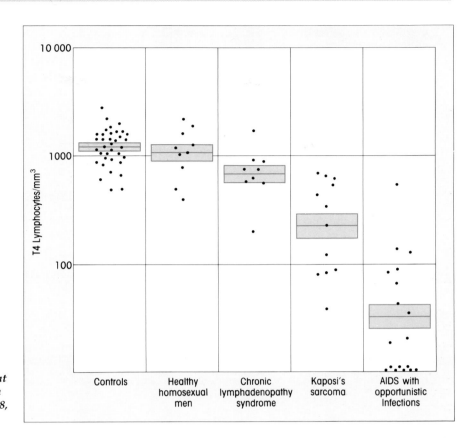

Figure 11.19. *Absolute levels of circulating CD4 (T4) positive lymphocytes in patients with AIDS, Kaposi's sarcoma and chronic lymphadenopathy syndrome. Each point represents an individual patient. (From Lane H.C. et al. (1985)* **Amer. J. Med. 78,** *417–22.)*

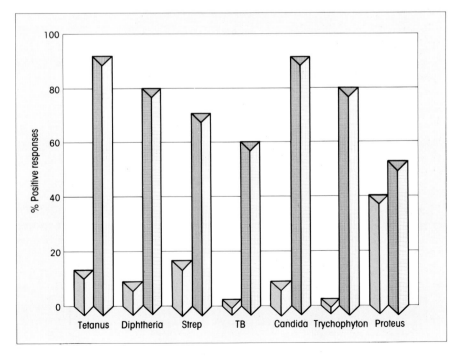

Figure 11.20. *Skin test reactivity to common microbial antigens among AIDS patients (; n = 20) and controls (; n = 10). Other studies with more advanced patients have reported completely negative skin tests. (Reproduced from Lane H.C. & Fauci A.S. (1985)* **Ann. Rev. Immunol. 3,** *477, with permission.)*

INFECTION — PROPHYLAXIS AND IMMUNODEFICIENCY

'immunoblotting' (cf. pp. 97 and 233). Positive isolation of HIV is it—finito.

The control of AIDS

Identifying protective responses

After inadvertent transfusion of infected plasma, the first antibodies to appear are directed to the gp120 envelope glycoprotein; antibodies to core proteins p24 and 18 may be seen later. Most antibodies are non-neutralizing in that they fail to prevent infection of susceptible cells in culture, and in the rare instances when they are neutralizing, the titres tend to be disappointingly low and usually type-specific. A single mutational change can make the virus resistant and it must be said that, the gp120 gene seems rather jumpy with respect to mutation, a feature of other lentiviruses with hypervariable envelope regions which prevent immunization with any one variant from protecting against the new variants which emerge rapidly during infection. The hypervariable region V3, in HIV-1 gp120 dominant for the development of type-specific neutralizing antibodies is located between residues 307—330 within a loop formed by two highly conserved cysteine residues. When attached to keyhole limpet haemocyanin (KLH), the V3 loop produced high and persistent levels of neutralizing antibody in chimpanzees which were resistant to infection several weeks later. Antibodies raised to a peptide representing the conserved domain binding gp120 to CD4 effectively blocked the interaction between the two molecules but failed to prevent infection, probably because of multiple binding sites. Very occasionally, human and chimpanzee sera with high titred antibodies which block binding and exhibit broad virus neutralizing activity have been encountered but their precise specificity is unknown at the time of writing.

Interest has also focused on the other surface protein, gp41. A transmembrane conserved region, 735—752, can induce antibodies which neutralize HIV and have a wide ability to block fusion. In view of its supposed location within the membrane, it is somewhat inconsistent to find that the epitope can be demonstrated by immunofluorescent staining of infected cells. When this region is inserted into the surface of polio virus, it induces antibody and, as an antigen, is said to remove a major fraction of the group specific neutralizing and fusion inhibiting antibodies from some sera. This has the makings of a dominant target.

One gallant human was immunized by i.v. injection of paraformaldehyde-fixed autologous cells infected *in vivo* with recombinant vaccinia expressing the complete gp160 (used by the virus to provide gp120 and gp41), followed by gp160 derived from an HIV-1 clone. High levels of neutralizing antibody and CMI to divergent HIV-1 strains developed, but naturally there was no rush to test for resistance to infection. For this reason animal models are vital.

The development of animal models

Rabbits can be infected with HIV but they do not develop disease though they are useful for testing the responses to recombinant vaccinia—HIV vaccines. Monkeys would seem likely candidates but they show no sign of disease after infection with HIV-1. The less pathogenic HIV-2 does produce lymphadenopathy but nothing more. Probably the best model is the AIDS-like disease produced by the simian immunodeficiency virus (SIV). Protection against intra-muscular infection could be induced in macaque monkeys by immunization with killed SIV mixed with threonyl MDP in a squalene-pluronic polymer emulsion. ISCOMs (p. 238) may hold a special value since envelope protein in an ISCOM evoked quite high titres of neutralizing antibody in rhesus monkeys and CD8+ cytotoxic cells in mice.

We have little data on the utility of the pussycat model involving feline immunodeficiency virus but there is a great deal of money riding on the SCID mouse reconstituted with human fetal liver and thymus as an *in vivo* system for studying the efficacy of treatments for AIDS which must closely parallel many of the interactions occurring in infected people.

Other therapeutic strategies

Immunological reconstitution with matched bone marrow only gives transient improvement. Trials are underway with recombinant immunostimulators, IL-2 and IFNγ. The reverse transcriptase enzyme is a potentially good target for anti-viral therapy and the drug AZT (zidovudine) give worthwhile if expensive remissions. AZT, 3'-azido-3'-deoxythymidine, is a thymidine analogue which is absorbed after oral administration and triphosphorylated within human cells to produce an active intermediate which prevents reversed transcription of the HIV viral genome. AZT was tested in SCID mice with human lymphoid tissue infected with

250

HIV. 100% of untreated mice showed viral replication in the thymus by 2 weeks as revealed using the polymerase chain reaction. None of the AZT-treated animals had viral genome detectable by PCR but rare cells harbouring viral RNA transcripts were found by *in situ* hybridization, i.e. protection was striking but not complete.

Soluble CD4 molecules bind robustly to HIV and block its infectivity but only have a short half-life. A classy recombinant molecule consisting of the binding CD4 domains linked to two Fcγ domains has been synthesized; it has a much longer half-life and could be a useful therapeutic agent. A new 'super-immunoadhesin' which is 1000-times more potent than soluble CD4 in syncitium inhibition assays has been created by stitching 10 CD4 domains into a single IgM chimaeric molecule. 'Intracellular immunization' represents another ingenious approach in which bone marrow cells are transfected with a sequence of the CD4 gene coding for an HIV blocking peptide; on regrafting, some of the stem cells will become CD4 positive T-cells which secrete a surrounding barrier of the blocking peptide which protects the lymphocyte from infection by the virus. A totally different therapeutic approach utilizes an inhibitor which selectively affects the synthesis of viral carbohydrate thus abrogating infectivity. As mentioned already, mice with severe combined immunodeficiency (SCID) can be reconstituted with a human immune system and infected with HIV, so providing a valuable model for trying out various therapeutic strategies. Despite this frantic activity a change in social behaviour patterns must make a difference to the spread of AIDS.

SUMMARY

Passive immunity can be acquired by maternal antibodies or from homologous pooled γ-globulin. Horse antisera are more restricted because of the danger of serum sickness. Antibodies are being constructed to order using recombinant DNA technology. Active immunization provides a protective state through contact with a harmless form of the disease organism. Killed bacteria and viruses are easy to obtain and have been used widely. However, in many cases live attenuated organisms have the advantages that by replication they provide the host with a bigger antigen challenge and by behaving as the natural infecting agent, the most useful type of response in the appropriate location in the body is achieved. Live viruses such as vaccinia can be used as a piggyback for immunizing with genes from other viruses which are more difficult to grow or are inherently dangerous. Attention has been focused on BCG as a vehicle for antigens required to evoke CD4 T-cell immunity. Oral immunization with attenuated *Salmonella* constructs may provide not only gut immunity but also systemic protection to a number of other organisms. Attenuated vaccines run the risk of reverting to the virulent form. They must not be used with immunocompromised hosts.

Whole organisms have a multiplicity of antigens some of which are not protective, may induce hypersensitivity or might even be frankly immunosuppressive. It makes sense in these cases to use purified components and there is greatly increased use of recombinant DNA technology to produce these antigens. There is great interest in the possibility of using either synthetic peptides or monoclonal internal image anti-idiotypes as vaccines. These have the advantage that they mimic single antigenic determinants and may avoid induction of T-suppression or even of autoimmunity when certain whole antigens are employed. Both approaches are still in the experimental stage so far as large-scale immunization of human populations is concerned. Peptides may only usefully mimic the native protein for vaccination to produce antibody if the epitope is linear and relatively unconstrained in structure. Linear peptides can mimic T-cell epitopes in the whole protein.

Adjuvants work by producing depots of antigen, and by activating macrophages; they sometimes have direct effects on lymphocytes. New methods of delivery include linking the antigen to small lipid membrane vesicles (liposomes) or a special glycoside matrix (ISCOM).

Primary immunodeficiency states in the human occur, albeit somewhat rarely, as a result of a defect in almost any stage of differentiation in the whole immune system. Defects in phagocytic cells, the complement pathways or the B-cell system lead in particular to infection with bacteria which are disposed of by opsonization and phagocytosis. Patients with T-cell deficiencies are susceptible to viruses and moulds which are normally eradicated by cell-mediated immunity. Severe combined immunodeficiency (SCID) arises from a defect in the mechanism for combinatorial joining of V, D and J genes for B- and T-cell receptors.

Immunodeficiency may arise as a secondary consequence of malnutrition, lymphoproliferative

251

disorders, agents such as X-rays and cytotoxic drugs and viral infections. The most notorious of these involves the LAV/HTLV-III (now called HIV-I) retrovirus which causes the acquired immunodeficiency syndrome (AIDS) in which attack by the virus on CD4 (T4) helper T-cells destroys the ability to give a cell-mediated immune response and leaves the patient open to infection with opportunist organisms such as *Pneumocystis carinii* and cytomegalovirus which can kill. κB-Binding proteins induced by an immune response or by TNFα in a CD4-cell latently infected with HIV, result in viral replication and cell death. Poor to non-existent neutralizing antibodies to the AIDS virus are made during an infection. The best model for studying candidate vaccines is infection of monkeys with simian immunodeficiency virus. SCID mice reconstituted with human lymphoid tissue can be infected by HIV and used to test therapies. The drug AZT acts to inhibit viral reverse transcriptase.

252

Further reading

Chandra R.K. (ed.) (1983) *Primary and Secondary Immunodeficiency Disorders*. Churchill Livingstone, Edinburgh, UK.

Chapel H. & Haeney M. (1988) *Essentials of Clinical Immunology*, 2nd edn. Blackwell Scientific Publications, Oxford.

Dick G. (1986) *Practical Immunization*. MTP Press, Lancaster, UK.

Lerner R.A. *et al.* (eds) (1989) Modern approaches to new vaccines including prevention of AIDS. Cold Spring Harbor Lab, New York.

Porter R. & Whelan J. (eds) (1986) Synthetic Peptides as Antigens. *Ciba Foundation Symposium*, **119**. Wiley, Chichester, UK.

Rosenberg Z.F. *et al.* (1990) Series: HIV and the immune system. *Immunology Today*, **11**, 176 onwards.

Seligmann M. (1989) Primary immunodeficiencies: current findings and concepts. In *Progress in Immunology*, 7, 509, F. Melchers *et al.* (eds). Springer Verlag, Berlin. (Excellent survey.)

Stiehm E.R. (ed.) (1989) *Immunologic Disorders in Infants and Children*, 3rd edn. W.B. Saunders, Philadelphia.

WHO/IUIS Report (1982) Appropriate uses of human Ig in clinical practice. *Bull. World Health Organisation*, **60**, 43.

HYPERSENSITIVITY

An inappropriate immune response can lead to tissue damage

When an individual has been immunologically primed, further contact with antigen leads to secondary boosting of the immune response. However, the reaction may be excessive and lead to gross tissue changes (*hypersensitivity*) if the antigen is present in relatively large amounts or if the humoral and cellular immune state is at a heightened level. It should be emphasized that the mechanisms underlying these inappropriate reactions are those normally employed by the body in combating infection as discussed in Chapter 10. We speak of *hypersensitivity reactions* and a state of *hypersensitivity*. Coombs and Gell defined four types of hypersensitivity, to which can be added a fifth, viz. 'stimulatory', which they mention. Types I, II, III and V depend on the interaction of antigen with humoral antibody and tend to be called 'immediate' type reactions although some are more immediate than others! Type IV involves receptors bound to the T-lymphocyte surface and because of the longer time course this has in the past been referred to as 'delayed-type sensitivity'.

TYPE I — ANAPHYLACTIC HYPERSENSITIVITY

The phenomenon of anaphylaxis

A single injection of 1 mg of an antigen such as egg albumin into a guinea-pig has no obvious effect. However, if the injection is repeated two to three weeks later, the sensitized animal reacts very dramatically with the symptoms of generalized anaphylaxis; almost immediately the guinea-pig begins to wheeze and within a few minutes dies from asphyxia. Examination shows intense constriction of the bronchioles and bronchi and generally there is (i) contraction of smooth muscle and (ii) dilatation of capillaries. Similar reactions can occur in human subjects and have been observed following wasp and bee stings or injections of penicillin in appropriately sensitive individuals. In many instances only a timely intravenous injection of adrenaline to counter the smooth muscle contraction and capillary dilatation can prevent death.

Sir Henry Dale recognized that histamine mimics the systemic changes of anaphylaxis and furthermore that the uterus from a sensitized guinea-pig releases histamine and contracts on exposure to antigen (Schultz—Dale technique). Serum from such an animal can passively sensitize the uterus from a normal guinea-pig so that it, too, will contract on addition of the specific antigen. Contraction is associated with an explosive degranulation of the mast cells (figure 1.13) which is responsible for the release of histamine and a number of other mediators (figure 1.14). Passive transfer of anaphylactic sensitivity can be observed locally in the skin using Ovary's *passive cutaneous anaphylaxis* (PCA) technique; high dilutions of guinea-pig serum containing anaphylactic antibodies may be injected into the skin of a normal animal and following the intravenous injection of antigen with a dye such as Evans' Blue, the

253

anaphylactic reaction in the skin will lead to release of vasoactive amines and hence a local 'blueing'.

Cross-linking of IgE receptors triggers mast cells

Two main types of mast cell have been recognized, exemplified in the rat by those in the intestinal mucosa and those in the peritoneum and other connective tissue sites. They differ in a number of respects, for example in the type of protease and proteoglycan in their granules, and in the proliferative response of the mucosal mast cell to the T-cell lymphokine IL-3 (table 12.1). This last point is made rather tellingly by the striking proliferation of mast cells in the intestinal mucosa during infection with certain parasites in intact, but not in T-depleted rodents, the effect being mediated by a combination of IL-3 and IL-4. The two types have common precursors and are interconvertible depending upon the environmental conditions, with mucosal MC_t phenotype favoured by IL-3 and that of connective tissue MC_{tc} being promoted by a fibroblast factor. However, both types display a high affinity receptor for the $C\varepsilon 2 : C\varepsilon 3$ junction region of IgE Fc (cf. figure 3.17a), a property shared with their circulating counterpart, the basophil. The strength of binding to the mast cell is evident from the retention of IgE antibodies at a site of intradermal injection for several weeks; IgG4 in the human also binds to the mast cell receptor but more weakly and disperses from the injection site within a day or so. It has long been established that the anaphylactic antibodies in the human are mainly of the IgE class.

Table 12.1. *Comparison of two types of mast cell.*

CHARACTERISTICS	MUCOSAL MAST CELL	CONNECTIVE TISSUE MAST CELL
GENERAL		
Abbreviation	MC_t	MC_{tc}
Distribution	Gut & lung	Most tissues
Differentiation favoured by	IL-3	Fibroblast factor
T-cell dependence	+	−
High affinity Fcε receptor	2×10^5/cell	3×10^4/cell
GRANULES		
Alcian blue and Safranin staining	Blue & brown	Blue
Ultrastructure	Scrolls	Gratings/lattices
Protease	Tryptase*	Tryptase & chymase†
Proteoglycan	Chondroitin sulphate	Heparin
DEGRANULATION		
Histamine release	+	+ +
$LTC_4 : PGD_2$ release	25 : 1	1 : 40
Blocked by disodium cromoglycate/theophylline‡	−	+

Cross-linking of IgE antibodies bound to a mast cell by a divalent hapten will trigger mediator release; trimers are more effective and tetramers even more so. Degranulation is also induced when the IgE is cross-linked with anti-IgE but univalent (Fab) anti-IgE is inactive. That the critical event is the cross-linking of the receptors themselves is clearly shown by the ability of antibodies raised against the receptor itself to trigger the mast cell (figure 12.1).

Bridging of receptors is rapidly followed by the breakdown of phosphatidyl inositol to inositol triphosphate (IP3), the generation of diacylglycerol and an increase in intracytoplasmic free calcium (figure 12.2). Since inhibitors of methyltransferases and serine esterases inhibit all these events and

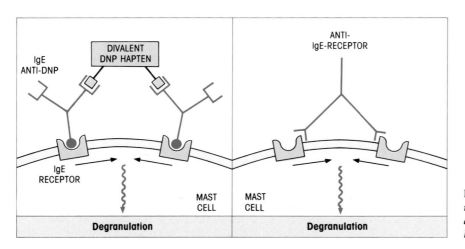

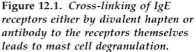

Figure 12.1. *Cross-linking of IgE receptors either by divalent hapten or antibody to the receptors themselves leads to mast cell degranulation.*

mediator release, it is assumed that activation of these enzymes by receptor bridging is the initial event. Phospholipase c activation generates both IP3 (cf. activation of B-cells, p. 118), which mobilizes intracellular Ca^{2+}, and diacylglycerol which in turn activates protein kinase C. The biochemical cascade produces membrane-active 'fusogens' such as lyso-phosphatidic acid which may facilitate granular membrane fusion and degranulation, and the series of arachidonic acid metabolites formed by the cyclo-oxygenase and lipoxygenase pathways (cf. figure 1.14). To recapitulate, the preformed mediators released from the granules include histamine, heparin, eosinophil and neutrophil chemotactic factors, and platelet activating factor, while leukotrienes LTB_4, LTC_4 and LTD_4, PGD_2 and thromboxanes are all newly synthesized. The role of cyclic AMP is uncertain: receptor bridging produces a short-lived rise in cAMP but a preformed high level of cAMP inhibits receptor-induced degranulation.

Under normal circumstances, these mediators help to orchestrate the development of a defensive acute inflammatory reaction (and in this context let us not forget that C3a and C5a can also trigger mast cells although not through IgE receptors). When there is a massive release of these mediators under abnormal conditions as in atopic disease, their bronchoconstrictive and vasodilatory effects predominate and become distinctly threatening.

Atopic allergy

Nearly 10% of the population suffer to a greater or lesser degree with allergies involving localized anaphylactic reactions to extrinsic allergens such as grass pollens, animal danders, the faeces from mites in house dust (figure 12.3) and so on. Contact of the allergen with cell-bound IgE in the bronchial tree, the nasal mucosa and the conjunctival tissues releases mediators of anaphylaxis and produces the symptoms of asthma or hay fever as the case may be (figure 12.4).

Awareness of the importance of sensitization to food allergens in the gut has increased dramatically. Contact of the food with specific IgE on mast cells in the gastro-intestinal tract may produce local reactions such as diarrhoea and vomiting or may allow the allergen to enter the body by causing a change in gut permeability through mediator release; the allergen may complex with antibodies and cause distal lesions by depositing in the joints, for example, or it may diffuse freely to other sensitized sites such as skin (figure 12.7b) or lungs where it will cause a further local anaphylactic reaction. Thus eating strawberries may produce urticarial reactions and egg may precipitate an asthmatic attack in appropriately sensitized individuals. The role of the sensitized gut acting as a 'gate' to allow entry of allergens is strongly suggested by experiments in

255

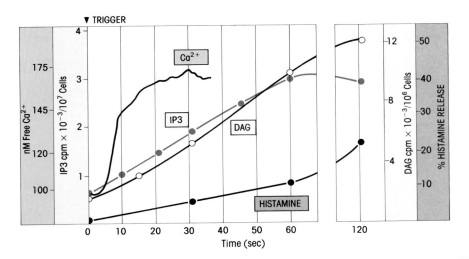

Figure 12.2. *Mast cell triggering: time course of changes in cytoplasmic Ca^{2+}, formation of diacylglycerol (DAG) and inositol triphosphate (IP3) and release of histamine from IL-3 dependent mouse mast cell line PT-18 sensitized with monoclonal IgE anti-DNP (dinitrophenyl) and triggered with a multivalent DNP-human serum albumin conjugate. (Combined data taken from Ishizaka T., White J.R. & Saito H. (1986) In Progress in Immunology VI, p. 870, Cinader B. and Miller R.G. (eds). Academic Press, with permission.)*

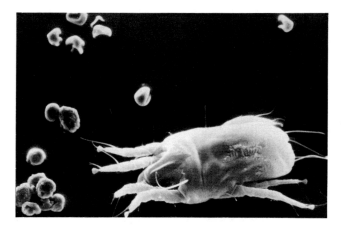

Figure 12.3. *House dust mite—a major cause of allergic disease. The electron micrograph shows the rather nasty looking mite graced by the name* **Dermatophagoides pteryonyssinus** *and faecal pellets on the bottom left which are the major source of allergen. The biconcave pollen grains (top left) shown for comparison indicate the size of particle which can become airborne and reach the lungs. The mite itself is much too large for that. (Reproduced by courtesy of Dr E. Tovey.)*

256

which oral sodium cromoglycate, a mast cell stabilizer, prevents subsequent asthma after ingestion of the provoking food (figure 12.5).

There is a strong familial predisposition to the development of atopic allergy (figure 12.6a) but although this is linked to inheritance of a given HLA haplotype within any one family, no association with specific HLA types has so far come to light. One factor seems to be the overall ability to synthesize the IgE isotype, the higher the level

of IgE in the blood the greater the likelihood of becoming atopic (figure 12.6b). Curiously, it is said that patients with allergy are less likely than their non-atopic counterparts to develop tumours.

Clinical tests for allergy

Sensitivity is normally assessed by the response to intradermal challenge with antigen. The release of histamine and other mediators rapidly produces a wheal and erythema (figure 12.7a), maximal within 30 minutes and then subsiding. The responsible IgE antibodies can be demonstrated by passive cutaneous anaphylaxis by testing the ability of patient's serum to passively sensitize the skin of normal humans (Praüsnitz−Kustner or 'P−K' test) or preferably of monkeys. This passive sensitization of human skin can be blocked most effectively by prior injection of a myeloma of IgE rather than of any other class. The interpretation is that the specialized sites on the skin mast cells become fully saturated by binding to the Fc regions of the IgE myeloma globulin which blocks the subsequent attachment of specific IgE antibodies.

There is an increasing recognition that immediate wheal and flare reactions may be followed by a late phase reaction (cf. figure 12.7a) which sometimes lasts for 24 hours; it is characterized by a dense cellular infiltrate and is more oedematous than the early reaction. The mechanism is unclear: it may be partially mediated by a high molecular weight neutrophil chemotactic factor released from the mast cell and involvement of T-cells has been tentatively mooted. These late phase reactions can also be seen

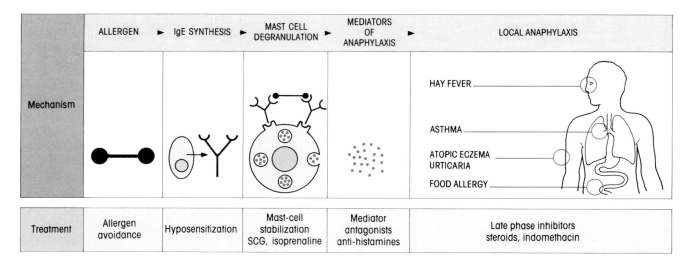

Figure 12.4. *Atopic allergies: sites of local anaphylaxis and possible therapies (SCG = sodium cromoglycate).*

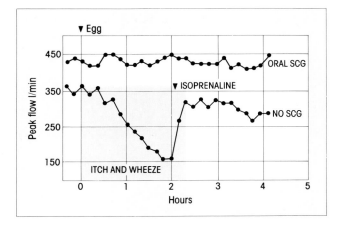

Figure 12.5. *The role of gut sensitivity in the development of asthma to food allergens. A patient challenged by feeding with egg developed asthma within hours as shown here by the depressed lung function test of measuring peak air flow; the symptoms at the end organ stage were counteracted by isoprenaline. However, oral sodium cromoglycate (SCG), which prevents antigen-specific mast cell triggering, also prevented the onset of asthma after oral challenge with egg. Note that SCG taken orally has no effect on the response of an asthmatic to inhaled allergen. (From Brostoff J.(1986) In* **Food Allergy,** *p.441, Brostoff J. and Challacombe S.J. (eds), Baillière Tindall, reproduced with permission.)*

following challenge of the nasal mucosa and bronchi of allergic subjects and may be of major importance in the development of chronic asthma. In this respect, it is worthy of note that the major basic protein of the eosinophil granule, which is present in high levels in the sputum of asthma patients, has been shown to cause damage to bronchial epithelium in organ culture which mimics that seen in bronchial asthma.

The correlation between skin prick test responses and the radioallergosorbent test (RAST, p. 94) for allergen-specific serum IgE is fairly good. In some instances, intranasal challenge with allergen may provoke a response even when both these tests are negative, probably as a result of local synthesis of IgE antibodies.

Therapy

If one considers the sequence of reactions from initial exposure to allergen right through to the production of atopic disease, it can be seen that several points in the chain provide legitimate targets for therapy (figure 12.4). Avoidance of contact with *potential* allergens is often impractical although, to

257

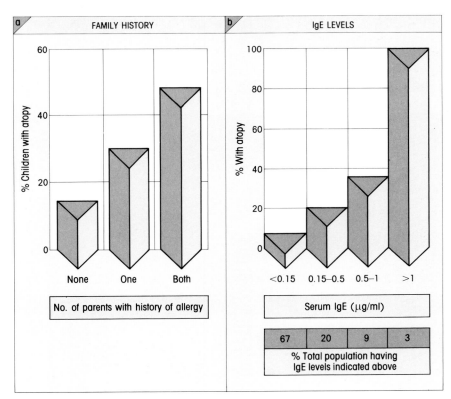

Figure 12.6. *Risk factors in allergy: (a) family history; (b) IgE levels—the higher the serum IgE concentration, the greater the chance of developing atopy.*

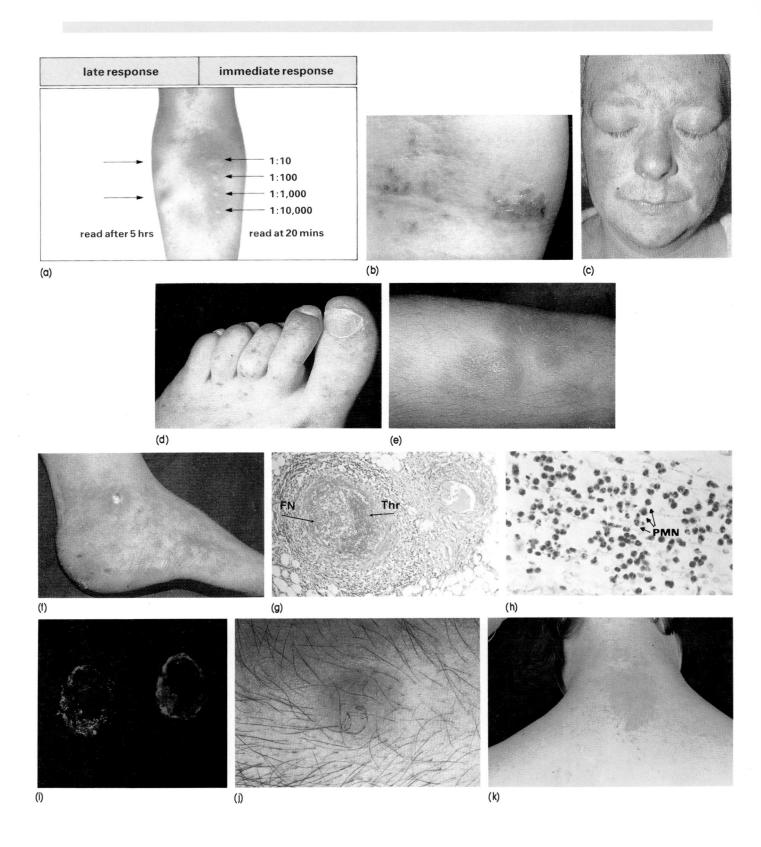

CHAPTER 12

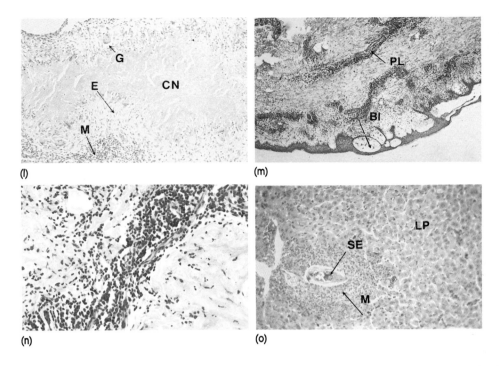

(l)   (m)

(n)   (o)

Figure 12.7 facing page and above. *Hypersensitivity reactions.*

Type I *(a) Skin prick tests with grass pollen allergen in a patient with typical summer hay fever. Skin tests were performed 5 hours (left) and 20 minutes (right) before the photograph was taken. The tests on the right show a typical end point titration of a type I immediate wheal and flare reaction. The late phase skin reaction (left) can be clearly seen at 5 hours especially where a large immediate response has preceded it. Figures for allergen dilution are given. (b) An atopic eczema reaction on the back of a knee of a child allergic to rice and eggs.*

Type III *(c) Facial appearance in systemic lupus erythematosus (SLE). Lesions of recent onset are symmetrical, red and oedematous. They are often most pronounced on the areas of the face which receive most light exposure, i.e. the upper cheeks and bridge of the nose, and the prominences of the forehead. (d) Vasculitic lesions in SLE. Small purpuric macules are seen. (e) Erythema nodosum leprosum, forearm. The patient has lepromatous leprosy with superimposed erythema nodosum leprosum. These acutely inflamed nodules were extremely tender and the patient was pyrexial. (f) Polyarteritis nodosa, ankle and foot. Livedo reticularis with chronic painful ulceration is sometimes seen in this disease. (g) Histology of acute inflammatory reaction in polyarteritis nodosa associated with immune complex formation with hepatitis B surface (HBs) antigen. A vessel showing thrombus (Thr) formation and fibrinoid necrosis (FN) is surrounded by a mixed inflammatory infiltrate, largely polymorphs. (h) High*

power view of acute inflammatory response in loose connective tissue of patient with polyarteritis nodosa — polymorphs (PMN) are prominent. (i) Immunofluorescence studies of immune complexes in the renal artery of a patient with chronic hepatitis B infection stained with fluoresceinated anti-hepatitis B antigen (left) and rhodaminated anti-IgM (right). The presence of both antigen and antibody in the intima and media of the arterial wall indicate the deposition of the complexes at this site. IgG and C3 deposits are also detectable with the same distribution.

Type IV *(j) Mantoux test showing cell-mediated hypersensitivity reaction to tuberculin, characterized by induration and erythema. (k) Type IV contact hypersensitivity reaction to nickel caused by the clasp of a necklace. (l) Chronic type IV inflammatory lesion in tuberculous lung showing caseous necrosis (CN), epithelioid cells (E), giant cells (G) and mononuclear inflammatory cells (M). (m) Perivascular lymphocytic infiltrates (PL) and blister (Bl) formation characterize a contact sensitivity reaction of the skin. (n) High power view to show the lymphocytic nature of the infiltrate in a contact hypersensitivity reaction. (o) Delayed-type hypersensitivity lesion of mononuclear inflammatory cells (M) around schistosome egg (SE) within the liver parenchyma (LP). ((a), (b) and (j) kindly provided by Dr J. Brostoff, (c), (d), (e) and (f) by Dr G. Levene, (g), (h), (m) and (n) by Prof. N. Woolf, (i) by Prof. A. Nowoslowski, (l) by Dr R. Barnetson and (o) by Dr M. Doenhoff; (k) reproduced from Brit. Soc. Immunol. teaching slides with permission of the Society and Dermatology Department, London Hospital.)*

give one example, feeding infants cow's milk at too early an age is discouraged. After sensitization, avoidance where possible is obviously worthwhile but the reluctance of some parents to dispose of the family cat to stop little Algernon's wheezing is sometimes quite surprising.

Attempts to desensitize patients immunologically by repeated treatment with allergen have at least the merit of a long history and in a significant but as yet unpredictable proportion of patients can lead to worthwhile improvement. It has generally been assumed that the purpose of these inoculations was to boost the synthesis of 'blocking' IgG antibody whose function was to divert the allergen from contact with tissue-bound IgE. This would be of unquestioned value were the increase in protective antibody (? particularly IgA) to occur locally at the sites vulnerable to allergen exposure. However, if T-lymphocyte cooperation is important for IgE synthesis, the beneficial effects of antigen injection may also be mediated through induction of tolerant or even suppressor T-cells. There was initial promise in the observation that IgE-producing cells or their precursors could be switched off with comparative ease by haptens coupled to thymus-independent carriers such as poly-D-Glu.Lys. or isologous IgG, or by substitution of the allergen by polyethylene glycol. Better results must ultimately be attainable when we understand the rationale of 'hyposensitization' through the use of purified allergens, assessment of T-cell reactivity and quantitative measurement of specific IgG, IgA and IgE antibodies in individuals undergoing treatment. The affinity of these antibodies and their availability at local sites of allergen challenge such as the nasal mucosa are also factors which cannot be ignored.

At the drug level, much relief has been obtained with agents such as isoprenaline and sodium cromoglycate which bind to different receptors on the mast cell surface and make it resistant to triggering. The symptoms of allergy are largely but not always controllable by anti-histamines, particularly when one is dealing with late phase reactions for which recourse to steroids may be necessary.

TYPE II — ANTIBODY-DEPENDENT CYTOTOXIC HYPERSENSITIVITY

Where an antigen is present on the surface of a cell, combination with antibody will encourage the demise of that cell by promoting contact with phagocytes either by reduction in surface charge, by opsonic adherence directly through the Fc, or by immune adherence through bound C3. Cell death may also occur through activation of the full complement system up to C8 and C9 producing direct membrane damage. Although in the case of haemolytic antibodies, the generation of a single active complement site is enough to cause erythrocyte lysis, other cells appear to have repair mechanisms and it is likely that several complement sites need to be recruited in order to overwhelm the cell's defences.

The operation of a quite distinct cytotoxic mechanism derives from the finding that target cells coated with low concentrations of IgG antibody can be killed 'non-specifically' through an extracellular non-phagocytic mechanism involving non-sensitized lymphoreticular cells which bind to the target by their specific receptors for the $C\gamma2$ and $C\gamma3$ domains of IgG Fc (figure 12.8). It should be noted that this so-called antibody-dependent cell-mediated cytotoxicity (ADCC) may be exhibited by both phagocytic and non-phagocytic myeloid cells (polymorphs and monocytes) and by large granular lymphocytes with Fc receptors dubbed 'K-cells' which are almost certainly identical with the natural killer (NK) cells (p. 14). Contact between the effector and target cells is essential and activity is inhibited by cytochalasin B which interferes with cell movement, and aggregated IgG which binds firmly to the Fc receptors and blocks their ability to interact with antibody on the surface of the target.

So far, ADCC has been studied exclusively as a phenomenon *in vitro*; to give examples, human K-cells have been shown to be strikingly unpleasant to chicken red cells coated with rabbit antibody and schistosomules coated with either IgG or IgE can be killed by eosinophils (cf. figure 10.16). Whether ADCC is merely a curiosity of the laboratory test-tube or plays a positive role *in vivo* remains an open question. Functionally, this extracellular cytotoxic mechanism would be expected to be of significance where the target is too large for ingestion by phagocytosis, e.g. large parasites and solid tumours. It could also act as a back-up system for T-cell killing when antibody production might otherwise lead to protection of the target from attack by T-cells through blocking of the surface antigens; the evolution of ADCC mechanisms would ensure that the antibody-coated target was still vulnerable.

The mechanisms leading to cell death in type II hypersensitivity are summarized in figure 12.9.

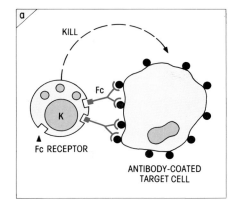
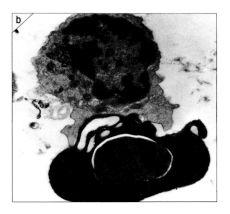

Figure 12.8. *Killing of antibody-coated target by antibody-dependent cell-mediated cytotoxicity (ADCC). The surface receptors for Ig Fc region bind the effector cell to the target which is then killed by an extracellular mechanism. Several different cell types may display ADCC activity: thus, human monocytes and IFNγ-activated neutrophils can kill antibody-coated tumour cells using their FcγRI and FcγRII receptors, and lymphocytes (NK cells) mediate killing of hybridoma targets through FcγRIII receptors. (a) Diagram of effector and target cells. (b) Electron micrograph of attack on antibody-coated chick red cell by a mouse large granular lymphocyte showing close apposition of effector and target and vacuolation in the cytoplasm of the latter (courtesy of P. Penfold).*

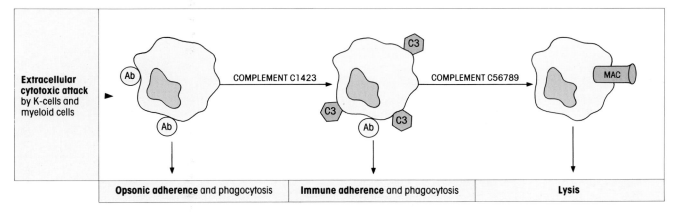

Figure 12.9. *Type II—antibody-dependent cytotoxic hypersensitivity. Antibodies directed against cell surface antigens cause cell death not only by C-dependent lysis but also by adherence reactions leading to phagocytosis or through non-phagocytic extracellular killing by certain lymphoreticular cells (antibody-dependent cell-mediated cytotoxicity).*

Type II reactions between members of the same species (isoimmune)

Transfusion reactions

Of the many different polymorphic constituents of the human red cell membrane, ABO blood groups form the dominant system. The antigenic groups A and B are derived from H substance (figure 12.10) by the action of glycosyl transferases encoded by A or B genes respectively. Individuals with both genes (group AB) have the two antigens on their red cells while those lacking these genes (group O) synthesize H substance only. Antibodies to A or B occur when the antigen is absent from the red cell surface; thus a person of blood group A will possess anti-B and so on. These *isohaemagglutinins* are usually IgM and are thought to arise through immunization against antigens of the gut flora which are similar to the blood group substances so that the antibodies formed cross-react with the appropriate red cell type. If an individual is blood group A, he will be tolerant to antigens closely similar to A and will only form cross-reacting antibodies capable of agglutinating B red cells; similarly an O individual

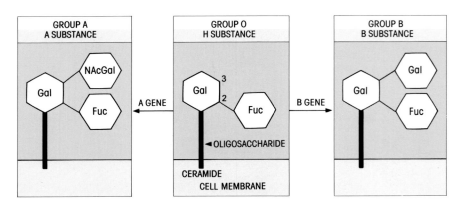

| GROUP A
A SUBSTANCE | GROUP O
H SUBSTANCE | GROUP B
B SUBSTANCE |

Figure 12.10. The ABO system. The allelic genes A and B code for transferases which add either N-acetylgalactosamine or galactose respectively to H substance. The oligosaccharide is anchored to the cell membrane by coupling to a sphingomyelin called ceramide. 85% of the population secrete blood group substances in the saliva where the oligosaccharides are present as soluble polypeptide conjugates formed under the action of a secretor (se) gene.

will make anti-A and anti-B (table 12.2). On transfusion, mismatched red cells will be coated by the isohaemagglutinins and cause severe reactions.

Rhesus incompatibility

The rhesus (Rh) blood groups form the other major antigenic system, the RhD antigen being of the most consequence for isoimmune reactions. A mother with an RhD negative blood group (i.e. dd genotype) can readily be sensitized by red cells from a baby carrying RhD antigens (DD or Dd genotype). This occurs most often at the birth of the first child when a placental bleed can release a large number of the baby's erythrocytes into the mother. The antibodies formed are predominantly of the IgG class and are able to cross the placenta in any subsequent pregnancy. Reaction with the D-antigen on the fetal red cells leads to their destruction through opsonic adherence giving haemolytic disease of the newborn (figure 12.11).

These anti-D antibodies fail to agglutinate RhD+ red cells *in vitro* ('incomplete antibodies') because the low density of antigenic sites does not allow sufficient antibody bridges to be formed between the negatively charged erythrocytes to overcome the electrostatic repulsive forces. Erythrocytes coated with anti-D can be made to agglutinate by

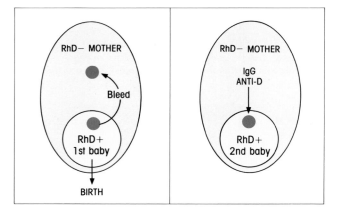

Figure 12.11. Haemolytic disease of the newborn due to rhesus incompatibility.

addition of albumin or of an anti-immunoglobulin serum (Coombs' reagent; figure 12.12).

If a mother has natural isohaemagglutinins which can react with any fetal erythrocytes reaching her circulation, sensitization to the D antigens is less likely due to 'deviation' of the red cells away from the antigen-sensitive cells. For example, a group O RhD−ve mother with a group A RhD+ve baby would destroy any fetal erythrocytes with her anti-A before they could immunize to produce anti-D. In an extension of this principle, RhD−ve mothers are now treated prophylactically with small amounts of avid IgG anti-D at the time of birth of the first child, and this greatly reduces the risk of sensitization. Another success for immunology.

Organ transplants

A long-standing homograft which has withstood the first onslaught of the cell-mediated reaction can evoke humoral antibodies in the host directed

Table 12.2. *ABO blood groups and serum antibodies.*

BLOOD GROUP (PHENOTYPE)	GENOTYPE	ANTIGEN	SERUM ANTIBODY
A	AA, AO	A	ANTI-B
B	BB, BO	B	ANTI-A
AB	AB	A and B	NONE
O	OO	H	ANTI-A ANTI-B

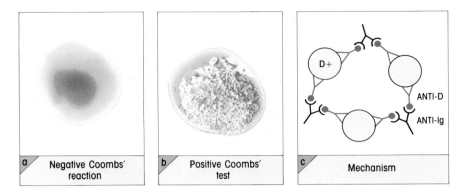

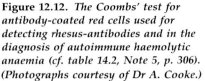

| a | Negative Coombs' reaction | b | Positive Coombs' test | c | Mechanism |

Figure 12.12. *The Coombs' test for antibody-coated red cells used for detecting rhesus-antibodies and in the diagnosis of autoimmune haemolytic anaemia (cf. table 14.2, Note 5, p. 306). (Photographs courtesy of Dr A. Cooke.)*

against surface transplantation antigens on the graft. These may be directly cytotoxic or cause adherence of phagocytic cells or 'non-specific' attack by K-cells. They may also lead to platelet adherence when they combine with antigens on the surface of the vascular endothelium (figure 13.7, p. 282). Hyper-acute rejection is mediated by preformed antibodies in the graft recipient.

Autoimmune type II hypersensitivity reactions

Autoantibodies to the patient's own red cells are produced in autoimmune haemolytic anaemia. They react at 37°C with epitopes on antigens of the Rhesus complex distinct from those which incite transfusion reactions. Red cells coated with these antibodies have a shortened half-life largely through their adherence to phagocytic cells in the spleen. Similar mechanisms account for the anaemia in patients with cold haemagglutinin disease who have monoclonal anti-I after infection with *Mycoplasma pneumoniae*, and in some cases of paroxysmal cold haemoglobinuria associated with the actively lytic Donath–Landsteiner antibodies specific for blood group P. These antibodies are primarily of IgM isotype and only react at temperatures well below 37°C.

The sera of patients with Hashimoto's thyroiditis contain antibodies which in the presence of complement are directly cytotoxic for isolated human thyroid cells in culture. In Goodpasture's syndrome (included here for convenience), antibodies to kidney glomerular basement membrane are present. Biopsies show these antibodies together with complement components bound to the basement membranes where the action of the full complement

system leads to serious damage (figure 12.13a). I suppose one could also include the stripping of acetylcholine receptors from the muscle end-plate by autoantibodies in myasthenia gravis as a further example of type II hypersensitivity.

263

Type II drug reactions

This is complicated. Drugs may become coupled to body components and thereby undergo conversion from a hapten to a full antigen which will sensitize certain individuals (we don't know which). If IgE antibodies are produced, anaphylactic reactions can result. In some circumstances, particularly with topically applied ointments, cell-mediated hypersensitivity may be induced. In other cases where coupling to serum proteins occurs, the possibility of type III complex-mediated reactions may arise. In the present context we are concerned with those instances where the drug appears to form an antigenic complex with the surface of a formed element of the blood and evokes the production of antibodies which are cytotoxic for the cell–drug complex. When the drug is withdrawn, the sensitivity is no longer evident. Examples of this mechanism have been seen in the *haemolytic anaemia* sometimes associated with continued administration of chlorpromazine or phenacetin, in the *agranulocytosis* associated with the taking of amidopyrine or of quinidine, and the now classic situation of *thrombocytopenic purpura* which may be produced by Sedormid, a sedative of yester-year. In the latter case, freshly drawn serum from the patient will lyse platelets in the presence, but not in the absence, of Sedormid; inactivation of complement by preheating the serum at 56°C for 30 minutes abrogates this effect.

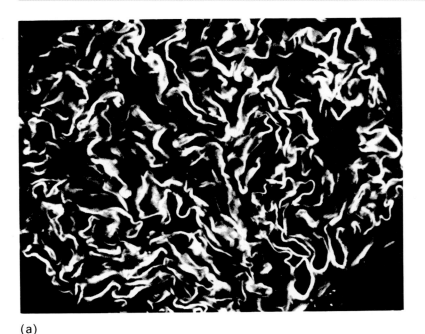

(a)

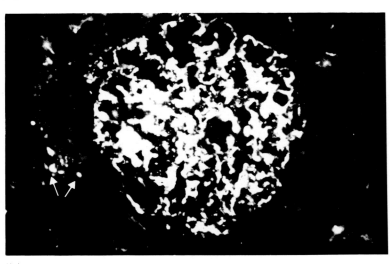

(b)

Figure 12.13. *Glomerulonephritis: (a) due to linear deposition of antibody to glomerular basement membrane here visualized by staining the human kidney biopsy with a fluorescent anti-IgG (courtesy of Dr F.J. Dixon) and (b) due to deposition of antigen–antibody complexes which can be seen as discrete masses lining the glomerular basement membrane following immunofluorescent staining with anti-IgG; patches of blue autofluorescence are present in the extraglomerular tissue (arrowed) (courtesy of Dr D. Doniach). Similar patterns to these are obtained with a fluorescent anti-C3.*

TYPE III—IMMUNE-COMPLEX-MEDIATED HYPERSENSITIVITY

The body may be exposed to an excess of antigen over a protracted period in a number of circumstances, persistent infection with a microbial organism, autoimmunity to self-components and repeated contact with environmental agents. The union of such antigens and antibodies to form an insoluble complex at fixed sites within the body may well give rise to acute inflammatory reactions (figure 12.14). If complement is fixed, anaphylatoxins will be released as split products of C3 and C5 and these will cause release of mast cell mediators with vascular permeability changes. The chemotactic factors also produced will lead to an influx of polymorphonuclear leucocytes which begin the phagocytosis of the immune complexes; this in turn results in the extracellular release of the polymorph granule contents, particularly when the complex is deposited on a basement membrane and cannot be phagocytosed (so-called 'frustrated phagocytosis'). The proteolytic enzymes (including neutral proteinases and collagenase), kinin-forming enzymes and polycationic proteins which are released will of course damage local tissues and intensify the inflammatory responses. Further damage may be mediated by reactive lysis in which activated C5,6,7 becomes adventitiously attached to the surface of nearby cells and binds C8,9. Under appropriate conditions, platelets may be aggregated with two consequences: they provide yet a further source of vasoactive amines and may also form microthrombi which can lead to local ischaemia. (The discerning reader will appreciate the need for the system of inhibitors present in the body.) Insoluble complexes taken up by macrophages cannot readily be digested and provide a persistent activating stimulus (figure 12.14).

The outcome of the formation of immune complexes *in vivo* depends not only on the absolute amounts of antigen and antibody, which determine the intensity of the reaction, but also on their *relative* proportions which govern the nature of the complexes (cf. precipitin curve, p. 86) and hence their distribution within the body. Between *antibody excess* and *mild antigen excess*, the complexes are rapidly precipitated and tend to be localized to the site of introduction of antigen, whereas in *moderate* to *gross antigen excess*, soluble complexes are formed.

The fate of these complexes is bound up closely with the operation of the classical complement pathway. Fixation of complement inhibits the precipitation of immune complexes by covalent attachment of C3b which prevents the Fc—Fc interactions required to form large insoluble aggregates (figure 12.15). These small complexes containing C3b bind by immune adherence to CR1 complement receptors on the human erythrocyte and are transported to fixed macrophages in the liver where they are safely inactivated. If there are defects in this system, for

example deficiencies in classical pathway components (cf. p. 266; figure 12.15) or perhaps if the system is overloaded, then the immune complexes are free in the plasma and widespread disease involving deposition in the kidneys, joints and skin may result.

Inflammatory lesions due to locally formed complexes

The Arthus reaction

Maurice Arthus found that injection of soluble antigen intradermally into hyperimmunized rabbits with high levels of precipitating antibody, produced an erythematous and oedematous reaction reaching a peak at 3—8 hours and then usually resolving. The lesion was characterized by an intense infiltration with polymorphonuclear leucocytes (cf. figure 12.7h). The injected antigen precipitates with antibody often within the venule, too fast for the classical complement system to prevent it; subsequently the complex binds complement and, using fluorescent reagents, antigen, immunoglobulin and complement components can all be demonstrated in this lesion (figure 12.7i). Anaphylatoxin is soon generated and causes mast cell degranulation. Local intravascular complexes will also cause platelet aggregation and vasoactive amine release and, as a result, erythema and oedema increase. The formation of chemotactic factors leads to the influx of polymorphs. The Arthus reaction can be blocked by depletion of complement or of the neutrophil polymorphs (by nitrogen mustard or specific antipolymorph sera).

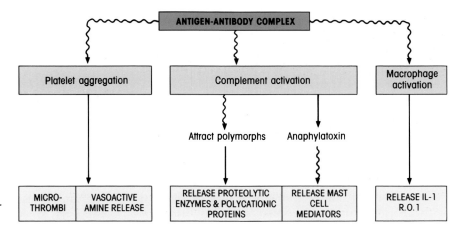

Figure 12.14. *Type III immune-complex-mediated hypersensitivity.*

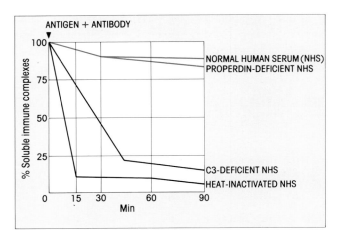

Figure 12.15. *Complement inhibits the formation of insoluble complexes as antigen and antibody combine. Serum deficient in C3 or in which complement had been inactivated by heating, failed to block the formation of precipitating complexes. Deficiency of the alternative pathway component properdin had no effect. (Data from Schifferli J.A., Ng Y.C. & Peters D.K. (1986) N. Engl. J. Med. 315, 488, reproduced with permission from the* **New England Journal of Medicine.***)*

Reactions to inhaled antigens

Intrapulmonary Arthus-type reactions to exogenous inhaled antigen appear to be responsible for a number of hypersensitivity disorders in man. The severe respiratory difficulties associated with farmer's lung occur within 6–8 hours of exposure to the dust from mouldy hay. The patients are found to be sensitized to thermophilic actinomycetes which grow in the mouldy hay, and extracts of these organisms give precipitin reactions with the subject's serum and Arthus reactions on intradermal injection. Inhalation of bacterial spores present in dust from the hay introduces antigen into the lungs and a complex-mediated hypersensitivity reaction occurs. Similar situations arise in pigeon-fancier's disease where the antigen is probably serum protein present in the dust from dried faeces, in rat handlers sensitized to rat serum proteins excreted in the urine (figure 12.16) and in many other quaintly named cases of extrinsic allergic alveolitis resulting from continual inhalation of organic particles, e.g. cheese washer's disease (*Penicillium casei* spores), furrier's lung (fox fur proteins) and maple bark stripper's disease (spores of *Cryptostroma*). Evidence that an immediate anaphylactic type I response may sometimes be of importance for the initiation of an Arthus reaction comes from the study of patients with allergic bronchopulmonary aspergillosis who have high levels of IgE and precipitating IgG antibodies to *Aspergillus* species.

Reactions to internal antigens

Type III reactions are often provoked by the local release of antigen from infectious organisms within the body; for example, living filarial worms such as *Wuchereria bancrofti* are relatively harmless, but the dead parasite found in lymphatic vessels initiates an inflammatory reaction thought to be responsible for obstruction of lymph flow and the ensuing, rather monstrous, elephantiasis. Chemotherapy may cause an abrupt release of microbial antigens in individuals with high antibody levels, producing quite dramatic immune complex-mediated reactions such as erythema nodosum leprosum in the skin of dapsone-treated lepromatous leprosy patients (figure 12.7e) and the Jarisch–Herxheimer reaction in syphilitics on penicillin.

An interesting variant of the Arthus reaction is seen in rheumatoid arthritis where complexes are formed locally in the joint due to the production of self-associating IgG anti-IgG by synovial plasma cells (cf. p. 334).

It has also been recognized that complexes could be generated at a local site by a quite different mechanism involving non-specific adherence of an antigen to tissue structures followed by the binding of soluble antibody—in other words, the antigen becomes fixed in the tissue *before* not *after* combining with antibody. Although it is not clear to what extent this mechanism operates in patients with immune complex disease, let me describe the experimental observation on which it is based. After injection with bacterial endotoxin, mice release DNA into their circulation which binds specifically to the collagen in the basement membrane of the glomerular capillaries: infusion of anti-DNA now gives rise to antigen–antibody complexes in the kidney.

Disease resulting from circulating complexes

Serum sickness

Injection of relatively large doses of foreign serum (e.g. horse anti-diphtheria) used to be employed for various therapeutic purposes. It was not uncommon for a condition known as 'serum sickness' to arise

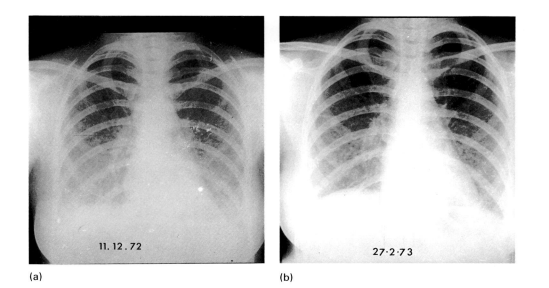

(a)   (b)

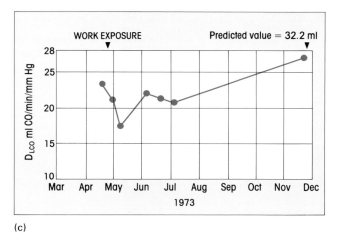

(c)

Figure 12.16. *Extrinsic allergic alveolitis due to rat serum proteins in a research assistant handling rats (type III hypersensitivity). Typical systemic and pulmonary reactions on inhalation and positive prick tests were elicited by rat serum proteins; precipitins against serum proteins in rat urine were present in the patient's serum. (a) Bilateral micronodular shadowing during acute episode. (b) Marked clearing within 11 days after cessation of exposure to rats. (c) Temporary fall in pulmonary gas exchange measured by DL_{co} (gas transfer, single breath) following a 3-day exposure to rats at work (arrowed). (From Carroll K.B., Pepys J., Longbottom J.L., Hughes D.T.D. & Benson H.G. (1975)* **Clin. Allergy** *5, 443; figures by courtesy of Prof. J. Pepys.)*

some eight days after the injection. A rise in temperature, swollen lymph nodes, a generalized urticarial rash and painful swollen joints associated with a low serum complement and transient albuminuria could be encountered. These result from the deposition of soluble antigen–antibody complexes formed in antigen excess.

Some individuals begin to synthesize antibodies against the foreign protein—usually horse globulin. Since the antigen is still present in gross excess at that time, circulating soluble complexes of composition Ag_2Ab, Ag_3Ab_2, Ag_4Ab_3, etc. will be formed

(cf. precipitin curve, figures 5.1 and 5.2). To be pathogenic, the complexes have to be of the right size—too big and they are snapped up smartly by the macrophages of the reticuloendothelial system, too small (<19S) and they fail to induce an inflammatory reaction. Even when they are the right size, it seems that they will only localize in vessel walls if there is a change in vascular permeability. This may come about through release of 5-hydroxytryptamine (5HT) from platelets reacting with larger complexes or through an IgE or complement-mediated degranulation of basophils and mast cells to produce histamine, leukotrienes and platelet activating factor. The effect on the capillaries is to cause separation of the endothelial cells and exposure of the basement membrane to which the appropriately sized complexes attach, the skin, joints, kidneys and heart being particularly affected. As antibody synthesis increases, antigen is cleared and the patient normally recovers.

Immune complex glomerulonephritis

The deposition of complexes is a dynamic affair and long-lasting disease is only seen when the antigen is persistent as in chronic infections and auto-immune diseases. Experimentally, Dixon produced chronic glomerular lesions by repeated administration of foreign proteins to rabbits. Not all animals showed the lesion and perhaps only those genetically capable of producing low affinity antibody (Soothill & Steward) or antibodies to a restricted number of determinants (Christian) formed soluble complexes in the right size range. The smallest complexes reach the epithelial side but progressively larger complexes are retained in or on the endothelial side of the glomerular basement membrane (figure 12.17). They build up as 'lumpy' granules staining for antigen, immunoglobulin and complement (C3) by immunofluorescence (figure 12.13b) and appear as large amorphous masses in the electron microscope (cf. figure 15.5).

Many cases of glomerulonephritis are associated with circulating complexes and biopsies give a fluorescent staining pattern similar to that of figure 12.13b which depicts DNA/anti-DNA/complement deposits in the kidney of a patient with systemic lupus erythematosus (cf. p. 264). Well known is the disease which can follow infection with certain strains of so-called 'nephritogenic' streptococci and the nephrotic syndrome of Nigerian children associated with quartan malaria where complexes with antigens of the infecting organism have been implicated. Immune complex nephritis can arise in the course of chronic viral infections; for example, mice infected with lymphocytic choriomeningitis virus develop a glomerulonephritis associated with circulating complexes of virus and antibody. This may well represent a model for many cases of glomerulonephritis in man.

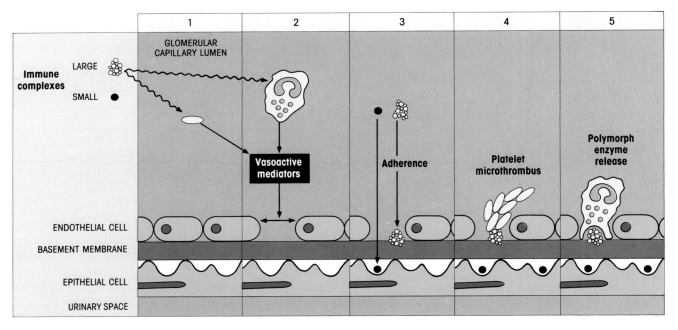

Figure 12.17. *Deposition of immune complexes in the kidney glomerulus. (1) Complexes induce release of vasoactive mediators from basophils and platelets which cause (2) separation of endothelial cells, (3) attachment of larger complexes to exposed basement membrane, smaller complexes passing through to epithelial side, (4) complexes induce platelet aggregation, (5) chemotactically attracted neutrophils release granule contents in 'frustrated phagocytosis' to damage basement membrane. Complex deposition is favoured in the glomerular capillary because it is a major filtration site and has a high hydrodynamic pressure. Deposition is greatly reduced in animals depleted of platelets or treated with vasoactive amine antagonists.*

Deposition of complexes at other sites

The choroid plexus being a major filtration site is also favoured for immune complex deposition and this could account for the frequency of central nervous disorders in systemic lupus. Neurologically affected patients tend to have depressed C4 in the cerebrospinal fluid (c.s.f.) and at postmortem, SLE patients with neurological disturbances and high titre anti-DNA were shown to have scattered deposits of immunoglobulin and DNA in the choroid plexus. Subacute sclerosing panencephalitis is associated with a high c.s.f. to serum ratio of measles antibody, and deposits containing Ig and measles Ag may be found in neural tissue.

The vasculitic skin rashes which are a major feature of serum sickness are also characteristic of systemic and discoid lupus erythematosus (figure 12.7c and d) and biopsies of the lesions reveal amorphous deposits of Ig and C3 at the basement membrane of the dermal−epidermal junction.

The necrotizing arteritis produced in rabbits by experimental serum sickness closely resembles the histology of polyarteritis nodosa (figure 12.7g and h) and it has recently been reported that in some of these patients (figure 12.7f), immune complexes containing the HBs antigen of hepatitis B virus are present in the lesions (figure 12.7i). Another example is the haemorrhagic shock syndrome found with some frequency in South-East Asia during a second infection with a dengue virus. There are four types of virus, and antibodies to one type produced during a first infection may not neutralize a second strain but rather facilitate its entry into, and replication within, human monocytes by attachment of the complex to Fc receptors. The enhanced production of virus leads to immune complex formation and a massive intravascular activation of the classical complement pathway. In some instances drugs such as penicillin become antigenic after conjugation with body proteins and form complexes which mediate hypersensitivity reactions.

It should be said that persistence of circulating complexes does not invariably lead to type III hypersensitivity (e.g. in many cancer patients and in individuals with idiotype−anti-idiotype reactions). Perhaps in these cases the complexes lack the ability to initiate the changes required for complex deposition, but some hold the view that complexes detected in the serum may sometimes be artefacts released from their *in vivo* attachment to the erythrocyte CR1 receptors by the action of factor I during processing of the blood.

Detection of immune complex formation

Tissue-bound complexes are usually visualized by the immunofluorescent staining of biopsies with conjugated anti-immunoglobulins and anti-C3 (cf. figure 12.13b).

Many techniques for detecting circulating complexes have been described and because of variations in the size, complement-fixing ability and Ig class of different complexes, it is useful to apply more than one method. Bearing in mind the caveat concerning the possibility of artefacts just mentioned, in our laboratory we tend to prefer:
1 precipitation of complexed IgG from serum at concentrations of polyethylene glycol which do not bring down significant amounts of IgG monomer, followed by estimation of IgG in the precipitate by single radial diffusion or laser nephelometry, and
2 binding of C3b-containing complexes to beads coated with conglutinin (cf. p. 204) and estimation of the bound Ig with enzyme-labelled anti-Ig.

Other techniques include (i) estimation of the binding of ^{125}I-Clq to complexes by co-precipitation with polyethylene glycol, (ii) inhibition by complexes of rheumatoid factor-induced aggregation of IgG-coated particles, and (iii) detection with radio-labelled anti-Ig of serum complexes capable of binding to bovine conglutinin or to the C3b (and to a lesser extent the Fc) receptors on the Raji cell line. Sera from patients with immune complex disease often form a cryoprecipitate when allowed to stand at 4°C. Measurement of serum C3 and its conversion product C3c are sometimes useful.

Treatment

The avoidance of exogenous inhaled antigens inducing type III reactions is obvious. Elimination of micro-organisms associated with immune complex disease by chemotherapy may provoke a further reaction due to copious release of antigen. Suppression of the accessory factors thought to be necessary for deposition of complexes would seem logical; for example, the development of serum sickness is prevented by histamine and 5HT antagonists. Disodium cromoglycate, heparin and salicylates are often used, the latter being an ef-

269

fective platelet stabilizer as well as a potent anti-inflammatory agent. Corticosteroids are particularly powerful inhibitors of inflammation and are immunosuppressive. In many cases, particularly those involving autoimmunity, conventional immunosuppressive agents may be justified. Where type III hypersensitivity is thought to arise from an inadequate immune response, the more aggressive approach of immunopotentiation to boost avidity is being advocated, but that is a path that will be trodden gently.

TYPE IV — CELL-MEDIATED (DELAYED-TYPE) HYPERSENSITIVITY

This form of hypersensitivity is encountered in many allergic reactions to bacteria, viruses and fungi, in the contact dermatitis resulting from sensitization to certain simple chemicals and in the rejection of transplanted tissues. Perhaps the best known example is the Mantoux reaction obtained by injection of tuberculin into the skin of an individual in whom previous infection with the mycobacterium had induced a state of cell-mediated immunity (CMI). The reaction is characterized by erythema and induration (figure 12.7j) which appears only after several hours (hence the term 'delayed') and reaches a maximum at 24–48 hours, thereafter subsiding. Histologically the earliest phase of the reaction is seen as a perivascular cuffing with mononuclear cells followed by a more extensive exudation of mono- and polymorphonuclear cells. The latter soon migrate out of the lesion leaving behind a predominantly mononuclear cell infiltrate consisting of lymphocytes and cells of the monocyte–macrophage series (figure 12.7l). This contrasts with the essentially 'polymorph' character of the Arthus reaction (figure 12.7h).

Comparable reactions to soluble proteins are obtained when sensitization is induced by incorporation of the antigen into complete Freund's adjuvant (p. 131). In some but not all cases, if animals are primed with antigen alone or in incomplete Freund's adjuvant (which lacks the mycobacteria), the delayed hypersensitivity state is of shorter duration and the dermal response more transient. This is known as 'Jones–Mote' sensitivity but has recently been termed *cutaneous basophil hypersensitivity* on account of the high proportion of basophils infiltrating the skin lesion.

The cellular basis of type IV hypersensitivity

Unlike the other forms of hypersensitivity which we have discussed, delayed-type reactivity cannot be transferred from a sensitized to a non-sensitized individual with serum antibody; lymphoid cells, in particular the T-lymphocytes, are required. Transfer has been achieved in the human using viable white blood cells and, interestingly, by a low molecular weight material extracted from them (Lawrence's transfer factor). The nature of this substance is, however, a mystery. The extracts contain a variety of factors which appear capable of stimulating pre-committed T-cells mediating delayed hypersensitivity, but whether there is also an informational molecule conferring antigen-specific reactivity is still a highly contentious issue.

It cannot be stressed too often that the hypersensitivity lesion results from an exaggerated interaction between antigen and the *normal* cell-mediated immune mechanisms (cf. p. 139). Following earlier priming, memory T-cells recognize the antigen together with class II MHC molecules on an antigen-presenting cell and are stimulated into blast cell transformation and proliferation. The stimulated T-cells release a number of soluble factors which function as mediators of the ensuing hypersensitivity response particularly by attracting and activating macrophages; they also help cytotoxic T-cell precursors to become killer cells which can cause tissue damage (figure 12.18).

Tissue damage produced by type IV reactions

Infections

The development of a state of cell-mediated hypersensitivity to bacterial products is probably responsible for the lesions associated with bacterial allergy such as the cavitation, caseation and general toxaemia seen in human tuberculosis and the granulomatous skin lesions found in patients with the borderline form of leprosy. When the battle between the replicating bacteria and the body defences fails to be resolved in favour of the host, persisting antigen provokes a chronic local delayed hypersensitivity reaction. Continual release of lymphokines from sensitized T-lymphocytes leads

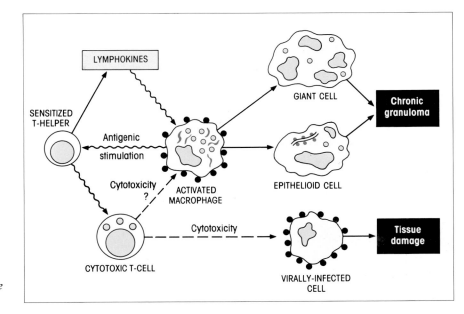

Figure 12.18. *The cellular basis of type IV hypersensitivity.*

to the accumulation of large numbers of macrophages, many of which give rise to arrays of epithelioid cells, while others fuse to form giant cells. Macrophages bearing bacterial antigen on their surface may become targets for killer T-cells and be destroyed. Further tissue damage will occur as a result of indiscriminate cytotoxicity by lymphokine-activated macrophages (and NK cells?) and perhaps lymphotoxin itself. Morphologically, this combination of cell types with proliferating lymphocytes and fibroblasts associated with areas of fibrosis and necrosis is termed a *chronic granuloma* and represents an attempt by the body to wall-off a site of persistent infection (figure 12.7l; figure 12.18). It should be noted that granulomas can also arise from the persistence of indigestible antigen—antibody complexes or inorganic materials such as talc within macrophages, although non-immunological granulomas may be distinguished by the absence of lymphocytes.

The skin rashes in smallpox and measles and the lesions of herpes simplex may be largely attributed to delayed-type allergic reactions with extensive damage to virally infected cells by cytotoxic T-lymphocytes. Cell-mediated hypersensitivity has also been demonstrated in the fungal diseases, candidiasis, dermatomycosis, coccidioidomycosis and histoplasmosis, and in the parasitic diseases, leishmaniasis and schistosomiasis where the pathology has been attributed to a reaction against soluble enzymes derived from the eggs which lodge in the liver capillaries (figure 12.7o).

Sarcoidosis is a disease of unknown aetiology affecting lymphoid tissue and involving the formation of chronic granulomas. Delayed-type hypersensitivity is depressed and the patients are anergic on skin testing with tuberculin; curiously they give positive responses if cortisone is injected together with the antigen and it has been suggested that cortisone-sensitive T suppressors might be responsible for the anergy. The patients develop a granulomatous reaction a few weeks after intradermal injection of spleen extract from another sarcoid patient—the Kweim reaction.

Contact dermatitis

The epidermal route of inoculation tends to favour the development of a T-cell response through processing by class II-rich dendritic Langerhans' cells (cf. figure 2.6i) which migrate to the lymph nodes and present antigen to T-lymphocytes. Thus, delayed-type reactions in the skin are often produced by foreign materials capable of binding to body constituents, possibly surface molecules of the Langerhans cell, to form new antigens. The reaction is characterized by a mononuclear cell infiltrate peaking at 12—15 hours, accompanied by oedema of the epidermis with microvesicle formation (figure 12.7m and n). Contact hypersensitivity can occur in people who become sensitized while working with chemicals such as picryl chloride and chromates, or who repeatedly come into contact with the substance urushiol from the poison ivy plant.

p-Phenylene diamine in certain hair dyes, neomycin in topically applied ointments, and nickel salts formed from articles such as nickel jewellery clasps (figure 12.7k), can provoke similar reactions.

Other examples

Delayed hypersensivity contributes significantly to the prolonged reactions which result from insect bites. The possible implication of homograft rejection by cytotoxic T-cells as a mechanism for the control of cancer cells is discussed in Chapter 13. The contribution made by cell-mediated hypersensitivity reactions to certain autoimmune diseases may be important (cf. p. 335).

TYPE V — STIMULATORY HYPERSENSITIVITY

Many cells receive instruction by agents such as hormones through surface receptors which specifically bind the external agent presumably through complementarity of structure. This combination may lead to allosteric changes in configuration of the receptor or of adjacent molecules which become activated and transmit a signal to the cell interior. For example, when thyroid stimulating hormone (TSH) of pituitary origin binds to the thyroid cell receptors, there appears to be an activation of adenyl cyclase in the membrane which generates cyclic-AMP from ATP and this 'second messenger' acts to stimulate activity in the thyroid cell. The thyroid stimulating antibody present in the sera of thyrotoxic patients (cf. p. 326) is an autoantibody directed against an antigen on the thyroid surface which stimulates the cell and produces the same changes as TSH, similarly utilizing the cyclic-AMP pathway. It is likely that the antibody combines with a site on the TSH receptor or an adjacent molecule to produce the changes required for adenyl cyclase activation. The situation is analogous to lymphocyte stimulation; B-lymphocytes with immunoglobulin surface receptors can be stimulated by changes induced through the receptor molecules either by binding of specific antigen or by an antibody to the immunoglobulin (even anti-Fc) as shown in figure 12.19. Intriguingly, there are indications that cimetidine-resistant duodenal ulcer patients may have stimulatory antibodies directed to H2-histamine receptors.

Other experimental examples of stimulation by antibodies to cell surface antigens may be cited: the

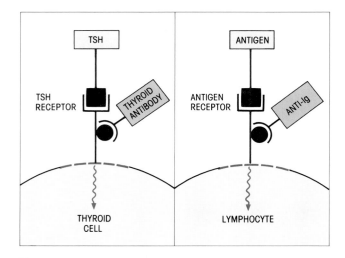

Figure 12.19. *Stimulation of thyroid cell and of lymphocyte by physiological agent or by antibody both of which cause comparable membrane changes leading to cell activation by reacting with surface receptors.*

transformation of human T-lymphocytes by monoclonal antibodies to the CD3 antigen; the production of cell division in thyroid cells by 'growth' autoantibodies; the induction of pinocytosis by anti-macrophage serum; and the mitogenic effect of antibodies to sea-urchin eggs. It is worthy of note that although antibodies to enzymes directed against determinants near to the active site can exert a blocking effect, combination with more distant determinants can sometimes bring about allosteric conformational changes which are associated with a considerable increase in enzymic activity as has been described for certain variants of penicillinase and β-galactosidase.

'INNATE' HYPERSENSITIVITY REACTIONS

Excessive activation of the alternative complement pathway can lead to tissue-damaging hypersensitivity reactions such as disseminated intravascular coagulation. A good model for this is the Shwartzmann reaction produced in rabbits by intravascular endotoxin. This activates the alternative pathway so that the endotoxin becomes coated with C3b and sticks to platelets by immune adherence; the C5,6,7 complexes generated cause platelet destruction by reactive lysis with release of clotting factors. Although in man, C3b adherence reactions involve red cells and leucocytes rather than platelets, somewhat similar mechanisms

272

associated with intense complement consumption underlie the disseminated intravascular coagulation seen in human patients with Gram-negative septicaemia or dengue haemorrhagic shock produced by a substantial viraemia occurring in the second infection of individuals with high titre antibodies. In a dog model of myocardial infarction, the resulting damage was reduced by 40% by dint of infusion of an antibody to the CR3 complement receptor (anti-CD11b) apparently by preventing complement-mediated neutrophil damage to the vasculature of the heart.

The reader's attention has already been drawn to the unusual susceptibility of the erythrocytes to lysis in paroxysmal nocturnal haemoglobinuria resulting from deficiency in C3b control proteins on the red cell surface (p. 240). Undue C3 consumption is associated with mesangiocapillary glomerulo-nephritis and partial lipodystrophy in patients with the so-called C3 nephritic factor which appears to be an IgG autoantibody capable of activating the alternative pathway by combining with and stabil-izing the C3bBb convertase.

We should include idiopathic pulmonary fibrosis in this section. It is a chronic fatal disorder charac-terized by diffuse fibrosis of the alveolar walls in which local macrophages play a central role. On activation they produce an early G1 competence growth signal such as platelet-derived growth factor and fibronectin, and then a late G1 progression growth signal such as insulin-like growth factor 1. As a result, the fibroblasts multiply and become embedded in a collagen matrix to the respiratory detriment of the host.

SUMMARY

The normal effector mechanisms for cell-mediated and humoral immunity are dependent upon the activation of T- and B-cells respectively. Excessive stimulation of these effector mechanisms by antigen in a sensitized host can lead to tissue damage and we speak of hypersensitivity reactions of which five main types can be distinguished.

Type 1 — anaphylactic hypersensitivity

This depends upon the reaction of antigen with specific IgE antibody bound through its Fc to the mast cell, leading to release from the granules of mediators including histamine, leukotrienes and platelet activating factor, plus eosinophil and neutrophil chemotactic factors. Hay fever and ex-trinsic asthma represent the most common atopic allergic disorders. The offending antigen is identified by intradermal prick tests giving im-mediate wheal and erythema reactions or by provocation testing. Late-stage cellular reactions may be important for the development of chronic bronchial asthma. There is a strong familial dis-position; the tendency to produce high levels of IgE is an important contributing factor. Symptomatic treatment involves the use of mediator antagonists or agents which stabilize the mast cell granules; steroids are effective against late reactions. Courses of antigen injection may desensitize by formation of blocking IgG or IgA antibodies or by turning off IgE production.

Type II — antibody-dependent cytotoxic hypersensitivity

This involves the death of cells bearing antibody attached to a surface antigen. The cells may be taken up by phagocytic cells to which they adhere through their coating of IgG or C3b or lysed by the operation of the full complement system. Cells bearing IgG may also be killed by polymorphs and macrophages or by K-cells through an extracellular mechanism (antibody-dependent cell-mediated cytotoxicity). Examples are: transfusion reactions, haemolytic disease of the newborn through rhesus incompatibility, antibody-mediated graft destruc-tion, auto-immune reactions directed against the formed elements of the blood and kidney glomerular basement membranes, and hypersensitivity re-sulting from the coating of erythrocytes or platelets by a drug.

Type III — complex-mediated hypersensitivity

This results from the effects of antigen—antibody complexes through (i) activation of complement and attraction of polymorphonuclear leucocytes which release tissue-damaging enzymes on contact with the complex, and (ii) aggregation of platelets to cause microthrombi and vasoactive amine release. Where circulating antibody levels are high, the antigen is precipitated near the site of entry into the body. The reaction in the skin is characterized by polymorph infiltration, oedema and erythema maximal at 3—8 hours (Arthus reaction). Examples are farmer's lung, pigeon fancier's disease and pulmonary aspergillosis where inhaled antigens provoke high antibody levels, reactions to an abrupt

273

increase in antigen caused by microbial cell death during chemotherapy for leprosy or syphilis, and an element of the synovial lesion in rheumatoid arthritis. In relative *antigen excess*, soluble complexes are formed which are removed by binding to the CR1 C3b receptors on red cells. If this system is overloaded or if the classical complement components are deficient, the complexes circulate in the free state and are deposited under circumstances of increased vascular permeability at certain preferred sites, the kidney glomerulus, the joints, the skin and the choroid plexus. Complexes can be detected in tissue biopsies by immunofluorescence and in serum by precipitation with polyethylene glycol, reaction with C1q, changes in C3 and C3c, and binding to the C3 receptor on the Raji cell line. Examples are: serum sickness following injection of large quantities of foreign protein, glomerulonephritis associated with systemic lupus or infections with streptococci, malaria and other parasites, neurological disturbances in systemic lupus and subacute sclerosing panencephalitis, polyarteritis nodosa linked to hepatitis B virus, and haemorrhagic shock in dengue viral infection.

Type IV — cell-mediated or delayed-type hypersensitivity

This is based upon the interaction of antigen with primed T-cells and represents tissue damage resulting from inappropriate cell-mediated immunity reactions. A number of soluble mediators (lymphokines) are released which acount for the events which occur in a typical delayed hypersensitivity response such as the Mantoux reaction to tuberculin, namely, the delayed appearance of an indurated and erythematous reaction which reaches a maximum at 24–48 hours and is characterized histologically by infiltration with mononuclear phagocytes and lymphocytes. Another subpopulation of T-cells is activated by class I major histocompatibility antigens to become directly cytotoxic to target cells bearing the appropriate antigen. *In vitro* tests for cell-mediated hypersensitivity include macrophage migration inhibition and assessment of blast cell transformation. Examples are: tissue damage occurring in bacterial (tuberculosis, leprosy), viral (smallpox, measles, herpes), fungal (candidiasis, histoplasmosis) and parasitic (leishmaniasis, schistosomiasis) infections, contact dermatitis from exposure to chromates and poison ivy, and insect bites. Continuing provocation of delayed hypersensitivity by persisting antigen leads to formation of chronic granulomata.

Type V — stimulatory hypersensitivity

This is where the antibody reacts with a key surface component such as a hormone receptor and 'switches on' the cell. An example is the thyroid hyper-reactivity in Graves' disease due to a thyroid-stimulating autoantibody.

Features of the five types of hypersensitivity are compared in table 12.3.

Table 12.3. *Comparison of different types of hypersensitivity.*

	I Anaphylactic	II Cytotoxic	III Complex-mediated	IV Cell-mediated	V Stimulatory
Antibody mediating reaction	Homocytotropic Ab Mast-cell binding	Humoral Ab ± CF*	Humoral Ab ± CF	Receptor on T-lymphocyte	Humoral Ab Non-CF
Antigen	Usually exogenous (e.g. grass pollen)	Cell surface	Extracellular	Associated with MHC antigens on macrophage or target cell	Cell surface
Response to intradermal antigen: Max. reaction Appearance	30 min (+ late reaction) Wheal and flare	—	3–8 hours Erythema and oedema	24–48 hours Erythema and induration	—
Histology	Degranulated mast cells; oedema; (late reaction cellular incl. eosinophils)	— —	Acute inflammatory reaction; predominant polymorphs	Perivascular inflammation: polymorphs migrate out leaving predominantly mononuclear cells	—
Transfer sensitivity to normal subject	◄——————————— Serum antibody ———————————►			Lymphoid cells Transfer factor	Serum antibody
Examples:	Atopic allergy, e.g. hay fever	Haemolytic disease of newborn (Rh)	Complex glomerulonephritis Farmer's lung	Mantoux reaction to TB Granulomatous reaction to schistosome eggs Contact sensitivity	Thyrotoxicosis

* CF = Complement fixation

'Innate' hypersensitivity reactions

These reactions involving excessive C3 activation are seen in disseminated intravascular coagulation produced by the Shwartzmann reaction, Gram-negative septicaemia and dengue haemorrhagic shock.

Further reading

Chapel H. & Mansell H. (eds) (1988) *Essentials of Clinical Immunology*, 2nd edn. Blackwell Scientific Publications, Oxford. (Very broad account of the diseases involving the immune system. Good illustration by case histories and the laboratory tests available. Also MCQ. One reviewer questions the adequacy of the treatment of allergy.)

Dale M.M. & Foreman J.C. (eds) (1989) *Textbook of Immunopharmacology*, 2nd edn. Blackwell Scientific Publications, Oxford.

Haeney M. (1985) *Introduction to Clinical Immunology*. Butterworths-Update, London. (In vivid technicolour; suitable for the busy clinician.)

Kazatchkin E.M. (ed.) (1989) *Bailliere's Clinical Immunology & Allergy*, vol.2, no.2. Complement and immunological disease. Academic Press, New York. (Excellent for clinician with special interest in complement and updates the non-clinical immunologist.)

Lachmann P. & Peters D.K. (eds) (1982) *Clinical Aspects of Immunology*, 4th edn. Blackwell Scientific Publications, Oxford.

Middleton E. *et al.* (eds) (1988) *Allergy: Principles and Practice*, 2nd edn. C.V. Mosby, Saint Louis, Mo.

Mygind N. (1986) *Essential Allergy*. Blackwell Scientific Publications, Oxford.

Samter M. *et al.* (eds) (1988) *Immunological Diseases*, 4th edn, vols I & II. Little Brown & Co., Boston. (Comprehensive and compendious tomes on clinical immunology by distinguished authors.)

Stiehm E.R. (ed.) (1989) *Immunologic Disorders in Infants and Children*, 3rd edn. W.B. Saunders Co., Philadelphia.

Thompson R.A. (ed.) (1985) Laboratory Investigation of Immunological Disorders. *Clinics in Immunology and Allergy*, 5. W.B. Saunders, London.

Thompson R.A. (series ed.) *Recent Advances in Clinical Immunology*. Churchill Livingstone, Edinburgh.

275

CHAPTER 13

TRANSPLANTATION

GRAFT REJECTION

The replacement of diseased organs by a transplant of healthy tissue has long been an objective in medicine but has been frustrated to no mean degree by the uncooperative attempts by the body to reject grafts from other individuals. Before discussing the nature and implications of this rejection phenomenon, it would be helpful to define the terms used for transplants between individuals and species:

Autograft — tissue grafted back on to the original donor.

Isograft — graft between syngeneic individuals (i.e. of identical genetic constitution) such as identical twins or mice of the same pure line strain.

Allograft (old term, homograft) — graft between allogeneic individuals (i.e. members of the same species but different genetic constitution), e.g. man to man and one mouse strain to another.

Xenograft (heterograft) — graft between xenogeneic individuals (i.e. of different species), e.g. pig to man.

It is with the allograft reaction that we have been most concerned although it should one day be possible to use grafts from other species. The most common allografting procedure is probably blood transfusion where the unfortunate consequences of mismatching are well known. Considerable attention has been paid to the rejection of solid grafts such as skin and the sequence of events is worth describing. In mice, for example, the skin allograft

settles down and becomes vascularized within a few days. Between three and nine days the circulation gradually diminishes and there is increasing infiltration of the graft bed with lymphocytes and monocytes but very few plasma cells. Necrosis begins to be visible macroscopically and within a day or so the graft is sloughed completely (figure 13.1).

Evidence that rejection is immunological

First and second set reactions

It would be expected, if the reaction has an immunological basis, that the second contact with antigen would represent a more explosive event than the first and indeed the rejection of a second graft from the same donor is much accelerated. The initial vascularization is poor and may not occur at all. There is a very rapid invasion by polymorphonuclear leucocytes and lymphoid cells including plasma cells. Thrombosis and acute cell destruction can be seen by three to four days.

Specificity

Second set rejection is not the fate of all subsequent allografts but only of those derived from the original donor or a related strain. Grafts from unrelated donors are rejected as first set reactions.

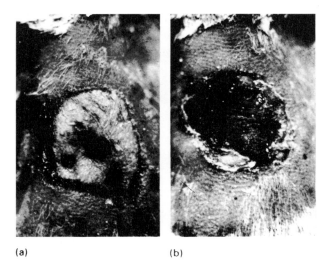

(a)   (b)

Figure 13.1. *Rejection of CBA skin graft by strain A mouse. (a) 10 days after transplantation; discoloured areas caused by destruction of epithelium and drying of the exposed dermis. (b) 13 days after transplantation; the scabby surface indicates total destruction of the graft. (Courtesy Prof. L. Brent.)*

Role of the lymphocyte

Neonatally thymectomized animals have difficulty in rejecting skin grafts but their capacity is restored by injection of lymphocytes from a syngeneic normal donor, suggesting that T-cells are implicated. The recipient of T-cells from a donor which has already rejected a graft will give accelerated rejection of a further graft of the same type (figure 13.2) showing that the lymphoid cells are primed and retain memory of the first contact with graft antigens.

Production of antibodies

After rejection, humoral antibodies with specificity for the graft donor may be recognized. In the mouse where the erythrocytes carry transplantation antigens, haemagglutination tests become positive; in the human, lymphocytotoxins are found. A Jerne plaque test using donor strain thymocytes in place of sheep erythrocytes will often demonstrate the presence of antibody-forming cells in the lymphoid tissues of grafted animals.

Genetic control of transplantation antigens

The specificity of the antigens involved in graft rejection is under genetic control. Genetically iden-

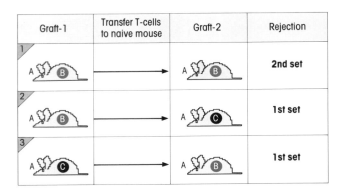

Figure 13.2. *Graft rejection induces memory which is specific and can be transferred by T-cells. In experiment 1, an A strain recipient of T-cells from another A strain mouse which had rejected a graft from strain B, will give accelerated (i.e. 2nd set) rejection of a B graft. Experiments 2 and 3 show the specificity of the phenomenon with respect to the genetically unrelated third party strain C.*

tical individuals such as mice of a pure strain or uniovular twins have identical transplantation antigens and grafts can be freely exchanged between them. The Mendelian segregation of the genes controlling these antigens has been revealed by interbreeding experiments between mice of different pure strains. Since these mice breed true within a given strain and always accept grafts from each other, they must be homozygous for the 'transplantation' genes. Consider two such strains A and B with allelic genes differing at one locus. In each case paternal and maternal genes will be identical and they will have a genetic constitution of, say, *A/A* and *B/B* respectively (by convention, the genes are expressed in italics and the antigens they encode in normal type). Crossing strains A and B gives a first familial generation (F1) of constitution *A/B*. Now all F1 mice accept grafts from either parent showing that they are tolerant to both A and B. By intercrossing the F1 generation one would expect an average distribution of genotypes for the F2s as shown in figure 13.3; only 1 in 4 would have no A genes and would therefore reject an A graft because of lack of tolerance, and 1 in 4 would reject B grafts for the same reason. Thus for each locus, 3 out of 4 of the F2 generation will accept parental strain grafts. Extending the analysis, if instead of one locus with a pair of allelic genes there were n loci, the fraction of the F2 generation accepting parental strain grafts would be $(3/4)^n$. In this way an estimate of the number of loci controlling transplantation antigens can be made.

In the mouse around 40 such loci have been

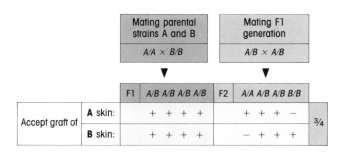

				F1	A/B	A/B	A/B	A/B	F2	A/A	A/B	A/B	B/B	
Accept graft of	**A** skin:				+	+	+	+		+	+	+	−	3/4
	B skin:				+	+	+	+		−	+	+	+	

Figure 13.3. *Inheritance of genes controlling transplantation antigens.* **A** *represents a gene expressing the A antigen and* **B** *the corresponding allelic gene at the same genetic locus. The pure strains are homozygous for* **A/A** *and* **B/B** *respectively. Since the genes are co-dominant, an animal with* **A/B** *genome will express both antigens, become tolerant to them and therefore accept grafts from either A or B donors. The illustration shows that for each gene controlling a transplantation antigen specificity, three-quarters of the F2 generation will accept a graft of parental skin. For* **n** *genes the fraction is* (3/4)^n. *If F1* **A/B** *animals are back-crossed with an* **A/A** *parent, half the progeny will be* **A/A** *and half* **A/B**; *only the latter will accept* **B** *grafts.*

established, but as we have seen much earlier, the complex locus termed H-2 predominates in the sense that it controls the 'strong' transplantation antigens which provoke intense allograft reactions and we have looked at the structure (cf. figure 3.18, p. 52) and biology of this *major histocompatibility locus* in some detail in previous chapters. The non-H-2 or 'minor' transplantation antigens such as the male H-Y are recognized as processed peptides in association with the MHC molecules on the cell surface by T-cells but not at all readily by B-cells. One should not be misled by the term 'minor' into thinking that these antigens do not give rise to serious rejection problems, albeit more slowly than the MHC.

Some other consequences of H-2 incompatibility

Class II MHC differences produce a mixed lymphocyte reaction (MLR)

When lymphocytes from strains of mice of different class II haplotype are cultured together, blast cell transformation and mitosis occurs (MLR), the T-cells of each population of lymphocytes reacting against MHC class II determinants on the surface of the other population. For the 'one-way MLR', the stimulator cells are made unresponsive by treatment with mitomycin C or X-rays and then added to

the responder lymphocytes from the other donor. The responding cells belong predominantly to a population of CD4 positive T-lymphocytes and are stimulated by the class II determinants present mostly on B-cells, macrophages and especially dendritic antigen-presenting cells. Thus, the MLR is inhibited by antisera to class II determinants on the stimulator cells.

Cell-mediated lympholysis (CML)

The involvement of class II MHC antigens in the provocation of transplantation rejection has been brought into some focus by the discovery of the phenomenon of CML which was developed as a possible test for histocompatibility. The principle is illustrated in figure 13.4. In short, responder cells activated by the class II-induced MLR help in the generation of cytotoxic T-cells directed to the H-2D/K determinants; in essence, the recognition of class II molecules helps to generate effectors against the class I molecules, in some ways reminiscent of the carrier-hapten system in T−B collaboration with class II equivalent to carrier and class I to hapten (cf. p. 121).

The graft-vs-host reaction (g.v.h.)

When competent T-cells are transferred from a donor to a recipient which is incapable of rejecting them,

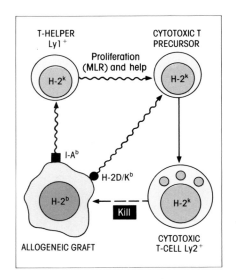

Figure 13.4. *Cell-mediated lympholysis: generation of H-2^k T-cells cytotoxic for H-2^b grafts. T-helpers respond to I-A^b on the graft cells by proliferating (mixed lymphocyte reaction) and are then able to help cytotoxic T-cell precursors specific for the H-2D^b or H-2K^b antigens of the graft to become cytotoxic effectors.*

the grafted cells survive and have time to recognize the host antigens and react immunologically against them. Instead of the normal transplantation reaction of host against graft, we have the reverse, the so-called graft-vs-host (g.v.h) reaction. In the young rodent there can be inhibition of growth (runting), spleen enlargement and haemolytic anaemia (due to production of red cell antibodies). In the human, fever, anaemia, weight loss, rash, diarrhoea and splenomegaly are observed with cytokines, especially TNF, being thought to be the major mediators of pathology. The 'stronger' the transplantation antigen difference, the more severe that reaction. Where donor and recipient differ at HLA or H-2 loci, the consequences can be fatal, although it should be noted that reactions to dominant minor transplantation antigens, or combinations of them, may be equally difficult to control.

Two possible situations leading to g.v.h. reactions are illustrated in figure 13.5. In the human this may arise in immunologically anergic subjects receiving bone marrow grafts, e.g. for combined immuno-deficiency (p. 243), for red cell aplasia after radiation accidents or as a possible form of cancer therapy. Competent T-cells in blood or present in grafted organs given to immunosuppressed patients may give g.v.h. reactions; so could maternal cells which adventitiously cross the placenta, although in this case there is as yet no evidence of diseases caused by such a mechanism in the human.

Mechanisms of graft rejection

Lymphocyte-mediated rejection

A great deal of the work on allograft rejection has involved transplants of skin or solid tumours because their fate is relatively easy to follow. In these cases there is little support for the view that humoral antibodies are instrumental in destruction of the graft although, as we shall see later, this is not necessarily so with transplants of other organs such as the kidney. Whereas passive transfer of *serum* from an animal which has rejected a skin allograft cannot usually accelerate the rejection of a similar graft on the recipient animal, injection of *lymphoid cells* (particularly recirculating small lymphocytes) is effective in shortening graft survival (cf. figure 13.2).

A primary role of lymphoid cells in first set rejection would be consistent with the histology of the early reaction showing infiltration by mononuclear

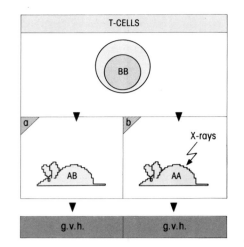

Figure 13.5. *Graft-vs-host reaction. When competent T-cells are inoculated into a host incapable of reacting against them, the grafted cells are free to react against the antigens on the host's cells which they recognize as foreign. The ensuing reaction may be fatal. Two of many possible situations are illustrated: (a) the hybrid AB receives cells from one parent (BB) which are tolerated but react against the A antigen on host cells; (b) an X-irradiated AA recipient restored immunologically with BB cells cannot react against the graft and a g.v.h. reaction will result.*

cells with very few polymorphs or plasma cells (figure 13.6). The dramatic effect of neonatal thymectomy on prolonging skin transplants, as mentioned earlier, and the long survival of grafts on children with thymic deficiencies implicate the T-lymphocytes in these reactions. In the chicken, homograft rejection and g.v.h. reactivity are influenced by neonatal thymectomy but not bursectomy. More direct evidence has come from *in vitro* studies showing that T-cells taken from mice rejecting an allograft could kill target cells bearing the graft antigens *in vitro*. Recent work on the importance of murine L3T4 and human CD4$^+$ cells as effectors has cast some doubt, probably wrongly, on the role of cytotoxic cells in graft rejection *in vivo*; although sometimes CD4 cells have cytotoxic potential for class II targets, as a rule they are associated with helper activity, in this case particularly for cytotoxic T-cell precursors, and with the production of lymphokines mediating delayed hypersensitivity reactions. Perhaps they act to encourage access of cytotoxic T-cells to their targets? We do know that IFNγ upregulates antigen expression on the target graft cell so increasing its vulnerability to CD8 cytotoxic cells.

Normal individuals have a very high frequency of alloreactive cells (i.e. cells which react with allografts) which presumably accounts for the intensity

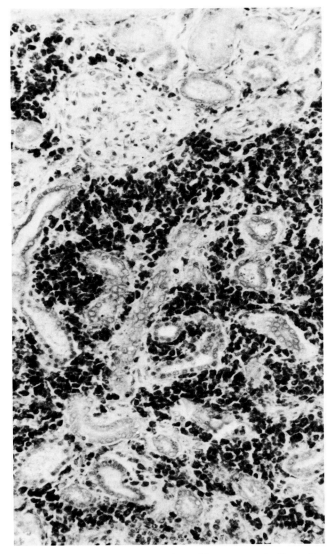

Figure 13.6. *Acute early rejection of human renal allograft 10 days after transplantation showing dense cellular infiltration of interstitium by mononuclear cells (pyronin stain). (Courtesy Prof. K. Porter.)*

The role of humoral antibody

It has long been recognized that isolated allogeneic cells such as lymphocytes can be destroyed by cytotoxic (type II) reactions involving humoral antibody. However, although earlier experience with skin and solid tumour grafts suggested that they were not readily susceptible to the action of cytotoxic antibodies, it is now clear that this does not hold for all types of organ transplants. Consideration of the different ways in which kidney allografts can be rejected illustrates the point.

1 *Hyperacute rejection* within minutes of transplantation, characterized by sludging of red cells and microthrombi in the glomeruli, occurs in individuals with pre-existing humoral antibodies— either due to blood group incompatibility or presensitization to class I MHC through blood transfusion.

2 *Acute early rejection* occurring up to 10 days or so after transplantation is characterized by dense cellular infiltration (figure 13.6) and rupture of peritubular capillaries and appears to be a cell-mediated hypersensitivity reaction involving T-lymphocytes probably compounded by CD8 cytotoxic attack on graft cells whose MHC antigen expression has been upregulated by γ-interferon.

3 *Acute late rejection*, which occurs from 11 days onwards in patients suppressed with prednisone and azathioprine, is probably caused by the binding of immunoglobulin (presumably antibody) and complement to the arterioles and glomerular capillaries where they can be visualized by immunofluorescent techniques. These immunoglobulin deposits on the vessel walls induce platelet aggregation in the glomerular capillaries leading to acute renal shutdown (figure 13.7). The possibility of damage to antibody-coated cells through antibody-dependent cell-mediated cytotoxicity must also be considered.

4 *Insidious and late rejection* associated with subendothelial deposits of immunoglobulin and C3 on the glomerular basement membranes which may sometimes be an expression of an underlying immune complex disorder (originally necessitating the transplant) or possibly of complex formation with soluble antigens derived from the grafted kidney.

The complexity of the action and interaction of cellular and humoral factors in graft rejection is therefore considerable and an attempt to summarize the postulated mechanisms involved is presented in figure 13.8.

There are also circumstances when antibodies

of MHC mismatched rejection. Now, do these alloreactive T-cells recognize just the foreign MHC molecules alone or do they respond to foreign MHC associated with a host of different peptides derived from the cytoplasmic proteins of the graft by normal processing? The latter seems to be true: alloreactive cytotoxic T-cells specific for H-2K^b expressed on the murine tumour EL-4, were unable to lyse human cells transfected with and expressing the H-2K^b molecules unless an extract of EL-4 cytoplasmic proteins, cleaved to peptides by cyanogen bromide, was added to the system. Thus, self-peptides expressed with MHC class I are responsible for allorecognition.

may actually *protect* a graft from destruction and this important phenomenon of *enhancement* will be considered further below.

THE PREVENTION OF GRAFT REJECTION

Matching tissue types on graft donor and recipient

Since MHC differences provoke the most vicious rejection of grafts, a prodigious amount of effort has gone into defining these antigen specificities in an attempt to minimize rejection by matching graft and recipient in much the same way that individuals are cross-matched for blood transfusions (incidentally, the ABO group provides strong transplantation antigens).

Methods for tissue typing

Alleles (tissue types) at the three class I loci, HLA-A, -B and -C (cf. figure 3.20, p. 54) are identified by complement-dependent cytotoxic reactions using operationally monospecific sera which are selected from patients transfused with whole blood and multigravidas who often become immunized with fetal antigens with specificities defined by paternally derived genes absent from the mother's genome. An individual is typed by setting up his lymphocytes against a panel of such sera in the presence of complement, cell death normally being judged by

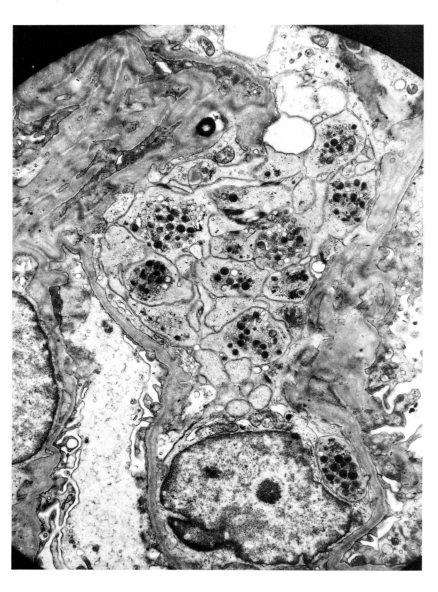

Figure 13.7. *Acute late rejection of human renal allograft showing platelet aggregation in a glomerular capillary induced by deposition of antibody on the vessel wall (electron micrograph). (Courtesy Prof. K. Porter.)*

the inability to exclude trypan blue or eosin (figure 13.9a). Each different antigen is arbitrarily assigned a numerical specificity (figure 13.10); an individual heterozygous at each locus must express four *major* class I HLA specificities and two minor ones (HLA-C) derived from both the maternal and paternal chromosomes.

The original class II locus, *HLA-D*, was defined by the mixed lymphocyte reaction (MLR) using homozygous stimulating cells for typing (figure 13.9b); if an individual fails to respond to a given typing cell then his lymphocytes must be tolerant to those specificities on the typing cells because they are already present on his own body cells. These specificities defined by T-cell recognition are designated by a Dw number (table 13.1). As serological reagents were developed it transpired that the *D* locus could be split into *DR* and *DQ* each encoding heterodimer class II molecules with homology for murine I-E and I-A respectively. Subsequently a new locus, *HLA-DP*, was discovered (figure 13.20).

HLA alleles are now defined by their gene sequences and individuals can now be typed by restriction fragment length polymorphism using DNA probes (figure 13.9c). However, it is vitally important to bear in mind the important distinction

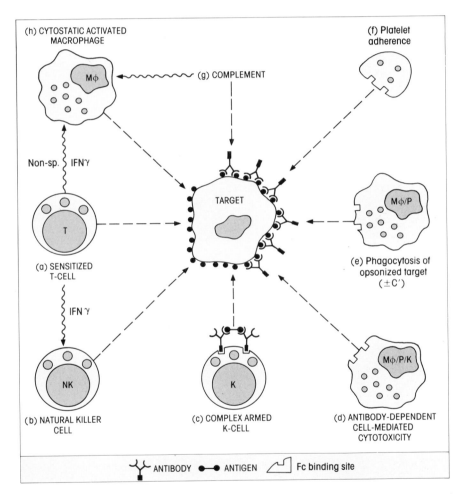

Figure 13.8. *Mechanisms of target cell destruction. Mφ = macrophage; P = polymorph; K = K cell. (a) Direct killing by cytotoxic T-cells binding through specific surface receptors. Indirect tissue damage through release of lymphokines from delayed-type hypersensitivity T-cells. (b) Killing by NK cells (p. 14) enhanced by interferon. (c) Specific killing by immune-complex-armed K-cell which recognizes target through free antibody valencies in the complex. (d) Attack by antibody-dependent cell-mediated cytotoxicity (in a—d the killing is extracellular). (e) Phagocytosis of target coated with antibody (heightened by bound C3b). (f) Sticking of platelets to antibody bound to surface of graft vascular endothelium leading to formation of microthrombi. (g) Complement-mediated cytotoxicity. (h) Macrophages activated non-specifically by agents such as BCG, endotoxin, poly-I: C, IFNγ and possibly C3b are cytostatic and sometimes cytotoxic for dividing tumour cells, perhaps through extracellular action of peroxide and O₂⁻-derived radicals generated at the cell surface (p. 7).*

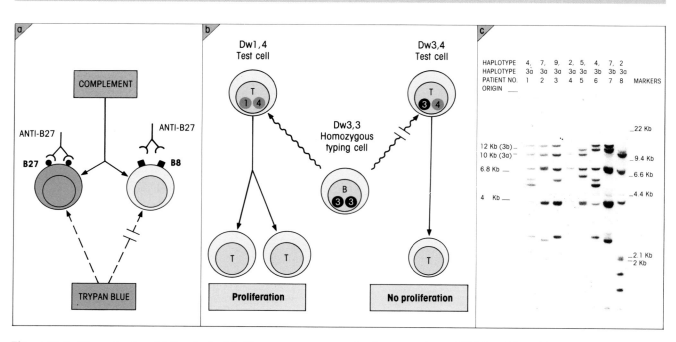

Figure 13.9. *Tissue typing. (a) Serological testing. Complement-mediated killing by mono-specific antibody allows entry of Trypan Blue. (b) Mixed lymphocyte reaction. Cells bearing the HLA-D specificity of the homozygous typing cell are tolerant to that antigen and do not respond. Cells lacking this specificity give a proliferative response measured by incorporation of [³H]thymidine. (c) Southern blot of DNA from heterozygous HLA-DR3 patients digested with TAQ1 endonuclease and hybridized with a DRβ probe showing different RFLP patterns produced by each gene. (Courtesy of R.W. Vaughan.)*

284

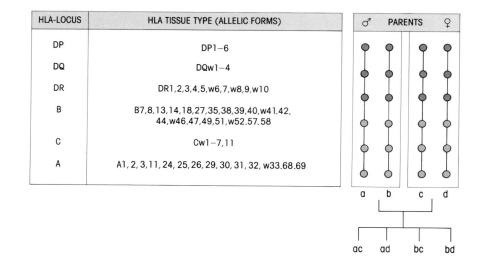

HLA-LOCUS	HLA TISSUE TYPE (ALLELIC FORMS)
DP	DP1-6
DQ	DQw1-4
DR	DR1,2,3,4,5,w6,7,w8,9,w10
B	B7,8,13,14,18,27,35,38,39,40,w41.42, 44,w46.47,49,51,w52.57.58
C	Cw1-7,11
A	A1,2,3,11,24,25,26,29,30,31,32,w33.68.69

Figure 13.10. *HLA specificities and their inheritance. The complex lies on chromosome 6, the DP locus being closest to the centromere. The numbers at the A and B loci do not overlap. For brevity, each number preceded by a stop has the w designation, e.g. w46.47, 49 ≡ w46, w47, 49. The small 'w' before a number stands for 'workshop' and indicates that the specificity concerned has not yet been characterized sufficiently for upgrading to full HLA-status. Since there are several possible alleles at each locus, the probability of a random pair of subjects from the general population having identical HLA specificities is low. However, there is a 1:4 chance that two* **siblings** *will be identical in this respect because each group of specificities on a single chromosome forms a haplotype which will be inherited* **en bloc** *giving four possible combinations of paternal and maternal chromosomes. Parent and offspring can only be identical (1:2 chance) if the mother and father have one haplotype in common.*

between typing based on T-cell discrimination and all other types of analysis because the important initial event for transplantation is the recognition of the graft antigens by *T-cells*, and antibodies do not necessarily define the same epitopes. Thus, individuals bearing the serologically defined DR4 specificities, can be subdivided by T-lymphocyte typing into several different subgroups (table 13.1). Ultimately these T-cell specificities are related to specific allelic gene sequences which encode the linear T-cell epitopes.

The polymorphism of the human HLA-system

With so many alleles at each locus and so many loci in each individual, it will readily be appreciated that this gives rise to an exceptional degree of polymorphism which is compounded further by the existence of multiple allotypic forms of the class III MHC complement components C2, C4A, C4B and factor B.

This remarkable polymorphism is of great potential value to the species since the need for T-cells to recognize their own individual specificities provides a defence against microbial molecular mimicry in which a whole species might be put at risk by its inability to recognize as foreign an organism which displays determinants similar in structure to these crucial MHC conformations. It is also possible that in some way the existence of a high degree of polymorphism helps to maintain the diversity of antigenic recognition within the lymphoid system of a given species and also ensures heterozygosity (hybrid vigour).

The value of matching tissue types

Improvements in operative techniques and the use of drugs such as cyclosporin A have greatly diminished the effects of mismatching HLA specificities on graft survival but, nevertheless, most transplanters favour a reasonable degree of matching especially at the DR locus (see figure 13.10). The consensus is that matching at the DR loci is of greater benefit than the B loci which in turn are of more relevance to graft survival than the A loci. In addition, the need for cross-matching to detect presensitized recipients is now taken very seriously.

Because of the many thousands of different HLA phenotypes possible (figure 13.10), it is usual to work with a large pool of potential recipients on a continental basis so that when graft material becomes available the best possible match be-

Table 13.1. *Subdivision of serologically-defined DR specificities using new nomenclature.*

HLA Alleles	HLA-DR specificities (antibody-defined)		HLA-D associated (T-cell defined)
	Old	New	
DRB1*0101	DR1	DR1	Dw1
DRB1*0102	DR1	DR1	Dw20
DRB1*0103	DR1	DR'BR'	Dw'BON'
DRB1*1501	DR2	DRw15	Dw2
DRB1*1502	DR2	DRw15	Dw12
DRB1*1601	DR2	DRw16	Dw21
DRB1*1602	DR2	DRw16	Dw22
DRB1*0301	DR3	DRw17	Dw3
DRB1*0302	DR3	DRw18	Dw'RSH'
DRB1*0401	DR4	DR4	Dw4
DRB1*0402	DR4	DR4	Dw10
DRB1*0403	DR4	DR4	Dw13
DRB1*0404	DR4	DR4	Dw14
DRB1*0405	DR4	DR4	Dw15
DRB1*0406	DR4	DR4	Dw'KT2'
DRB1*0407	DR4	DR4	Dw13
DRB1*0408	DR4	DR4	Dw14
DRB1*1101	DR5	DRw11	Dw5
DRB1*1102	DR5	DRw11	Dw'JVM'
DRB1*1103	DR5	DRw11	—
DRB1*1104	DR5	DRw11	Dw'FS'
DRB1*1201	DR5	DRw12	Dw'DB6'
DRB1*1301	DRw6	DRw13	Dw18
DRB1*1302	DRw6	DRw13	Dw19
DRB1*1303	DRw6	DRw13	Dw'HAG'
DRB1*1401	DRw6	DRw14	Dw9
DRB1*1402	DRw6	DRw14	Dw16
DRB1*0701	DR7	DR7	Dw17
DRB1*0702	DR7	DR7	Dw'DB1'
DRB1*0801	DRw8	DRw8	Dw8.1
DRB1*0802	DRw8	DRw8	Dw8.2
DRB1*0803	DRw8	DRw8	Dw8.3
DRB1*0901	DR9	DR9	Dw23
DRB1*1001	DRw10	DRw10	—

DRB1*0302 = *HLA-DR β-chain locus no. 1* main gene sequence no. 3, minor sequence variant no. 2. The specificities apply to the peptide gene products.*

made. The position will be improved when the pool of available organs can be increased through the development of long-term tissue storage banks but techniques are not good enough for this at present except in the case of bone marrow cells which can be kept viable even after freezing and thawing. With a paired organ such as the kidney, living donors may be used; siblings provide the best chance of a good match (cf. figure 13.10). However, the use of living donors poses difficult ethical problems and there has been encouraging progress in the use of cadaver material. Some groups are looking at the possibility of animal organs or mechanical substitutes while some are even trying to prevent the disease in the first place!

Agents producing general immunosuppression

Graft rejection can be held at bay by the use of agents which non-specifically interfere with the induction or expression of the immune response. Because these agents are non-specific, patients on immunosuppressive therapy tend to be susceptible to infections; they are also more prone to develop lymphoreticular cancers.

Targetting lymphoid populations

Anti-CD3 monoclonals are in widespread use as anti-T-cell reagents to successfully reverse acute graft rejection. They produce a complex flu-like clinical syndrome which includes fever, chills, headache and gastrointestinal discomfort associated with an increase in serum IFNγ, TNFα and often IL-2, presumably resulting from T-cell activation. Like other monoclonal antibodies reacting with cell-surface antigens, the anti-CD3 immunoglobulins have a propensity to evoke neutralizing anti-idiotypes, but this problem can be circumvented by using a succession of different anti-CD3s. Xenosensitization to the mouse monoclonal can be avoided either by 'humanizing' the antibody (p. 139) or by injecting under an umbrella of anti-CD4 which allows the host to become tolerant to the murine Ig epitopes.

The IL-2 receptor β-chain represents another potential target and attachment of a chelate containing β-emitting isotopes to monoclonal anti-IL-2R gave marked prolongation of heart xenografts in monkeys. Results with conjugates of the monoclonal with ricin A-chain toxin are not too encouraging because, although the molecule is internalized slowly in coated pits and thence into endosomic vesicles, it does not pass easily into the cytosol where it has its toxic action on elongation of factor-2. A somewhat similar strategy is to construct a fusion protein of IL-2 itself with PE-40, the truncated pseudomonas exotoxin which should be taken up selectively by cells bearing IL-2 receptors. Following the relative ease of engraftment of allogeneic bone marrow in patients with a deficiency of the 'adhesin' molecule LFA-1 (p. 119), attention is now turning to the use of anti-LFA-1 as an immunosuppressant for such grafts.

Total lymphoid irradiation (TLI)

Fractionated irradiation focused on the lymphoid tissues with shielding of marrow, lungs and other vital non-lymphoid tissue, has been used in humans to treat Hodgkin's disease for over 20 years. When mice given similar treatment are injected with allogeneic bone marrow, they fully accept the graft and show no signs of graft-vs-host disease which would normally occur. Furthermore, the chimaerism (co-existence of both donor and host cells) is permanent and such mice will accept grafts of other tissue from the bone marrow donor strain. The irradiation induces the formation of large granular lymphocytes lacking T, B and macrophage markers which non-specifically suppress the antigen-specific cytolytic arm of allogeneic immune reactions while at the same time facilitating the development of antigen-specific suppressors which maintain tolerance. That TLI can induce true transplantation tolerance to renal allografts in the human is suggested by the fact that three patients receiving this form of therapy prior to engraftment had still not rejected their kidneys after 6 years without any further immunosuppression.

Immunosuppressive drugs

The development of an immunological response requires the active proliferation of a relatively small number of antigen-sensitive lymphocytes to give a population of sensitized cells large enough to be effective. Many of the immunosuppressive drugs now employed were first used in cancer chemotherapy because of their toxicity to dividing cells. Aside from the complications of blanket immunosuppression mentioned above, these antimitotic drugs are especially toxic for cells of the bone marrow and small intestine and must therefore be used with great care.

One of the most commonly used drugs in this field is *azathioprine* which has a preferential effect on T-cell mediated reactions. It is broken down in the body first to 6-mercaptopurine and then converted to the active agent, the ribotide. Because of the similarity in shape (figure 13.11), this competes with inosinic acid for enzymes concerned in the synthesis of guanylic and adenylic acids; it also inhibits the synthesis of 5-phosphoribosylamine, a precursor of inosinic acid, by a feedback mechanism. The net result is inhibition of nucleic acid synthesis. Another drug, methotrexate, through its

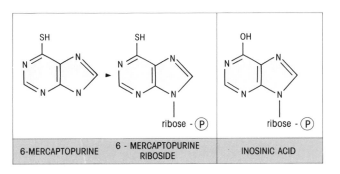

Figure 13.11. *Metabolic conversion of azathioprine through 6-mercaptopurine to the ribotide: similarity to inosinic acid with which it competes.*

action as a folic acid antagonist also inhibits synthesis of nucleic acid. The N-mustard derivative cyclophosphamide probably attacks DNA by alkylation and cross-linking so preventing correct duplication during cell division. These agents appear to exert their damaging effects on cells during mitosis and for this reason are most powerful when administered after presentation of antigen at a time when the antigen-sensitive cells are dividing.

Cyclosporin A, a neutral hydrophobic cyclical peptide containing 11 amino acids, represents an exciting and entirely new class of compound which is having a dramatic impact on the human transplantation scene. It is an extremely insoluble fungal metabolite which is of particular interest since it penetrates antigen-sensitive T-cells in the G_0 to G_1 phase and selectively blocks the transcription of lymphokine mRNA, perhaps through binding with high affinity to cytophilin, which has been identified as peptidyl-prolyl isomerase, an enzyme involved in protein folding. Resting cells which carry the vital memory for immunity to microbial infections are spared and there is little toxicity for dividing cells in gut and bone marrow. Some studies also point to an 'exquisite' sensitivity of the dendritic antigen-presenting cells to the drug. What is really striking is that in some cases it has been possible to show that cyclosporin treatment has led to the development of *specific* T-suppressor cells which could actively maintain tolerance (see figure 13.15 for an experimental example). Benefits of cyclosporin in diseases such as idiopathic nephrotic syndrome, type 1 insulin-dependent diabetes and psoriasis have been interpreted to suggest or confirm a pathogenic role for the immune system. However, effects not only on Langerhans dendritic cells but also on proliferation of normal and transformed

keratinocytes *in vitro* may contribute to the favourable outcome in psoriasis. A rapid onset of benefit, and relapse when treatment is stopped, are common features of cyclosporin therapy.

There are, of course, side-effects. It has to be used at doses below those causing nephrotoxicity so that blood levels have to be monitored regularly by radioimmunoassay. There is also some cause for concern that cyclosporin may make patients susceptible to EB virus-induced lymphomas since the drug inhibits T-cells which control EB virus transformation of B-cells *in vitro*; however, the latest results suggest that the incidence of lymphoma is relatively low in comparison with that reported for allografted patients on conventional immunosuppressive therapy. Cyclosporin is proving to be of great clinical value (see figure 13.12 as an example of its use in cardiac transplantation).

Another T-cell-specific immunosuppressive drug, FK-506 (figure 13.13), recently isolated from a species of streptomyces, synergizes with cyclosporin in blocking lymphokine production. It has a greatly superior potency to cyclosporin on a molar basis but is seriously toxic in non-human primates. Although structurally distinct from cyclosporin, FK-506 also binds to and inhibits a peptidyl-prolyl

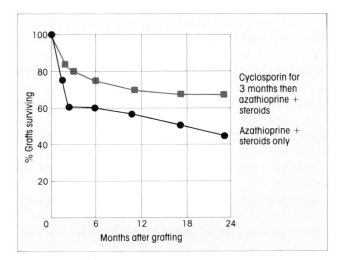

Figure 13.12. *Efficacy of initial short-term treatment with cyclosporin for the survival of cardiac allografts. After 3 months on cyclosporin A, the first group were then switched to the conventional therapy of azathioprine and steroids used throughout for the control group; 54 patients on cyclosporin, 60 in the other group. Some transplanters use cyclosporin alone as the only form of immunosuppression. (Reproduced from Morris P.J. (1985)* **Transplantation Proceedings XVII,** *1153, with permission.)*

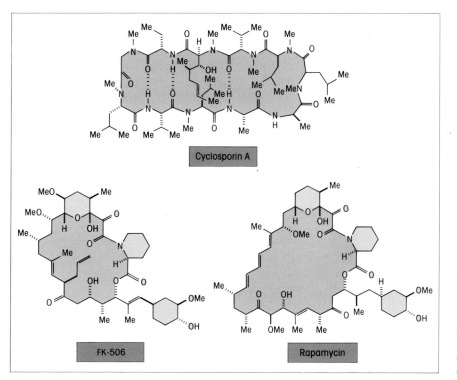

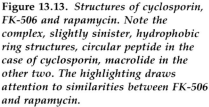

Figure 13.13. *Structures of cyclosporin, FK-506 and rapamycin. Note the complex, slightly sinister, hydrophobic ring structures, circular peptide in the case of cyclosporin, macrolide in the other two. The highlighting draws attention to similarities between FK-506 and rapamycin.*

isomerase but this is not the same protein as that which reacts with cyclosporin and neither do both drugs show cross-inhibition. It must be admitted that the relevance of this enzymic proclivity to T-cell activation remains obscure. None the less, a new door has been opened with respect to the development of agents with selective action against T-lymphocytes. The latest addition to the stable is rapamycin, a product of the fungus *Streptomyces hygroscopicus*, which is a macrolide like FK-506, and is more active than cyclosporin when given by the intraperitoneal route post-transplant.

Steroids such as prednisone intervene at many points in the immune response, affecting lymphocyte recirculation and the generation of cytotoxic effector cells, for example; in addition, their outstanding anti-inflammatory potency rests on features such as inhibition of neutrophil adherence to vascular endothelium in an inflammatory area and suppression of monocyte/macrophage functions such as microbicidal activity and response to lymphokines. Corticosteroids form complexes with intracellular receptors which then bind to regulatory genes and block transcription of TNF, IFNγ, IL-1, IL-2, IL-3, IL-6 and MHC class II, i.e. they block expression of lymphokines and monokines whereas cyclosporin has its main action on lymphokines. In another twist to the tale, one of the corticosteroids was idiosyncratic in its ability to block angiogenesis in chronic granulomatous reactions without any effect on the chronic inflammatory response; anti-inflammatory steroids usually show the converse.

Strategies for antigen-specific depression of allograft reactivity

If the disadvantages of blanket immunosuppression are to be avoided, we must aim at knocking out only the reactivity of the host to the antigens of the graft, leaving the remainder of the immunological apparatus intact. One approach is through the induction of tolerance. Total lymph node irradiation plus bone marrow (*vide supra*) is known to induce T-suppression in mice, and grafts of skin and heart from the same donor enjoy prolonged survival. As cloned histocompatibility antigens are available, it should ultimately not be beyond the wit of *Homo sapiens* to juggle the relative timing and dosages of antigen and various immunosuppressants to produce a specific hyporesponsive state.

One hopeful strategy seems to be emerging. The object must be to manipulate peripheral tolerance—inducing mechanisms for T-cells since it is not possible in the adult to induce central, i.e. thymic, tolerance except perhaps to bone marrow transplants. Let us start with the observation that xenogeneic rat anti-CD4 induces tolerance in mice to rat immunoglobulin and other antigens injected at the same time. This is not due to ablation of CD4 T-cells and therefore we must deduce that antigen provides a tolerogenic signal when presented to helper T-cells whose CD4 molecules have reacted with antibody. The same must apply to CD8 cells since 3 weeks' therapy with a mixture of rat IgG anti-CD4 and anti-CD8 monoclonals permitted an $H-2^k$ mouse to retain an $H-2^b$ skin allograft for a prolonged period (figure 13.14)—quite a feat! Second set skin grafts in these tolerant donors were slowly rejected, perhaps indicating that processed cyto-plasmic peptides are presented in the period after new grafting but disappear in longer term grafts. This tolerogenic regimen also permitted the survival of second set grafts involving multiple minor trans-plantation antigens in mice already sensitized by a first graft. These non-depleting immunosuppressive monoclonals induce unresponsiveness in those T-cells which specifically interact with antigen during the period of treatment, leaving the remainder of the T-cell population free to react with infectious agents subsequently. The specifically anergic cells also appear to induce tolerance in newly emerging antigen-specific cells arising in the thymus pro-viding the presence of antigen is maintained. Looking ahead to possible use in human transplants, it is envisaged that the body T-cell mass would be 'debulked' by repeated injection of humanized Campath 1 (anti-CDw52), an anti-lymphocyte monoclonal, so that only a relatively small number of remaining lymphocytes would need to be toler-ized. One is inclined to bet that this whole approach will become one of the most important therapeutic strategies.

Full-frontal attack by antigen itself is also possible provided it is presented in a tolerogenic form. Thus, syngeneic mouse tumour cells transfected with the $H-2K^b$ antigen were able to prolong the survival of $H-2^b$ heart allografts in $H-2^k$ mice. Autologous bone marrow stem cells would be possible targets for transfection by genes coding for the intended graft antigens, perhaps under a safety umbrella of non-depleting anti-CD4. Needless to say, we have much more to learn about the consequences of such ma-

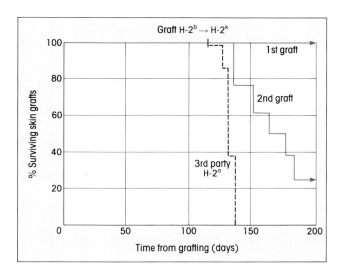

Figure 13.14. *Tolerance of CBA/Ca mice to skin grafts from H-2 + minor mismatched donors (C57/BL.10 to CBA/Ca) induced by concurrent injection of anti-CD4 and anti-CD8. CBA/Ca (H-2^k) mice received tail skin from C57/BL.10 (H-2^b) mice under cover of CD4 and CD8 monoclonal antibody therapy. Test groups received 2 depleting doses of the rat IgG2b CD4 and CD8 synergistic sets (800μg total Mab per mouse), followed by the non-depleting rat IgG2a Mabs up to 3 weeks. All animals received fresh grafts after 4 months. All the first B10 grafts have remained intact (>200 days). Second B10 grafts have rejected at a relatively slow rate (median survival time {MST} = 44 days). Third party BALB/c grafts were rejected promptly (MST = 13 days). (From Waldmann H., Cobbold S.P. & Qin S. (1989)* **Progress in Immunology,** 7, 147. Melchers F. et al. (eds). Springer Verlag, Berlin.)*

nipulations in model systems before contemplating intervention in human subjects, let alone over-coming the technical difficulties in the actual trans-fection of stem cells.

On rather a different tack, it has been reported that tolerance between rodent strains can be estab-lished by deliberate autoimmunization with the idiotype of the host receptor for donor transplan-tation antigens. It now appears that the same effect can be achieved more reliably and somewhat unexpectedly by cyclosporin A treatment of rats receiving kidney allografts. The experiments de-scribed in figure 13.15a show that spleen T-cells from cyclosporin-A-treated rats bearing a long-standing kidney allograft can suppress graft rejec-tion in a naïve animal. The suppressors proliferate *in vitro* when stimulated by blast cells generated by exposure of host strain T-cells to graft antigens and it is concluded that the suppressors are directed to the idiotype of the cells capable of recognizing the graft (figure 13.15c). Another important feature of

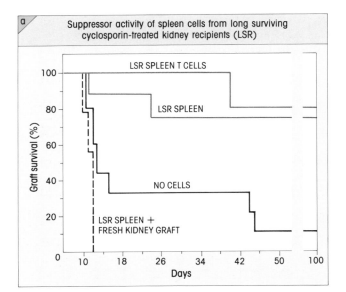

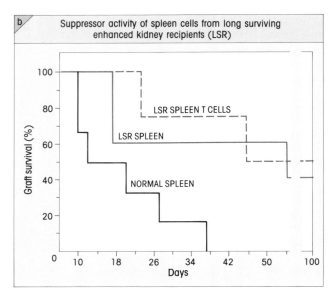

Figure 13.15. *Long-term survival of kidney grafts maintained by T-suppressors induced by enhancement or cyclosporin. Naïve rats were injected with spleen cells from rats treated with cyclosporin (a) or enhancing antibodies (b), carrying long-standing kidney allografts. Unless stated as 'fresh', the grafts had been 'parked' in a cyclosporin or enhanced animal to eliminate immunogenic passenger cells. The mechanism (c) is thought to involve loss of passenger cells and generation of anti-idiotypic T-suppressors. (Data in (a) and (b) reproduced from Batchelor J.R. & Ch. Y.L. (1986) In **Progress in Immunology VI** p. 1002, Cinader B. and Miller R.G. (eds), Academic Press, with permission.)*

290

these experiments is that suppression is only effective when the grafted kidney is one which has been 'parked' for some time in a cyclosporin-treated recipient; fresh kidneys are rejected normally. A likely interpretation is that passenger B-lymphocytes and dendritic accessory cells rich in class II Ia antigens which are far and away the most immunogenic cells in tissue grafts, are eliminated from the 'parked' kidney graft by the cyclosporin. The argument would be that graft antigens presented on donor dendritic cells provoke powerful rejection by direct stimulation of the appropriate T-helpers, whereas in the absence of dendritic cells, the graft antigens would have to be presented after

processing by host cells in association with host class II and under the influence of cyclosporin this allows a build-up of inhibitory anti-idiotype T-suppressors.

Rather comparable mechanisms operate in the survival of kidney grafts produced by the technique of *immunological enhancement*. It has long been recognized that deliberate immunization of animals with irradiated tumour cells produces enhancing antibodies which prolong the life of the tumour. Somewhat comparable manipulations can also enhance the survival of kidney grafts and again it transpires that, as with cyclosporin, two major events occur, the elimination of immunogenic passenger cells and the generation of anti-idiotype suppressors (figure 13.15b).

It is relevant that thyroid, parathyroid and islets of Langerhans, after culture for several days in 95% oxygen, are readily accepted as allografts and this has been attributed to loss of Ia-positive dendritic cells; such grafts are rapidly rejected if the recipient is injected with as few as 10^3 peritoneal cells of donor origin which potently present allogeneic class I in the context of allogeneic class II.

CLINICAL EXPERIENCE IN GRAFTING

Privileged sites

Corneal grafts survive without the need for immunosuppression. Because they are avascular they do not sensitize the recipient although they become cloudy if the individual has been pre-sensitized. Grafts of cartilage are successful in the same way but an additional factor is the protection afforded the chondrocytes by the matrix. With bone and artery it doesn't really matter if the grafts die because they can still provide a framework for host cells to colonize.

Kidney grafts

Thousands of kidneys have been transplanted and with improvement in patient management there is a high survival rate (figure 13.16). Matching at the HLA-D locus has a strong effect on graft survival but in the long term (5 years or more) the desirability of reasonable HLA-B, and to a lesser extent HLA-A, matching also becomes apparent. It has now been firmly established that multiple blood transfusions prior to grafting have a significant beneficial effect on survival (figure 13.16) presumably due to tolerance induction of some kind.

DRw6-positive individuals are rather intriguing. They are relatively poor at accepting DRw6-negative grafts while their kidneys survive relatively well as grafts (table 13.2). The conjecture is that in the recipient, DRw6 is a good immune response (Ir) gene for class II antigens and that when DRw6 is present on a graft it is a good inducer of T-suppression.

Patients are partially immunosuppressed at the time of transplantation because uraemia causes a degree of immunological anergy. The combination of azathioprine and prednisone is commonly employed in the long-term management of kidney grafts but replacement of the azathioprine with cyclosporin A looks very promising. If kidney function is poor during a rejection crisis renal dialysis can be used. When transplantation is performed because of immune complex induced glomerulonephritis, the immunosuppressive treatment used may help to prevent a similar lesion developing in the grafted kidney. Patients with glomerular basement membrane antibodies (e.g. Goodpasture's syndrome) are likely to destroy their renal transplants unless first treated with plasmapheresis and immunosuppressive drugs.

Table 13.2. *HLA-DRw6 and graft survival two years post-transplant.*

RECIPIENT	DR MISMATCHES	DONOR DRw6 POSITIVE	DONOR DRw6 NEGATIVE
DRw6	0	80%	—
POSITIVE	1	78%	50%
(n = 303)	2	—	50%
DRw6	0	—	71%
NEGATIVE	1	75%	63%
(n = 852)	2	81%	62%

Note DRw6+ grafts do better than DRw6−, and DRw6− grafts do worse in DRw6+ than in DRw6− unmatched recipients.

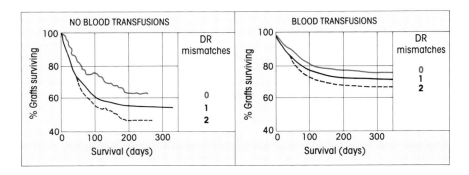

Figure 13.16. *Effect of DR mismatches and of prior blood transfusions on the survival of cadaver renal transplants. (Reproduced from Opelz G. (1985) Transpl. Proc. XVII, 1015, with permission.) Most centres now report very high survival rates of 85−90% at one year even in high risk situations.*

291

Heart transplants

The 1-year survival figure for heart transplants has moved up to around the 80% mark (figure 13.17), helped considerably by the introduction of cyclosporin A therapy. Its nephrotoxicity is a drawback, however, and some groups switch over to conventional treatment with azathioprine plus steroids (cf. figure 13.14). Full HLA matching is of course not practical but single DR mismatches gave 90% survival at 3 years compared with a figure of 65% for two DR mismatches. Aside from the rejection problem it is likely that the number of patients who would benefit from cardiac replacement is much greater than the number dying with adequately healthy hearts. More attention will have to be given to the possibility of xenogeneic grafts and mechanical substitutes.

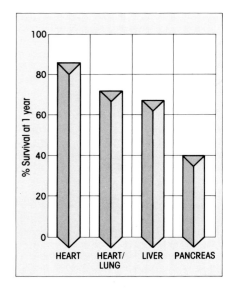

Figure 13.17. *Survival of organ allografts at 1 year. (Data from Batchelor J.R. & Ch. Y.L. (1986) In* **Progress in Immunology VI,** *p.1002, Cinader B. and Miller R.G. (eds), Academic Press, with permission.)*

Liver transplants

Survival rates for orthotopic liver grafts are broadly in line with those receiving heart transplants (figure 13.17), particularly using combined cyclosporin/steroid therapy. Rejection crises are dealt with by high dose steroids and if this proves ineffective, anti-lymphocyte globulin. The use of a totally synthetic colloidal hydroxyethyl starch solution containing lactobionate as a substitute for chloride, allows livers to be preserved for 24 hours or more and has revolutionized the logistics of liver transplantation. To improve the prognosis of patients with primary hepatic or bile duct malignancies which were considered to be inoperable, transplantation of organ clusters with liver as the central organ has been designed, e.g. liver and pancreas, or liver, pancreas, stomach and small bowel or even colon. None the less the outcome is not very favourable in that up to three-quarters of the patients transplanted for hepatic cancer have had recurrence of their tumour within one year.

Experience with liver grafting between pigs revealed an unexpected finding. Many of the animals retained the grafted organs in a healthy state for many months without any form of immunosuppression. The transplanted liver represented a large antigen pool which induced a state of unresponsiveness to grafts of skin or kidney from the same donor. The mechanism is not clear but may involve true tolerance or enhancement. There is as yet no evidence that this highly desirable state can be established by a hepatic transplant in man.

Work is in progress on the transfer of isolated hepatocytes attached to collagen-coated microcarriers injected i.p. for the correction of isolated deficiencies such as albumin synthesis. This attractive approach could have much wider applications although in the distant future it will presumably run into competition from gene therapy.

Bone marrow grafting

Patients with certain immunodeficiency disorders and aplastic anaemia are obvious candidates for treatment with bone marrow stem cells as are acute leukaemia patients treated radically with intensive chemotherapy and possibly whole body irradiation in attempts to eradicate the neoplastic cells (table 13.3). Successful results with bone marrow transfers require highly compatible donors if fatal graft-vs-host reactions are to be avoided, and here siblings offer the best chance of finding a matched donor (figure 13.10). Matching for antigens quite distinct from those controlled by the major HLA loci may prove to be essential. The incidence of chronic graft-vs-host disease is reduced if T-cells in the grafted marrow are first removed by a cytotoxic cocktail of anti-T-cell monoclonals and significant improvements have also been reported both for success of primary engraftment and the

DISEASE		PROBABILITY	
TYPE	STAGE	LONG-TERM SURVIVAL	DISEASE RECURRENCE
Acute leukaemia	Relapse	0.1–0.3	0.60
Acute non-lymphocytic leukaemia	1st remission	0.6	0.25
Acute lymphocytic leukaemia	2nd remission	0.3	0.25
Chronic granulocytic leukaemia	Blastic phase	0.2	0.70
Chronic granulocytic leukaemia	Accelerated phase	0.2	0.50
Chronic granulocytic leukaemia	Chronic phase	0.6	0.30
Severe combined immunodeficiency	—	0.5	—
Severe aplastic anaemia	—	0.8	—
Thalassemia major	—	0.7	0.3

Table 13.3. *Bone marrow transplants: summary of survival and relapse data from many centres.*

prevention of g.v.h. disease when patients are treated with cyclosporin A. However, g.v.h. disease could arise by a curious mechanism involving the sneaking through of autoreactive T-cells which fail to be deleted in the thymus possibly because of thymic damage due to pre- or post-transplant therapy, e.g. associated viral infection, irradiation or even cyclosporin itself. It may be significant that cyclosporin inhibits the programmed cell death of immature thymocytes which occurs on activation by anti-CD3 and it is known that an autologous 'g.v.h.' supervenes on termination of prolonged cyclosporin administration to young irradiated rats which had received syngeneic bone marrow. A curious effect that requires further exploration is the observation that leukaemia patients with g.v.h. disease have a lower incidence of relapse. An interesting practical point: cord blood contains sufficient haemopoietic stem cells for bone marrow transplantation.

Other organs

It is to be expected that improvement in techniques of control of the rejection process will encourage transplantation in several other areas — not cases of endocrine disorders where exogeneous replacement therapy is convenient, but, for example, in diabetes the number of transplants recorded is rising rapidly and the current success rate is around 40% (figure 13.17. There is talk of prolonged survival of xenogeneic islets given with immunosuppressive monoclonal anti-CD4. One looks forward in particular to the successful transplantation of skin for lethal burns.

ASSOCIATION OF HLA TYPE WITH DISEASE

Linkage disequilibrium and disease susceptibility

An impressive body of data is accumulating which links specific HLA antigens with particular disease states in the human (table 13.4) and even more striking relationships may be uncovered as the complexity of the HLA-D region is unravelled. The relationships are influenced by *linkage disequilibrium*, a state where closely linked genes on a chromosome tend to remain associated rather than undergo genetic randomization in a given population, so that the frequency of a pair of alleles occurring together is greater than the product of the individual gene frequencies (figure 13.18a). This could result from natural selection favouring a particular haplotype or from insufficient time elapsing since the first appearance of closely located alleles to allow them to become randomly distributed throughout the population. Be that as it may, a significant association between a disease and a given HLA specificity does not imply that we have identified the disease susceptibility gene because we might find an even better correlation with another HLA gene in linkage disequilibrium with the first. To take an example: in multiple sclerosis, an association with the B7 allele was first established but when patients were typed for the D locus, a much stronger correlation with DR2 emerged (figure 13.18b). The initial correlation with B7 resulted from linkage disequilibrium between B7 and DR2. We

293

Table 13.4. *Association of HLA with disease.*

DISEASE	HLA ALLELE	RELATIVE RISK
a Class II associated		
Hashimoto's disease	DR5	3.2
Rheumatoid arthritis	DR4	5.8
Dermatitis herpetiformis	DR3	56.4
Chronic active hepatitis (autoimmune)	DR3	13.9
Coeliac disease	DR3	10.8
Sjögren's syndrome	DR3	9.7
Addison's disease (adrenal)	DR3	6.3
Insulin-dependent diabetes	DR3	5.0
	DR4	6.8
	DR3/4	14.3
	DR2	0.2
Thyrotoxicosis (Graves')	DR3	3.7
Primary myxoedema	DR3	5.7
Goodpasture's syndrome	DR2	13.1
Tuberculoid leprosy	DR2	8.1
Multiple sclerosis	DR2	4.8
b Class I, HLA-B27 associated		
Ankylosing spondylitis	B27	87.4
Reiter's diesase	B27	37.0
Post-salmonella arthritis	B27	29.7
Post-shigella arthritis	B27	20.7
Post-yersinia arthritis	B27	17.6
Post-gonococcal arthritis	B27	14.0
Uveitis	B27	14.6
Amyloidosis in rheumatoid arthritis	B27	8.2
c Other class I associations		
Subacute thyroiditis	Bw35	13.7
Psoriasis vulgaris	Cw6	13.3
Idiopathic haemochromatosis	A3	8.2
Myasthenia gravis	B8	4.4

(Data mainly from Ryder et al.: see legend to figure 13.18.)

still cannot be sure that DR2 itself is the disease susceptibility gene since, carrying the argument a stage further, one cannot exclude the possibility of finding an even greater association with another closely linked gene especially since 17 new genes have been described in the region between the complement and HLA-B loci.

Ethnic studies may help by making available recombination events which alter haplotypes and permit the identification of susceptibility determinants outside their normal context. Thus, the DQα linked to DR7 on the Caucasian haplotype has a neutral effect on diabetes susceptibility but, in the black population, DR7 is associated with a different DQα and now becomes a susceptibility haplotype.

Association with immunological diseases

With the odd exception such as idiopathic haemochromatosis and congenital adrenal hyperplasia resulting from a 21-hydroxylase deficiency, HLA-linked diseases are intimately bound up with immunological processes. By and large, the HLA-D related disorders are autoimmune with a tendency for DR3 to be associated with organ-specific diseases involving cell surface receptors. The question of some link between DR3 and these receptors has been mooted, though not with much confidence. It

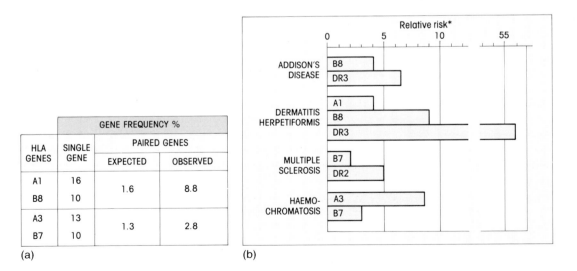

(a)　　　　　　　　　　　　　　　(b)

Figure 13.18. *Linkage disequilibrium and the association between HLA and disease. (a) Two examples of linkage disequilibrium. The expected frequency for a pair of genes is the product of each individual gene frequency. B8 and DR3 are in linkage disequilibrium as are B7 and DR2; thus the haplotypes A1, B8, DR3 and A3, B7, DR2 are* **relatively**

common. (b) Influence of linkage disequilibrium on disease association. * Relative risk: the increased chance of contracting the disease for individuals bearing the antigen relative to those lacking it. (Data from Ryder L.P., Andersen E. & Svejgaard A. (1979) HLA and disease Registry 1979. **Tissue Antigens, Supplement.)**

has also been suggested that HLA antigens might also affect the susceptibility of a cell to viral attachment or infection, thereby influencing the development of autoimmunity to associated surface components.

Inevitably, because class II genes tend to be dominant in these relationships (for the time being), the temptation is to think in terms of immune response genes controlling the nature of the reaction to the relevant autoantigen or to whatever might be a causative agent. On this basis, DR3 and DR4 must influence separate but synergistic immune responses which mediate the onset of insulin-dependent diabetes. Actually, susceptibility in DR4 subjects is more closely related to the DQB.3.2 gene which is in linkage disequilibrium with DR4 and like the class II I-Aβ gene in the non-obese diabetic (NOD) mouse which spontaneously models the pancreatic islet cell autoimmunity of the patients, residue 57 is a serine instead of the aspartic acid present in nearly all normal individuals. The importance of this residue for disease production is clearly brought out by the observation that transgenic mice carrying an NOD I-Aβ gene in which aspartic is substituted for serine do not develop diabetes. The orientation of the aspartic residue in the class II α-helix suggests that it may form a salt bridge with a side-chain at position 79 on the opposing α-helix and that its replacement may influence the binding of an antigenic peptide to the groove.

DR4 and to a lesser extent DR1 are risk factors for rheumatoid arthritis in white Caucasians. Analysis of DR4 subgroups, and of other ethnic populations where the influence of DR4 is minimal, has identified a particular linear T-cell epitope as the disease susceptibility element and the variations observed are based on sharing of this epitope with other HLA-DR specificities which presumably arose from the recombination and gene conversion events responsible for MHC polymorphism. Unlike the situation in diabetes, these susceptibility residues are in positions on the α-helix which contact T-cells.

In both diabetes and in rheumatoid arthritis, the DR2 allele is under-represented and DR2-positive patients have less severe disease, implying that DR2 might be considered a poor-responder gene. In the case of multiple sclerosis where DR2 is a major risk factor, it is conceivable that these individuals are poor T-cell responders to measles since defective cell-mediated immunity to this virus is to date the only major immunological abnormality recognized. Direct associations with responses to infection have

been documented. A rather complex example is provided by a single antigen from *Schistosoma japonicum* where, in a given haplotype, the DR molecule is implicated in proliferative T-cell responses while the DQ1 element controls a dominant non-responsive state. However, the B7 allele which we have seen contributes to the multiple sclerosis susceptibility haplotype also correlates positively with an increased incidence of paralytic polio and with relatively poor T-cell activity *in vitro* for heterologous target cells. This raises another interpretation of this phenomenon, which does not necessarily exclude some contribution from immune response genes, in which it is postulated that individual DR alleles or even the whole MHC 'superhaplotype' of which they are part, control overall cellular interactions and reactivity rather than individual antigenic specificities. In this connection it is worthy of note that the relationship of MHC to disease resistance and vaccine efficacy in farm animals is beginning to preoccupy veterinary scientists; it is known for instance, that susceptibility to Marek's disease in White Leghorn chickens is associated with distinct MHC haplotypes.

The association with HLA in ankylosing spondylitis is quite extraordinary; up to 95% of patients are of B27 phenotype as compared with around 5% in controls. The incidence of B27 is also markedly raised in other conditions when accompanied by sacro-iliitis, e.g. Reiter's disease, acute anterior uveitis, psoriasis and other forms of infective sacro-iliitis such as yersinia, gonococcal and salmonella arthritis. The very close association with B27 makes it unlikely that as good a correlation with any other gene will be found. The involvement of infective agents may provide a clue: does molecular similarity to B27 imply a tolerance to certain microbial antigens, or is there some more subtle interaction with microbial products? Reports by Ebringer and colleagues of a cross-reaction of B27 with *Klebsiella pneumoniae* is certainly provocative in this respect and controversial in its interpretation, as is the homology between the urease of *Proteus mirabilis* and DR4.

Deficiencies in C4 and C2, which are MHC class III molecules, clearly predispose to the development of immune complex disease (p. 265) and so it would be expected that the inheritance of null genes or alleles coding for the less active complement allotypes would increase the risk of rheumatological disorders and add yet further complexity to the correlations between HLA types and disease.

295

THE IMMUNOLOGICAL RELATIONSHIP OF MOTHER AND FETUS

A further consequence of polymorphism in an outbred population is that mother and fetus will almost certainly have different MHCs. Some examples of selection for heterozygotes (where maternally and paternally derived haplotypes are different) over homozygotes (both fetal haplotypes identical with the mother's) in viviparous animals suggest that this is beneficial. Likewise, the placentae of F1 offspring are larger than normal when mothers are preimmunized to the paternal H-2 haplotype and smaller when mothers are tolerant to these antigens.

The threat posed to the fetus as a potential graft due to the possession of paternal transplantation antigens so intrigued Lewis Thomas that he was moved to suggest that rejection of the fetus might initiate parturition, although it would be difficult to account for the normal birth of female offspring to pure-strain mating pairs where fetus and mother would have identical histocompatibility antigens without further postulating a placenta-specific surface antigen.

None the less, in the human haemochorial placenta, maternal blood with immunocompetent lymphocytes does circulate in contact with the fetal trophoblast and we have to explain how the fetus avoids allograft rejection, despite the development of an immunological response in a proportion of mothers as evidenced by the appearance of anti-HLA antibodies and cytotoxic lymphocytes. In fact, prior sensitization with a skin graft fails to affect a pregnancy, showing that trophoblast cells are immunologically protected and indeed they are resistant to most cytotoxic mechanisms although susceptible to IL-2 activated NK cells. Some of the many speculations which have been aired on this subject are summarized in figure 13.19.

Undoubtedly, the most important factor is the well-documented lack of both class I and class II MHC antigens on the placental villous trophoblast which protects the fetus from allogeneic attack. It has recently been shown that certain human cytotrophoblast populations in the smooth part of the chorion (chorion laeve), and invasive cytotrophoblasts in the placental bed, throughout gestation express unusual class I MHC-related molecules which are products of genes distinct from HLA-A or -B. They could be the human homologue of the Qa-Tla genes in the mouse. They could be

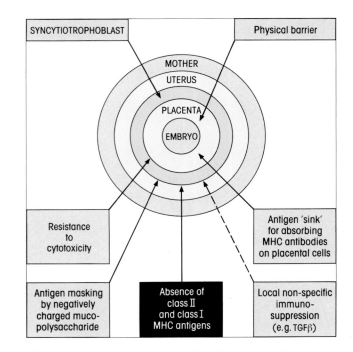

Figure 13.19. *Mechanisms postulated to account for the survival of the fetus as an allograft in the mother. (After L. Brent.)*

involved in suppression of maternal responses by localized small non-B, non-T granular lymphocytes making TGFβ. Cytokines seem to have a role in post-implantation pregnancy given the production of factors such as GM-CSF and TGFβ by the maternal endometrium and the presence of receptors on the trophoblast.

IS THE CANCER CELL LIKE AN ALLOGRAFT?

The ability to reject transplants of tissue may be traced back a long way down the evolutionary tree — back even as far as the annelid worms. Long before the studies on the involvement of self-MHC in immunological responses, Lewis Thomas suggested that the allograft rejection mechanism represented a means by which the body's cells could be kept under *immunological surveillance* so that altered cells with a neoplastic potential could be identified and summarily eliminated. For this to operate, cancer cells must display some new surface structure which can be recognized by the lymphoid cells and examples have been discovered although the phenomenon is not universal.

Changes on the surface of tumour cells (figure 13.20)

(a) Virally controlled antigens

Cells infected with oncogenic viruses usually display two new antigens on their surface, one (V) identical with an antigen on the isolated virion and the other (T), also a product of the viral genome, present only on infected cells, presumably a viral peptide associated with MHC since it behaves as a strong transplantation antigen and generates haplotype-restricted cytotoxic T-cells. All syngeneic tumours induced by a given virus carry the same surface antigen, irrespective of their cellular origin, so that immunization with any one of these tumours confers resistance to subsequent challenge with the others.

(b) Expression of embryonic genes

If the uncontrollable cell division of a cancer cell is attributable to the constitutive expression of one of a number of normal genes (so-called cellular oncogenes), their products or the products encoded by other genes which secondarily might become derepressed could be differentiation antigens normally associated with an earlier fetal stage. Thus tumours derived from the same cell type are often found to express such oncofetal antigens which are also present on embryonic cells. Examples would be α-fetoprotein in hepatic carcinoma and carcinoembryonic antigen (CEA) in cancer of the intestine. Certain monoclonal antibodies raised against human melanoma cells also react with tumours of neural crest origin and fetal melanocytes. Another monoclonal antibody defines the SSEA-1 antigen found on a variety of human tumours and early mouse embryos but absent from adult cells with the exception of human granulocytes and monocytes.

(c) MHC molecules

Changes have quite frequently been observed in the expression of class I MHC molecules. Diminished or absent expression has been reported, in most cases associated with increased metastatic potential. In breast cancer, for example, around 60% of metastatic tumours lack class I. On the other hand, expression of class II with adhesion molecules such as ICAM-1 on primary melanoma cells are predictors for early metastasis. Sometimes it has

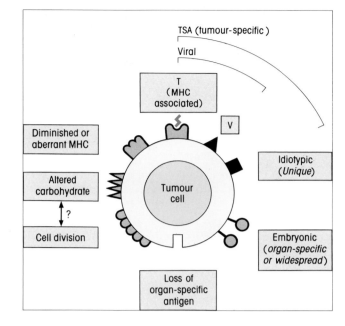

Figure 13.20. *Tumour-associated surface changes. Even virally induced tumours may possess idiotypic specificities.*

proved possible to identify an alien specificity not present on the host class I molecules and attributed by some to gene conversion events with silent class I genes somewhere in the Qa/Tla region in the mouse; there is even evidence that such genes themselves may be transcribed to replace the normal class I expression, but this is a highly controversial area.

(d) Changes on the surface of cycling cells

The carbohydrate moiety of surface membrane glycoproteins may change during cell division. For example, Thomas found that the density of surface sugar determinants cross-reacting with blood group H fell as murine mastocytoma cells moved into the G_1 phase of the division cycle while, reciprocally, group B determinants increased. Surface components binding the lectin, wheat-germ agglutinin are poorly represented on resting T- and B-cells, but within 24 hours of stimulation by lymphocyte polyclonal activators and before DNA synthesis begins, high concentrations of lectin binding sites appear on the surface. Transferrin receptors are also abundant on dividing cells which presumably are keen to take more iron on board. Indeed many tumour antigens turn out to be normal molecules expressed in unduly large amounts or which are suppressed in normal cells.

(e) Unique ('idiotypic') determinants

Tumours induced by chemical agents, benzopyrene for example, also possess specific transplantation antigens, but each tumour produced by a given chemical carcinogen has its own individual idiotypic antigen; even when a carcinogen produces two different primary tumours in the same animal, they do not exhibit the same antigenic specificities and do not confer cross-resistance by immunization. The antigens are associated with surface stress proteins of 96 kDa but although the antigens are tumour-specific, no sequence differences have yet been uncovered. It could be that their role is to present some tumour related peptide (e.g. derived from p21 ras proteins, *v. infra*) to effectors such as a γδ-T-cell subset, but that is still idle speculation. One gets nearer to really tumour-specific antigens with the Ig idiotype on the surface of chronic lymphocytic leukaemic cells and the p21 oncogenic proteins. Three members of the murine *ras* gene family, encoded by *ras* genes, *Harvey, Kirsten* and *N-ras* encode p21 proteins which bind guanine nucleotides, possess GTPase activity and are localized to the cytoplasmic surface of the plasma membrane. Certain oncogenic sequences from human tumour cells are homologous with these *ras* genes, and the oncogenic forms, termed activated p21, differ from their normal counterpart by point mutations usually leading to single amino acid substitutions in positions 12, 13 or 61. Such mutations have been recorded in 40% of human colorectal cancers and their pre-neoplastic lesions, in more than 90% of pancreatic carcinomas, in acute myelogenous leukaemia and in preleukaemic syndromes, and in tumours induced by chemical carcinogens. A number of monoclonal antibodies specific for activated p21 ras proteins with particular amino acid substitutions have been raised; they do not react with the normal protein.

Immune response to tumours

When present, many of these antigens can provoke immune responses in experimental animals which lead to resistance against tumour growth but they vary tremendously in their efficiency and in their ability to activate T-suppressors. Powerful antigens associated with tumours induced by oncogenic viruses or ultraviolet light generate strong resistance while the recently discovered gp 96 family of transplantation antigens on chemically induced tumours are weaker and somewhat variable; disappointingly, tumours which arise spontaneously in animals produce little or no response. This would seem to reason against the immune surveillance theory, although it might be argued that most tumours were silenced at their inception by immunological control and that only the very few which lacked a provocative surface component were 'successful'. However, athymic nude mice have a normal incidence of spontaneous tumours and this makes a single, exclusively T-cell surveillance system most unlikely. Furthermore, the only increase in cancer reported in immunosuppressed patients was related to the lymphoreticular system which could have been the direct target for the drugs employed. None the less, there are exceptions. One exception was the considerable increase in skin cancer in immunosuppressed patients living in high sunshine regions north of Brisbane and we have already noted the 'antigen strength' of such tumours provoked in experimental animals. It is also relevant that most of the B-cell lymphomas arising under immunosuppression and in children with T-cell deficiency linked to Wiskott—Aldrich syndrome or ataxia telangiectasia, express Epstein-Barr virus genes; they show unusually restricted expression of EBV latent proteins which are the major potential target epitopes for immune recognition, and cellular adhesion molecules such as ICAM-1 and LFA-3 which mediate conjugate formation with cytolytic T-cells (CTL) cannot be detected on their surface. Knowing that most normal individuals have highly efficient EBV-specific CTLs, this must be telling us that only by downregulating appropriate surface molecules can the lymphoma cells escape even the limited T-cell surveillance operating in these patients. So don't let us throw the baby out with the bathwater; let's take it that some tumours, perhaps a minority, can come under T-cell control.

Returning to the idea of cancer as a potential allograft, it has been argued that since normal class I MHC molecules would be needed to present neo-antigens on tumours to cytotoxic T-cells, their absence from the cell surface may enable the tumours to escape from surveillance. Accordingly, one group transfected a functional class I gene into highly tumorigenic adenovirus-transformed cells which originally failed to express class I antigens; the treated cells not only expressed the H-2L^d transfected gene but also were no longer oncogenic.

Perhaps in speaking of immunity to tumours, one too readily thinks in terms of acquired responses whereas it is highly possible that innate mechan-

298

isms will prove to be of greater significance. Macrophages taken from BCG-infected animals, or activated by a diversity of factors, bacterial lipopolysaccharide, double-stranded RNA, T-cell lymphokine and so forth, destroy tumour cells in tissue culture through the copious production of hydrogen peroxide, a cytolytic protease and tumour necrosis factor (TNF).

There is an uncommon flurry of interest in the natural killer (NK) cells which are spontaneously cytolytic for certain, but by no means all, tumour lines in culture. They commonly express the low affinity FcγRIII receptor, CD16, and the NKH-1/Leu-19 marker on human cells. Low NK cytotoxic activity correlates with decreased survival and earlier appearance of metastases in patients with solid cancers. Powerful evidence implicating these cells in protection against cancer is provided by the beige mice which congenitally lack type I NK cells. Mice of this strain die with spontaneous tumours earlier than their non-deficient +/bg litter mates and the incidence of radiation induced leukaemia is reduced by prior injection of cloned isogeneic NK cells which could be suppressing pre-leukaemic cells. Tumours induced chemically or with murine leukaemia virus were handled normally. On activation by IL-2, NK cells are capable of killing a variety of fresh tumour cells *in vitro*. The range of specificity for tumours and the ability to kill *fresh* cancer cells distinguish these so-called 'lymphokine-activated killer' (LAK) cells from the resting NK set. Their use in the therapy of cancer will be discussed below. It is surmised that the target of NK and LAK cells might be altered carbohydrates on the surface membrane glycoproteins, but there is no hard evidence to substantiate this.

Approaches to cancer immunotherapy

On one point all are agreed, if immunotherapy is to succeed, it is essential that the tumour load should first be reduced by surgery, irradiation or chemotherapy, since not only is it unreasonable to expect the immune system to cope with a large tumour mass, but considerable amounts of antigen released by shedding would tend to prevent the generation of any significant response in some cases due to the stimulation of T-suppressors. This leaves the small secondary deposits as the proper target for immunotherapy.

Exploitation of acquired immune responses

For active immunization we need antigen. Based on the not unreasonable belief that certain forms of cancer (e.g. lymphoma) are caused by oncogenic viruses, attempts are being made to isolate the virus and prepare a suitable vaccine from it. In fact, large-scale protection of chickens against the development of Marek's disease lymphoma has been successfully achieved by vaccination with another herpes virus native to turkeys. In human Burkitt's lymphoma work is in progress to develop a vaccine to exploit the ability of cytotoxic T-cells to target EBV related antigens on the cells of all Burkitt tumours. It may be an advantage to treat the patient at the same time with cytokines to upregulate the expression of ICAM-1, LFA-3 and possibly of the virus itself. The unique idiotype on monoclonal B-cell tumours with surface Ig also offers a potentially feasible target for immunotherapy and successful treatment of one patient has had wide publicity. Melanomas display high levels of gangliosides on their surface and monoclonal antibodies have been used to affinity purify them to use as potential vaccines in combination with BCG.

Another line of attack is to expand the lymphocytes infiltrating a tumour by treatment *in vitro* with IL-2 and then introduce a gene such as IL-4 with neomycin resistance and an incomplete murine retroviral vector; reinjection should take these smartly to the site of the tumour. The strategy rests on the fond hope that the tumour-infiltrating population contains some antigen-specific cytolytic T-cells. This does seem to be the case with a number of melanomas but in a series of other solid tumours the infiltrating cells were CD3+ T− lymphocytes with NK-like unrestricted cytotoxicity.

Immunologists have for long been bemused by the idea of eliminating tumour cells by specific antibody linked to a killer molecule. Not surprisingly, the 'magic bullet' devotees were greatly encouraged by experiments in which guinea-pig B lymphoma cells were killed *in vitro* by anti-idiotype conjugated with ricin, a toxin of such devastating potency that one molecule entering the cell is lethal (those readers who still maintain contact with the outside world will recollect that minute amounts of ricin on the end of a pointed walking stick provide a favourite weapon for the liquidation of unwanted intelligence agents). There is optimism that by using monoclonal antibodies, it may be feasible to apply this approach to the human but the pathway to success is not without its difficulties.

299

The immunotoxins must have a reasonable half-life in the circulation, penetrate into tumours and not bind significantly to non-tumour cells; they must also be internalized efficiently and delivered to the correct intracellular department, e.g. ricin must go to the transgolgi network or a postgolgi compartment. Another problem, and this is true for all antibody-targetting gambits, is the heterogeneity of tumours with respect to the putative antigen.

Nothing daunted, there is a plethora of ingenious initiatives. For example, a mixture of two bispecific heteroconjugates of anti-tumour/anti-CD3 and anti-tumour/anti-CD28 should act synergistically to induce contact between a T-cell and the tumour to activate direct cytotoxicity even though the T-cell itself will not have conventional specificity for the tumour target. Radioimmunoconjugates which carry a radiation source such as Tc-99 and In-111 to the tumour site for therapy or diagnosis are being intensively developed and a bright new idea is to inject specific antibody coupled to alkaline phosphatase followed later by phosphorylated derivatives of three anti-cancer drugs. A general point: specific antibody, or its more diffusible and penetrative small fragments Fab' or DAB (cf. p. 139), can be deployed to maximum advantage relative to control Ig for imaging and therapy, if the tumour is small or a cluster of cells.

It should be mentioned that differentiation antigens present on leukaemic cells but absent from bone-marrow stem cells, even though not tumour-specific, can be used to prepare tumour-free autologous stem cells to restore function in patients treated with chemotherapy or X-irradiation which destroys both their tumour cells and their haematopoietic tissue (figure 13.21). Recombinant GM-CSF, G-CSF and IL-3, which enhance haemopoiesis, are of great value in shortening the period of neutropenia following chemotherapy. The difficulty is to cope with the few remaining tumour cells and autologous grafts do not provide the little understood beneficial 'graft-versus-leukaemia' effect obtained with allogeneic marrow mentioned earlier, albeit the potential is there for more generalized g.v.h. disease.

Despite reports of cytotoxic antibodies in a proportion of patients with malignant melanoma and cytotoxic leucocytes from patients with neuroblastoma or bladder cancer, which indicate that some form of immunological response to tumour antigens is possible, it must be said that attempts to control human cancer by immunization still have a long way to go. Many attempts are being made to boost

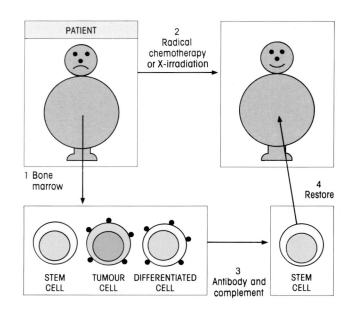

Figure 13.21. *Treatment of leukaemias by autologous bone marrow rescue. By using cytotoxic antibodies to a differentiation antigen (●) present on leukaemic cells and even on other normal differentiated cells, but absent from stem cells, it should be possible to obtain a tumour-free population of the latter which can be used to restore haematopoietic function in patients subsequently treated radically to destroy the leukaemic cells. However, techniques to clean up the marrow effectively are still improving.*

the inherently weak autoantigenicity of tumour cells by infection with viruses, membrane insertion of chemical haptens or fusion with highly immunogenic, allogeneic or xenogeneic normal cells. One hope is that xenogeneic antibodies combining with a tumour cell would be endocytosed and possibly represented as a peptide on the cell surface thus serving as a target for cytolytic T-cells. Another interesting attack is suggested by the finding of different groups that a proportion of tumour cells after treatment with mutagenic drugs and cloning can be shown to have acquired new antigens (tum⁻) which induce an immunological response in syngeneic recipients and may confer resistance to the parent tumour.

Harnessing innate immunity

With respect to putatively non-antigenic tumours, there have been numerous, not very successful, attempts to boost 'non-specific' effector mechanisms mediated by macrophages and NK cells through the injection of BCG or *C. parvum*. Intimate contact of the adjuvant with the tumour itself can produce dramatic results and one hopeful study records the beneficial effects of intrathoracic BCG in lung cancer. However, significant advances are undoubtedly being made as a result of the availability of recombinant tumour necrosis factor and biological response modifiers such as IL-2, IFNγ and colony stimulating factors.

Immunotherapy based on systemic administration of lymphokine-activated killer (LAK) cells and recombinant interleukin-2

Patients are leucopheresed and the cells cultured for several days with IL-2 to allow LAK cells to develop. Administration of autologous LAK cells together with high doses of IL-2 has led, in one study, to more than 50% reduction in evaluable tumour in 14 out of 41 cancer patients. Renal cancers (figure 13.22), some melanomas and some colorectal cancers are sensitive to this treatment whereas sarcomas appear to be unresponsive (figure 13.23). Although the treatment is cumbersome, gruesome for the patient, and has significant side-effects, there is some promise in this approach.

The combination of IL-2 with IFNα showed synergy in murine studies and is now being applied to cancer patients with initially encouraging results.

By injecting IL-4 daily it is expected that tumour infiltrating lymphocytes will be expanded and cause tumour regression.

Interferon therapy

In trials using IFNα and IFNβ, a 10–15% objective response rate was seen in patients with renal carcinoma, melanoma and myeloma, an approximate 20% response rate among patients with Kaposi's sarcoma, about 40% positive responders in patients with various lymphomas and a remarkable response rate of 80–90% among patients with hairy cell leukaemia and mycosis fungoides.

With regard to the mechanisms of the antitumour effects, in certain tumours interferons may serve primarily as anti-proliferative agents; in others, activation of NK cells and macrophages may be important, while augmenting the expression of class I MHC molecules may make the tumours more susceptible to control by immune effector mechanisms. In some circumstances the anti-viral effect could be contributory.

For diseases like renal cell cancer and hairy cell leukaemia, IFNs have induced responses in a significantly higher proportion of patients than

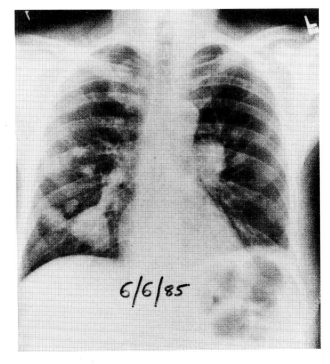

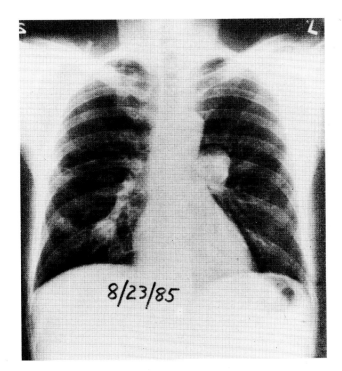

Figure 13.22. *Regression of renal-cell cancer metastases in the lung following treatment with autologous LAK cells and rIL-2. X-ray films of multiple pulmonary nodules before (left) and after (right) treatment. All nodules regressed markedly, and most resolved completely. The remaining lesions were continuing to regress at $3\frac{1}{2}$ months. (Reproduced from Rosenberg S.A. et al. (1985) N. Eng. J. Med. 313, 1485, with permission from the New England Journal of Medicine.)*

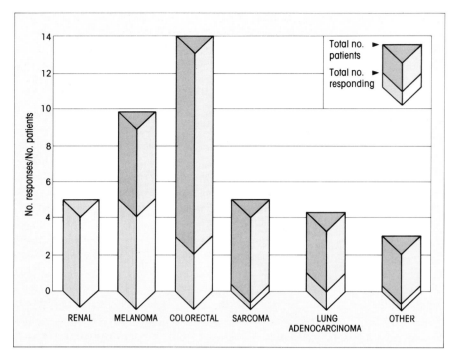

No. responses/No. patients

14

12

10

8

6

4

2

0

RENAL   MELANOMA   COLORECTAL   SARCOMA   LUNG ADENOCARCINOMA   OTHER

Total no. patients ►
Total no. responding ►

Figure 13.23. *Response of cancer patients to therapy with autologous LAK cells and IL-2. Other cancers included 1 oesophageal adenocarcinoma, 1 lymphoma and 1 gastrinoma. A positive response was reduction of tumour size by ≥50%. (Data from Rosenberg S.A. et al. (1986)* **Surgery 100, 262.)**

conventional therapies. However, in the wider setting, most investigators consider that their role will be in combination therapy, e.g. with various chemotherapeutic agents where synergistic action has been observed in murine tumour systems. IFNα and β synergize with IFNγ and the latter synergizes with tumour necrosis factor. α-Interferon acts as a radiation sensitizer and its ability to increase the expression of oestrogen receptors on cultured breast cancer cells suggests the possibility of combining IFN with anti-oestrogens in this disease.

Colony stimulating factors

Normal cell development proceeds from an immature stem cell with the capacity for unlimited self-renewal, through committed progenitors to the final lineage-specific differentiated cells with little or no potential for self-renewal. Therapy aimed at inducing tumour cell differentiation is founded on the idea that the induction of cell maturation decreases and possibly abrogates the capacity of the malignant clone to divide. Along these lines, the colony stimulating factor which promotes the formation of granulocyte/macrophage colonies in bone marrow cultures (GM-CSF) has been shown to enhance the differentiation, decrease the self-renewal capacity and suppress the leukaemogenicity of murine myeloid leukaemias. Recombinant human products are now undergoing trials.

Immunodiagnosis

Analysis of blood for the oncofetal antigens, α-fetoprotein in hepatoma and carcinoembryonic antigen in tumours of the colon has provided valuable diagnostic information, but enthusiasm has been slightly curtailed by the knowledge that there is a high incidence of so-called 'false positives'. Reappearance of these proteins after surgical removal of the primary is strongly indicative of fresh tumour growth. The GM1 monosialoganglioside has been demonstrated in the blood of 96% of patients with pancreatic carcinoma and 64% of colorectal carcinomas as against 2% in normal subjects. Identification of the cell type by surface markers is of increasing value for the diagnosis and treatment of childhood leukaemias such as non-T, non-B-ALL (p. 191).

We have already discussed some of the issues concerned in the localization of tumours *in vivo* by radiolabelled monoclonal antibodies for either therapy or imaging but one further crafty scheme is worthy of mention. A bifunctional antibody consisting, say, of anti-carcinoembryonic antigen and anti-isotope acceptor is injected followed 24–120 hours later by the acceptor chelate containing In-111. This allows clearance of non-targetted primary antibody and produces good tumour localization with reduced liver and bone marrow uptake. It has been suggested that the antibody imaging technique is more likely to challenge the computerized axial tomography (CAT) scans for tumours of the abdomen than the lungs where there is high density contrast.

SUMMARY

Graft rejection is an immunological reaction: it shows specificity, the second set response is brisk, it is mediated by lymphocytes, and antibodies specific for the graft are formed. In each vertebrate species there is a major histocompatibility complex (MHC) which is responsible for provoking the most intense graft reactions.

Class II MHC molecules provoke a mixed lymphocyte reaction of proliferation and blast transformation when genetically dissimilar lymphocytes interact; this reaction stimulates the formation of helper T-cells required for the generation of cytotoxic T-cells directed against class I determinants (cf. T−B cooperation with carrier-hapten). Class II differences are largely responsible for the reaction of tolerated grafted lymphocytes against host antigen (g.v.h.). The MHC in man (HLA) consists of three loci (HLA-A, B and C) for class I antigens and three (HLA-DP, DQ and DR) for the class II. Individuals are typed by cytotoxic antisera, the mixed lymphocyte reaction and Southern blot RFLPs. The very high degree of polymorphism of the MHC may protect a species from molecular mimicry by parasites, maintain diversity of antigenic recognition and ensure heterozygosity ('hybrid vigour'). Siblings have a 1:4 chance of identity with respect to MHC.

Grafts are rejected either by sensitized T-cells or by antibody inducing platelet aggregation or type II hypersensitivity reactions (e.g. antibody-dependent cell-mediated cytotoxicity). Rejection may be prevented by: (i) tissue matching including the DR-locus, (ii) anti-mitotic drugs (e.g. azathioprine), anti-inflammatory steroids and anti-lymphocyte monoclonals which produce general immunosuppression, and a new series of drugs, cyclosporin A, FK-506 and rapamycin which are selective for T-cells (iii) antigen-specific depression through tolerance induction under an anti-CD4 'umbrella' or enhancement by deliberate immunization.

Cornea and cartilage grafts are avascular and comparatively well tolerated. Kidney grafting gives excellent results and has been the most widespread although immunosuppression must normally be continuous. High success rates are also being achieved with heart and liver transplants particularly helped by the use of cyclosporin. Bone marrow grafts for immunodeficiency and aplastic anaemia are accepted from matched siblings but it is difficult to avoid g.v.h. disease with allogeneic marrow although this can be kept more under control with cyclosporin A.

HLA specificities are often associated with particular diseases, e.g. HLA-B27 with ankylosing spondylitis, B8 with myasthenia gravis, DR3 with autoimmune chronic active hepatitis, DR4 with rheumatoid arthritis and DR2 with multiple sclerosis.

Differences between MHC of mother and fetus may be beneficial to the fetus but as a potential graft it must be protected against transplantation attack by the mother; suggested defence mechanisms are (i) most importantly lack of class I and II MHC antigens on syncytiotrophoblast, (ii) mucopolysaccharide coat around trophoblast, and (iii) local production of immunosuppressant.

The immune surveillance theory of cancer postulates that changes in the surface of the neoplastic cell are recognized by the immune system and eliminated. However, although virally coded, idiotypic and oncofetal antigens may be detected on experimentally induced tumour cells together with components linked to cell division, the incidence of spontaneous cancers in immunosuppressed individuals is only higher than normal with respect to lymphomas and, in regions of high sunshine, skin. Examples of immune responses to tumours in human cancer are known but attempts at control by immunization with tumour antigens are still in their infancy. Other strategies involving non-specific immune mechanisms are looking more promising. These include treatment with autologous lymphokine activated killer (LAK) cells plus recombinant IL-2, interferons and colony stimulating factors. Monoclonal antibodies to tumour-associated antigens are proving to be of increasing value for diagnosis including imaging.

Further reading

Borel J.F. *et al.* (1989) Cyclosporin. *Pharmacol. Rev.* **41**, 239, (Series of reviews on every aspect of cyclosporin with exhaustive bibliographies.)
Hogarth P.J. (1982) *Immunological Aspects of Mammalian Reproduction.* Praeger, New York.
Mason D.W. & Morris P.J. (1986) Effector mechanisms in allograft rejection. *Ann. Rev. Immunol.*, **4**, 119.

Mitchison N.A. (1982) Protective immunity (to tumours) *in vivo*. In *Clinical Aspects of Immunology*, 4th edn. P Lachmann & D.K. Peters (eds). Blackwell Scientific Publications, Oxford.

Slavin S. (1987) Total lymphoid irradiation. *Immunology Today*, **8**, 88.

Waldmann H. (1989) Manipulation of T-cell responses with monoclonal antibodies. *Ann. Rev. Immunol.*, **7**, 407.

W.H.O. (1990) Nomenclature for factors of the HLA system, 1989. *Immunogenetics*, **31**, 131. (An up-to-date reference source for HLA specificities.)

AUTOIMMUNE DISEASES
I – Scope and Aetiology

The monumental repertoire of the adaptive immune system has evolved to allow it to recognize and ensnare virtually any shaped microbial molecules either at present in existence or yet to come, and in so doing, has been unable to avoid the generation of lymphocytes which react with the body's own constituents. We have already discussed the mechanisms which exist to prevent these self-components from provoking an adaptive immune response but, as with all machinery, there is always a chance that these systems might break down, and the older the individual, the greater the chance of a breakdown. Notwithstanding the IgM low affinity *autoantibodies* (i.e. antibodies capable of reacting with 'self' components) produced by CD5 + B-cells as part of the 'natural' antibody spectrum which we will discuss later, we are here concerned more with autoimmune phenomena which appear in relation to certain defined human diseases. Ideally we wish to apply the term 'autoimmune disease' to those cases where it can be shown that the autoimmune process contributes to the pathogenesis of the disease rather than situations where apparently harmless autoantibodies are formed following tissue damage, e.g. heart antibodies appearing after a myocardial infarction. Yet the role of autoimmunity in many disorders is still not clearly defined, and it is as a matter of convenience that we will refer to all maladies firmly associated with autoantibody formation as 'autoimmune diseases', except where it can be shown that the immunological phenomena are purely secondary findings.

These disorders may be looked upon as forming a spectrum. At one end we have *'organ-specific diseases'* with organ-specific autoantibodies. Hashimoto's disease of the thyroid is an example: there is a specific lesion in the thyroid involving infiltration by mononuclear cells (lymphocytes, histiocytes and plasma cells), destruction of follicular cells and germinal centre formation, accompanied, as we showed originally, by the production of circulating antibodies with absolute specificity for certain thyroid constituents (Roitt, Doniach & Campbell).

Moving towards the centre of the spectrum are those disorders where the lesion tends to be localized to a single organ but the antibodies are non-organ specific. A typical example would be primary biliary cirrhosis where the small bile ductule is the main target of inflammatory cell infiltration but the serum antibodies present—mainly mitochondrial—are not liver specific.

At the other end of the spectrum are the *'non-organ-specific diseases'* broadly belonging to the class of rheumatological disorders, exemplified by systemic lupus erythematosus (SLE) where both lesions and autoantibodies are not confined to any one organ. Pathological changes are widespread and are primarily lesions of connective tissue with fibrinoid necrosis. They are seen in the skin (the 'lupus' butterfly rash on the face is characteristic), kidney glomeruli, joints, serous membranes and blood vessels. In addition, the formed elements of the blood are often affected. A bizarre collection of autoantibodies are found, some of which react with the DNA and other nuclear constituents of all cells in the body.

An attempt to fit the major diseases considered to be associated with autoimmunity into this spectrum is shown in table 14.1.

Table 14.1. *Spectrum of autoimmune diseases.*

ORGAN SPECIFIC	Hashimoto's thyroiditis
	Primary myxoedema
	Thyrotoxicosis
	Pernicious anaemia
	Autoimmune atrophic gastritis
	Addison's disease
	Premature meno-pause (few cases)
	Male infertility (few cases)
	Myasthenia gravis
	Juvenile diabetes
	Goodpasture's syndrome
	Pemphigus vulgaris
	Pemphigoid
	Sympathetic ophthalmia
	Phacogenic uveitis
	(?? Multiple sclerosis ??)
	Autoimmune haemolytic anaemia
	Idiopathic thrombocytopenic purpura
	Idiopathic leucopenia
	Primary biliary cirrhosis
	Active chronic hepatitis HB$_S$-ve
	Cryptogenic cirrhosis (some cases)
	Ulcerative colitis
	Sjögren's syndrome
	Rheumatoid arthritis
	Scleroderma
	Wegener's granulomatosis
	Poly/ Dermatomyositis
	Discoid LE
NON-ORGAN SPECIFIC	Systemic lupus erythematosus (SLE)

Notes to table 14.2:
1 *Two major types of antibody to intrinsic factor are detected, viz. blocking and binding (figure 14.2). Binding antibody combines with preformed Int.Fact.—radioactive B$_{12}$(*B$_{12}$) complex which can then be precipitated at 50% ammonium sulphate (cf. figure 5.12) and the radioactivity in the precipitate counted. Blocking antibody prevents binding of *B$_{12}$ to Int.Fact. and the uncombined *B$_{12}$ can then be adsorbed to charcoal and counted.*
2 *Antibodies occur in the minority of patients with associated Addison's disease.*
3 *Only small percentage show agglutinins. Spermatozoa may be agglutinated head to head, tail to tail or joined through their mid-piece. Seen also in small percentage of infertile women.*
4 *Most if not all insulin-dependent diabetics have islet cell antibodies at some stage during the first year of onset. In contrast islet cell antibodies in diabetic patients with an associated autoimmune polyendocrinopathy persist for many years.*
5 *The Coombs' test involves the demonstration of bound antibody on the washed red cell by agglutination with an antiglobulin (cf. figure 12.12). Erythrocyte autoantibodies, which bind well over the temperature range $0-37°C$ ('warm' Ab), are mostly IgG, approximately 60 per cent of cases are primary, the remainder being associated with other autoimmune disorders, e.g. SLE, ulcerative colitis. 'Cold' Ab, which react best over the range $0-20°C$, are mostly IgM and red cells coated with this Ab can often be agglutinated by anticomplement sera; approximately half are primary, the others being associated with* **Mycoplasma pneumoniae** *infection or generalized neoplastic disease of the lymphoreticular tissues.*
6 *Antibodies specifically reacting with the epithelium of salivary gland excretory ducts are demonstrable by immunofluorescence in over half the cases of secondary Sjögren's associated with RA or SLE. SS-A and SS-B antibodies give a speckled nuclear fluorescence pattern.*
7 *The main antiglobulin factors react with the Fc portion of IgG which is usually adsorbed on to latex particles (human IgG) or present in an antigen—antibody complex (sheep red cells coated with sub-agglutinating dose of rabbit antibody). In the radioassay test, rabbit IgG is bound to a plastic tube, patient's serum added and the antiglobulin bound assessed by subsequent binding of labelled anti-human IgG or IgM (cf. p. 94). Rheumatoid factors specific for human IgG can be detected by this test using human Ecγ to coat the tubes and labelled anti-human Fdγ or IgM for the final stage.*
8 *In scleroderma (progressive systemic sclerosis) antinucleolar antibodies are frequently found. Scl-70 is topoisomerase 1.*
9 *Jo-1 is histidine tRNA synthetase.*
10 *This-syndrome combines features of scleroderma, rheumatoid arthritis, SLE and dermatomyositis. The antigen is an extractable nuclear antigen which gives speckled fluorescence and RNase-sensitive precipitation by counter-current electrophoresis.*
11 *Antibodies to single or double-stranded DNA are assayed by the salt copptn. test (cf. figure 5.12) using labelled Ag, or by a DNA-coated tube test similar to the radioassay for antiglobulins (note 7 above).*
12 *When blood from an SLE patient is incubated at 37°C, some white cells are damaged and allow the entry of antibodies. Certain of the antibodies combining with the nuclear surface bind complement and attract polymorphs which strip away the cytoplasm and engulf the nucleus. The polymorph containing the engulfed homogenized nucleus is called an LE-cell.*
13 *Component of 1° granule, probably serine proteinase III gives cytoplasmic staining. In periarteritis nodosa, antibodies to myeloperoxidase give perinuclear staining in alcohol fixed PMNs.*

Table 14.2. *Autoantibodies in human disease. (IFT = immunofluorescent test; CFT = complement fixation test.)*

DISEASE	ANTIGEN	DETECTION OF ANTIBODY
Hashimoto's thyroiditis Primary myxoedema	Thyroglobulin	Precipitins; passive haemagglutination
	2nd colloid Ag (CA2)	IFT on fixed thyroid
	Thyroid peroxidase: Cytoplasmic Cell surface	IFT on unfixed thyroid; passive haemagglutination IFT on viable thyroid cells; C'-mediated cytotoxicity
Thyrotoxicosis	Cell surface TSH receptors	Bioassay — stimulation of mouse thyroid *in vivo*; blocking combination TSH with receptors; stimulation adenyl cyclase
	'Growth' receptors	Induction of cell division in thyroid fragments
Pernicious anaemia[1]	Intrinsic factor	Neutralization; blocking combination with vit-B_{12}; binding to Int.Fact-B_{12} by coprecipitation
	Parietal cell gastrin receptors	IFT on unfixed gastric mucosa: block gastrin action
Addison's disease	Cytoplasm adrenal cells	IFT on unfixed adrenal cortex
Premature onset of menopause[2]	Cytoplasm steroid-producing cells	IFT on adrenal and interstitial cells of ovary and testis
Male infertility (some)[3]	Spermatozoa	Sperm agglutination in ejaculate
Insulin-dependent (juvenile) diabetes[4]	Cytoplasm of islet cells	IFT on unfixed human pancreas
	Cell surface	IFT on isolated cells
Type B insulin resistance c̄ acanthosis nigricans	Insulin receptor	Block hormone binding to receptor
		Radioimmunoassay with purified receptor
Atopic allergy (some)	β-Adrenergic receptor	Blocking radioassay with hydroxybenzylpindolol
Myasthenia gravis	Skeletal and heart muscle	IFT on skeletal muscle
	Acetyl choline receptor	Blocking or binding radioassay with α-bungarotoxin
Eaton–Lambert syndrome	Ca^{2+} channels in nerve endings	IgG produces neuromuscular defects in mice
(Multiple sclerosis)	Brain	Cytotoxic effects on cerebellar cultures by serum and lymphocytes (? secondary to disease)
Goodpasture's syndrome	Glomerular and lung basement membrane	Linear staining by IFT of kidney biopsy with fluorescent anti-IgG Radioimmunoassay with purified Ag
Pemphigus vulgaris	Desmosomes between prickle cells in epidermis	IFT on skin
Pemphigoid	Basement membrane	IFT on skin
Phacogenic uveitis	Lens	Passive haemagglutination
Sympathetic ophthalmia	Uvea	(Delayed skin reaction to uveal extract)
Autoimmune haemolytic anaemia[5]	Erythrocytes	Coombs' antiglobulin test
Idiopathic thrombocytopenic purpura	Platelets	Shortened platelet survival *in vivo*
Primary biliary cirrhosis	Mitochondria (pyruvate dehydrogenase)	IFT on mitochondria-rich cells (e.g. distal tubules of kidney)
Active chronic hepatitis (HB_S−ve)	Smooth muscle / nuclear lamins / nuclei Cell surface lipoproteins	IFT (e.g. on gastric mucosa) Immunoblotting
Ulcerative colitis	Colon 'lipopolysaccharide'	IFT; passive haemagglutination (cytotoxic action of lymphocytes on colon cells)
	Colon epithelial cell surface protein	ADCC on colon cancer cell line Ab data in this disease not universally accepted
Sjögren's syndrome[6]	SS-A(Ro) SS-B(La)	IFT; gel precipitation
	Ducts / mitochondria / nuclei / thyroid	IFT
	IgG	Antiglobulin (rheumatoid factor) tests
Rheumatoid arthritis[7]	IgG	Antiglobulin tests: latex agglutination, red sheep cell aggln. test (SCAT; commercial product, RAHA test) and radioassay
	Collagen	Passive haemagglutination
Discoid lupus erythematosus	Nuclear / IgG	IFT / antiglobulin tests
Scleroderma[8]	Nuclear / IgG / centromere	IFT
	Nuclear / IgG / Sc-70	IFT; countercurrent electrophoresis
Dermatomyositis[9]	Nuclear / IgG / Jo-1	IFT; countercurrent electrophoresis
Mixed connective tissue disease[10]	Extractable nuclear	IFT; countercurrent electrophoresis
Systemic lupus erythematosus	DNA	Radioassay[11]; pptn
	Sm ribonucleoprotein	IFT; gel precipitation techniques
	Nucleoprotein	IFT; L.E. cells[12]
	Cytoplasmic sol.Ag	'Non-organ sp.C'-fixation test
	Array of other Ag incl. formed elements of blood / clotting factors / IgG	
	Cardiolipin	Radioassay
Wegener's granulomatosis	Neutrophil cytoplasm (ANLA)[13]	IF on alcohol fixed polymorphs

AUTOIMMUNE DISEASES — SCOPE

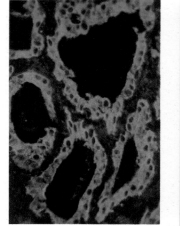

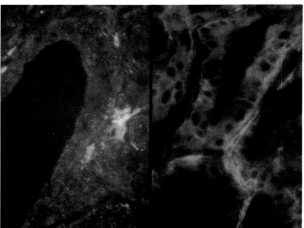

(a)

(b)

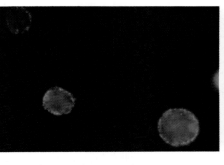

(c)

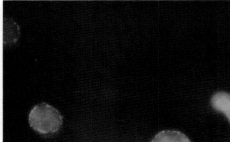

(d)

(e)

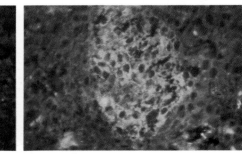

(f)

Figure 14.1 above and facing page. *Fluorescent antibody studies in autoimmune diseases. (a) Thyroid microsomal (thyroid peroxidase) antibodies staining cytoplasm of acinar cells. (b) Human thyroid sections stained for MHC class II: LHS—normal thyroid with unstained follicular cells and an isolated strongly MHC class II positive dendritic cell; RHS— thyrotoxic (Graves' disease) thyroid with abundant cytoplasmic MHC class II indicative of active synthesis. (c) Viable suspension of islet cells from the diabetic-prone BB/ E/ H rat stained for surface MHC class II induced by treatment with recombinant IFNγ, then fixed, cytocentrifuged and stained with fluorescein labelled antibodies to reveal intracytoplasmic insulin. Three cells showing abundant induction of surface class II. (d) That these are insulin-producing cells is shown by simultaneous intracytoplasmic green staining for the hormone. (e) Fluorescence of cells in the pancreatic islets of Langerhans stained with serum from insulin-dependent diabetic. (f) The same, showing cells stained simultaneously for somatostatin (the yellow cells are stained with rhodamine antisomatostatin and fluorescein anti-human IgG which localizes the bound patient's autoantibody). (g) Serum of patient with Addison's disease staining cytoplasm of monkey adrenal granulosa cells. (h) Fluorescence of distal tubular cells of the kidney after reaction with mitochondrial autoantibodies. (i) Diffuse nuclear staining on a thyroid section obtained with nucleoprotein antibodies from an SLE patient. (j) Serum of a scleroderma patient staining the nucleoli of SV-40-transformed human keratinocytes (K14) in monolayer culture. ((a), (e), (f), (g), (h) and (i) kindly provided by Dr F. Bottazzo, (b) by Dr R. Pujol-Borrell, (c) and (d) by Dr A. Cooke and (j) by Dr F.T. Wojnarowska.)*

308

CHAPTER 14

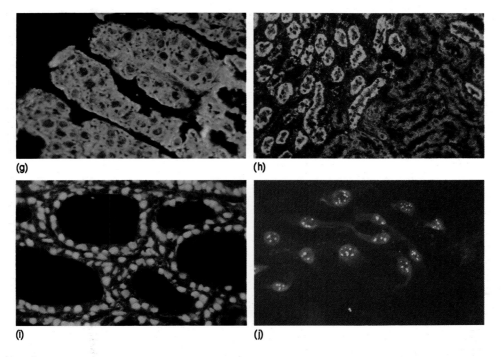

(g)

(h)

(i)

(j)

Figure 14.1 continued

Autoantibodies in human disease

At this stage in the discussion it may be of value to have a more precise account of the major autoantibodies detected in the different diseases to provide a framework for reference. Table 14.2 documents a list of these antibodies and the methods employed in their detection. The notes following the table amplify specific points while some of the tests are illustrated in figures 14.1, 14.2, 5.15 and 5.16.

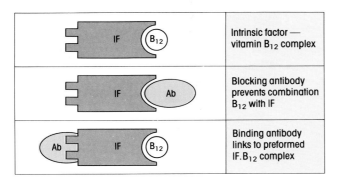

	Intrinsic factor — vitamin B_{12} complex
	Blocking antibody prevents combination B_{12} with IF
	Binding antibody links to preformed IF.B_{12} complex

Figure 14.2. *Intrinsic factor autoantibodies: sites of determinants for binding and blocking. Similar considerations apply to the acetyl choline receptor and its antibodies. (Roitt I.M., Doniach D. & Shapland C. (1964) Lancet ii, 469.)*

Overlap of autoimmune disorders

There is a tendency for more than one autoimmune disorder to occur in the same individual and when this happens the association is often between diseases within the same region of the autoimmune spectrum (cf. table 14.1). Thus patients with autoimmune thyroiditis (Hashimoto's disease or primary myxoedema) have a much higher incidence of pernicious anaemia than would be expected in a random population matched for age and sex (10% as against 0.2%). Conversely, both thyroiditis and thyrotoxicosis are diagnosed in pernicious anaemia patients with an unexpectedly high frequency. Other associations are seen between Addison's disease and autoimmune thyroid disease and in the rare cases of juveniles with pernicious anaemia and polyendocrinopathy which includes Addison's disease, hypoparathyroidism, diabetes and thyroiditis.

There is an even greater overlap in serological findings. 30% of patients with autoimmune thyroid disease have concomitant parietal cell antibodies in their serum. Conversely, thyroid antibodies have been demonstrated in up to 50% of pernicious anaemia patients. It should be stressed that these are not cross-reacting antibodies. The thyroid-specific antibodies will not react with stomach and vice versa. When a serum reacts with both organs it means that two populations of antibodies are present, one with specificity for thyroid and the other for stomach.

At the non-organ-specific end of the spectrum, SLE is clinically associated with rheumatoid arthritis and several other diseases which are themselves uncommon: haemolytic anaemia, idiopathic leucopenia and thrombocytopenic purpura, dermatomyositis and Sjögren's syndrome. Antinuclear antibodies, non-organ-specific complement fixation reactions, and anti-globulin (rheumatoid) factors are a general feature of these disorders.

Sjögren's syndrome occupies an interesting position (table 14.3); aside from the clinical and serological features associated with non-organ-specific disease mentioned above, characteristics of an organ-specific disorder are evident. Antibodies reacting with salivary ducts are demonstrable and there is an abnormally high incidence of thyroid autoantibodies; histologically the affected lacrimal and salivary glands reveal changes of a similar nature to those seen in Hashimoto's disease, namely a replacement of the glandular elements by patchy lymphocytic and plasma cell granulomatous tissue. Associations between diseases at the two ends of the spectrum have been reported, but, as might be predicted from the serological data (table 14.3), they are not common.

There is still no entirely satisfactory explanation to account for the rare tendency to develop hypogammaglobulinaemia and the increased incidence of certain cancers occurring in autoimmune disease. Patients with organ-specific disorders are slightly more prone to develop cancer in the affected organ whereas generalized lymphoreticular neoplasia shows up with uncommon frequency in non-organ-specific disease.

Genetic factors in autoimmune disease

Autoimmune phenomena tend to aggregate in certain families. For example, the first degree relatives (sibs, parents and children) of patients with Hashimoto's disease show a high incidence of thyroid autoantibodies (figure 14.3) and of overt and subclinical thyroiditis. Interestingly there is also an increased frequency of 'non-immunological' thyroid disorders, such as non-toxic nodular goitre. The proportion with autoantibodies is higher in those families where more than one member is clinically affected. Parallel studies have disclosed similar relationships in the families of pernicious anaemia patients in that gastric parietal cell antibodies are prevalent in the relatives who are wont to develop achlorhydria and atrophic gastritis. Familial aggregation of mitochondrial antibodies has been observed, albeit to a lesser extent, in primary biliary cirrhosis. Turning to SLE, disturbances of immunoglobulin synthesis and a susceptibility to develop 'connective tissue diseases' have been reported but there are some conflicting accounts still not resolved.

These familial relationships could be ascribed to environmental factors such as infective microorganisms, but there is evidence that one or more genetic components must be given serious consideration. In the first place, when thyrotoxicosis occurs in twins there is a greater concordance rate (i.e. both twins affected) in identical than in nonidentical twins. Secondly, thyroid autoantibodies are more prevalent in individuals with ovarian dysgenesis having X-chromosome aberrations such as XO and particularly the iso-chromosome X abnormality. Furthermore, there are strong associations between several autoimmune diseases and particular HLA specificities, e.g. DR3 in Addison's disease and DR4 in rheumatoid arthritis (table 13.4, p. 294). Figure 14.4 shows a multiplex family, with insulin-dependent diabetes in which the disease is linked to a particular HLA-haplotype. Only very restricted determinants on the autoantigenic molecules evoke autoantibodies (e.g. thyroglobulin of molecular weight 650 000, has an effective valency of only 4), and it will be important to see whether the same holds true for T-cell epitopes since it is precisely

DISEASE	% POSITIVE REACTIONS FOR ANTIBODIES TO:			
	THYROID*	STOMACH*	NUCLEI*	IgG†
Hashimoto's thyroiditis	99.9	32	8	2
Pernicious anaemia	55	89	11	
Sjögren's syndrome	45	14	56	75
Rheumatoid arthritis	11	16	50	75
SLE	2	2	99	35
Controls‡	0–15	0–16	0–19	2–5

Table 14.3. *Organ-specific and non-organ-specific serological interrelationships in human disease.*
* *Immunofluorescence test*
† *Rheumatoid factor classical tests*
‡ *Incidence increases with age and females > males.*

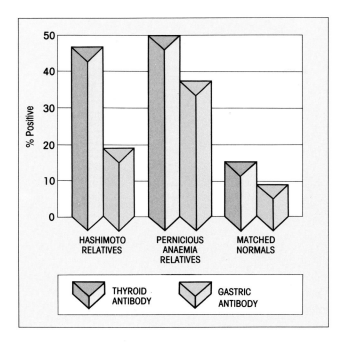

Figure 14.3. *The high incidence of thyroid and gastric autoantibodies in the first degree relatives of patients with Hashimoto's disease or pernicious anaemia. Note the overlap of gastric and thyroid autoimmunity and the higher incidence of gastric autoantibodies in pernicious anaemia relatives. (Data from Doniach D. & Roitt I.M. (1964) Semin. Haematol. I, 313.)*

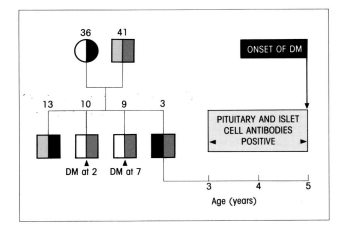

Figure 14.4. *HLA-haplotype linkage and onset of insulin-dependent diabetes (DM). Haplotypes: □ A3, B14, DR6; ■ A3, B7, DR4; ▨ A28, B51, DR4; and ▨ A2, B62, C3, DR4. Disease is linked to possession of the A2, B62, C3, DR4 haplotype. The 3-year-old brother had complement-fixing antibodies to the islet cell surface for 2 years before developing frank diabetes. (From Gorsuch A.N. et al. (1981) Lancet ii, 1363.)*

under such circumstances that the class II MHC-related immune response effects (Ir genes, p. 165) operate. Another pointer to the central role of class

II structure in determining T-cell responsiveness to self derives from the inability of the non-obese diabetic mouse to develop pancreatic autoimmunity when just a single amino acid residue in the α-helix of the I-Aβ chain is altered.

It is also worthy of note that lines of animals have been bred which spontaneously develop auto-immune disease. In other words, the autoimmunity is genetically programmed. There is an Obese line of chickens with autoimmune thyroiditis and the New Zealand Black (NZB) mouse with autoimmune haemolytic anaemia. The hybrid of NZB with another strain, the New Zealand White (B × W hybrid), actually develops LE-cells, antinuclear antibodies and a fatal immune complex induced glomerulonephritis. Suitable intercross and back-cross breeding of these mice has established that a *minimum* of three genes determines the expression of autoimmunity and that the production of both red cell and nuclear antibodies may be under sep-arate genetic control, i.e. there may be different factors predisposing to aggressive autoimmunity on the one hand, and to the selection of antigen on the other. This view finds support in the genetic analysis of Obese chickens which has delineated an influence of the MHC, abnormalities in T-cell con-trol and a defect in the thyroid gland.

The facts presented by human autoimmune dis-ease also attest to multifactorial control. The over-laps in autoantibodies and disease discussed above point to a general tendency to develop autoimmunity in these individuals and further, the factors which predispose to organ-specific disease must be different from those in non-organ-specific disorders (as judged by the minimal overlap between them). There must be additional factors which are organ related in that relatives of patients with pernicious anaemia are more prone to gastric autoimmunity than members of Hashimoto families (figure 14.3).

Autoantibodies, invariably IgM, are demon-strable in comparatively low titre in the general population and the incidence of positive results increases steadily with age (figure 14.5) up to around 60–70 years. In the case of the thyroid and stomach at least, biopsy has indicated that the presence of raised titres of antibody, especially of the IgG class is almost invariably associated with minor thyroid-itis or gastritis lesions (as the case may be), and it is of interest that post-mortem examination has ident-ified 10% of middle-aged women with significant degrees of lymphadenoid change in the thy-roid similar in essence to that characteristic of Hashimoto's disease.

311

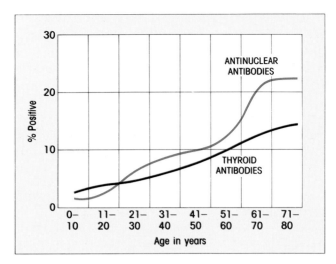

Figure 14.5. *Incidence of autoantibodies in the general population. A serum was considered positive for thyroid antibodies if it reacted at a dilution of 1/10 in the tanned red cell test or neat in the immunofluorescent test and positive for antinuclear antibodies if it reacted at a dilution of 1/4 by immunofluorescence.*

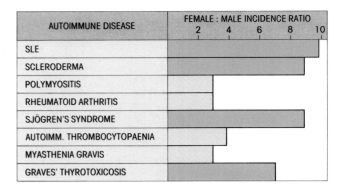

Figure 14.6. *Increased incidence of autoimmune disease in females.*

Sex influences in autoimmunity

These changes recorded in middle-aged females represent just one example of the general trend for autoimmune disease to occur far more frequently in women than in men (figure 14.6). The reasons for this are still unresolved. There is a suggestion that higher oestrogen levels are found in patients and mice with SLE. Pregnancy is often associated with amelioration of disease severity, particularly in rheumatoid arthritis, and there is sometimes a striking relapse after giving birth, a time at which there are drastic hormonal changes, not forgetting the loss of the placenta. We should also note the frequent development of post-partum hypothyroidism in women with pre-existing thyroid autoimmunity.

Does the environment contribute?

Twin studies

The 50% concordance rate for the development of the autoimmune disease insulin-dependent diabetes mellitus (IDDM; type I diabetes) in identical twins is considerably higher than that in dizygotic twins; this suggests a strong genetic element but still leaves 50% unaccounted for. This is not necessarily all due to environment since although monozygotic twins have identical germ line immunoglobulin and T-cell receptor genes, the processes of diversification of receptors and of internal anti-idiotype interactions are so complex that the resulting receptor repertoires will be extremely plastic and unlikely to be identical. None the less, a later study on concordance rates for IDDM in monozygotic twins gave the extraordinarily high figure of 70% if they were DR3/DR4 heterozygotes, but only 40% if they were not. Thus, in the same disease, the genetic element can be almost completely dominant or be a significant but minor factor in determining the outcome. As we turn to the non-organ specific diseases such as SLE we find an even lower genetic contribution with a concordance rate of only 23% in same sex monozygotic twins compared with 9% in same sex dizygotic twins. There are also many examples where clinically unaffected relatives of patients with SLE have a higher incidence of nuclear autoantibodies if they are household contacts than if they live apart from the proband. However, within a given home, the spouse is less likely to develop autoantibodies than blood relatives. Summing up, in some disorders the major factors are genetic, whereas in others, environmental influences seem to dominate.

Non-microbial factors

What environmental agents can we identify? Diet could be one—fish oils containing long chain, highly polyunsaturated omega-3 fatty acids are reputed to be beneficial for patients with rheumatoid arthritis; someone must know whether rheumatologists in Greenland are underworked. Sunshine is an undisputed trigger of the skin lesions in SLE.

Exposure to organic solvents can initiate the basement membrane autoimmunity which results in Goodpasture's syndrome—witness the high-incidence of this disease in HLA-DR2 individuals who work in dry-cleaning shops or syphon petrol from other people's petrol tanks. A more contrived situation is the production of a similar disease in Brown Norway rats by injection of mercuric chloride, but it makes its point, and there are several drug induced diseases such as SLE, myasthenia gravis, autoimmune haemolytic anaemia, and so on.

Microbes

Of course everyone's favourite environmental agent has to be an infectious micro-organism and we do have some clearcut examples of autoimmune disease following infection, usually in genetically predisposed individuals: acute rheumatic fever follows group A streptococcal pharyngitis in 2–3% of patients with a hereditary susceptibility, B1 Coxsackie virus produces autoimmune myositis in certain mouse strains, reactive arthritis can arise as a consequence of infection with Yersinia in HLA-B27 subjects, and so on.

In most cases of human chronic autoimmune disease, the problem is the long latency period which makes it difficult to track down the initiating event and, secondly, viable organisms usually cannot be isolated from the affected tissues (although a recent report identified type A retroviral particles in two Sjögren salivary gland biopsies). This forces us into looking for circumstantial evidence such as that linking Epstein-Barr virus (EBV) to Sjögren's syndrome. In this disease, the epithelial cells of the patients' salivary glands can be stained by immunofluorescence for the EBV diffuse early antigen, a result not obtained with tissue from control subjects. Furthermore, EBV DNA has been demonstrated in extracts of diseased glands by hybridization techniques. It may also not be fortuitous that EBV RNA EBER1 and EBER2 bind to the SS-B (La) protein, an RNP to which all cellular RNAs transcribed by RNA polymerase III bind and which induces antibodies which are a diagnostic marker of the disease. The report that one-third of primary Sjögren's patients have antibodies reacting with the p24 gag protein of HIV-1 would seem to provide us with a surfeit of microbial candidates for this disease, but embarrassment will probably be avoided by the assignation of the affected patients to a subset lacking anti-SS-A and -SS-B. In the sections that follow we will discuss the variety of mechanisms by which infectious agents could trigger autoimmunity, but that does not mean that they necessarily are the initiators of the human diseases.

AETIOLOGY OF AUTOIMMUNE RESPONSES

Autoreactivity is natural

Tolerance mechanisms do not destroy all self-reactive lymphocytes. The reader will recall the B-cell population bearing the T-cell marker CD5, which starts off early in life by forming a network connected by germ-line idiotypes. The cells are stimulated by the idiotypic interactions to produce so-called 'natural antibodies', a term applied to those serum antibodies thought to be present before external antigen challenge and therefore to arise independently of conventional antigen stimulation. These antibodies are IgM and include a basic set of autoantibodies with low affinity reactivity for multiple specificities and which cross-react with common bacterial antigens usually of a carbohydrate nature. One can see this as a strategy which ensures that preliminary excitation of cells by autoantigens (including idiotypes) will provide bacterial protection especially since the polymeric nature of the carbohydrate antigens will mean that the IgM antibodies, even though of low affinity, will bind with high avidity to the microbes.

Other functions for these natural antibodies have been proposed which are not mutually exclusive: Grabar viewed them as transporting agents responsible for scavenging effete body components while others envisage a role in which they actually prevent stimulation of autoreactive cells in the conventional CD5 negative B-cell population. This raises an important issue. The IgM autoantibodies produced by the CD5$^+$ B-subset are harmless in the sense that they do not cause tissue-damaging hypersensitivity reactions; but under abnormal circumstances, do they give rise to cells which produce the high affinity IgG antibodies characteristic of most autoimmune diseases? This question is difficult to resolve but we will return to it later.

As enthusiasts for symmetry and order might have predicted, there appears to be an analogous T-cell population, of phenotype CD3$^+$T4$^-$T8$^-$ bearing the B-cell marker B220, containing large internally

313

activated cells which react strongly with self-T-cells and are expanded in early life. It is likely that they connect to the CD5$^+$ B-cells through idiotype interactions. Again, it will be important to know whether this T-cell population provides the autoreactive clones which can be isolated from patients or animal models of autoimmune disease, which react specifically with myelin basic protein, thyroglobulin, thyroid surface antigens and other autoantigens such as collagen. The reader may be surprised to learn that in generating T-cell lines it is not an uncommon experience to isolate cells which proliferate and release IL-2 in response to autologous class II positive feeder cells; even allowing for the fact that the presence of these feeders in the cultures will tend to select for such autoreactive cells, it would not have been predicted that cells with these specificities would be permitted to roam around freely in the body unless constrained in some way. It is also of interest that self-reactive effector T-cells have been generated when lymphocytes have been cultured with a variety of autologous tissues in the presence of an agent such as a mitogenic lectin or fetal calf serum.

Whatever their precise lineage, much evidence suggests that the effector cells of autoimmune disease are present in normal individuals, although abnormal conditions must be required for their stimulation. In experimental models of organ-specific disease such as that induced in the thyroid by injection of thyroglobulin in complete Freund's adjuvant, the effector T-cells and the plasma cells making high affinity IgG autoantibodies are generated in normal animals. Complete Freund's will not produce antibodies to double-stranded DNA, the Sm or other autoantigens typical of non-organ-specific disorders and this may be telling us that the appropriate antigen-specific T-cells are not available in the normal repertoire. However, if T-cells are stimulated by radically different approaches, non-organ specific antibodies can be coaxed out of normal animals; in one system, allogeneic T-cells inducing a graft-v-host reaction are stimulated by, and thence polyclonally activate, class II-bearing B-cells, while the other, still to be confirmed, involves immunization with a public anti-DNA idiotype (16/6) in complete Freund's.

Is autoimmunity driven by antigen?

This is not such a silly question as it might appear since lymphocytes can be stimulated by polyclonal activators and anti-idiotypes as well as by antigen. And if the answer is in the affirmative, is the self molecule an auto-immunogen or just an auto-antigen, i.e. does it drive the autoimmune response or is it merely recognized by its products?

First, some direct evidence straight from the shoulder. The Obese strain (OS) chicken spontaneously develops precipitating IgG autoantibodies to thyroglobulin and a chronic inflammatory anti-thyroid response which destroys the gland so causing hypothyroidism. If the source of antigen is removed by neonatal thyroidectomy, no autoantibodies are formed. Injection of these animals with normal thyroglobulin then induces antibodies. Thyroidectomy of chickens with established thyroiditis is followed by a dramatic fall in antibody titre. Conclusions: the spontaneous antithyroglobulin immunity is initiated and maintained by auto-antigen from the thyroid gland. Furthermore, since the response is completely T-cell dependent, we can infer both B- and T-cells are driven by thyroglobulin in this model.

By establishing T-cell lines from experimental and human diseases, it has been possible to show direct stimulation by autoantigen, but in the case of B-cells, it is necessary to call upon indirect evidence. This usually takes the form of looking for high affinity IgG autoantibodies with evidence for somatic mutation. The reason for this, simply, is that high affinity IgG antibodies only arise through mutation and selection by antigen (cf. p. 135). Suffice it to say that ample evidence for somatic mutation and high affinity antibodies has been reported. More indirect is the argument that when antibodies are regularly formed against a cluster of antigens such as those in the nucleosome, it is difficult to propose a hypothesis independent of stimulation by antigen.

Do these autoantigens normally meet their lymphocyte counterparts? Our earliest view, with respect to organ-specific antibodies at least, was that the antigens were sequestered within the organ, and through lack of contact with the lymphoreticular system failed to establish immunological tolerance. Any mishap which caused a release of the antigen would then provide an opportunity for autoantibody formation. For a few body constituents this holds true, and in the case of sperm, lens and heart for example, release of certain components directly into the circulation can provoke autoantibodies. But, in general, the experience has been that injection of

314

unmodified extracts of those tissues concerned in the organ-specific autoimmune disorders does not readily elicit antibody formation. Indeed detailed investigation of the thyroid autoantigen, thyroglobulin, has disclosed that it is not completely sequestered within the gland but gains access to the extracellular fluid around the follicles and leaves via the thyroid lymphatics (figure 14.7) reaching the serum in normal human subjects at concentrations of approximately 0.01−0.05 μg/ml. In fact, in the majority of cases—e.g. red cells in autoimmune haemolytic anaemia, DNA released from dying cells in SLE and surface receptors in many cases of organ-specific autoimmunity—the autoantigens are accessible to circulating lymphocytes. None the less, with respect to T-cell recognition, accessibility is not sufficient; there must be an adequate association with class II MHC. Thus, the question must be raised whether these circulating components can achieve a high enough concentration on antigen-presenting cells to be perceived by T-helpers, and indeed whether potential autoantigens on the surface of cells not expressing class II can remain other than silent (cf. p. 188).

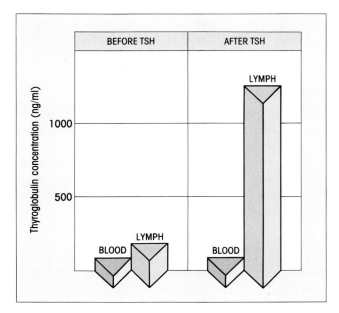

Figure 14.7. *Thyroglobulin in the cervical lymph draining the thyroid in the rat. The concentration of thyroglobulin is increased after injection of pituitary thyroid stimulating hormone (TSH) suggesting that the release from thyroid follicles is linked to the physiological activity of the acinar cells. (From Daniel P.N., Pratt O.E., Roitt I.M. & Torrigiani G. (1967)* **Quart. J. Exp. Physiol. 52, 184.)**

The T-helper cell is pivotal for control

The message then is that we are all sitting on a minefield of self-reactive cells, with potential access to their respective autoantigens, but since autoimmune disease is more the exception than the rule, the body must have homeostatic mechanisms to prevent them being triggered under normal circumstances. Accepting its limitations, figure 14.8 provides a framework for us to examine ways in which these mechanisms may be circumvented to allow autoimmunity to develop. It is assumed that the key to the system is control of the autoreactive T-inducer/helper cell since the evidence heavily favours the T-dependence of virtually all autoimmune responses, so that interaction between the T-cell and MHC-associated antigen peptide becomes the core consideration. Presumably these cells are unresponsive because of clonal deletion, clonal anergy, T-suppression or inadequate autoantigen presentation.

Figure 14.8. *Autoimmunity arises through bypass of the control of autoreactivity. The constraints on the stimulation of self-reactive inducer/ helper T-cells by autoantigen can be circumvented either through bypassing the helper cell or by disturbance of the regulatory mechanisms.*

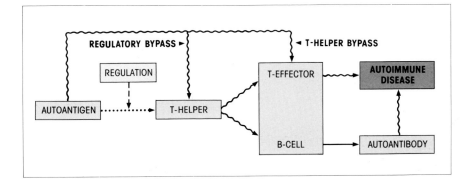

T-helper bypass mechanisms leading to autoimmunity

Provision of new carrier determinant

Allison and Weigle argued independently that if autoreactive T-cells are tolerized and thereby unable to collaborate with B-cells to generate autoantibodies, provision of new carrier determinants to which no self-tolerance had been established would bypass this mechanism and lead to autoantibody production (figure 14.9).

(i) Modification of the autoantigen

A new carrier could arise through some modification to the molecule, for example by defects in synthesis or by an abnormality in lysosomal breakdown yielding a split product exposing some new groupings. Experimentally it has been found that large proteolytic fragments of thyroglobulin are autoantigenic when injected alone but no evidence for such a mechanism has yet been uncovered in man. In fact many studies on spontaneous autoimmune disease have failed to reveal an abnormality in the antigen. Remember the experiment in which neonatal thyroidectomized Obese strain chickens make

autoantibodies if injected with thyroglobulin prepared from *normal* chickens suggesting that the immunological response rather than the antigen is abnormal. None the less, there may be defects in the iodine metabolism of the gland itself in this strain and recent work has shown that the severity of thyroiditis is ameliorated when the birds are put on a low iodine diet. There might also be more subtle changes in glycosylation patterns which are not picked up by the available serological reagents, the most exciting example being the defect in galactosylation of the Fcγ sugar chains in rheumatoid arthritis, to be discussed later.

Incorporation into Freund's complete adjuvant frequently endows many autologous proteins with the power to induce autoallergic disease in laboratory animals. It is conceivable that the physical constraints on the proteins at the water—oil interface of the emulsion provide the required alteration in configuration of the 'carrier portions' of the molecules.

Modification can also be achieved through combination with a drug. The autoimmune haemolytic anaemia associated with administration of α-methyl dopa might be attributable to modification of the red-cell surface in such a way as to provide a carrier for stimulating B-cells which recognize the rhesus *e* antigen. This is normally regarded as a 'weak'

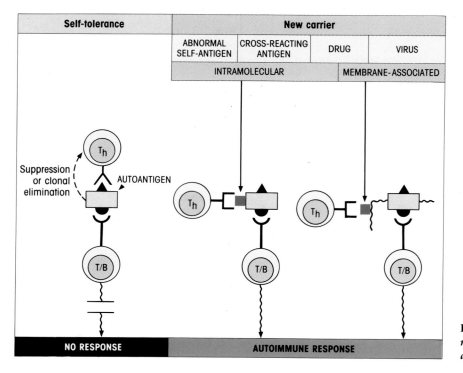

Figure 14.9. *T-helper bypass through new carrier determinant generates autoimmunity.*

antigen and would be less likely to induce B-cell tolerance than the 'stronger' antigens present on the erythrocyte. Isoniazid may produce arthritis associated with nuclear antibodies and unlike most other cases of drug-induced autoimmunity, synthesis of these antibodies is said to continue after cessation of drug therapy. A high proportion of patients on continued treatment with procainamide develop nuclear antibodies and 40% present with clinical signs of SLE. Myasthenia gravis and symptoms of pemphigus have been described in some patients on penicillamine. It is not clear in every case whether the drug provides carrier help through direct modification of the autoantigen or of some independent molecule concerned in associative recognition.

(ii) Cross-reactions of B-cell epitopes

Many examples are known in which potential auto-antigenic determinants are present on an exogenous cross-reacting antigen which provides the new carrier that provokes autoantibody formation. Post-rabies vaccine encephalitis is thought to result from an autoimmune reaction to brain initiated by heterologous brain tissue in the vaccine (cf. experimental allergic encephalomyelitis below). Some microorganisms carry determinants which cross-react with the human and this may prove to be an important way of inducing autoimmunity. In rheumatic fever, antibodies produced to the streptococcus also react with heart, and the sera of 50% of children with the disease who develop Sydenham's chorea give neuronal immunofluorescent staining which can be absorbed out with streptococcal membranes. Colon antibodies present in ulcerative colitis have been found to cross-react with *Escherichia coli* 014. There is also some evidence for the view that antigens common to *Trypanosoma cruzi* and cardiac muscle and peripheral nervous system provoke some of the immunopathological lesions seen in Chagas' disease.

(iii) Cross-reactions of T-cell epitopes

The drawback with the Allison—Weigle model of cross-reaction of B-cell epitopes and provision of a new T-cell carrier is that once the cross-reacting agent is eliminated from the body, and with it the T-cell epitope, there is no way that the auto-immunity can be sustained. The same, however, need not be true for T-cell cross-reactions and, to understand why, we need to start with some

experimental data on the experimental allergic encephalomyelitis model (EAE) in which demyelinating lesions in the brain are induced by immunizing with myelin basic protein (MBP) in complete Freund's adjuvant. Autoreactive T-cells are produced which react with antigen-presenting cells in the brain which have processed self-MBP and the resulting chronic inflammatory attack leads to destruction of myelinated nerve fibres. Murine MBP induces EAE in mice unless they are first tolerized to the N-terminal 11-mer peptide sequence (peptide I; figure 14.10a); heterologous MBP from guinea pigs is able to induce EAE even in tolerized mice (figure 14.10b). Further analysis revealed that in the latter case, EAE was induced by sensitization to a second peptide sequence (peptide II') which cross-reacted with the mouse peptide II although it was not completely identical in sequence. The naïve T-cells had sufficient avidity for antigen-presenting cells with the processed guinea-pig peptide II'/MHC class II complex on their surface and were primed; the processing of autologous MBP peptide II is clearly inadequate to prime these naïve T-cells since the protein was unable to immunize tolerized mice. Now this is the critical point, although processing of autologous peptide II was inadequate for priming of naïve cells, it was sufficient for stimulation of cells already activated and primed by the heterologous peptide II', witness the ability of peptide II'-primed cells to recognize the mouse's own processed peptide II on brain antigen-presenting cells and cause EAE (figure 14.10c). The reason for this is the greater avidity of primed, as distinct from naïve, cells due to selection for higher affinity receptor and the much greater density of accessory molecules, such as CD2 and LFA-1 which assist binding to antigen-presenting cells. Thus, molecules with cross-reacting T-cell epitopes can prime naïve autoreactive T-cells which cannot react with the self-epitope and, once primed, they can then be stimulated by the self-peptide which can theoretically perpetuate the autoimmune process even after elimination of the cross-reacting agent.

A large number of microbial peptide sequences with varying degrees of homology with human proteins have been identified (table 14.4) but it should be emphasized at this stage that they only provide clues for further study. The mere existence of a homology is no certainty that infection with that organism will necessarily lead to autoimmunity because everything depends on the manner in

317

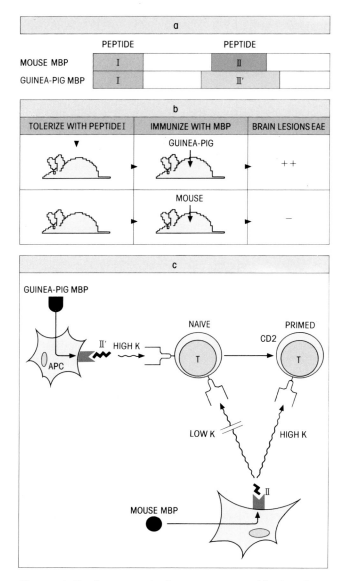

Table 14.4. *Homologies between microbes and body components as potential cross-reacting T-cell epitopes.*

Microbial molecule	Body component
Bacteria:	
Arthritogenic *Shigella flexneri*	HLA-B27
Klebsiella nitrogenase	HLA-B27
Proteus mirabilis urease	HLA-DR4
Coxsackie B VP1	Myocardium
Mycobact. tuberculosis 65 kDa h.s.p.	Joint (adjuvant arthritis)
Viruses:	
EBV gp 110	Dw4 T-cell epitope
HBV octamer	Myelin basic protein
HSV glycoprotein	Acetyl choline receptor
measles haemagglutinin	T-cell subset
retroviral gag p32	U-1 RNA

Figure 14.10. *Cross-reaction between two peptides in guinea-pig and mouse myelin basic protein (MBP) induces autoimmunity to self T-cell epitope. (a) The N-terminal peptide sequence 1–11 is the same in both proteins. Peptides II and II' are similar but not identical. (b) Immunization with peptide II' (whole MBP to mouse tolerized to peptide I) induces autoimmunity to mouse's own peptide II on antigen-presenting cells (APC) in brain. (c) The mechanism: peptide II cannot stimulate the naïve T-cell but peptide II' with a higher affinity can; the primed cell with increased expression of adhesion molecules now has a higher affinity and can react with self peptide II.*

which the proteins are processed by the antigen-presenting cells and we cannot predict, as yet, which peptides will be presented and in what concentration.

(iii) Associative recognition

I have applied the term in the present context to the phenomenon in which one membrane component may provide help for the immune response to another. In the context of autoimmunity, a new helper determinant may arise through drug modification as mentioned above, or through the insertion of viral antigen into the membrane of an infected cell (figure 14.11d). That this can promote a reaction to a pre-existing cell component is clear from the studies in which infection of a tumour with influenza virus elicited resistance to uninfected tumour cells. The appearance of cold agglutinins often with blood group I specificity after *Mycoplasma pneumonia* infection could have a similar explanation. For this mechanism to work, the helper component must still be attached to the membrane fragment bearing the B-cell epitope which is recognized by the B-cell receptor; in this way the helper component will be processed and presented as an epitope for recognition by T-cells (cf. intrastructural as distinct from intramolecular links between B- and T-cell epitopes, p. 123).

Idiotype bypass mechanisms

A substantial body of evidence argues for the view that a regulatable idiotype network appears early in life, possibly related to Ly1+ B-cells and to auto-antibody formation (cf. p. 184 and 185). This raises the possibility of involving autoreactive lymphocytes with responses to exogenous agents through idiotype network connections, particularly since most autoimmune diseases are characterized by major cross-reactive idiotypes.

Thus, knowing that T-helpers with specificity for the idiotype on a lymphocyte receptor can be

319

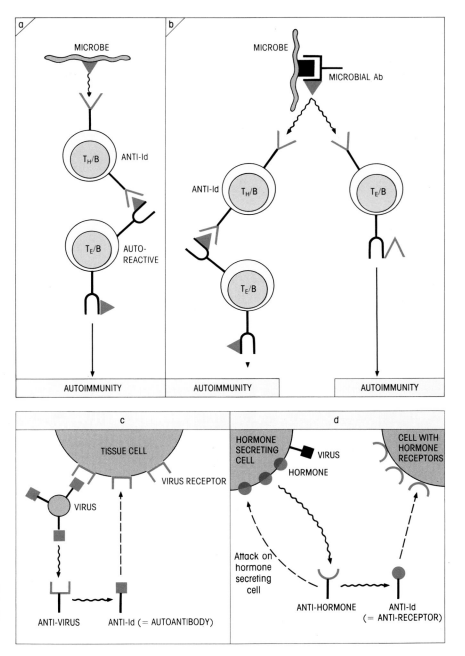

Figure 14.11. *Idiotypic mechanisms leading to autoimmunity. (a) Microbial antigen cross-reacts with autoreactive lymphocyte Id. (b) Microbial antibodies either share Ids with or are anti-Id to autoreactive lymphocytes. (c) Anti-virus generates anti-Id which is autoantibody to viral receptor (Plotz). (d) Viral protein provides T-help to activate anti-hormone/anti-receptor network.*

instrumental in the stimulation of that cell, it is conceivable that an environmental agent such as a parasite or virus which triggered antibody carrying a public idiotype (CRI) which happened to be shared with the receptor of an autoreactive T- or B-cell, could provoke an autoimmune response (figure 14.11b). Similarly, if it is correct that the germ-line idiotypes on autoantibodies generate a whole range of anti-idiotypes which mediate the response to exogenous antigens, then by the same token, it is conceivable that antibodies produced in

response to an infection may react with the corresponding idiotype on the autoreactive lymphocyte (figure 14.11b). For example, a hybridoma from a myasthenia gravis patient secreted an anti-Id to an acetylcholine receptor autoantibody; this anti-Id was found to react with the bacterial product 1,3-dextran. Similarly, immunization with rheumatoid factor (autoantibody to IgG) gave rise to peptidoglycan antibodies although this could also be explained by an alternative mechanism in which the microbial epitope would be assumed to be similar in shape to the autoantibody Id (figure 14.11a). Finally, it is possible for Id network interactions to allow a viral infection to give rise to autoantibodies reacting with the viral receptor (figure 14.11c). Since viruses all bind to specific complementary receptors on the cells they infect, this sequence of events may have serious consequences; we note for example that β-adrenergic receptors are the surface targets for certain reoviruses and that rabies virus binds to the acetylcholine receptor.

Polyclonal activation

Microbes often display adjuvant properties through their possession of polyclonal lymphocyte activators such as bacterial endotoxins which act by providing a non-specific inductive signal for B-cell stimulation, so bypassing the need for specific T-cell help (figure 14.12). This can occur by direct interaction with the B-lymphocyte or indirectly through stimulating the secretion of non-specific factors from T-cells or macrophages. A good example is the thymus-dependent production of autoantibodies by injection of mice with thyroglobulin and endotoxin lipopolysaccharide (LPS) although we are still not sure whether specific T-cells are induced. The variety of autoantibodies detected in cases with infectious mononucleosis must surely be attributable to the polyclonal activation of B-cells by EB virus. They are seen also in lepromatous leprosy where the abundance of mycobacteria reproduces some of the features of Freund's adjuvant. However, unlike the usual situation in human autoimmune disease, these autoantibodies tend to be IgM and, in addition, do not persist when the microbial components are cleared from the body. The bet is that the reactions largely involve CD5$^+$ B-cells.

Curiously, lymphocytes from mice with spontaneous autoimmunity (e.g. NZB and BXSB) produce abnormally large amounts of IgM when cultured *in vitro* as if they were under polyclonal activation; so do lymphocytes from many patients with SLE. On the other hand, the failure of neonatally thyroidectomized Obese strain chickens to make thyroglobulin autoantibodies (p. 314) implies that autoantigen itself is needed for the induction of autoimmunity, in organ-specific disease at least, although the possible requirement for spontaneous production of accessory signals as in the thyroglobulin/LPS experiment just cited, cannot be excluded.

Non-organ-specific autoantibodies directed to autoantigens like DNA and red cells which have repeating antigenic determinants capable of cross-linking surface Ig receptors, are produced by a graft-vs-host reaction in which allogeneic T-cells react with host class II molecules on the B-cell. This form of cooperative polyclonal activation could arise if the self-reactive class II specific T-cells mentioned earlier took the place of the allogeneic T-cells (figure 14.12).

Autoimmunity arising through bypass of regulatory mechanisms

Suppressor circuits may not work

It should be emphasized that these T-helper bypass mechanisms for the induction of autoimmunity do not by themselves ensure the continuation of the response, since normal animals have been shown to be capable of damping down autoantibody production through T-suppressor interactions as, for

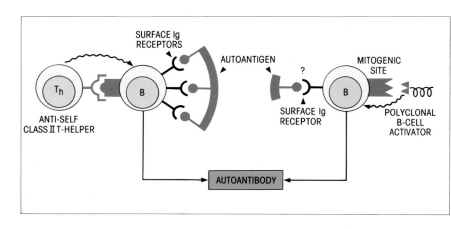

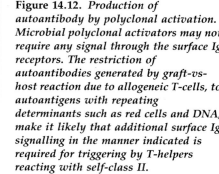

Figure 14.12. *Production of autoantibody by polyclonal activation. Microbial polyclonal activators may not require any signal through the surface Ig receptors. The restriction of autoantibodies generated by graft-vs-host reaction due to allogeneic T-cells, to autoantigens with repeating determinants such as red cells and DNA, make it likely that additional surface Ig signalling in the manner indicated is required for triggering by T-helpers reacting with self-class II.*

example, in the case of red cell autoantibodies induced in mice by injection of rat erythrocytes (figure 14.13). When T-suppressor activity is impaired by low doses of cyclophosphamide or if strains like the SJL which have prematurely ageing suppressors are used, autoimmunity is prolonged and more severe.

In general, manipulations which reduce T-suppressors encourage the development of auto-antibodies. Thymectomy within a narrow window of 2–4 days after birth in the mouse is quite startling in that it gives rise to widespread organ-specific autoimmune disease affecting mainly stomach, thyroid, ovary, prostate and sperm; circulating antibodies are frequently detected and deposits of Ig and complement are frequently seen around the basement membranes. High levels of T-cells with the T-cell receptor Vβ11 family are retained by this neonatal thymectomy in animals in which they would otherwise be eliminated by intrathymic deletion and one must suppose that autoreactive cells are being produced. Spleen cells from intact adult females but not males injected into these 3-day thymectomized mice cannot prevent the development of prostatitis although they do prevent gastritis, from which one concludes that the normal male has additional suppressor T-cells specific for prostate and activated by prostate antigens. Presumably the thymus is producing potential organ-specific suppressors between days 2–4 and at that time thymectomy upsets the balance between auto-reactive and suppressor cells.

Neonatal thymectomy which greatly depletes the T-suppressor population, induces or exacerbates spontaneous autoimmune states in susceptible animals—autoimmune haemolytic anaemia in NZB mice and thyroiditis in Obese strain chickens and Buffalo rats. Coombs' positivity (i.e. the state in which circulating red cells are coated with antibody) can be transferred with the spleen cells of a Coombs' positive NZB to a young negative mouse of the same strain, but the continued production of red cell antibodies is short lived unless the recipient's T-cells are first depleted by pretreatment with anti-lymphocyte serum. Other changes seen with age in the NZB are an increasing resistance to the induction of tolerance to soluble proteins and a sudden fall in the plasma concentration of the thymic peptide thymulin before the onset of disease (note: thymulin is said to inhibit the autoreactive response of spleen cells to syngeneic fibroblasts in culture). Thus, there is a widely held view that one defect in the NZB is a progressive loss of T-suppressors with age

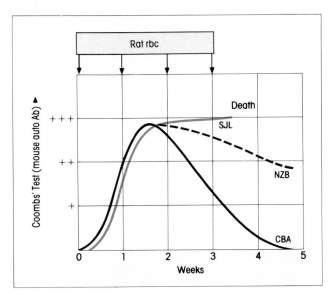

Figure 14.13. *Regulation of self-reactivity. When CBA mice are injected with rat red cells, autoantibodies are produced by this cross-reacting antigen (p. 317) which coat the host erythrocytes and are detected by the Coombs' test (p. 263). The SJL strain, in which suppressor activity declines rapidly with age, is unable to regulate the autoimmune response and develops particularly severe disease. The response is also prolonged in the autoimmune NZB strain (after A. Cooke & P. Hutchings).*

(figure 14.13) and it may be relevant that CD8 cells which may be required for suppression are low in diseased mice.

Defects are possible at various other control points in the regulatory mechanism: for example, the NOD mouse which spontaneously develops autoimmune diabetes fails to express I-E. Cross-breeding with the C3H strain shows the failure to be recessive and linked to the development of disease. It could be that T-suppressors are generated by a response to I-E in this system (cf. p. 158) and fail to develop if it is not expressed, or perhaps that a critical TCR Vβ family is eliminated intrathymically by exposure to I-E derived peptides presented by 1-A^{NOD} (or conversely by 1-A^{NOD} peptides presented by I-E?). Another mutant mouse strain with a spontaneous SLE-like syndrome, the MRL/lpr, has ample numbers of effective CD8 cells but CD4 helpers are reported to be resistant to their suppressor action due, it is said, to excessive *contrasuppressor* activity by a subpopulation of Ly1$^+$2$^-$ T-cells with binding sites for the lectin *Vicia villosa*. While this area is still relatively woolly, it requires no gigantic leap of imagination to realize that undue activity by such cells will lower the threshold for autoimmunity (figure 14.14).

AUTOIMMUNE DISEASES — SCOPE

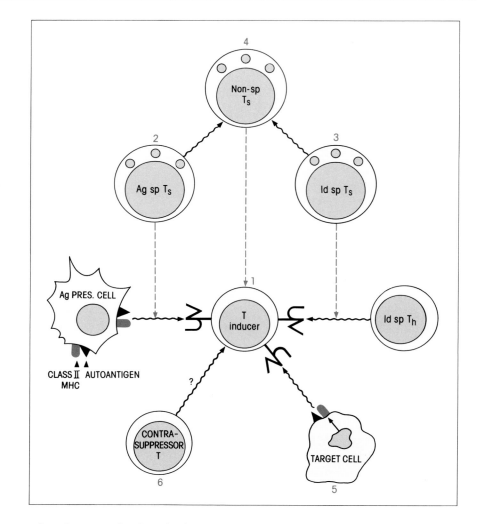

Figure 14.14. *Bypass of regulatory mechanisms leads to triggering of autoreactive T-helper cells through defects in (1) ability to respond to or induce T-suppressors, or (2) expression of antigen-specific, (3) idiotype-specific or (4) non-specific T-suppressors, or through (5) imbalance of the cytokine network producing derepression of class II genes with inappropriate cellular expression of class II and presentation of antigen on target cell, stimulation of antigen-presenting cell, and possible activation of anergic T-helper, or (6) through stimulation of the infamous contrasuppressor cell.*

We have previously drawn attention to the distinctive properties of the CD5$^+$ B population with respect to its propensity to synthesize IgM auto-antibodies and its possible intimate relationship to the setting up of the regulatory idiotype network (cf. p. 159) and one must seriously entertain the hypothesis that unregulated activity by these cells could be responsible for certain autoimmune disorders. The pitifully named moth-eaten strain is heavily into autoimmunity, and the mice make masses of anti-DNA and anti-polymorphs and die with intense pneumonitis, often before they have tasted the fruits of life. Their IgM levels rise to a staggering level of 25–50 times normal and—this is quite bizarre—their B-cells are nearly all CD5

positive. This population is also raised in the NZB and largely accounts for the production of the IgM autoantibodies in this strain. Since pathogenic auto-antibodies often tend to be IgG, one is prompted to ask whether these CD5$^+$ B-cells have escaped regulatory control and undergo an unrestrained isotype switch to IgG as a basis for production of disease. Indirect evidence for their participation in the disease process comes from breeding experiments with CBA/N mice with the X-linked immune deficiency (xid) trait which includes an inability to develop CD5$^+$ B-cells. Crossing a female CBA/N with a male NZB gives F1 animals which do express the xid defect and *do not* develop autoimmune haemolytic anaemia, whereas (male CBA/N × female

NZB) F1s do not have the xid defect, do make CD5$^+$ B-cells and do develop autoimmune disease.

In man, a high proportion of CD5$^+$ B-cells make IgM rheumatoid factors (anti-Fcγ) and anti-DNA using germ-line genes. In rheumatoid arthritis patients, although there are increased numbers of circulating CD5$^+$ B-cells, the polyclonal rheumatoid factors synthesized do not by and large, bear the public idiotypes of the CD5$^+$ set nor show somatic mutation. SLE could be different because the 16/6 public idiotype associated with germ-line genes encoding anti-DNA is found on a significant fraction of the IgG anti-DNA in patients' sera. Gene sequencing is required to establish the relationship between CD5$^+$ B-cells and IgG autoantibody synthesis, particularly since CD5$^+$ B-cells lose their surface marker as they mature after activation.

Less is known of regulatory circuits in man although there is increasing evidence that non-specific T-suppressor function in SLE may be poorly regulated. B-lymphocytes from patients with active disease secrete larger amounts of Ig when cultured *in vitro* than normal B-cells. Concanavalin-A-induced non-specific suppressors are reduced or absent and T-cells with Fcγ receptors, which suppress pokeweed mitogen-stimulated lymphocytes (p. 155) are low, the defect being greater the more active the disease. The production of thymulin and of interleukin-2 is also depressed in these patients. A significant proportion of clinically un-affected close relatives also demonstrate abnormally low levels of non-specific suppressors indicating that the deficit in SLE patients is not a consequence of the illness or its treatment and that additional factors must be implicated in the causation of disease.

In any case, it is difficult to account for the antigenic specificity of different autoimmune disorders on the basis of a generalized depression of non-specific suppressors alone, without invoking defects in either antigen- or idiotype-specific suppressor T-cells (p. 158). There is, however, a further possibility which has aroused much interest.

Inappropriate expression of class II molecules

The majority of organ-specific autoantigens normally appear on the surface of the cells of the target organ in the context of class I but not class II MHC molecules. As such they cannot communicate with T-helpers and are therefore immunologically silent. Pujol-Borrell, Bottazzo and colleagues reasoned that if the class II genes were somehow derepressed and class II molecules were now synthesized, they would endow the surface molecules with potential autoantigenicity (figure 14.14). Indeed, they have been able to show that human thyroid cells in tissue culture can be persuaded to express HLA-DR (class II) molecules on their surface after stimulation with γ-interferon, and, further, that the cytoplasm of epithelial cells from the glands of patients with Graves' disease (thyrotoxicosis) stains strongly with anti-HLA-DR reagents, indicating active synthesis of class II polypeptides (figure 14.2b). Inappropriate class II expression has also been reported on the bile ductules in primary biliary cirrhosis and on endothelial cells and some β-cells in the diabetic pancreas both in the human and in the BB rat model (figure 14.2c and d). Whether adventitious expression of class II on these cells by something like virally induced interferon is responsible for *initiating* the autoimmune process by priming autoreactive T-helpers, or whether reaction with *already activated* T-cells induces class II by release of IFNγ and makes the cell a more attractive target for provoking subsequent tissue damage, is still an unresolved issue.

Transfection of mice with the class II I-A gene linked to the insulin-promoter led to expression of class II on the β-islet cells of the pancreas and did *not* induce autoimmunity although it did cause insulin exhaustion by a non-immunological mechanism. On the other hand transfection with the IFNγ gene under the same circumstances produced a local inflammatory reaction in the pancreas with aberrant expression of class II and diabetes; this may have been a result of autoimmunity since a normal pancreas grafted into the same animal suffered a similar fate.

Cytokine imbalance may induce autoimmunity

This last experiment implies that unregulated cytokine production producing a local inflammatory reaction may initiate autoimmunity perhaps by upregulating MHC expression, increasing the available concentration of processed intracellular autoantigens, increasing the avidity of antigen-processing cells for naïve T-cells by upregulating adhesion molecules, or even by making previously anergic cells responsive to antigen. We can correct some spontaneous models of autoimmune disease by injection of cytokines: IL-1 cures the diabetes of

NOD mice and TNF prevents the onset of SLE symptoms in NZB × W hybrids.

Detailed studies have been made of cytokine synthesis in the battleground of the joint in rheumatoid arthritis. Cultures of synovial T-cells spontaneously produced high levels of TNFα and of GM-CSF which strongly activate macrophages, but very little IFNγ or TNFβ even though mRNA was present (perhaps due to TGF?). Does this hot-bed of chronic inflammation nurture the seeds of persistent autoimmune reactivity?

Autoimmune disorders are multifactorial

I must come back to this. Undoubtedly, the autoimmune diseases have a multifactorial aetiology. Perhaps most, if not all, the defects we have discussed may contribute in different combinations to different disorders. Although these defects individually may be not uncommon, their origin remains obscure. Superimposed upon a genetically complex susceptibility, we might be dealing with some ageing process affecting the thymus or the lymphoid stem cells and their internal control of self-reactivity. Sex hormones may contribute. Now throw into this melange a panoply of environmental factors particularly microbial agents which could have a variety of effects on the target organs, the lymphoid system and the cytokine network.

SUMMARY

Autoimmunity is associated with certain diseases which form a spectrum. At one pole, exemplified by Hashimoto's thyroiditis, the autoantibodies and the lesions are *organ specific* with the organ acting as the target for autoimmune attack; at the other pole are the *non-organ-specific* diseases such as systemic lupus erythematosus where the autoantibodies have widespread reactivity and the lesions resemble those of serum sickness relating to deposition of circulating immune complexes. There is a tendency for organ-specific disorders such as thyroiditis and pernicious anaemia to overlap in given individuals while overlap of rheumatological disorders is greater than expected by chance. Multifactorial genetic factors increase predisposition to autoimmune

disease: these include HLA tissue type and factors affecting the immune system and possibly the potential autoantigens.

Autoantigens are for the most part accessible to circulating lymphocytes which normally include autoreactive T- and B-cells. It is assumed that the key to the system is control of autoreactive T-inducer/helper cells which are normally unresponsive because of clonal deletion, clonal anergy, T-suppression or inadequate autoantigen processing. Autoimmunity might arise by several mechanisms involving bypass of these key T-helper cells. These would include the provision of new carrier determinants on the autoantigen either through abnormal modification through synthesis or breakdown, through cross-reaction with exogenous antigens, or by associative recognition with viral or administered drug determinants. T-helpers could also be bypassed by idiotype network interactions with cross-reactions between public idiotypes on autoantibodies and microbial antibodies or microbes themselves, or by antibodies formed to anti-viral idiotypes which behaved as internal images of the virus and reacted with the cell surface viral receptor. Finally, B-cells can be stimulated directly by polyclonal activators such as EB virus or lipopolysaccharides, or by an expansion of naturally occurring autoreactive anti-self class II T-helpers.

T-helper bypass alone may be insufficient to *maintain* autoimmunity and it is generally considered that, in addition, a regulatory defect is required. This could occur through an inability of the central T-helper cell to respond to or induce T-suppressors. It could also arise through defects in the antigen-specific, idiotype-specific and non-specific T-suppressor systems. Other possibilities would be a stimulation of contrasuppressor cells, the derepression of class II genes giving rise to inappropriate cellular expression of class II so breaking the 'silence' between cellular autoantigen and autoreactive T-inducer, and cytokine imbalance.

Given the genetic predisposition, these changes could come about by some spontaneous internal dysregulation related perhaps to ageing, and/or through environmental factors, particularly microbes, which could act in an uncomfortably large number of different ways.

Suggestions for further reading are given at the end of the following chapter.

CHAPTER 15

AUTOIMMUNE DISEASES
II – Pathogenesis, Diagnosis and Treatment

PATHOGENIC MECHANISMS IN AUTOIMMUNE DISEASE

We have mentioned that despite certain exceptions as, for instance, myocardial infarction or damage to the testis, traumatic release of organ constituents does not in general elicit antibody formation. Destruction of thyroid tissue by therapeutic doses of radio-iodine does not initiate thyroid auto-immunity, nor does damage to the liver in alcoholic cirrhosis result in the synthesis of mitochondrial antibodies, to give but two examples. We should now look at the evidence which bears directly on the issue of whether autoimmunity, however it arises, plays a *primary* pathogenic role in the production of tissue lesions in the group of diseases labelled as 'autoimmune'.

Effects of humoral antibody

Blood

The erythrocyte antibodies play a role in the destruction of red cells in autoimmune haemolytic anaemia. Normal red cells coated with autoantibody eluted from Coombs' positive erythrocytes have a shortened half-life after reinjection into the normal subject. Platelet antibodies are apparently responsible for idiopathic thrombocytopenic purpura (ITP). IgG from a patient's serum when given to a

normal individual causes a depression of platelet counts and the active principle can be absorbed out with platelets. The transient neonatal thrombocytopenia which may be seen in infants of mothers with ITP is explicable in terms of transplacental passage of IgG antibodies to the child.

Some children with immunodeficiency associated with very low white cell counts have a serum lymphocytotoxic factor which requires complement for its activity. Lymphopenia occurring in patients with SLE and rheumatoid arthritis may also be a direct result of antibody since non-agglutinating antibodies coating the white cells have been reported in such cases.

Thyroid

Cytotoxic antibodies

The serum of patients with Hashimoto's disease is cytotoxic for human thyroid cells growing in monolayer culture after dispersal by trypsin. This is a typical complement-mediated antibody reaction directed against a cell surface antigen which is identical with the thyroid peroxidase antigen revealed by intracytoplasmic staining of thyroid sections with sera from Hashimoto patients. Curiously, this antigen is expressed only on the apical portion of the follicular cells in contact with the colloid so that it is not normally accessible to circulating antibody. This explains why simple fragments of thyroid which have intact follicles are unaffected by incubation in the presence of medium containing cytotoxic antibody and complement, and also why there is no evidence that infants born to Hashimoto mothers have defective thyroid function despite the presence of the antibody in their serum. None the less, antibody can be detected on the inner surface of thyroid follicles in tissue removed from patients with autoimmune thyroiditis, and it seems necessary to postulate that thyroid damage only occurs when there is collaboration with other factors such as immune complex deposition, sensitized T-cell effectors or mechanisms which bring about a reversal of polarity of the epithelial cells.

Thyroid-stimulating antibodies

Under certain circumstances antibodies to the surface of a cell may stimulate rather than destroy (cf. type V sensitivity; Chapter 12). This would seem to be the case in thyrotoxicosis (Graves' or Basedow's disease). There has long been indirect evidence suggesting a link between autoimmune processes and this disease: thyroid antibodies are detectable in up to 85% of thyrotoxic patients and histologically the majority of the glands removed at operation show varying degrees of thyroiditis and local antibody formation in addition to the characteristic acinar cell hyperplasia; thyrotoxicosis is found with undue frequency in the families of Hashimoto patients; there is an association with gastric autoimmunity in that 30% have gastric antibodies and up to 10% pernicious anaemia. The direct link came with the discovery by Adams and Purves of thyroid stimulating activity in the serum of thyrotoxic patients. Using a new bioassay they found that the serum caused a stimulation of the thyroid gland of the recipient animal which was considerably prolonged relative to the time course of action

of the physiological thyroid stimulating hormone (TSH) from the pituitary; it was ultimately shown that this was due to the presence of thyroid stimulating antibodies (TSAb). These antibodies can block the binding of TSH to thyroid membranes and seem to act in the same manner as TSH, probably by stimulating the identical receptors (cf. figure 12.20). Both operate through the adenyl cyclase system as indicated by the potentiating effect of theophylline, and both produce similar changes in ultrastructural morphology in the thyroid cell, but it is one of Nature's 'passive transfer experiments' which links TSAb most directly with the pathogenesis of Graves' disease. When TSAb from a thyrotoxic mother crosses the placenta it is associated with the production of neonatal hyperthyroidism (figure 15.1), which resolves after a few weeks as the maternal IgG is catabolized.

There is a good correlation between the titre of TSAb and the severity of hyperthyroidism. Because TSAb act independently of the pituitary–thyroid axis, iodine uptake by the gland is unaffected by administration of thyroxine or tri-iodothyronine, whereas normally this would cause feedback inhibition and suppression of uptake; this forms the basis of an important diagnostic test for thyrotoxicosis.

There is reason to believe that enlargement of the thyroid in this disorder is due to the action of antibodies which react with a 'growth' receptor and directly stimulate cell division as distinct from metabolic hyperactivity, (figure 15.2a). In contrast, sera from patients with primary myxoedema contain antibodies capable of blocking the mitogenic action of TSH (figure 15.2b) thereby preventing the regeneration of follicles which is a feature of the enlarged Hashimoto goitre. We see now that there is considerable diversity in the autoimmune response to the thyroid leading to tissue destruction, metabolic stimulation, growth promotion or mitotic inhibition

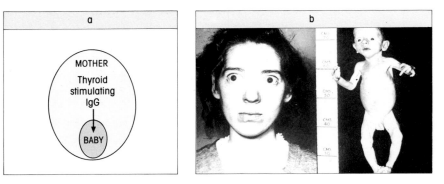

Figure 15.1. *Neonatal thyrotoxicosis. (a) The autoantibodies which stimulate the thyroid through the TSH-receptors are IgG and cross the placenta. (b) The thyrotoxic mother therefore gives birth to a baby with thyroid hyperactivity which spontaneously resolves as the mother's IgG is catabolized. (Photograph courtesy of Dr A. MacGregor.)*

326

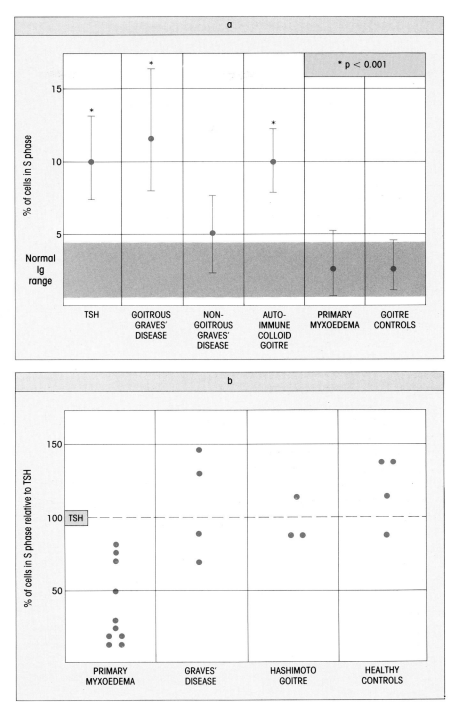

Figure 15.2. *Autoantibodies affecting thyroid growth. (a) Stimulating antibodies in goitrous Graves' disease and autoimmune colloid goitre shown by the increase of cells entering the DNA synthetic (S) phase of the cell cycle in thyroid fragments treated with IgG from the patient's serum. p values relate to differences from results with normal Ig. (b) Blocking antibodies in primary myxoedema revealed by the ability of patient's IgG to inhibit the growth stimulation caused by TSH. Each point represents the value for an individual patient's serum. (Data from Drexhage H.A., Bottazzo G.F., Doniach D., Bitensky L. & Chayen J. (1980) Lancet ii, 287 and from (1981) Nature 289, 594.)*

which in different combinations account for the variety of forms in which autoimmune thyroid disease presents (figure 15.3).

Stomach

Autoantibodies to intrinsic factor, a product of gastric mucosal secretion were first demonstrated in

pernicious anaemia patients by oral administration of intrinsic factor, vitamin B_{12} and the serum from a patient with this disease. The serum was found to prevent intrinsic factor from mediating the absorption of B_{12} into the body, and further studies showed the active principle to be an antibody. Circulating antibody does not seem to be capable of neutralizing the physiological activity of intrinsic

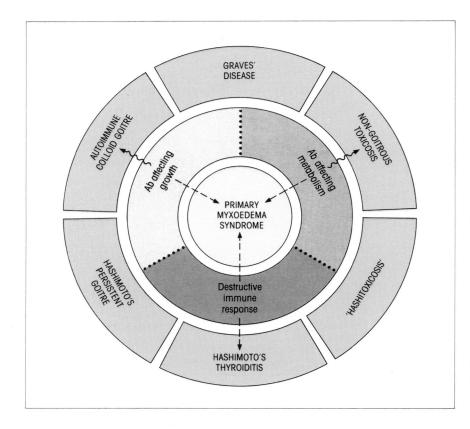

Figure 15.3. *Relationship of different autoallergic responses to the circular spectrum of autoimmune thyroid diseases. Responses involving thyroglobulin and the thyroid peroxidase microsomal surface microvillous antigen lead to tissue destruction whereas other autoantibodies can stimulate or block metabolic activity or thyroid cell division. 'Hashitoxicosis' is the down-to-earth term used by our Scots' colleagues to describe a gland showing Hashimoto's thyroiditis and thyrotoxicosis simultaneously (courtesy of Prof. D. Doniach and Dr G.F. Bottazzo).*

factor; a patient immunized parenterally with hog intrinsic factor in complete Freund's adjuvant had high serum antibody levels and good cell-mediated skin responses but still absorbed B_{12} well when fed with hog intrinsic factor. These data imply that the antibodies have to be present within the lumen of the gastro-intestinal tract to be biologically effective, and indeed they can be identified in the gastric juice of these patients, synthesized by plasma cells in the gastric lesion.

While there is no evidence that antibodies which can block the gastrin receptor on parietal cells are capable of tissue destruction, it is odds on that they contribute to the hypo- and achlorhydria seen in pernicious anaemia and atrophic gastritis especially when there are residual parietal cells in the gastric mucosa. The idea that some cases of gastric ulcer may result from stimulation of acid secretion by activation through antibodies to histamine receptors is appealing and we await the further work required to establish its validity.

Sperm

In some infertile males, agglutinating antibodies cause aggregation of the spermatozoa and interfere with their penetration into the cervical mucus.

Glomerular basement membrane (gbm)

With immunological kidney disease the experimental models preceded the finding of parallel lesions in the human. Injection of cross-reacting heterologous gbm preparations in complete Freund's adjuvant produces glomerulonephritis in sheep and other experimental animals. Antibodies to gbm can be picked up by immunofluorescent staining of biopsies from nephritic animals with anti-IgG. The antibodies are largely, if not completely, absorbed out by the kidney *in vivo* but they appear in the serum on nephrectomy and can passively transfer the disease to another animal of the same species.

An entirely analogous situation occurs in man in certain cases of glomerulonephritis, particularly those associated with lung haemorrhage (Goodpasture's syndrome). Kidney biopsy from the patient shows *linear* deposition of IgG and C3 along the basement membrane of the glomerular capillaries (figure 12.13a). After nephrectomy, gbm antibodies can be detected in the serum. Lerner and his colleagues eluted the gbm antibody from a diseased kidney and injected it into a squirrel monkey. The antibody rapidly fixed to the gbm of the recipient animal and produced a fatal nephritis

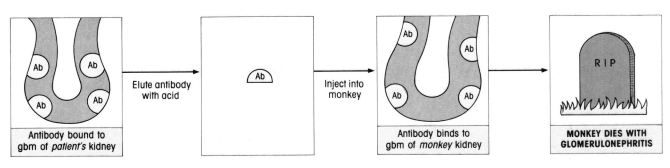

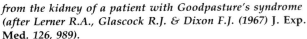

Figure 15.4. *Passive transfer of glomerulonephritis to a squirrel monkey by injection of antiglomerular basement membrane (anti-gbm) antibodies isolated by acid elution* *from the kidney of a patient with Goodpasture's syndrome (after Lerner R.A., Glascock R.J. & Dixon F.J. (1967) J. Exp. Med. 126, 989).*

(figure 15.4). It is hard to escape the conclusion that the lesion in the human was the direct result of attack on the gbm by these complement-fixing antibodies. The lung changes in Goodpasture's syndrome are attributable to cross-reaction with some of the gbm antibodies.

Muscle

The transient muscle weakness seen in a proportion of babies born to mothers with myasthenia gravis calls to mind neonatal thrombocytopenia and hyperthyroidism and would certainly be compatible with the transplacental passage of an IgG capable of inhibiting neuromuscular transmission. Strong support for this view is afforded by the consistent finding of antibodies to muscle acetylcholine receptors in myasthenics and the depletion of these receptors within the motor end-plates. In addition, myasthenic symptoms can be induced in animals by injection of monoclonal antibodies to acetylcholine receptors or by active immunization with the purified receptors themselves. None the less, the majority of babies with myasthenic mothers do not display muscle disease and it transpires that they are protecting themselves by producing antibodies directed to idiotypes on the maternal autoantibodies.

Table 15.1 summarizes these direct pathogenic effects of humoral autoantibodies.

329

DISEASE	AUTOANTIGEN	LESION
Autoimmune haemolytic anaemia	Red cell	Erythrocyte destruction
Lymphopenia (some cases)	Lymphocyte	Lymphocyte destruction
Idiopathic thrombocytopenic purpura	Platelet	Platelet destruction
Male infertility (some cases)	Sperm	Agglutination of spermatozoa
Pernicious anaemia	Intrinsic factor	Neutralization of ability to mediate B_{12} absorption
Hashimoto's disease	Thyroid peroxidase surface antigen	Cytotoxic effect on thyroid cells in culture
Primary myxoedema	TSH receptor	Blocking of thyroid cell
Thyrotoxicosis	TSH receptor	Stimulation of thyroid cell
Goodpasture's syndrome	Glomerular basement membrane	Complement-mediated damage to basement membrane
Myasthenia gravis	Acetylcholine receptor	Blocking and destruction of receptors
Acanthosis nigricans (type B) and ataxia telangiectasia with insulin resistance	Insulin receptor	Blocking of receptors
Atopic allergy (some cases)	β-Adrenergic receptors	Blocking of receptors

Table 15.1. *Direct pathogenic effects of humoral antibodies.*

Systemic lupus erythematosus (SLE)

Where autoantibodies are formed against soluble components to which they have continual access, complexes may be formed which can give rise to lesions similar to those occurring in serum sickness especially when defects in the early classical complement components prevent effective clearance (cf. p. 265). In SLE, complexes of DNA and other nuclear antigens, together with immunoglobulin and complement, can be detected by immunofluorescent staining of kidney biopsies from patients with evidence of renal dysfunction. The staining pattern with a fluorescent anti-IgG or anti-C3 is punctate or 'lumpy-bumpy' as some would describe it (figure 12.13b) in marked contrast with the linear pattern caused by the gbm antibodies in Goodpasture's syndrome (figure 12.13a; p. 264). The complexes grow in size to become large aggregates visible in the electron microscope as amorphous humps on the epithelial side of the glomerular basement membrane (figure 15.5). During the active phase of the disease, serum complement levels fall as components are affected by immune aggregates in the kidney and circulation. Attempts to detect autoantigens in the circulating complexes have not been conspicuously successful; immunoglobulins and complement components make up the usual tally of constituents which can be identified. Although in a way negative evidence, this is consistent with the possibility that anti-idiotype may perpetuate an autoimmune state once it is initiated (i.e. acts as a surrogate autoantigen) and generate circulating idiotype—anti-idiotype complexes.

Immunofluorescent studies on skin biopsies from patients with the related disease discoid lupus erythematosus also reveal the presence of immune complexes.

Rheumatoid arthritis

Morphological evidence for immunological activity

The joint changes in rheumatoid arthritis are in essence produced by the malign growth of the synovial cells as a pannus overlaying and destroying cartilage and bone (figure 15.6a—f). The synovial membrane which surrounds and maintains the joint space becomes intensely cellular as a result of considerable immunological hyper-reactivity as evidenced by large numbers of T-cells, mostly CD4, in various stages of activation, usually associated with dendritic cells and macrophages; clumps of plasma cells are frequently observed and sometimes even secondary follicles with germinal centres are present as though the synovium had become an active lymph node (figure 15.6g, h and i). Indeed it has been estimated that the synthesis of immunoglobulins by the synovial tissue ranks with that of a stimulated lymph node. There is widespread expression of surface HLA-DR (class II); T- and B-cells, dendritic and synovial lining cells and macrophages are all positive, indicative of some pretty lively action (figure 15.6k). The thesis is that this fiery immunological reactivity provides an intense stimulus to the synovial lining cells which undergo a Dr Jeckyll to Mr Hyde transformation into the invasive pannus which brings about joint erosion through the release of destructive mediators.

What is provoking this immunological activity?

From the T-cell standpoint, no conventional antigens have yet been identified. There are currently reports of the isolation of T-cell lines from the joint which are driven by EB virus transformed B-cell lines derived from the same lymphocyte populations. This suggest perhaps four main possibilities for the T-cell-line specificities: anti-B-cell idiotype, and anti-self class II MHC either alone or associated with processed EBV protein or stress (heat shock) proteins. Synthesis of the latter increases in response to external 'insults' such as a rise in temperature, viral infection, cytokine stimulation, or may be even shear forces in joints which are active. Although it should not be too difficult to sort out this matter, at the time of writing I do not have the required data. For argument's sake let me plump for the possibility that there are significant numbers of T-cells which react with autologous class II determinants bearing peptides derived from stress proteins. The reader should be warned that the disproportionate amount of space devoted to the next few sections reflects the author's idiosyncratic view of the subject.

IgG autosensitization

By utilizing the mechanism set out in figure 14.12 (p. 320), these T-cells could stimulate joint B-lymphocytes expressing stress protein peptides which have reacted with autoantigens bearing

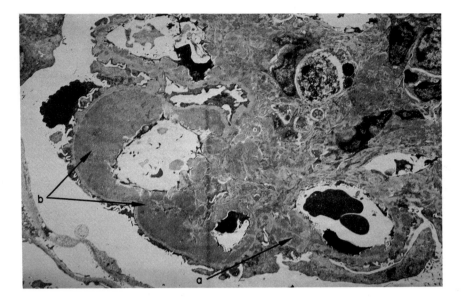

Figure 15.5. *Renal biopsy of SLE patient with severe immune complex glomerulonephritis and proteinuria. Electron micrograph showing irregular thickening of glomerular capillary walls by subepithelial complexes (a) and subendothelial complexes (b). The mesangial region shows abundant (probably phagocytosed) complexes. (Courtesy of Dr A. Leatham.)*

repeating determinants; in particular, in the context of rheumatoid arthritis, these might be the multiple Fc regions of IgG within a soluble immune complex. This would lead to the synthesis of autoantibodies to the IgG Fc region, known as antiglobulins or rheumatoid factors. These are the hallmark of the disease, being demonstrable in virtually all patients with rheumatoid arthritis. The majority have IgM antiglobulins which react in the classical latex and sheep cell agglutination tests (table 14.2; note 7) and both they and the 'seronegative' patients who fail to react in these tests can be shown to have elevated levels of IgG antiglobulins detectable by solid phase immunoassay (cf. p. 94; figure 15.7).

If, therefore, autosensitization to IgG is an almost universal feature of the disease, most of the plasma cells in the synovium should be synthesizing antiglobulins. But in fact only a relative minority of the plasma cells (say 10−20%) bind fluoresceinated IgG, either in the form of heat-aggregated material (figure 15.6j) or immune complexes (rheumatoid factor is a low affinity antibody and good binding is only seen when multivalent IgG is used as antigen). However, we must take into account a strange and unique feature of IgG antiglobulins; because they are both antigen and antibody at the same time, they are capable of self-association (figure 15.8b) and this hides the majority of free antiglobulin valencies. Cleverly realizing that destruction of the Fc regions by pepsin would liberate these hidden binding sites (figure 15.8c), Munthe & Natvig observed that as many as 40−70% of the plasma

cells in the synovium displayed an anti-IgG specificity following treatment with this enzyme.

IgG aggregates, presumably products of these plasma cells, can be regularly detected in the synovial tissues and in the joint fluid where they give rise to typical acute inflammatory reactions with fluid exudates. Analysis shows them to consist almost exclusively of immunoglobulins and complement while a major proportion of the IgG is present as self-associated antiglobulin as shown by binding to an Fcγ immunosorbent after treatment with pepsin.

Abnormal glycosylation

One of the most recent events in the rheumatoid arthritis saga has been the discovery that the patients' IgG is abnormally glycosylated. The two C_H2 domains in the Fc region are held apart (cf. p. 44) by two asparagine-linked sugars of the general structure shown in figure 15.9a. The 1,3 arms from each sugar provide a bridge between the domains while the 1,6 sugars are directed towards the protein surface where the terminal sialic acid−galactose lies in a special 'lectin-like' pocket (figure 15.9b and c). Some chains end in N-acetyl-glucosamine and lack the terminal sialic acid−galactose sugars. In normal individuals, some 14% of the IgG Fc sugar groups lack the terminal galactose on *both* chains. What is extraordinary is that the percentage of sugars completely lacking galactose in the IgG of rheumatoid arthritis patients is always higher than

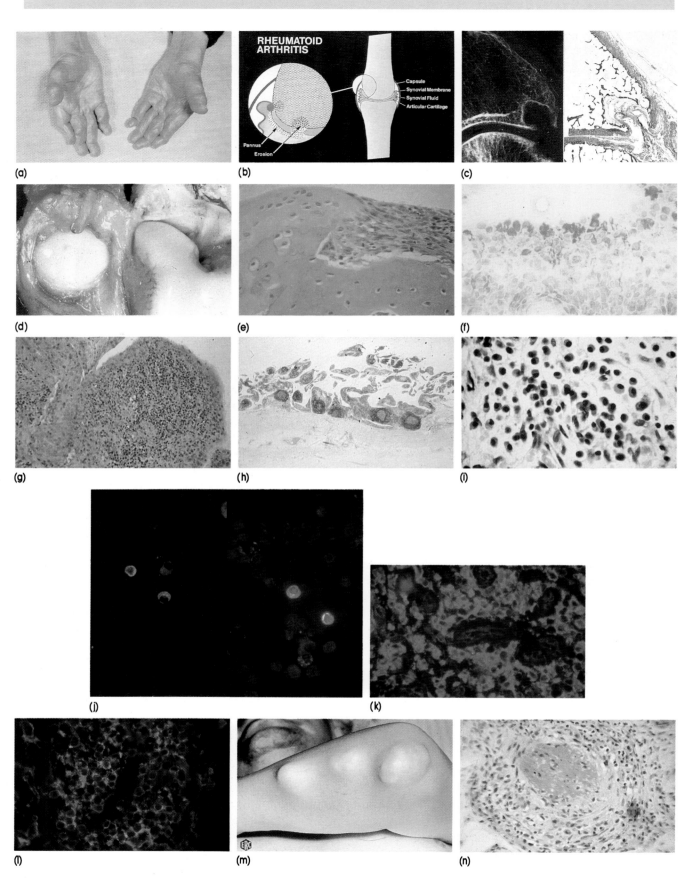

(a)

(b) RHEUMATOID ARTHRITIS
Capsule
Synovial Membrane
Synovial Fluid
Articular Cartilage
Pannus
Erosion

(c)

(d)

(e)

(f)

(g)

(h)

(i)

(j)

(k)

(l)

(m)

(n)

CHAPTER 15

in the controls and can go as high as 60% (figure 15.10). This glycosylation defect could lead to conformational change in the Fc structure with two possible consequences:

1 the Fc may have increased autoantigenicity, and
2 self-associated IgG complexes (figure 15.8) would be held together more strongly if the terminal sialic acid—galactose on the Fab sugar of one IgG fits into the lectin site on C_H2 left vacant by the lack of galactose on the Fc sugar. The glycosylation defect is not seen in SLE but is every bit as abnormal in tuberculosis!

The production of tissue damage

As explained in the legend to figure 15.8, the complexes can be stabilized by the multivalent Fcγ-binding molecules, IgM rheumatoid factor and Clq, and when present in the joint space they may initiate an Arthus reaction leading to an influx of polymorphs with which they react to release lysosomal enzymes. These include neutral proteinases and collagenase which can damage the articular cartilage by breaking down proteoglycans and collagen fibrils. More damage results if the complexes are adherent to the cartilage since the polymorph binds but is unable to internalize them ('frustrated phagocytosis'); as a result the lysosomal hydrolases are released extracellularly into the space between the cell and the cartilage where they are protected from enzyme inhibitors such as α_2-macroglobulin.

The aggregates may also stimulate the macrophage-like cells of the synovial lining, either directly through their surface receptors or indirectly through phagocytosis and resistance to intracellular digestion. The release of lymphokines such as TNFα and GM-CSF from activated T-cells provides further potent macrophage stimulators.

The activated synovial cells grow out as a malign pannus (cover) over the cartilage (figure 15.7d) and at the margin of this advancing granulation tissue breakdown can be seen (figure 15.7e), almost certainly as a result of the release of enzymes, reactive oxygen intermediates and especially of interleukin-1, IL-6 and TNFα. Activated macrophages also secrete plasminogen activator and the plasmin formed as a consequence activates a latent collagenase produced by synovial cells. Sensitization to partially degraded collagen may occur and this could lead secondarily to amplification of the lesion. The secreted products of the stimulated macrophage, can activate chondrocytes to exacerbate cartilage breakdown, and osteoclasts to bring about bone resorption which is a further complication of severe disease. Subcutaneous nodules are granulomata (figure 15.6m and n) possibly formed through local production of insolubilized self-associating antiglobulins.

The rheumatological pulse quickened perceptibly a few years ago with the discovery that a high proportion of patients with rheumatoid arthritis have elevated titres of circulating antibodies to a nuclear antigen present in EB virus transformed but absent from normal lymphocytes. This led to the finding that the T-cells in these patients are deficient in the γ-interferon-mediated control of EB virus transformation of B-lymphocytes. Although it is unlikely that this signifies a primary aetiological role for EB virus infection, it could represent a basic

333

Facing page

Figure 15.6. *Rheumatoid arthritis (RA). (a) Hands of a patient with chronic RA showing classical swan-neck deformities. (b) Diagrammatic representation of a diarthrodial joint showing bone and cartilagenous erosions beneath the synovial membrane derived pannus. (c) Proximal interphalangeal joint depicting marked bony erosion and marginal erosion of the cartilage. (d) Early pannus of granulation tissue growing over the patella. (e) Histology of pannus showing clear erosion of bone and cartilage at the cellular margin. (f) Histology of the pannus stained for macrophage non-specific esterase; note long stained dendritic processes. (g) Chronic inflammatory cells in the deeper layers of the synovium in RA. (h) A hypervillous synovium with well-formed secondary follicles with germinal centres (relatively rare occurrence). (i) A high power view of an area of diseased synovium showing collections of classical plasma cells. (j) Plasma cells isolated from a patient's synovial tissue stained simultaneously for IgM (with fluorescein-labelled F(ab')₂ anti-μ) and rheumatoid factor (with rhodamine-labelled aggregated Fcγ). Two of the four IgM-positive plasma cells appear to be synthesizing rheumatoid factors. (k) Rheumatoid synovium showing large numbers of cells stained by anti-HLA-DR (anti-class II). (l) Rheumatoid synovium showing class II positive accessory cells (green) in intimate contact with CD4 positive T-cells (orange). (m) Large rheumatoid nodules on the forearm. (n) Granulomatous appearance of the rheumatoid nodule with central necrotic area surrounded by epithelioid cells, macrophages and scattered lymphocytes. Plasma cells making rheumatoid factor are often demonstrable and the lesion probably represents a response to the formation of insoluble anti-IgG complexes. ((a) kindly given by Dr D. Isenberg, (c), (d), (e), (g), (h) and (i) by Dr L.E. Glynn, (f) by Dr J. Edwards, (j) by Drs P. Youinou and P. Lydyard and (k) and (l) by Prof. G. Janossy.)*

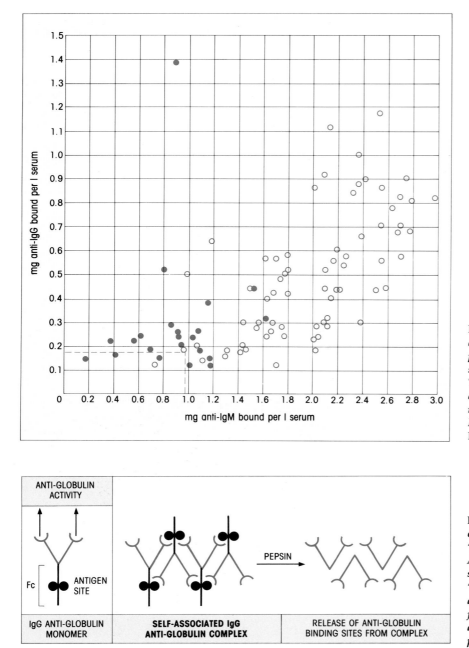

Figure 15.7. *IgM and IgG antiglobulins determined by tube radioassay in patients with seropositive (○) and seronegative (●) rheumatoid arthritis. The dotted lines indicate the 95% confidence limits (mean + 2 S.D.) of the normal group. (From Nineham L., Hay F.C. & Roitt I.M. (1976) J. Clin. Path. 29, 1121.)*

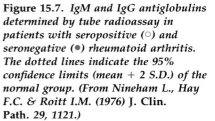

Figure 15.8. *Self-associated complexes of IgG antiglobulins and the exposure of 'hidden' binding sites by pepsin. Although of relatively low affinity, the strength of binding is boosted by the 'bonus effect' of the mutual attachment and, furthermore, such complexes in the joint may be stabilized by IgM antiglobulin and Clq which have polyvalent binding sites for IgG.*

regulatory abnormality which results in defective handling of some initiating micro-organism and possibly allows the emergence of the autoreactive T-cells. An overview of the pathogenesis of the disease and speculation on its aetiology are presented in figure 15.11, but it should be emphasized that there are many other conceivable hypotheses, including cross-reactions between microbes and IgG and generation of T-helper anti-Ids, to account for the development of IgG autosensitization.

Systemic vasculitis

Traditionally, these disorders have been linked with an immune complex mediated pathogenesis but the true factors causing vascular damage remain elusive. They are frequently associated with the presence of circulating antibodies to components of the polymorph primary granule, a serine protease III in the case of Wegener's granulomatosis and myeloperoxidase in some patients with polyarteritis nodosa.

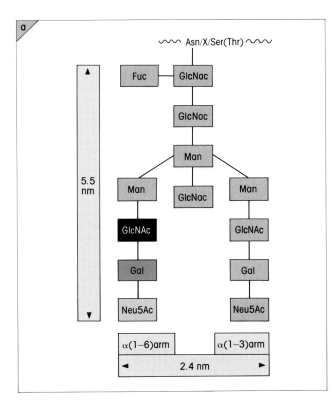

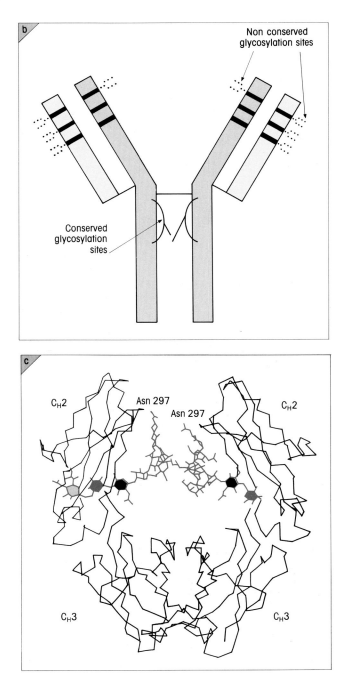

Figure 15.9. *The Fc sugars and their role in bridging the two C$_H$2 domains. (a) Typical structure of each N-linked sugar. Some chains lack terminal galactose—sialic acid. (b) Position of sugar chains in C$_H$2 domains. (c) Structure of the C$_H$2 regions and the association between the terminal galactose—sialic acid on the 1,6 arm and the protein surface. The 1,3 arms, one of which must lack galactose, bridge the two domains. (GlcNAc, N-acetylglucosamine; Man, mannose; Gal, galactose; Neu5Ac, sialic acid; Fuc, fucose.)*

Cellular hypersensitivity

The inflammatory infiltrate in organ-specific auto-immune disease such as thyroiditis, pernicious anaemia and type I diabetes is usually essentially mononuclear in character and, although not an infallible guide, this has been taken as an expression of cell-mediated hypersensitivity. Firm evidence for a direct participation of T-lymphocytes in any of these reactions has yet to be provided although the recent demonstration of the expression of class II molecules on cells in affected organs and the presence of antigen-specific T-cells would accord with an involvement of these cells. So would the beneficial effect of cyclosporin A in early insulin-dependent diabetes at levels which have little effect on antibody production, since this agent targets so specifically on T-cell lymphokine synthesis. As we shall see, pathogenic T-cells play a primary role

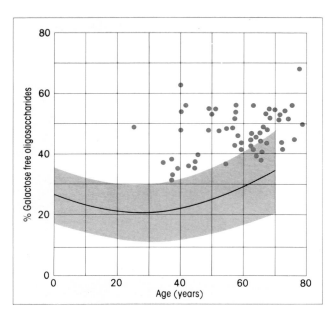

Figure 15.10. *Plots of the percentage of IgG sugars which completely lack terminal galactose showing the abnormal glycosylation of IgG in patients with rheumatoid arthritis. The shaded area indicates the mean ± S.D. of the normal controls. There is preliminary evidence that the defect is less marked when the disease is inactive. (Data from Parekh R.B., Isenberg D.A., Rook G.A.W., Roitt I.M., Dwek R.A. and Rademacher T.W. (1989) J. Autoimmunity, 2, 101.)*

336

in many of the animal models of organspecific autoimmune disease, encouraging the view that comparable processes are implicated in the corresponding human disorders.

Indirect evidence for a destructive role of the inflammatory cells comes from the observation that high doses of steroids may restore gastric function in certain patients with pernicious anaemia. In one such case studied, biopsy after intensive treatment with prednisone showed a diminution in the cellular infiltrate and new formation of parietal and chief cells in the gastric mucosa; acid and intrinsic factor were now produced after histamine stimulation and the ability to absorb vitamin B_{12} assessed by the Schilling test was restored to near normal values. The most likely explanation is that attack by the inflammatory cells and attempts to regenerate by mucosal cells were more or less in balance in the atrophic mucosa. Elimination of inflammatory cells by the prednisone allowed the regeneration of gastric mucosal cells to become dominant.

Our views on the pathogenesis of pernicious anaemia may be stated as follows. Autoimmune attack based on the parietal cell antigen gives rise to an atrophic gastritis which in many cases settles down to a dynamic equilibrium where the rate of destruction roughly balances the rate of regeneration; the loss of capacity to make intrinsic factor is evident in tests showing defective B_{12} absorption but sufficient vitamin is absorbed to keep the body in balance. These patients often have parietal cell antibodies and go on for 15 years or so without developing megaloblastic anaemia. However, if they should produce antibodies to intrinsic factor in the lumen of the gastro-intestinal tract, these will neutralize the small amount of intrinsic factor still available and the body will move into negative balance for B_{12}. The symptoms of B_{12} deficiency will then appear some considerable time later as the liver stores become exhausted (figure 15.12). A similar long latent period before the onset of clinical disease is evident in the prospective study of a family with insulin-dependent diabetes documented in figure 14.4 (p. 311) where complement-fixing islet-cell antibodies were detected two years before overt signs of pancreatic deficiency were apparent. Note also that the disease occurs after the autoimmunity pointing yet again to a primary pathogenetic role for the immune process.

One also cannot ignore the possibility of ADCC mechanisms. For example, the destruction of isolated liver cells by leucocytes from patients with HBs-negative active chronic hepatitis can be blocked by antigen (hepatic lipoprotein) or by aggregated normal IgG (which would bind to K-cell Fc receptors), but is not affected by removal of T-cells.

The nature of the cellular attack in organ-specific disorders is still not resolved but it is not improbable that cell-mediated hypersensitivity, antibody-mediated cytotoxicity and inflammatory reactions due to immune complexes may operate alone or in concert.

Experimental models of autoimmune disease

If autoimmune processes are pathogenic in human diseases we would expect that the production of autoimmunity should lead to comparable lesions in experimental animals.

Experimental autoallergic disease

When animals are injected with extracts of certain organs emulsified in oil containing killed tubercle

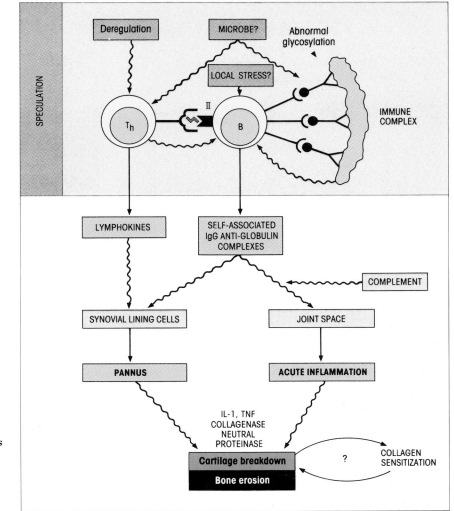

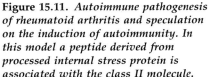

Figure 15.11. *Autoimmune pathogenesis of rheumatoid arthritis and speculation on the induction of autoimmunity. In this model a peptide derived from processed internal stress protein is associated with the class II molecule.*

bacilli (i.e. in complete Freund's adjuvant), auto-antibodies and destructive inflammatory lesions specific to the organ used for immunization result. Thus, Rose and Witebsky found that rabbits receiving rabbit thyroglobulin in Freund's adjuvant developed antibodies to thyroglobulin and thyroiditis involving invasion of the gland by mononuclear cells of lymphocytic and histiocytic types with destruction of the normal follicular architecture. Histologically there are many points of similarity between this experimental auto-allergic lesion and human autoimmune thyroiditis (figure 15.13).

In some of the earliest work in this field it was shown that injection of central nervous tissue produced encephalomyelitis and paralysis in monkeys and guinea-pigs; the parallel with post-rabies vaccine encephalitis is clear since the vaccine con-tains brain extracts, and optimistic comparisons with multiple sclerosis have been made. Just as with the thyroid, the most convenient model for the production of allergic encephalomyelitis involves immunization with the antigen, in this case myelin basic protein, incorporated in complete Freund's adjuvant. If one uses myelin from peripheral nerve instead of the central nervous system, an experimental autoimmune neuritis resembling the Guillain-Barré syndrome develops. Similar lesions can be induced in the adrenal (cf. Addisonian idiopathic adrenal atrophy) and the testis (? model for granulomatous orchitis), while experimental myasthenia gravis can be induced by immunization with acetylcholine receptor. Heterologous glomeruli stimulate the formation of glomerular basement membrane autoantibodies which localize in the kidney of the host to cause severe glome-

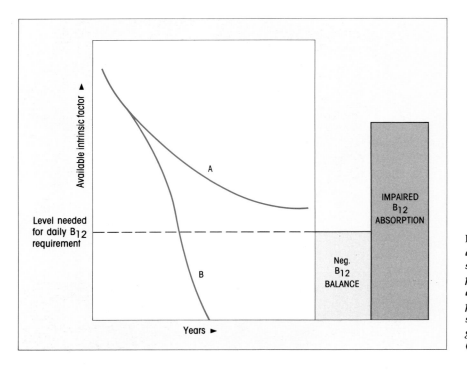

Figure 15.12. *Pathogenesis of pernicious anaemia. Group A: patients with long-standing atrophic gastritis having parietal cell but no intrinsic factor antibodies. Group B: pernicious anaemia patients with intrinsic factor antibodies superimposed upon the atrophic gastritis. (After Doniach D. & Roitt I.M. (1964)* **Semin. Hematol.** *I, 313.)*

338

rulonephritis (Steblay model) resembling closely that seen in Goodpasture's syndrome.

The experimental disease can usually be transmitted to syngeneic animals by lymphoid cells from immunized donors and occasionally by serum. In the case of experimental autoallergic orchitis, a synergism between cell-mediated hypersensitivity and antibody was recognized in the transfer studied. Allergic encephalomyelitis can be induced in syngeneic animals by injection of purified T-cells from sensitized donors and in particular by T-cell lines and clones which respond *in vitro* to myelin basic protein. On the other hand, transfer of monoclonal autoantibodies raised to acetylcholine receptors produces the muscle weakness characteristic of myasthenia. To produce a full-blown demyelinative lesion like that in multiple sclerosis requires the further synergistic action of antibodies to other myelin antigens such as galactocerebroside or myelin-oligodendrocyte glycoprotein which induce antibody-dependent macrophage mediated myelinolysis.

Experimental autoallergic thyroiditis and adjuvant arthritis represent other models where the central lesions have been successfully transferred with sensitized T-cells. In the latter, Freund's adjuvant alone without any added antigen produces a migratory polyarthritis in rats, and it has proved possible to transmit the disease to naïve animals by injecting a T-cell clone specific for the 65 kDa heat shock protein component of the mycobacterium which is said to cross-react with the core protein of cartilage proteoglycan. Clearly in those models where the disease can be transferred by antibody, the T-cells will be playing back-stage as helpers for B-cell stimulation.

The pre-eminent ability of Freund's complete adjuvant to enhance the production of experimental autoallergic disease may depend upon several factors acting concomitantly: modification of antigen, activation of cellular heat shock (stress) proteins(?), stimulation of T-helpers and effectors and (more controversially) disruption of normal T-suppressor feedback perhaps through priming of contrasuppressor cells. Although the precise nature of the events leading to tissue damage has yet to be resolved, it is abundantly clear that the deliberate provocation of an autoallergic state can produce lesions which closely mimic those seen in human organ-specific autoimmune disease and add weight to the notion that the immunological events are directly concerned in the pathogenesis of these disorders.

Spontaneous autoimmune disease

The message from animal models in which autoimmune desease develops spontaneously is the same. Neonatal bursectomy largely prevents the appearance of thyroglobulin antibodies and

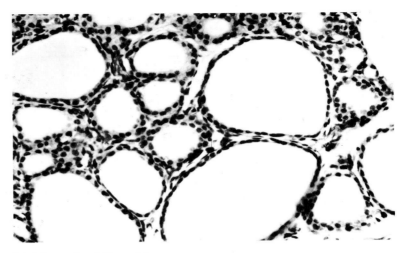

(a) Normal rat thyroid

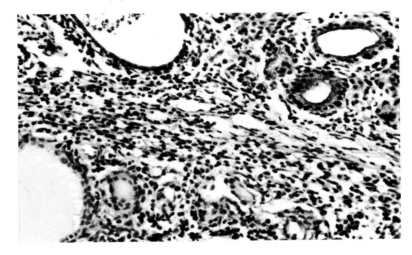

(b) Thyroiditis in the rat

Figure 15.13. *Similarity of lesions in spontaneous human autoimmune thyroiditis and the experimental disease produced by injection of rats with homologous thyroid in complete Freund's adjuvant. Other features of Hashimoto's disease such as the eosinophilic metaplasia of acinar cells (Askenazy cells) and local lymphoid follicles are not seen in this experimental model although the latter occur in the spontaneous thyroiditis of Obese strain chickens.*

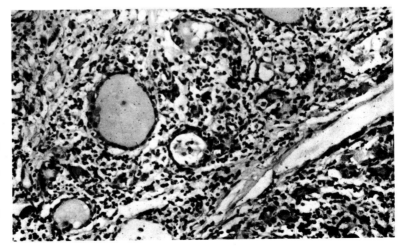

(c) Spontaneous human autoimmune thyroiditis

thyroiditis in Obese strain chickens, so pointing to a primary involvement of thyroid antibodies in the tissue lesions. Immunological control is also implicated by the exacerbation of disease caused by neonatal thymectomy.

Very informative models of spontaneous insulin-dependent diabetes mellitus (IDDM) are provided by the BB rat and the non-obese diabetic (NOD) mouse (cf. p. 323); the disease involves production of islet cell antibodies, mononuclear cell infiltration of the islets and finally selective destruction of the insulin-producing β-cells. T-cell depletion prevents the onset of disease and in the NOD, both CD4 and CD8 cells from diabetic animals are required for the most vicious transfer of disease to young syngeneic mice. The dramatic announcement that disease could be induced in prediabetic NOD mice by T-cell clones from diabetic animals specific for a 65 kDa heat shock protein, has accelerated a number of cerebral circuits. Furthermore, prediabetic mice immunized with the 65 kDa protein in *incomplete* Freund's adjuvant (lacking the mycobacterium) are resistant to attack by the pathogenic T-cells and do not go on to develop spontaneous diabetes. For the clones to target on the islet β-cells, there must be some tissue-specific changes leading to expression of stress-protein antigens. A-type retroviral particles are said to be associated with the β-cells and it will be recalled that the β-cells of diabetes-prone BB, but not diabetes-resistant or normal strains of rat, express class II MHC on their surface in response to INFγ (cf. figure 14.2c).

The now famous strain of mouse, the New Zealand Black (NZB), consistently develops an autoimmune haemolytic anaemia with positive Coombs' tests (agglutination of antibody-coated erythrocytes by an antiglobulin serum). As discussed earlier, the disease can be provoked in young unaffected NZBs by transfer of spleen cells from a Coombs' positive donor suggesting that it is the production of red cell antibodies which leads to shortened erythrocyte survival and consequent anaemia. A high proportion of these mice, and especially their hybrids with the partially related New Zealand White, (NZB x W)F1, have circulating antinuclear antibodies and an immune complex induced glomerulonephritis. Several other mutant mouse strains which have SLE-like symptoms are also positive for anti-DNA and die with type III hypersensitivity kidney lesions.

DIAGNOSTIC VALUE OF AUTOANTIBODY TESTS

Serum autoantibodies frequently provide valuable diagnostic markers. The most useful routine test is screening of the serum by immunofluorescence on a frozen section prepared from a composite block of unfixed human thyroid and stomach, and rat kidney and liver. This is supplemented by agglutination tests for rheumatoid factors and for thyroglobulin, thyroid microsome and red cell antibodies and by radioassay for antibodies to intrinsic factor, DNA and IgG (see table 14.2). The salient information is summarized in table 15.2.

The tests will also prove of value in screening for people at risk, e.g. relatives of patients with autoimmune disease, thyroiditis patients for gastric autoimmunity and vice versa and ultimately the general population.

TREATMENT OF AUTOIMMUNE DISORDERS

Metabolic control

The majority of approaches to treatment, not unnaturally, involve manipulation of immunological responses (figure 15.14). However, in many organ-specific diseases, metabolic control is usually sufficient, e.g. thyroxine replacement in primary myoedema, insulin in juvenile diabetes, vitamin B_{12} in pernicious anaemia, anti-thyroid drugs for Graves' disease, and so forth. Anticholinesterase drugs are commonly used for long-term therapy in myasthenia gravis; thymectomy is of benefit in most cases and it is conceivable that the gland contains ACh receptors in a particularly antigenic form(? associated with HLA-D expression).

Anti-inflammatory drugs

Patients with severe myasthenic symptoms respond well to high doses of steroids and the same is true for serious cases of other autoimmune disorders such as SLE and immune complex nephritis where the drug helps to suppress the inflammatory lesions.

DISEASE	ANTIBODY	COMMENT
Hashimoto's thyroiditis	Thyroid	Distinction from colloid goitre, thyroid cancer and subacute thyroiditis Thyroidectomy usually unnecessary in Hashimoto goitre
Primary myxoedema	Thyroid	Tests +ve in 99% of cases. If suspected hypothyroidism assess 'thyroid reserve' by TRH stimulation test
Thyrotoxicosis	Thyroid	High titres of cytoplasmic Ab indicate active thyroiditis and tendency to post-operative myxoedema: anti-thyroid drugs are the treatment of choice although HLA-B8 patients have high chance of relapse
Pernicious anaemia	Stomach	Help in diagnosis of latent PA, in differential diagnosis of non-autoimmune megaloblastic anaemia and in suspected subacute combined degeneration of the cord
Idiopathic adrenal atrophy	Adrenal	Distinction from tuberculous form
Myasthenia gravis	Muscle	When positive suggests associated thymoma (more likely if HLA-B12)
	ACh receptor	Positive in >80%
Pemphigus vulgaris and pemphigoid	Skin	Different fluorescent patterns in the two diseases
Autoimmune haemolytic anaemia	Erythrocyte (Coombs' test)	Distinction from other forms of anaemia
Sjögren's syndrome	Salivary duct cells SS-A, SS-B	
Primary biliary cirrhosis (PBC)	Mitochondrial	Distinction from other forms of obstructive jaundice where test rarely +ve Recognize subgroup within cryptogenic cirrhosis related to PBC with +ve mitochondrial Ab
Active chronic hepatitis	Smooth muscle anti-nuclear and 20% mitochondrial	Smooth muscle Ab distinguish from SLE
Rheumatoid arthritis	Antiglobulin, e.g. SCAT and latex fixation	High titre indicative of bad prognosis
SLE	High titre antinuclear, DNA	DNA antibodies present in active phase Ab to double-stranded DNA characteristic; high affinity complement-fixing Ab give kidney damage, low affinity CNS lesions
	Phospholipid	Thrombosis, recurrent fetal loss and thrombocytopaenia
Scleroderma	Nucleolar	
Wegener's granulomatosis	Neutrophil cytoplasm	Anti-serine protease closely associated with disease; treatment urgent

Table 15.2 *Autoantibody tests and diagnosis.*

341

In rheumatoid arthritis, apart from steroids, anti-inflammatory drugs such as salicylates and innumerable synthetic prostaglandin inhibitors are widely used. Penicillamine, gold salts and anti-malarials such as chloroquine all find an important place in therapy but their mode of action is unknown.

Therapeutic blocking of other mediators directly concerned in immunological tissue damage will be feasible if lymphokine and complement antagonists become available.

Immunosuppressive drugs

In a sense, because it blocks lymphokine secretion by T-cells, cyclosporin A is an anti-inflammatory drug and since lymphokines like IL-2 are also obligatory for lymphocyte proliferation, cyclosporin is also an anti-mitotic drug. It is of proven efficacy in uveitis, early type I diabetes, nephrotic syndrome and psoriasis and of moderate efficacy in idiopathic thrombocytopenic purpura, SLE, polymyositis,

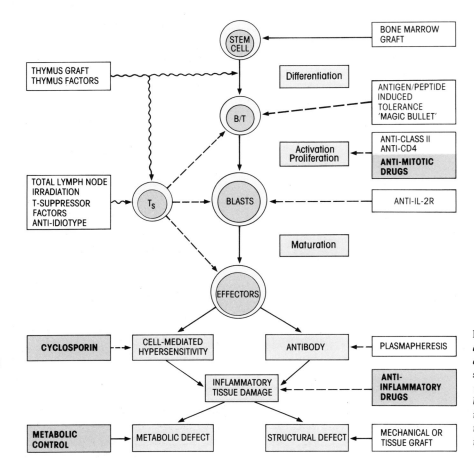

Figure 15.14. *The treatment of autoimmune disease. Current conventional treatments are in bold type; some feasible approaches are given in white boxes. (In the case of a live graft, bottom right, the immunosuppressive therapy used may protect the tissue from the autoimmune damage which affected the organ being replaced.)*

Crohn's disease, primary biliary cirrhosis and my-asthenis gravis. In a double-blind randomized control trial, cyclosporin demonstrated significant though not complete disease suppression over 12 months in a group of previously refractory rheumatoid arthritis patients. There is no evidence yet that administration of the drug during an ongoing autoimmune response is likely to establish the type of T-suppression seen in kidney grafting (cf. p. 290).

While awaiting more selective therapy, conventional non-specific anti-mitotic agents such as azathioprine, cyclophosphamide and methotrexate, usually in combination with steroids, have been used effectively in SLE, rheumatoid arthritis, chronic active hepatitis and autoimmune haemolytic anaemia for example. High dose i.v. cyclophosphamide plus ACTH or total lymph node irradiation through its effect on the peripheral immune system either slowed or stopped the advance of disease in approximately two-thirds of progressive multiple sclerosis patients for 1−2 years, a strong indication that the disease is mediated by immune mechanisms. This is further supported by the unfortunate finding that IFNγ exacerbates disease in the majority.

Immunological control strategies

Cellular manipulation

It should one day be practical to correct any relevant defects in stem cells or in thymus processing by bone marrow or thymus grafting or perhaps, in the latter case, by thymic hormones.

Injection of monoclonal anti-class II and anti-CD4 successfully fends off lupus in spontaneous mouse models and it is relevant to record the preliminary clinical observations that injection of immunoglobulins eluted from placentae, and shown to contain anti-allo-class II, significantly ameliorate the symptoms of rheumatoid arthritis.

Some take the anti-IL-2 receptor approach to deplete activated T-cells but I would like to refer back to our discussion of the long-lasting effect of *non-depleting* anti-CD4 for the induction of tolerance particularly when reinforced by repeated exposure to antigen (cf. p. 289). Antigen reinforcement of course is an obvious continuing feature in autoimmune disease so that anti-CD4 should be ideal as a therapy in disorders where the natural 'switch-off' tolerogenic signals are still accepted by the CD4 cells; this may not be so in every case but the treatment should be a good way to test whether the CD4 read-out mechanism is still normal. Back up with non-depleting anti-LFA-1 should improve efficacy even more.

We can manage perfectly well in life without a complete set of our T-cell receptor Vβ genes; after all wild mice, and presumably ourselves, delete large tracts of Vβ families during thymic differentiation and it does not seem to do them much harm. So, the argument runs, if the autoimmune T-cell clones specific for the autoantigen in a given disease happen to be restricted to membership of a particular Vβ family, we could delete all members of that family *in vivo* with the appropriate antiserum and yet not make irreparable holes in the host's defences. In PL mice immunized with the N-terminal peptide of myelin basic protein, anti-Vβ8 eliminated experimental autoallergic encephalitis almost entirely, so the strategy can work. Not so good with SJL mice which respond to peptide 89−101 with 50% of the T-cells using Vβ17 receptors; in this case, anti-Vβ17 did not block disease. Clearly, until we have wider knowledge of the extent of Vβ restriction for each antigen and also for each individual, we must suspend judgement on the general feasibility of the strategy.

Idiotype control

With antibody

The powerful immunosuppressive action of anti-idiotype antibodies has led to much rumination on the feasibility of controlling autoantibody production by provoking appropriate interactions within the immune network. The ability of the newborn children of myasthenic mothers to defend themselves against the pathogenetic effects of maternal acetylcholine receptor antibodies by synthesizing anti-idiotypes, encourages the view that idiotype manipulation might prove to be effective. We have focused previously on the intimate network interactions between hormone receptors, hormones and their respective antibodies (cf. p. 161) and it might be that the autoimmune disorders involving these receptors prove to be especially amenable to idiotype control. There is a growing realization that, in general, more fundamental suppression can be achieved by utilizing the internal elements of the idiotype network rather than anti-idiotype reagents raised in other species. Thus, xenogeneic anti-idiotypes have only achieved transient and partial improvement in the spontaneous thyroiditis of the Buffalo rat and the autoimmune lupus of NZB × W mice presumably due to compensation by idiotype negative clones. On the other hand, much more profound changes have been achieved by treatment with monoclonal autoantibodies (idiotypes) derived from the autoimmune strain in question.

Curiously, intravenous injection of Ig pooled from many normal donors is said to have a beneficial effect in a number of autoimmune blood diseases, recurrent abortions associated with cardiolipin antibodies and patients with autoantibodies to procoagulant factor VIII. The latter has been studied in some detail and the inhibitory effects of $F(ab')_2$ fractions from the normal Ig pool suggests that we are dealing with anti-idiotypic reactions; it is as though the normal pool was re-establishing a properly controlled network.

With T-cells

It is possible to protect animals against the induction of experimental allergic encephalomyelitis by immunization with an attenuated T-cell clone specific for myelin basic protein. This must be mediated by the induction of suppressor T-cells specific for the effector cell receptor idiotype. Confirmation has come from experiments showing that the encephalitis can be prevented if mice are first immunized with synthetic peptide from the Vβ chain of the encephalitogenic clone; this procedure generates CD8 T-cells specific for the receptor peptide presented by class I MHC, and which transfer protection against induction of encephalitis. Is it strange that exogenous peptide becomes inserted into the class I pathway?

T-cell vaccination has been used to protect against the spontaneous development of diabetes in NOD mice and the production of arthritis following sensitization with type II collagen. It has also proved possible to switch off Freund-adjuvant-induced arthritis with an attenuated clone of T-cells generated in response to the 65 kDa mycobacterial heat shock protein.

This adjuvant model has been looked at in depth (I. Cohen). Perversely, the earliest T-cell responses preceding the adjuvant-induced arthritis were antigen-specific suppression and anti-idiotypic reactivity; responses to the antigen itself emerged a few days before the appearance of clinical arthritis.

T-cell vaccination accelerated the kinetics of the antigen response, abolished antigen-specific suppression, activated anti-idiotypic T-cells and inhibited arthritis. The extremely rapid appearance of anti-idiotype and antigen-specific suppressors so soon after immunization with the 65 kDa heat shock protein strongly suggests a pre-existing network linked to epitopes on this antigen. This could serve two functions. One, to prevent autoimmune disease; malfunctioning of the network would then produce disease. Secondly, the network might cause the autoimmune response to be focused on a particular antigen so that if autoimmunity were triggered it would be expressed against a chosen antigen which could be well controlled. In this respect it is notable that certain autoantigens dominate similar diseases across species, for example myelin basic protein in autoallergic encephalitis, ACh receptor in myasthenia gravis and in SLE, the DNA and Sm antigens. On this view, vaccination with T-cell receptor epitopes is an attempt to re-establish a natural network.

Manipulation by antigen

The object is to present the offending antigen in sufficient concentration and in the form which will turn off an ongoing autoimmune response. Since T-cells have been accorded such a pivotal role, it is natural to devise the strategy in terms of T-cell epitopes rather than whole antigen, obviously a far more practical proposition because this reduces the problem to dealing with relatively short peptides. One strategy is to design peptide analogues which will bind obstinately to the appropriate MHC molecule and block the response to autoantigen. Since we express several different MHC molecules, this should not impair microbial defences unduly. However, we are now talking of patients not mice and this could involve very high doses of peptide. If possible I would prefer a strategy of actively stimulating peptide-specific unresponsiveness, say under an umbrella of anti-CD4.

Another potentially valuable approach for the future involves 'switching off' primed B-cells by presenting hapten linked to a thymus-independent carrier like the copolymer of D-glutamic and D-lysine (D-GL) or isologous IgG particularly when given with high cortisone doses. This has certainly worked well in NZB hybrid mice where anti-DNA levels have been reduced using nucleosides as the haptens: we shall have to see whether man and mouse really are that different.

And last, back to the Holy Grail business, several groups are trying to evolve a strategy based upon the 'magic bullet', the essence of which is to fashion different types of cytotoxic weaponry by coupling bacterial toxins or lots of radioactivity to the antigen which selectively homes on to the lymphocytes bearing specific surface receptors. Something good has got to come out of all this!

Plasmapheresis

Plasma exchange to lower the rate of immune complex deposition in SLE provides only temporary benefit although it may be of value in life-threatening cases of arteritis. Successful results have been obtained in Goodpasture's syndrome when the treatment has been applied in combination with anti-mitotic drugs (figure 15.15), the rationale being an increased tendency for antigen-reactive cells to divide as the negative feedback effect of IgG is lowered following removal of plasma proteins.

Longer shots

We have already discussed the possible role of thymic factors in maintaining T-suppressor control of autoimmunity and one anticipates some interesting advances now that purified materials are available. Hybridoma technology or even gene cloning might ultimately provide the clinician with antigen-specific suppressor factors. In the meantime, exploration of the therapeutic benefits of total lymph node irradiation (cf. p. 286) is being cautiously undertaken.

Other features of regulatory bypass mechanisms such as excessive contrasuppressor activity or inappropriate HLA-DR expression may also become feasible targets for therapy one day.

SUMMARY

There are many examples which would attribute the pathogenesis of autoimmune disorders to the autoimmune response. Antibodies to erythrocytes and to platelets shorten the half-lives of these cells and transplacental passage of platelet antibodies produces a transient neonatal thrombocytopenia. Different thyroid autoantibodies can cause tissue destruction, stimulation or suppression of thyroid hormone production and stimulation or suppression of thyroid cell division; the various forms in which thyroid autoimmunity presents can be

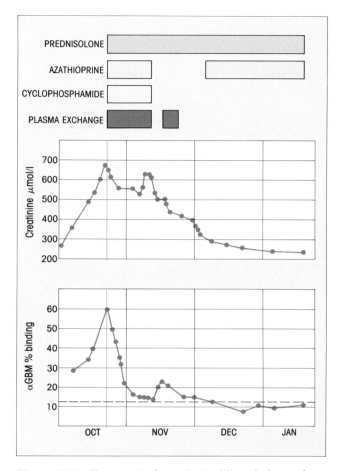

Figure 15.15. *Treatment of a patient with anti-glomerular basement membrane (α-GBM) nephritis with plasma exchange, steroids and immunosuppressive drugs. Kidney function is here monitored by the serum creatinine level. The treatment leads to loss of autoantibody (the dashed line represents the amount of GBM antigen bound in the assay by normal serum) and restoration of kidney function (courtesy of Dr C.M. Lockwood).*

interpreted in terms of different combinations of these antibodies. Antibodies to intrinsic factor and to sperm inhibit their biological actions. Elution of glomerular basement membrane autoantibodies from the kidney of a patient with Goodpasture's syndrome produced a fatal glomerulonephritis when injected into monkeys. Acetylcholine receptor autoantibodies evoke a transient neonatal muscle weakness in a proportion of babies born to myasthenic mothers.

Immune complexes, usually with bound complement, appear in the kidneys, skin and joints of patients with SLE, associated with lesions in the corresponding organs. Most patients with rheumatoid arthritis produce autoantibodies to IgG (rheumatoid factors) as a result of immu-

nological hyper-reactivity in the deeper layers of the synovium. The IgG rheumatoid factors self-associate to form complexes. These give rise to acute inflammation in the joint space and, together with activated T-cells (? anti-self heat shock proteins), stimulate the synovial lining cells to grow as a malign pannus which produces erosions in the underlying cartilage and bone through the release of interleukin-1, IL-6, TNFα, PGE$_2$, collagenase, neutral proteinase and reactive oxygen intermediates. The IgG in rheumatoid arthritis shows defective galactosylation of the Fc sugars.

Cellular hypersensitivity must play a role in the chronic inflammatory changes of many autoimmune disorders, particularly if one considers the phenomena of inappropriate class II MHC expression and the beneficial effects of cyclosporin A.

Autoallergic disease can be deliberately induced in the thyroid, brain, adrenal, testis and joints of rodents by immunization with the relevant antigen in complete Freund's adjuvant. Spontaneous thyroiditis, diabetes, haemolytic anaemia and lupus have all been observed in certain pure-bred animal strains and the importance of autoimmunity for pathogenesis is shown by the amelioration of symptoms whenever the immune response is suppressed.

A wide range of serum autoantibodies now provide valuable diagnostic markers. Routine immunofluorescent screening is carried out on composite sections of human thyroid and stomach and rat kidney and liver, supplemented by agglutination tests for rheumatoid factors, thyroid and red cell antibodies, and by radioassays for intrinsic factor, DNA and IgG antibodies.

Therapy conventionally involves metabolic control and the use of anti-inflammatory and immuno-suppressive drugs. Plasma exchange may be of value especially in combination with anti-mitotic drugs. A whole variety of potential immunological control therapies are under intensive investigation. These include antibody and T-cell idiotype manipulations and attempts to induce antigen-specific unresponsiveness particularly to T-cells using peptides.

The accompanying comparison of organ-specific and non-organ-specific autoimmune disorders (table 15.3) gives an overall view of many of the points raised in these last two chapters.

ORGAN-SPECIFIC (e.g. THYROIDITIS, GASTRITIS, ADRENALITIS)	NON-ORGAN SPECIFIC (e.g. SYSTEMIC LUPUS ERYTHEMATOSUS)
DIFFERENCES	
Antigens only available to lymphoid system in low concentration	Antigens accessible at higher concentrations
Antibodies and lesions organ-specific	Antibodies and lesions non-organ-specific
Clinical and serologic overlap — thyroiditis, gastritis and adrenalitis	Overlap SLE, rheumatoid arthritis, and other connective tissue disorders
Familial tendency to organ-specific autoimmunity	Familial connective tissue disease
Lymphoid invasion, parenchymal destruction by ? ± cell-mediated hypersensitivity ? ± antibodies	Lesions due to deposition of antigen– antibody complexes
Therapy aimed at controlling metabolic deficit	Therapy aimed at inhibiting inflammation and antibody synthesis
Tendency to cancer in organ	Tendency to lymphoreticular neoplasia
Antigens evoke organ-specific antibodies in normal animals with complete Freund's adjuvant	No antibodies produced in animals with comparable stimulation
Experimental lesions produced with antigen in Freund's adjuvant	Diseases and autoantibodies arise spontaneously in certain animals (e.g. NZB mice and hybrids) or after injection of parental lymphoid tissue into F_1 hybrids
SIMILARITIES	
Circulating autoantibodies react with normal body constituents	
Patients often have increased immunoglobulins in serum	
Antibodies may appear in each of the main immunoglobulin classes	
Greater incidence in women	
Disease process not always progressive; exacerbations and remissions	
Association with HLA	
Spontaneous diseases in animals genetically programmed	
Autoantibody tests of diagnostic value	

Table 15.3. *Comparison of organ-specific and non-organ-specific diseases.*

Further reading

Bottazzo G.F., Pujol-Borrell R., Hanafusa T. & Feldmann M. (1983) Hypothesis: role of aberrant HLA-DR expression and antigen presentation in the induction of endocrine autoimmunity. *Lancet*, ii 1115.

Brochier J., Clot J. & Sany J. (eds) (1986) Anti-Ia antibodies in treatment of autoimmune disease. *Immune Intervention*, **2**. Academic Press, London.

Haeney M. (1985) *Introduction to Clinical Immunology.* Butterworths-Update, London. (In vivid technicolour; suitable for the busy clinician.)

Ivanyi L. (ed.) (1986) *Immunological Aspects of Oral Disease.* MTP Press, Lancaster, UK.

Lachmann P.J. & Peters D.K. (eds) (1982) *Clinical Aspects of Immunology*, 4th edn. Blackwell Scientific Publications, Oxford.

McGregor A.M. (ed.) (1986) *Immunology of Endocrine Diseases.* MTP Press, Lancaster, UK.

Morrow J. & Isenberg D.A. (1987) *Autoimmune Rheumatic Disease.* Blackwell Scientific Publications, Oxford.

Parekh R.B. *et al.* (1989) A comparative analysis of disease associated changes in the galactosylation of serum IgG. *J. Autoimmunity*, **2**, 101.

Roitt I.M. & Cooke A. (1987) Idiotypes and autoimmunity. In *Progress in Immunology*, VI. Cinader B. & Miller R.G.(eds). Academic Press, Orlando,USA.

Selimena M. *et al.* (1990) Autoantibodies to GABA-ergic neurones and pancreatic β-cells in stiff man syndrome. *N. Eng. J. Med.*, **322**, 1555. (Fun to read just for the title!)

Shoenfeld Y. & Isenberg D. (1989) *The Mosaic of Autoimmunity (the Factors associated with Autoimmune Disease).* Elsevier, Amsterdam. (An excellent account.)

Stites D.P., Stobo J.D. & Wells J.V. (eds) (1987) *Basic and Clinical Immunology*, 6th edn. Appleton & Lange, Norwalk, Conn.

Thompson R.A. (ed.) (1985) Laboratory Investigation of Immunological Disorders. *Clinics in Immunol. & Allergy*, 5. W.B. Saunders, London.

Thompson R.A. (series ed.) *Recent Advances in Clinical Immunology.* Churchill Livingstone, UK.

Triger D.R. (ed.) (1986) *Clinical Immunology of Liver and Gastrointestinal Tract.* Wright, Bristol, UK.

INDEX

Page references in *italics* refer to figures, tables, or
the legends accompanying them.

INDEX

limulin 14
linkage disequilibrium 293–4
lipoarabinomannan 209
lipocortin 157
lipomodulin 157
liposomes, antigen presentation by 238
Listeria monocytogenes 209
livedo reticularis *258*
liver
  B-cell development in 183
  transplants 292
luciferase 95
Ly1 *see* CD5
Ly2 117, 199
lymph node 107–8, 109
  B-cell areas 108–10
  T-cell areas *109*, 110
lymphoblasts *21*
lymphocytes *21*
  and acquired memory 25–6, *27*
  clonal selection 24, 25
  effects of adjuvant on 238
  role in antibody production 20–4
  traffic between lymphoid tissues
    106–7
  'trapping' 106
  see also specific cell types
lymphoid tissue 107–12, *113*
  distribution *106*
  functional organization *105*
  lymphocyte traffic between 106–7
lymphokine-activated killer cells 299, 301,
  302
lymphokines 28, *29*, 139
  in chronic inflammatory, response
    146–7
  in clonal expansion of activated B-cells
    123–4
  in control of haemopoiesis 144
  in maturation of effector B-cells 124–5
  in parasitic infections 218–19
  as part of cytokine network 141–4
  secretion phenotypes 143
  synthesis failure 243
lymphomas
  chromosome translocation in 189
  immunodeficiency in 195–6
  immunohistological diagnosis 192–3,
    194
  incidence after cyclosporin A therapy
    287
  maturation arrest in 190–1
  see also specific disorders
lymphopenia 325
lymphoplasmacytoid cells *193*
lymphoproliferative disorders
  chromosome translocations in 189–90
  c-*myc* deregulation in 188–9
  immunodeficiency secondary to 195–6
  immunohistological diagnosis 191–4
  maturation arrest in 190–1
lymphotoxin 15, *142*
  in viral infection 147
lysozyme 13, 30

MAC 9, *10*, 11
  in the acute inflammatory response 12
MAC inhibitory factor (MACIF), defects

in 240, *241*
Mackaness phenomenon 209–10, 211,
  212
macrophages 2, *3*, 4, 30
  activation 210–12
  in the acute inflammatory response
    12–13
  as antigen-presenting cells 113–14
  bacterial invasion 208–9
  parasites in 220
  'sentinel' 175
'magic bullet' 299, 344
major basic protein 15, 257
major histocompatibility complex *see*
  MHC
malnutrition, effect on the immune
  response 169–70, 244
MALT 110, 112, *113*
  vascular addressin on 107
mannose-binding protein 14
mantle zone lymphoma 194
Mantoux reaction *258*, 270
maple bark stripper's disease 266
Marek's disease
  susceptibility to 295
  vaccination 299
mast cells *3*
  in the acute inflammatory response 12
  in anaphylactic hypersensitivity 253,
    254–5
  mediator release from *10*, 11
maternal/fetal immunological relationship
  296
MBP 15, 257
M-CSF *142*
  gene 141
  in haemopoiesis 144
MDP 238
membrane attack complex 9, *10*, 11
  in the acute inflammatory response 12
memory cells *27*, 125, *126*, 148–50
mesangial cells 4
methotrexate 286–7, 342
MHC 28, 31, 63
  in antigen recognition by T-cells 75–6,
    77–9, 117, 159
  Class I molecules 28, 63
    binding to peptide antigens 77–8
    in cytotoxic T-cell activity 159
    expression in tumours 297
    gene map 51, *54*
    and restriction of cytotoxic T-cells
      74–5
    structure 51, *52–3*
    tissue distribution 56
  Class II molecules 28, 63
    and antigen presentation to T-cells
      75–6
    in autoimmune disorders 310–11,
      323
    binding to peptide antigens 77–8
    and cell-mediated lympholysis 279
    expression in tumours 297
    gene map 51, *54*
    high/low responsiveness 167
    and mixed lymphocyte reaction 279
    and restriction of T-suppressor cells
      155–6
    structure 51, *52–3*

  in T-helper and -suppressor activity
    159
    tissue distribution 56
  Class III genes 51, 63
    map 51, *54*
  and disease associations 293–5
  and disease resistance 295
  functions 56
  genes
    co-dominant expression 56
    conversion 54, *56*
    mapping 51, 54
    polymorphism 51, 54
  and graft rejection 279–80, 283–5
  influence on the immune response
    165–7
  inheritance 56
  molecular structures 51, *52–3*
  nomenclature 55
  polymorphism 285
  tissue distribution 56
  and tissue typing 283–5
microbial antagonism 2
microbial vectors, in vaccine production
  229–30
microglia 4
microphages 2, *3*, 4, *5*, 30
migration inhibition factor (MIF) 141
  deficiency 243
mixed lymphocyte reaction (MLR) 279,
  283
molecular mimicry 220
monoclonal antibodies 36, 136, 138
  applications *138*
  genetically engineered variants 139,
    140
  human 139, 226
  as immunosuppressive agents 286
  production *136–7*
  specificity 74
monocyte *3*, 4, *5*
monokines 141
  see also cytokines
mononuclear phagocyte system 4
moth-eaten mouse strain 322
mucosal-associated lymphoid tissue 110,
  112, *113*
  vascular addressin on 107
mucus, as barrier to infection 2
multiple myeloma 36, 194–5, *196*
multiple sclerosis, HLA association
  293–4, 295
multivalency, 'bonus effect' of 19, 72–3
muramyl dipeptide 238
muscle weakness, transient neonatal 329
Mycobacterium tuberculosis 209
myeloma proteins 36, 194–5
myeloperoxidase deficiency 240
myositis, autoimmune 313

NAP-1 13
natural killer cells *see* NK cells
'natural suppressor cells' 158
N-CAM 196, 199, 200
NCF 13
necrotizing arteritis 269
negative selection 181
Neisseria gonorrhoeae 208

vaccines
  complications 230
  conditions for success 227
  containing individual antigens 231−7
  killed 227−8
  live attenuated 228−31
  oral 229−30
  storage 230
vaccinia virus, as vector in vaccine
      production 229, *230*
Van der Waals forces, in antigen/antibody
      binding 70−1
vascular addressins 106−7
vasculitis, systemic 334
vasoactive intestinal peptide 168
Vβ genes, deletion 343
VDJ combinations 59, *61*, 63, 198

'veiled' cells 115
V genes 57−8
  in lower vertebrates 198
  somatic mutation 61−2
Vibrio cholerae 208
VIP 168
viral infection
  cytokines in 147
  cytotoxin T-cells in 147−8, 159
  immunity to 212−16
  immunosuppressive effects 244−5
viral interference 14
VLA subfamily 199
v-*raf* oncogene 189
V region 36, *37*, 62
  amino acid variability *38*
  and antigen recognition 40−1, *43, 44*

Waldenström's macroglobulinaemia *193*, 195
Wegener's granulomatosis 334
Western blot analysis 96, *97*
wheal and flare reactions 256
Wiskott−Aldrich syndrome 243

X-chromosome aberrations in autoimmune
      disorders 310
xenograft 277
Xenopus, immune responses 197

Zidovudine 250−1
zinc deficiency 169

356

INDEX